Textbook of Hand Eczema

Ali Alikhan • Jean-Marie Lachapelle
Howard I. Maibach
Editors

Textbook of Hand Eczema

[illegible]

Springer

Editors
Ali Alikhan, MD
Department of Dermatology
Mayo Clinic
Rochester, MN
USA

Howard I. Maibach, MD
Department of Dermatology
University of California
San Francisco, CA
USA

Jean-Marie Lachapelle, MD, PhD
Department of Dermatology
Catholic University of Louvain
Brussels, Belgium

ISBN 978-3-642-39545-1 ISBN 978-3-642-39546-8 (eBook)
DOI 10.1007/978-3-642-39546-8
Springer Heidelberg New York Dordrecht London

Library of Congress Control Number: 2014931986

Printed on acid-free paper

Springer is part of Springer Science+Business Media (www.springer.com)

To my grandmother, Amma, for teaching me the meaning of love and sacrifice. Without her selflessness, kindness, and generosity, I would have never made it this far in life.

To my mother and father, who have been loving, supportive parents and incredible role models. Their passion, honesty, and perseverance provided me with a foundation to build upon.

To my fiancée, Sara, the love of my life, my soul mate, and my better half. I am truly blessed to have your love, support, and patience, all of which helped me complete this book.

Ali Alikhan

To Torkil Fischer, Arthur Rook, and Jean Foussereau

Jean-Marie Lachapelle, Howard I. Maibach

Preface

Hand eczema is a ubiquitous problem, affecting many people worldwide and resulting in lost work productivity and diminished quality of life.

Fortunately, we are continuing to learn more about the hand and more about hand eczema. Hand eczema is far more heterogeneous than originally thought, and this heterogeneity has implications for management.

Moreover, it is important to be aware of the various causes of hand eczema, diagnostic modalities, and the populations most predisposed to develop the disorder.

Advances in treatment of hand eczema have provided physicians with more tools to improve their patients' lives. Nonetheless, appropriate education is the cornerstone to any treatment plan.

It is our hope that this volume stimulates thought and discussion on hand eczema and provides a unique resource to allow for better understanding of disease heterogeneity, current management options, and future avenues for advancement.

Rochester, USA — Ali Alikhan
Brussels, Belgium — Jean-Marie Lachapelle
San Francisco, USA — Howard I. Maibach

Abbreviations

2-HEMA	2-Hydroxyethyl methacrylate
2-HPA	2-Hydroxypropyl acrylate
8-MOP	8-Methoxypsoralen
ACD	Allergic contact dermatitis
ACU	Allergic contact urticaria
AE	Atopic eczema
AHA	Alpha-hydroxy acids
AMP	Antimicrobial peptide
BBUVB	Broadband ultraviolet B (320–270 nm)
BCC	Basal cell carcinoma
BHT	Butylated hydroxytoluene
BIT	Benzisothiazolinone
BP	Bullous pemphigoid
BTK	Behind-the-knee test
BTX-A	Botulinum toxin type A
CARD	Contact allergen replacement database
CBS	N-Cyclohexyl-2-benzothiazolesulfenamide
CHD	Chronic hand dermatitis
CHE	Chronic hand eczema
CIM	Colorimetric indices of mildness
CSM	Corneosurfametry
CSSS	Cyanoacrylate skin surface stripping
CTCL	Cutaneous T-cell lymphoma
CU	Contact urticaria
CUS	Contact urticaria syndrome
CXM	Corneoxenometry
DBTU	Dibutylthiourea
DCR	Dental composite resin
DEA	Diethanolamine
DETU	Diethylthiourea
DGEBA	Diglycidyl ether of bisphenol A
DHA	Dehydroabietic acid
DIDP	Di-isodecyl phthalate
DLQI	Dermatology life quality index
DMTU	Dimethylthiourea
DNFB	Dinitrofluorobenzene

DPG	1,3-Diphenylguanidine
DPTD	Dipentamethylenethiuram disulfide
DPTU	Diphenylthiourea
DSCG	Disodium cromoglycate
DTDM	Dithiodimorpholine
ECM	Extracellular matrix
EDEN	European Dermato-Epidemiology Network
EDTA	Edetic acid
EGDMA	Ethylene glycol dimethacrylate
ETU	Ethylenethiourea
FDA	Food and Drug Administration
FIOH	Finnish Institute of Occupational Health
FLG	Filaggrin
FROD	Finnish Register of Occupational Diseases
GTP	Guanosine triphosphate
Gy	Gray
HDSS	Hyperhidrosis disease severity scale
HECSI	Hand eczema severity index
HHIQ	Hyperhidrosis impact questionnaire
HRIPT	Human repeated insult patch test
HRQOL	Health-related quality of life
HVL	Half value layer
ICD	Irritant contact dermatitis
IGA	Investigator's global assessment
IMPDH	Inosine monophosphate dehydrogenase
IPDA	Isophorone diamine
IPPD	N-Isopropyl-N′-phenyl-p-phenylene diamine
J/cm^2	Joules per centimeter squared
LDI	Laser Doppler imaging
LD-RT	Low-dose radiation therapy
LDF	Laser Doppler flowmetry
LE	Lupus erythematosus
LFA-3	Leukocyte-function-associated antigen 3
LUH	Localized unilateral hyperhidrosis
MBTS	Dibenzothiazyl disulfide
MCI/MI	Methylchloroisothiazolinone/methylisothiazolinone
MDA	4,4′-Methylenedianiline
MDI	Diphenylmethane-4,4′-diisocyanate
MEA	Monoethanolamine
MF	Mycosis fungoides
MI	Methylisothiazolinone
MMA	Methyl methacrylate
MMBT	Morpholinomercaptobenzothizole
MWF	Metalworking fluid
MXDA	m-Xylidenediamine
NACDG	North American Contact Dermatitis Group
NBR	Nitrile butadiene rubber
NBUVB	Narrowband ultraviolet B (313–308 nm)
nm	Nanometer

NMF	Natural moisturizing factor
NMSC	Non-melanoma skin cancers
NO	Nitrous oxide
NOSQ-2002	Nordic occupational skin questionnaire
NRL	Natural rubber latex
OCD	Occupational contact dermatitis
OCD	Occupational dermatitis
OHSI	Osnabrueck hand eczema severity index
OIT	Octylisothazolinone
OSD	Occupational skin disease
PAAB	p-Aminoazobenzene
PCD	Protein contact dermatitis
PCT	Porphyria cutanea tarda
PGE	Phenylglycidylether
PML	Progressive multifocal leukoencephalopathy
PMMA	Polymethyl methacrylate
PPD	p-Phenylenediamine
PPE	Personal protective equipment
PUVA	Psoralen plus UVA
PVC	Polyvinyl chloride
ROAT	Repeated open application test
SACD	Self-adhesive-coated disc
SC	Stratum corneum
SCC	Squamous cell carcinoma
SCORAD	Scoring of atopic dermatitis scale
SLS	Sodium lauryl sulfate
SPT	Skin prick test
TAC	Tacrolimus
TBTD	Tetrabutylthiuram disulfide
TCI	Topical calcineurin inhibitor
TCs	Topical corticosteroids
TEA	Triethanolamine
TETD	Tetraethylthiuram disulfide
TEWL	Transepidermal water loss
TMTD	Tetramethylthiuram disulfide
TMTM	Tetramethylthiuram monosulfide
TNF-α	Tumor necrosis factor α
TREGDA	Triethyleneglycol diacrylate
TREGDMA	Triethyleneglycol dimethacrylate
TRITs	Tandem repeated irritation tests
TU	Thiourea
UEDMA	Urethane dimethacrylate
UVA	Long-wave ultraviolet irradiation (400–320 nm)
UVB	Short-wave ultraviolet irradiation (320–270 nm)
wb MWF	Water-based MWF
ZDBC	Zinc dibutyldithiocarbamate
ZDEC	Zinc diethyldithiocarbamate
ZMBT	Zinc 2-mercaptobenzothiazole
$ZnSO_4$	Zinc sulfate

Contents

Contributors

Tove Agner, M.D., M.Sc. Department of Dermatology, Bispebjerg Hospital, University of Copenhagen, Copenhagen, Denmark

Iris S. Ale, M.D. Departments of Dermatology and Allergology, Universidad de la República del Uruguay, Montevideo, Uruguay

Ali Alikhan, M.D. Department of Dermatology, Mayo Clinic Rochester, Rochester, MN, USA

Flemming Andersen, M.D., Ph.D. Department of Dermato-venerology and the Allergy Centre, Odense University Hospital, Odense, Denmark

Klaus Ejner Andersen, M.D., Dr., Med., Sc. Department of Dermato-venerology and the Allergy Centre, Odense University Hospital, Odense, Denmark

Irena Angelova-Fischer, M.D., Ph.D. Department of Dermatology, University of Lübeck, Lübeck, Germany

Robert Baran, M.D. Nail Disease Center, Cannes, France

Richard Brans, M.D. Department of Dermatology, Environmental Medicine and Health Theory, University of Osnabrueck, Osnabrueck, Germany

Magnus Bruze, M.D., Ph.D. Department of Occupational and Environmental Dermatology, Skåne University Hospital, Lund University, Malmö, Sweden

Valeska Katinka Buder, M.D. Institute for Health Service Research in Dermatology and Nursing Clinical Research-Health Care Research-Health Economics, University Medical Center Hamburg-Eppendorf, Hamburg, Germany

Mark D.P. Davis, M.D. Department of Dermatology, Mayo Clinic Rochester, Rochester, MN, USA

Philippe O.R. Delvenne, M.D., Ph.D. Department of Dermatopathology, University Hospital of Liège, Liège, Belgium

Thomas L. Diepgen, M.D., Ph.D. Department of Social Medicine, University Hospital Heidelberg, Heidelberg, Baden-Württemberg, Germany

Peter Elsner, M.D., Ph.D. Department of Dermatology, University Hospital Jena, Jena, Germany

Malin Engfeldt, M.Sc.(Chem Eng), Ph.D. Department of Occupational and Environmental Dermatology, Skåne University Hospital, Lund University, Malmö, Sweden

Steven R. Feldman, M.D., Ph.D. Dermatology, Wake Forest School of Medicine, Winston-Salem, NC, USA

Gianfranco A. Frojo, BS University of Alabama at Birmingham, Birmingham, AL, USA

Johannes Geier, M.D. Information Network of Department of Dermatology (IVDK), University of Goettingen, Goettingen, Germany

Ana M. Giménez-Arnau, M.D., Ph.D. Department of Dermatology, Hospital del Mar, Universitat Autònoma i Pompeu Fabra, Barcelona, Spain

Anthony T.J. Goon, MBBS, MRCP, FRCP, Ph.D. National Skin Centre, Singapore

James L. Griffith Jr., M.S. School of Medicine, University of Mississippi, Jackson, MS, USA

Curtis P. Hamann, M.D. SmartPractice, Phoenix, AZ, USA

Sarah Hannam, M.B.B.S. Occupational Dermatology Research and Education Centre, Skin and Cancer Foundation, Inc, Melbourne, VIC, Australia

John Hassani, BA, MA New York Institute of Technology College of Osteopathic Medicine, Northern Boulevard, Old Westbury, NY, USA

Majken G. Hougaard, M.D. The National Research Centre for Allergy, University Hospital Gentofte, Gentofte, Denmark

Marléne A.I. Isaksson, M.D., Ph.D. Department of Occupational and Environmental Dermatology, Lund University, Skåne University Hospital, Malmö, Sweden

Swen Malte John, M.D. Department of Dermatology, Environmental Medicine and Health Theory, University of Osnabrueck, Osnabrueck, Germany

Alexandra Katsarou, M.D., Ph.D. Department of Dermatology, A. Sygros Hospital, University of Athens School of Medicine, Athens, Greece

Sanja Kezic, Ph.D. Coronel Institute of Occupational Health, Academic Medical Center, Amsterdam, The Netherlands

Jean-Marie Lachapelle, M.D., Ph.D. Department of Dermatology, Catholic University of Louvain, Brussels, Belgium

Antti Lauerma, M.D., Ph.D. Department of Dermatology, University of Helsinki, Helsinki, Finland

Sari J. Lehtimäki, Ph.D. Unit of Immunotoxicology, Finnish Institute of Occupational Health, Helsinki, Finland

Marie Lodén, Ms Pharm Sci, Dr Med Sci Research and Development, Eviderm Institute, Solna, Sweden

Howard I. Maibach, M.D. Department of Dermatology, University of California in San Francisco, San Francisco, CA, USA

Laura Malinauskiene, M.D. Allergologist and Clinical Immunologist, Allergy Center, Vilnius University Antakalnio Hospital, Vilnius, Lithuania

Birgitta Meding, M.D., Ph.D. Unit of Occupational and Environmental Dermatology, Institute of Environmental Medicine, Karolinska Institute, Stockholm, Sweden

Jean-François Nicolas, M.D., Ph.D. Department of Allergology and Immunology, Centre Hospitalier Lyon-Sud, Hospices Civils de Lyon, Pierre-Bénite, France

Rosemary L. Nixon, M.D. Occupational Dermatology Research and Education Centre, Skin and Cancer Foundation, Inc, Carlton, Melbourne, VIC, Australia

Audrey Nosbaum, M.D. Department of Allergology and Immunology, Centre Hospitalier Lyon-Sud, Hospices Civils de Lyon, Pierre-Bénite, France

Michal Wen Sheue Ong, BSc, MBBS Department of Dermatology, University of California, San Francisco, San Francisco, CA, USA

Konstantina Papagiannaki, M.D. Department of Dermatology, A. Sygros Hospital, University of Athens School of Medicine, Athens, Greece

Gérald E. Piérard, M.D., Ph.D. Department of Dermatopathology, University Hospital of Liège, Liège, Belgium

Sébastien Piérard Montefiore (Intelsig), University of Liège, Liège, Belgium

Claudine F. Piérard-Franchimont, M.D., Ph.D. Department of Dermatopathology, University Hospital of Liège, Liège, Belgium

Mark R. Pittelkow, M.D. Departments of Dermatology and Biochemistry and Molecular Biology, Mayo Clinic College of Medicine, Rochester, MN, USA

Denis Sasseville, M.D., FRCPC Division of Dermatology, Department of Medicine, McGill University Health Centre, Royal Victoria Hospital, Montreal, QC, Canada

Sibylle Schliemann, M.D. Department of Dermatology, University Hospital Jena, Jena, Germany

Christoph Skudlik, M.D. Department of Dermatology, Environmental Medicine and Health Theory, University of Osnabrueck, Osnabrueck, Germany

Kim M. Sullivan, B.A. SmartPractice, Phoenix, AZ, USA

Arash Taheri, M.D. Dermatology, Wake Forest School of Medicine, Winston-Salem, NC, USA

Dominique Tennstedt, M.D. Department of Dermatology, Catholic University of Louvain, Brussels, Belgium

Jacob P. Thyssen, M.D., Ph.D., DmSci The National Research Centre for Allergy, University Hospital Gentofte, Gentofte, Denmark

Niels K. Veien, M.D., Ph.D. Dermatology Clinic, Aalborg, Denmark

Henk B. van der Walle, M.D., Ph.D. Center of Occupational Dermatology, President Kennedylaan 100, The Netherlands

Michael R. Webster, M.B.B.S., FACD Radiotherapy Department, Skin and Cancer Foundation of Victoria, Carlton, VIC, Australia

Elke Weisshaar, M.D., Ph.D. Department of Clinical Social Medicine, Occupational and Environmental Medicine, Heidelberg University Hospital, Heidelberg, Germany

Annika Wilke Department of Dermatology, Environmental Medicine and Health Theory, University of Osnabrueck, Osnabrueck, Lower Saxony, Germany

Richard R. Winkelmann, DO Intern, O'Bleness Memorial Hospital, Athens, OH, USA

Karin Wrangsjö, M.D., Ph.D. Unit of Occupational and Environmental Dermatology, Institute of Environmental Medicine, Karolinska Institute, Stockholm, Sweden

Peggy Wright SmartPractice, St. Paul, MN, USA

Cooper C. Wriston, M.D. Department of Dermatology, Mayo Clinic College of Medicine, Rochester, MN, USA

Britta Wulfhorst, Ph.D. Department of Dermatology, Environmental Medicine and Health Theory, University of Osnabrueck, Osnabrueck, Germany

1 The Hand: An Anatomoclinical Approach

Jean-Marie Lachapelle

Contents

J.-M. Lachapelle, M.D., Ph.D.
Department of Dermatology,
Catholic University of Louvain,
10, Avenue Hippocrate, Brussels 1200, Belgium
e-mail: jean.marie.lachapelle@uclouvain.be

1.1 Introduction

The hand has always fascinated humanity, due to its unique characteristics. On the walls of Cosquer Cave, an underwater cave in Marseilles, France, prehistoric paintings include mysterious stencils of human hands.

Painters and sculptors have devoted their time to accurate reproductions of the hand.

In this respect, there is a wonderful museum in Lausanne (Switzerland) that is entirely dedicated to all sociocultural aspects of the hand [1].

The hand is well defined in Wikipedia (the free encyclopedia) [2]. It represents a very stimulating approach to this chapter. It is defined as a prehensile, multi-fingered extremity located at the end of an arm or forelimb of primates such as humans, chimpanzees, monkeys, and lemurs. Interestingly enough, a few other vertebrates, such as the koala (which has two opposable thumbs on each "hand" and fingerprints remarkably similar to human fingerprints), are often described as having either "hands" or "paws" on their front limbs.

1.2 The Human Hand: A Unique Structure

As far as we are concerned, the human hand is a unique structure, when compared to other parts of the body, and it is closely related to our environment. For example:

A. Alikhan et al. (eds.), *Textbook of Hand Eczema*,
DOI 10.1007/978-3-642-39546-8_1, © Springer-Verlag Berlin Heidelberg 2014

- The hands are used for both gross motor skills (such as grasping a large object) and fine motor skills (such as picking up a small pebble).
- As explained later on, the fingertips contain some of the densest areas of nerve endings on the body and are, therefore, the richest source of tactile feedback.

It is generally accepted that each hand is dominantly controlled by the opposing brain hemisphere, so that handedness (i.e., the preferred hand choice for single-handed activities, such as writing) reflects individual brain functioning.

This chapter is exclusively devoted to skin characteristics of the hand and is focused on some particularities that deserve special attention for an accurate understanding of lesions encountered in hand eczema.

There are hundreds of publications referring to the skeleton, the muscles, the tendons, the joints, the topography of vessels and nerves, and so forth, but they are beyond the scope of the current textbook.

1.3 Some Anatomical Remarks About the Fingers

A few observations about the five digits of the hand will help one to comprehend some characteristics of hand eczema, which is fully explained in the next chapters.

The terminology related to fingers is universally accepted. The thumb is located on one of the sides, parallel to the arm. A reliable way of identifying "true" hands is from the presence of opposable thumbs. Opposable thumbs are identified by the ability to be brought opposite to the fingers, a muscle action known as opposition.

The four other fingers can be folded over the palm, which allows the grasping of objects. Each finger, starting with the one closest to the thumb, has a colloquial name to distinguish it from the others:

- Index finger, pointer finger, or forefinger
- Middle finger or long finger
- Ring finger
- Little finger, pinky finger, or small finger

As far as the length of fingers is concerned, there is a dimorphism between males and females. The ring finger is proportionally longer than the index finger in men, whereas the index finger is proportionally longer than the ring finger in women. This is a very old observation. We have confirmed it in a recent study conducted in a cohort of 100 males and 100 females. The mean length of the ring finger was 7.96 ± 0.11 cm in men and 7.46 ± 0.17 cm in women. The mean length of the index finger was 7.64 ± 0.13 cm in men and 7.93 ± 0.08 cm in women (unpublished data).

Although correlation studies suggest that digit ratios reflect prenatal exposure to androgens, the developmental mechanism underlying sexually dimorphic digit development remains unknown. Nevertheless, recent studies have identified previously undescribed molecular dimorphisms between male and female limb buds and have provided experimental evidence that the digit ratio is a lifelong signature of prenatal hormonal exposure [3].

In another paper from the United Kingdom [4], it was demonstrated that men with index fingers longer than their ring fingers (inverted ratio) had a lower prostate cancer risk [5].

1.4 The Hand: A Mosaic of Various Juxtaposed Skin Structures

It is obvious that the skin of the hand is a very complex anatomoclinical entity. Other areas of the body share similar skin differences – for instance, the feet and the face. But, due to its vulnerability to aggressive agents, the hand deserves special attention. It is an important issue for dermatologists, occupational physicians, general practitioners, and nursing personnel. The term "mosaic" is most probably appropriate and of great help for a better understanding of various characteristics of hand eczema. When tracking fundamentals of occupational dermatology, it is important to focus on these anatomical aspects for a better understanding of several pathologies.

Most physicians divide the hand into two skin structures: the dorsum (back) of the hand and the palm. The fingers are considered separately. While this view is basically correct, it is an oversimplification of the entity. An extended view is fully explained in the next sections.

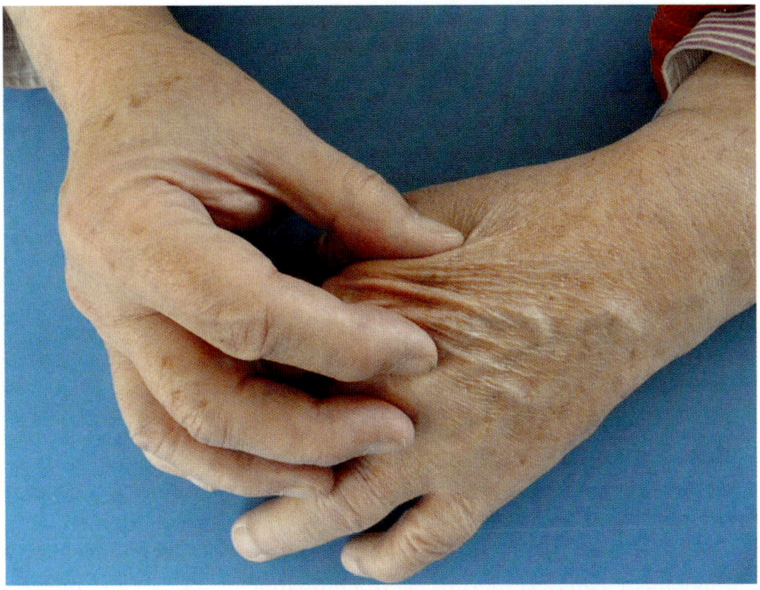

Fig. 1.1 The skin of the dorsum of the hand is thin, soft, and pliable

1.5 The Dorsum of the Hand

1.5.1 Clinical Aspects

The skin of the dorsum of the hand is generally considered very similar to the skin of the extensor aspect of the forearm.

The skin is thin, soft, and pliable so that it can recoil when the fingers are stretched. In young adults, veins may be apparent or not (Fig. 1.1).

Some areas may be hairy, mainly the latero-external sides of the hand and the back of the fingers. In occupational dermatology, when mineral oils were extensively used in many factories, these areas were classical sites for the occurrence of comedones and the so-called oil folliculitis, a rare condition nowadays [6].

1.5.2 Histological Features

The histological pattern of the dorsum of the hand and the dorsal aspect of the fingers, in formalin (or Bouin's solution)-fixed specimens, can be described as follows (Fig. 1.2):

- The rete ridges are prominent, as compared to the forearm skin, where they are flatter.
- The stratum granulosum is thick, usually three or four layers.

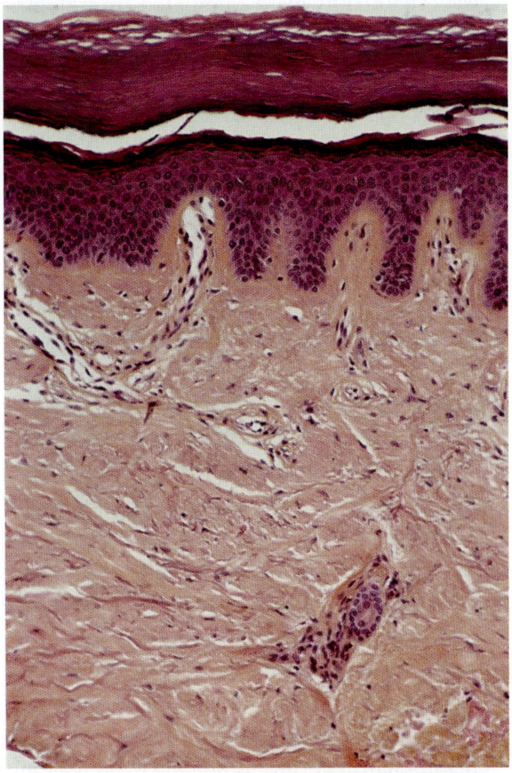

Fig. 1.2 Histological pattern of the skin of the dorsum of the hand (see text). Hematoxylin-eosin-saffron stain × 100

- The stratum corneum appears compact, often artificially separated from the stratum granulosum, due to fixations.

- Sometimes, the "basket-weave" architecture is observed in its upper layers.
- The dermis does not present specific features. Capillaries are abundant in the subepidermal area. Numerous elastic fibers play an important role in the flexibility of the skin in children and young adults. Sebaceous glands are absent. There are no corpuscular nerve endings.

The skin thickness of the dorsal hand has been precisely evaluated by histological measurements [7]. The thickness of the skin (epidermis plus dermis) ranged from 138 to 189 μm, and the thickness of the epidermis accounted for 3.6–16.8 % of the entire skin, as in most other body regions.

In a recent study, based on multiphoton laser tomography, the thicknesses of the total epidermis, viable epidermis, and stratum corneum and depth of papillary dermis were compared at the dorsal forearm and the dorsum of the hands. The results were calculated from depth-resolved intensity curves after correlation with multiphoton images [8]. They showed consistently that in all age groups, the four morphometric parameters were significantly higher on the hand compared to the forearm, while, surprisingly enough, there were no differences between age groups.

1.5.3 Some Regional Particularities

Regional particularities are important to be mentioned for a better comprehension of some characteristics of hand eczema:

- The skin covering the metacarpodigital joints is prominent when the hand is being flexed and, therefore, highly susceptible to mechanical and/or chemical aggressions. This involves rugosity and eventually crevices.
- The same remark can be applicable to the skin covering the interdigital proximal joints. But there is an additional anatomical feature worth noting. When the hand is being extended, this area is like a volcanic crater (i.e., a circular depression surrounded by skin pads). It is an ideal reservoir to store fluids or dust particles and is therefore a site of predilection for irritant contact dermatitis (Fig. 1.3).

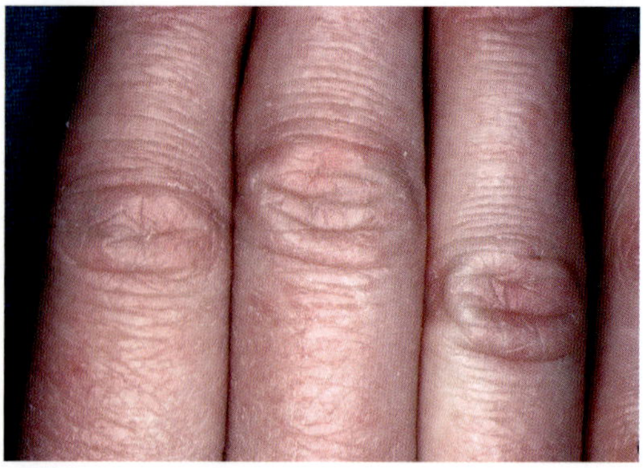

Fig. 1.3 The skin of the dorsum of the fingers covering the interdigital proximal joints. When the skin is being extended, this area is like a volcanic crater (i.e., a circular depression surrounded by skin pads) (see text)

- The eponychium is a fragile area at the extremity of the fingers. Its anatomical features are described in Chap. 4.

1.5.4 Aging and Photoaging

Like other sun-exposed areas of the skin, the dorsum of the hands is subjected to important anatomical alterations in the older population, due to the combined action of intrinsic aging and cumulative photoaging.

The main structural changes are as follows:

- Epidermal atrophy. The rete ridges disappear progressively. The stratum granulosum is thin, and the stratum corneum remains compact.
- The dermal tissue is completely disorganized. The elastic fibers are scarce; the collagen fibers become elastotic. These changes lead to an increased fragility of the skin. Fingers are less affected by the evolutive process.
- The clinical consequences are obvious: the veins are very apparent and dilated; minor traumas induce hemorrhages (Bateman's purpura) (Figs. 1.4 and 1.5). Actinic keratoses and lentigines are common in older people.

1.6 The Palm of the Hand

For clarity, the anatomoclinical features of the palm are described separately from those specifically characteristic of the pulps of the fingers.

1.6.1 Clinical Aspects

Several clinical features of the hand deserve attention.

In contrast to the skin of the dorsum of the hand, the palm is firm, sticky, and not easily pliable, particularly on the thenar and hypothenar areas.

There are very pronounced palmar creases, well delineated, horizontal, or oblique, with individual variances, most probably linked with genetic factors.

The dermatoglyphics (dermatoglyphs or fingerprints) are the hallmark of palmar skin. The term "dermatoglyphics" refers to the friction ridge formations that appear on the palm of the hands and soles. The ridging formations serve well to increase contact and aid in the prevention of slippage. All studies of the dermal ridge arrangements, including genetics and anthropology, are classified under the term "dermatoglyphics" [9].

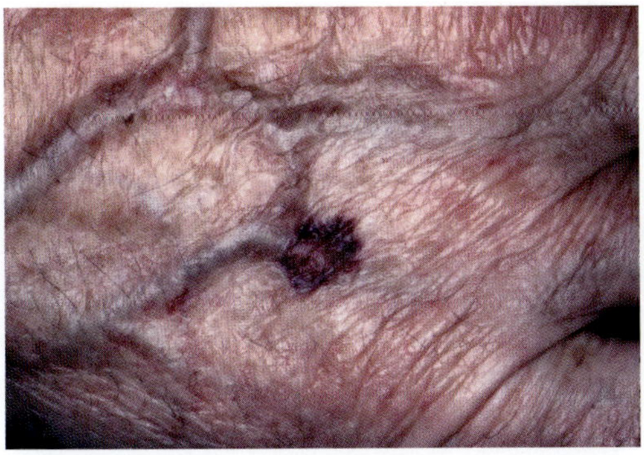

Fig. 1.4 The skin of the dorsum of the hand in aged people. The cumulative effect of aging and photoaging is clearly illustrated: skin atrophy, prominent veins, and Bateman's purpura

Although dermatoglyphics structure has been mechanistically related to fingerprint formation, a separate mechanism for fingerprint maintenance must exist, or prints would be lost by friction.

Indeed, a new mechanism of fingerprint maintenance was predicted theoretically and confirmed experimentally, as emphasized in a recent paper [10]. It is achieved by an organization of the print corneum, which ensures its continuous separation over the whole of the undulating print surface, even when friction is applied only to the tips of the ridges; the preferred route of separation of print keratinocytes runs up and down the print ridges and troughs and thereby maintains them and is presumably ordered by predominantly horizontal intercellular attachments between print keratinocytes.

This stimulating study is important because it sheds some light on the field of frictional and/or chemical irritant dermatitis of the palms and flexural aspects of the fingers, including the pulps. It is noteworthy that when dermatitis occurs, fingerprints momentarily disappear [11], but they recover when the disease is under control [10].

The proximal and middle palmar parts of the fingers share the same anatomical characteristics as those of the palmar hand skin.

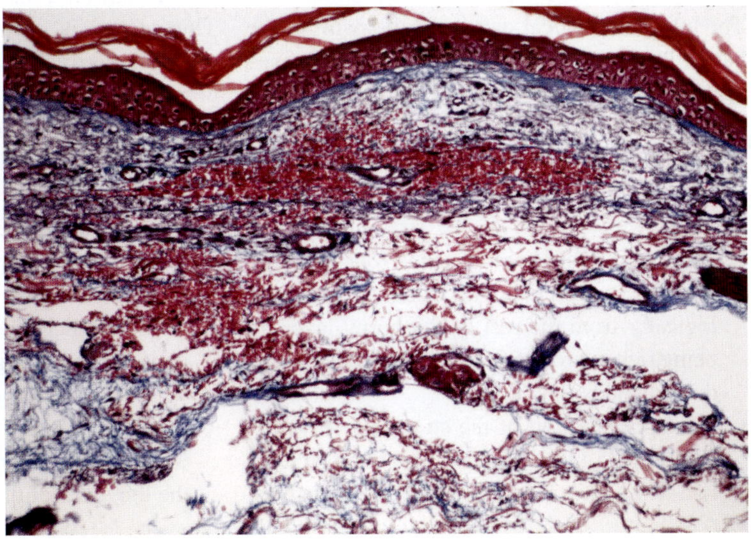

Fig. 1.5 Histological features of aged skin of the dorsum of the hand. Epidermis is linear, elastotic fibers are prominent, and dermal hemorrhages are typical of Bateman's purpura. Masson's Trichrome Blue stain × 100

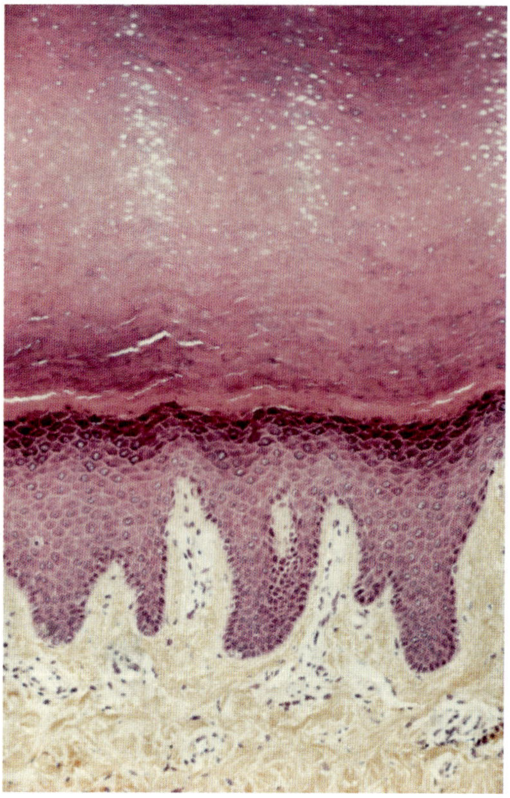

Fig. 1.6 Histological pattern of the skin of the palm of the hand. Hematoxylin-eosin-saffron stain × 100

People from African ancestry display reduced skin pigmentation in the designated locations.

1.6.2 Histological Features

The histopathological pattern of the palm of the hand, in formalin (or Bouin's solution)-fixed specimens, can be described as follows (Fig. 1.6):

- The epidermis is very thick. Rete ridges are elongated and the stratum granulosum is conspicuous.
- The lowest portion of the stratum corneum appears as a thin homogeneous zone, referred to as the stratum lucidum, which differs histologically from the rest of the horny layer by being rich in protein-bound lipids contained in the Odland bodies.
- The upper portion of the stratum corneum is compacted and thickened, as compared to non-acral sites. It is crossed by vertical sweat ducts, at regular intervals, either rectilinear or coiled.
- All of these epidermal features are similar to those encountered on the soles.
- Eccrine sweat glands, which, incidentally, are distributed ubiquitously over the body surface, exhibit higher density in the soles and the forehead, followed by the palms and the cheeks (see Chap. 34).
- Apocrine sweat glands, hairs, and sebaceous glands are totally absent.
- Special nerve endings—Meissner and Vater-Pacini corpuscles [12–14]—are present on the palm of the hand but are far more concentrated on the distal pulps of the fingers (for their description, see later). Of note, they are also encountered in the modified hairless skin at the mucocutaneous junctions, namely, the glans penis, prepuce, clitoris, labia minora, perianal region, and vermilion border of the lip.

In one of the studies quoted earlier [7], the thickness of the palm of the hand has been precisely evaluated. When considering the entire skin (epidermis plus dermis), the thickness ranged from 1318 to 1586 μm, whereas the thickness of the epidermis ranged from 601 to 637 μm and accounted for 40.6–44.6 % of the entire skin.

1.7 Special Nerve Endings: Meissner and Vater-Pacini Corpuscles

This section is devoted to some specific nerve endings, referred to as Meissner and Vater-Pacini corpuscles:

- Meissner corpuscles are located in the dermal papillae (Fig. 1.7) and mediate a sense of touch. At the site of their greatest concentration (i.e., the fingertips), approximately every fourth papilla contains a Meissner corpuscle. Their size averages 30–80 μm in diameter. Owing to their size and their elongated shape, they occupy the greatest part of the papilla where they are located. They possess a capsule composed of several layers of flattened Schwann cells that are arranged transverse to the long axis of the corpuscle [12, 13].

- Vater-Pacini corpuscles are large nerve end organs that are located in the subcutis and mediate a sense of pressure (Fig. 1.8). They measure up to 1 mm in diameter and are easily detected by light microscopy. They are formed most commonly below the skin of the volar aspects of the palms and soles, showing their greatest concentration at the tips of the fingers and toes. They vary in shape. Some are ovoid; others have the appearance of a flattened sphere, and still others have an irregular shape.

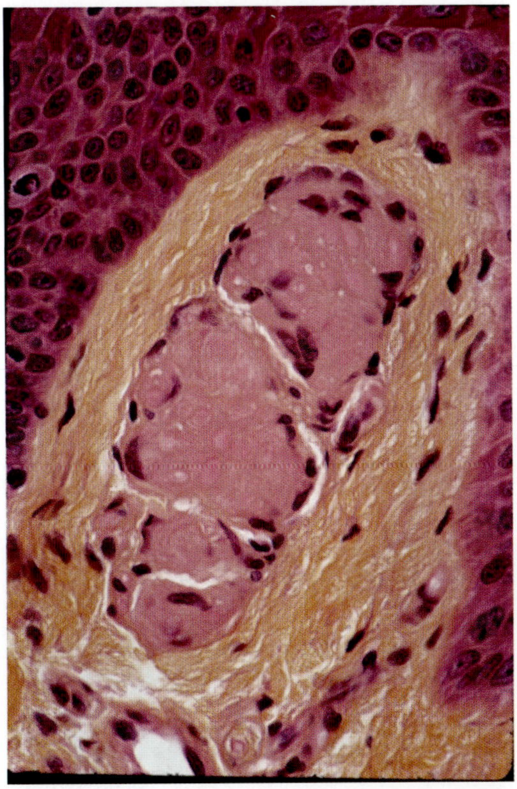

Fig. 1.7 Meissner corpuscles. Hematoxylin-eosin-saffron stain × 200

For further information, including ultrastructural aspects, one can refer to classical publications in the field [14].

1.8 Pulps of the Fingers (Fingertips)

The pulps of the fingers (or fingertips) represent a very unique entity, displaying particular clinical and histological features, as compared to other sites of palmar skin. These features clearly explain the specific characteristics of a variety of hand eczema (i.e., fingertip dermatitis) (see Chap. 3).

1.8.1 Clinical Aspects

Some specific clinical aspects can be described as follows:

- In most Caucasian individuals, the fingertips are reddish, whereas the palmar proximal and middle parts of the fingers are white. This can be related to marked differences in the microvasculature.

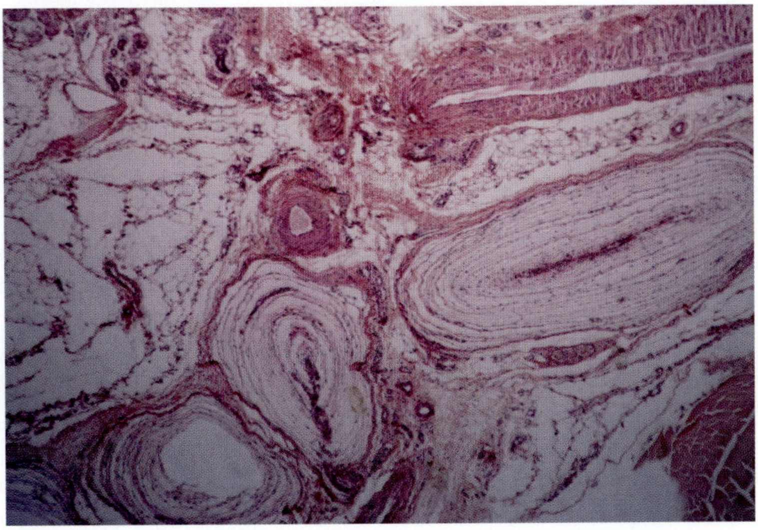

Fig. 1.8 Vater-Pacini corpuscles. Hematoxylin-eosin stain × 100

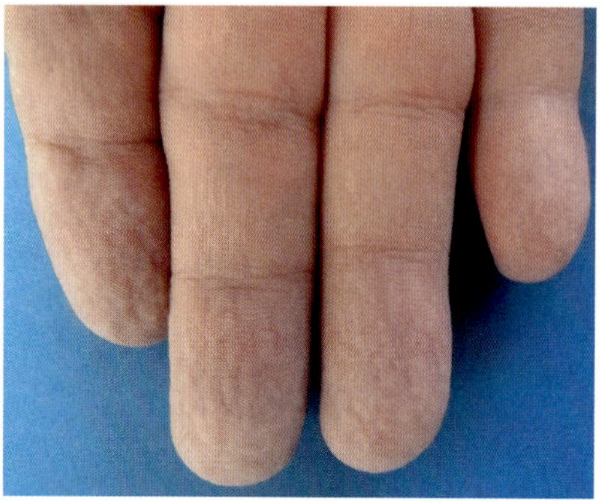

Fig. 1.9 Physiological wrinkling of the fingertips, after immersion in water (40°C) for 20 min

- Dermatoglyphs (fingerprints) are conspicuous. They disappear when fingertip dermatitis occurs, but they are restored when treatment has been successfully achieved.
- Physiological wrinkling of the fingertips after immersion in water (Fig. 1.9) is not fully understood. Entry of water into keratinocytes is partly responsible [15–17] but also depends on an intact sympathetic nervous system [17]. A proposed mechanism is that water enters the sweat glands, producing altered electrolyte concentrations, and the afferent message then triggers autonomic fibers to mediate vasoconstriction [17, 18].
- Apart from these (potentially combined) osmotic and/or sympathetic theories to explain physiological wrinkling of the fingers, a new theory, which has been called "mechanistic," has been advocated in a recent paper [19]. Evidence is provided that, rather than being an accidental side effect of wetness, wet-induced wrinkles have been selected to enhance grip in wet conditions. Their morphology has the signature properties of drainage networks, enabling efficient removal of water from the gripped surface.

  This can be compared to the grooved face of winter tires, which adhere more firmly to the road [19].

  Physiological wrinkling has to be distinguished from pathological conditions, such as aquagenic syringeal acrokeratoderma (see Chap. 5).

  Wrinkling may extend to other parts of the palms.

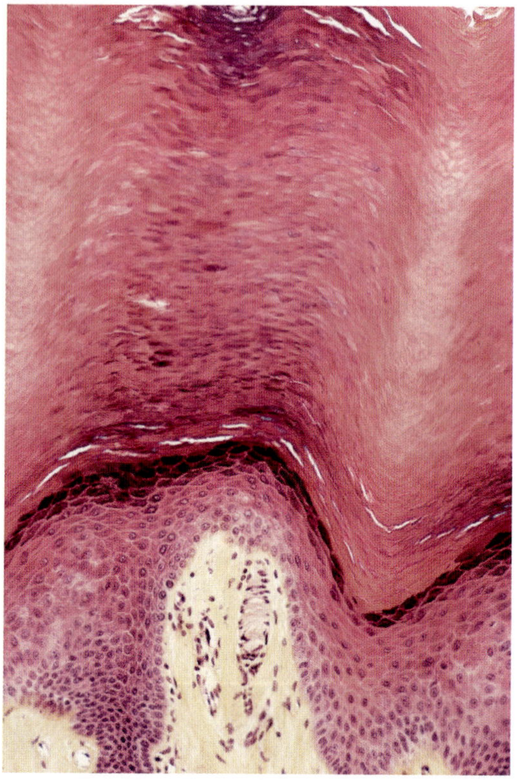

Fig. 1.10 Histological features of the fingertips (see text). Hematoxylin-eosin-saffron stain × 100

1.8.2 Histological Features

The fingertips have specific anatomical characteristics that can be summarized as follows:

- The pulp spaces of the palmar side of the tips of the fingers and thumb contain fatty tissue (pulp means "fleshy skin") that is divided into numerous compartments by fibrous septa that pass between the distal phalanx and the skin. Terminal branches of the digital vessels course through the spaces, and some of them supply the end of the distal phalanx. The pulp space is limited proximally by the firm adherence of the skin of the distal flexion crease to the underlying tissue; this prevents skin infection from spreading proximally along the finger.
- The epidermis is very thick and the rete ridges are prominent. The stratum granulosum is conspicuous, and the stratum corneum is compacted and very similar to that of the palmar hand skin, except that it is undulating, most probably characteristically related to repeated gripping (Figs. 1.10 and 1.11).

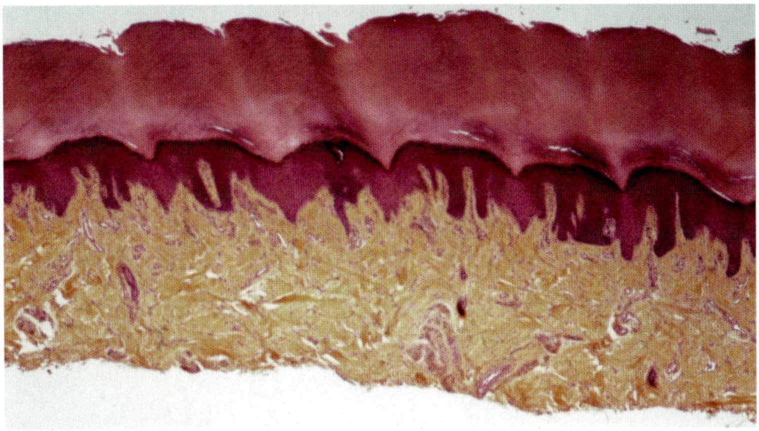

Fig. 1.11 Histological features of the fingertips: closer view. Hematoxylin-eosin-saffron stain × 100

- Meissner corpuscles are numerous in dermal papillae, as explained earlier in the text.
- Glomus cells (cutaneous glomus, Sucquet-Hoyer canal) are of smooth muscle origin and polyhedral in shape. These cells comprise specialized vascular structures called glomus formations that are abundant in the distal pads and nail beds of the fingers and to a lesser degree on the volar aspect of the palms and feet. They play an important role in thermoregulation [20].

1.9 Lateral Aspects of the Fingers

Lateral aspects of the fingers are a transitional zone between dorsal and palmar skin of the hand. There is a progressive evolution from the lower to the upper parts of the fingers, but it is generally acknowledged that the lower two-thirds of the fingers reproduce the pattern of palmar skin, whereas the upper third is similar to the skin of the dorsal hand.

These anatomoclinical particularities are worth mentioning when considering variants of hand eczema. The classical example is the burst of pompholyx (see Chaps. 3 and 13), which, at its onset, is strictly localized on the palms of the hand but also on the lower two-thirds of the lateral aspects of the fingers. Later on, pompholyx can eventually be widespread over the dorsum of the hand.

Conclusion

This chapter can be summarized as follows:

- The skin of the hand is considered a "mosaic" of different juxtaposed skin structures.
- It is obvious that the dorsum and the palm of the hands are structurally quite different; moreover, they exhibit some specific subunits.
- Consequently, it is obvious that hand eczema offers a multitude of clinical facets, directly linked with the anatomoclinical characteristics of the skin of the hand.

References

1. Verdan C. La main: cet univers. Donges, Switzerland; Editions du Verseau. Fondation du Musée de la Main; 1994: 223 pages.
2. Hand. Available from: http://en.wikipedia.org/wiki/Hand
3. Zheng Z, Cohn MJ. Developmental basis of sexually dimorphic digit ratios. Proc Natl Acad Sci USA. 2011; 108:16289–94.
4. Khaïrullin R. Segmental 2:4 digit ratio. Unilateral, bilateral and hand-type differences in man. Homo. 2011;62:478–86.
5. Rahman AA, Lophatananon A, Stewart-Brown S, Harriss O, Anderson J, Parker T, et al. Hand pattern indicates prostate cancer risk. Br J Cancer. 2011;104: 175–7.
6. Lachapelle J-M, Frimat P, Tennstedt D, Ducombs G. Précis de dermatologie professionnelle et de l'environnement. Paris: Masson; 1992. p. 372.
7. Lee Y, Hwang K. Skin thickness of Korean adults. Surg Radiol Anat. 2002;24:183–9.
8. Koehler MJ, Vogel T, Elsner P, König K, Bückle R, Kaatz M. In vivo measurement of the human epidermal thickness in different localizations by multiphoton laser tomography. Skin Res Technol. 2010;16:259–64.
9. Loomis CA. Development and morphogenesis of the skin. Adv Dermatol. 2001;17:183–210.
10. Shuster S. Fingerprint maintenance: a new dermatoglyphic mechanism. Br J Dermatol. 2011;164:738–42.
11. Lee CK, Chang CC, Johar A, Puwirr O, Roshidah B. Fingerprint changes and verification failure among patients with hand dermatitis. Arch Dermatol. 2012;17: 1–6.

12. Cauna N, Ross LL. The fine structure of the Meissner's touch corpuscles of human fingers. J Biophys Biochem Cytol. 1960;8:467–82.
13. Hashimoto K. Fine structure of Meissner corpuscle of human palmar skin. J Invest Dermatol. 1973;60:20–8.
14. Pease DC, Quilliam TA. Electron microcopy of the Pacinian corpuscle. J Biopohys Biochm Cytol. 1957;3: 331–44.
15. Braham J, Sadeh M, Sarova-Pinhas I. Skin wrinkling on immersion of hands. Arch Neurol. 1979;36: 113–4.
16. Tsai N, Kirkham S. Fingertip skin wrinkling – the effect of varying tonicity. J Hand Surg (Br). 2005;30:273–5.
17. Wilder-Smith EP, Chow A. Water-immersion wrinkling is due to vasoconstriction. Muscle Nerve. 2003;27: 307–11.
18. Wilder-Smith EP. Water-immersion wrinkling – physiology and use as an indication of sympathetic function. Clin Anatom Res. 2004;14:125–31.
19. Changizi M, Weber R, Kotecha R, Palazzo J. Are wet-induced wrinkled fingers prime rain treads? Brain Behav Evol. 2011;77:286–90.
20. Elder DE, Elenitsas R, Johnson BL, Murphy GF, editors. Lever's histopathology of the skin. 9th ed. Philadelphia: Lippincott, Williams and Wilkins; 2005. p. 1229.

Hand Dermometrology

2

Gérald E. Piérard, Sébastien Piérard,
Claudine F. Piérard-Franchimont,
and Philippe O.R. Delvenne

Contents

G.E. Piérard, M.D., Ph.D. (✉)
C.F. Piérard-Franchimont, M.D., Ph.D.
P.O.R. Delvenne, M.D., Ph.D.
Department of Dermatopathology,
University Hospital of Liège,
Boulevard de L' Hopital, Liège 4000, Belgium
e-mail: gerald.pierard@ulg.ac.be;
claudine.franchimont@ulg.ac.be;
p.delvenne@ulg.ac.be

S. Piérard
Montefiore (Intelsig), University of Liège,
Grand Traverse, Liège 4000, Belgium
e-mail: sebastien.pierard@ulg.ac.be

2.1 Introduction

Skin covering the hands is typically partitioned into two distinct and sharply demarcated structures corresponding to the palms and the dorsum, respectively. Inflammatory skin diseases affect one or the other anatomic aspect, or both. The response to treatments is not expected to be synchronous and similar on both aspects of the hands. In health and disease, most of the physical attributes of the skin on the back side of the hands closely resemble those of the dorsal forearm. By contrast, the physical properties of the palms are quite distinct. The differences result from specific structural and functional aspects of the skin tissues, including the stratum corneum (SC), the stratum Malpighi, and the dermal extracellular matrix (ECM). In addition, the physiologic activity of the eccrine sweat glands is clearly distinct on these respective skin areas [1].

A. Alikhan et al. (eds.), *Textbook of Hand Eczema*,
DOI 10.1007/978-3-642-39546-8_2, © Springer-Verlag Berlin Heidelberg 2014

Anywhere on the body, the intact SC prevents any uncontrolled loss of water and electrolytes from the skin. In addition, it attempts to protect the underlying living cells from daily exogenous threats, including physical insults, (immuno-) reactive chemicals, toxic/corrosive xenobiotics, and intruding microorganisms. Nevertheless, hands are particularly exposed to exogenous insults responsible for dermatoses. Their high prevalence is commonly due to some initial alterations taking place in the topmost SC layers. In addition, hand contact dermatoses, either primarily allergic or irritant in nature, are far from being trivial [2, 3]. They are responsible for both physical and psychological morbidity.

This chapter reviews a series of bioinstrumental methods relevant to the objective noninvasive characterization of hand dermatoses. A key feature is the structure and functional properties of the SC.

2.2 The Stratum Corneum: The Ultimate Barrier

In spite of its minimal intrinsic metabolic activity, the regular SC represents a highly specialized structure that is subject to continuous renewal while keeping an almost steady state in its architecture and thickness. However, some ultrastructural, molecular, and physical heterogeneity is present in the SC [4, 5]. In addition, the SC serves as a biosensor signaling the underlying living epidermis about a series of external stimuli and threats. Accordingly, the SC is intimately involved in the process of sensory irritation [6] and allergic/irritant contact dermatitis.

According to the hand side and the expected specific functions, two different aspects of SC are distinguished, namely, (1) the palms adapted for weight bearing and friction and (2) the dorsum, where the thin membranous SC exhibits high flexibility and relatively waterproof attributes. A 40-fold difference in average thickness distinguishes the thick, horny palms and the thin, membranous SC (about 600 μm vs. 15 μm, respectively). On the dorsum of the hands, the regular SC is typically composed of 12–20 layers of flattened polyhedral corneocytes, about 1 μm thick and approximately 1,000 μm^2 in exposed surface area. Of note, the average corneocyte area appears to be age dependent and influenced by any alteration in the SC turnover.

Each single corneocyte is composed of a water-insoluble protein complex forming a highly structured keratin microfibrillar scaffold. This structure is encapsulated in a protein- and lipid-enriched shell exhibiting variable maturation among corneocytes. Two distinct types of corneocyte envelopes were identified as the fragile/immature type, contrasting with the rigid/mature type [7]. Each corneocyte is further embedded in a wrap of hydrophobic lipid bilayers that preserves the SC water-holding capacity. This structure hinders the outward trans-SC water flux and prevents any tissue desiccation. Both the SC structure and the transepidermal water loss (TEWL) result from dynamic processes that are possibly altered in health and disease [1]. In these instances, the SC homeostasis is altered.

Palms are partitioned by shallow hollow creases delimiting dermatoglyphics (Fig. 2.1). Compared to the hand back side, corneocytes of the palms contain about half the amount of water-soluble compounds, and they become easily brittle upon dehydration. They are more permeable to water and chemicals. Any peculiar physical protection by the palms is almost entirely related to the prominent SC thickness. However, corneocytes of the palms prove to be more easily dissociated by rubbing and abrasive chemicals. In addition, the corneocyte envelopes are more easily altered by alkali than those forming the membranous SC.

The lamellar lipids in the SC play a key role in the skin permeability barrier function. Their organization is mainly due to three types of lipids, namely, the ceramides, cholesterol, and free fatty acids. Both the physical structure and the molecular composition of the SC contribute to this property, which is of vital importance to survival. The SC barrier function is of the utmost importance for the regulation of the epidermal biology. Constant renewal of the outermost layer of the epidermis and its orderly desquamation control this physiologic function.

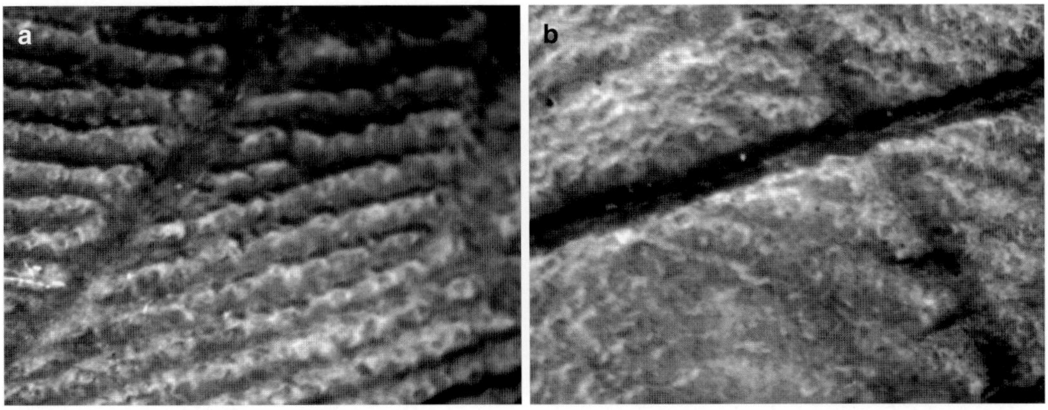

Fig. 2.1 Typical ridged pattern on the palmar aspect of the hand. (**a**) Parallel ridges, regularly spaced by shallow hollows. (**b**) Shallow and deeper creases

2.3 Objective Assessments in Occupational Dermatology

The SC is a repository for the end stage of many events that previously altered the underlying living epidermis. The ethnic and genetic background, age, nutritional status, some physical agents, and environmental factors, as well as a series of drugs, cosmetics, toiletries, and other chemical xenobiotics, represent major modulators of the SC structure [8, 9]. The appearance and performance of the SC are directly associated with its structural organization [10]. In particular, the complex biologic features of the epidermis govern the response to medical therapies and cosmetic management. It is thus important to control the nature, severity, and extent of any functional SC disturbance.

The diversity of hand dermatoses is large, but most of them are the expression of allergic contact dermatitis and irritant dermatitis [2, 3]. The disease history, as well as the clinical and histopathologic aspects, commonly helps to establish the accurate diagnosis. However, in some instances, the relative subjectivity linked to the clinical assessments is open to bias and to large interobserver variations. A growing demand is currently witnessed for objective, controlled, and standardized assessments of both the skin condition and therapeutic monitoring. In addition, measuring the skin biophysical properties appears valuable for predicting hand dermatosis risks following detection of subclinical signs [11, 12].

Dermometrology hardly distinguishes irritant from nonirritant reactions. Rather, dermometrology methods are crucial for validation of clinical scoring systems and for quantifying the dynamics of development and resolution phases of the inflammatory process. The choice of the bioinstrumentation remains primordial, depending on both the expected tissue level of skin alterations and the nature of the disturbed physiopathologic parameters. Indeed, it is quite easy to set down a probe onto the skin and display a computer reading. However, it is more important to generate meaningful information.

2.4 Skin Bioinstrumentation in Perspective

Dermometrology allows one to objectively assess clinical inflammatory signs, including erythema, scaling, and infiltration [13]. The methods characterize both functional and structural aspects of the skin. The most relevant analytic measurements deal with TEWL, SC moisture, SC cohesiveness, SC water-holding capacity, SC pH, capillary blood flow, and skin colors. Any of the bioinstrumental assessments have to be carried out under controlled and reasonably similar environmental conditions including the relative humidity (40–60 %), temperature (20–23°C), and dew-point values [14]. Ideally, in a given clinical setting, a dedicated, trained evaluator/investigator should perform all instrumental assessments in a similar controlled environment. For any dermometrology method, it is wise to rule out any interference of a formulation (topical medication, cosmetics, etc.) on the measurements.

The clinical evaluation usually relies on defined grading scales. However, these evaluations are negatively influenced by ordinal semiquantitative grading scales based on imprecise and blurred definitions. Indeed, any ordinal grade should fit with distinctive clinical descriptions similarly interpreted by different well-trained clinicians and investigators. Indistinct gradient categories are further clouded by introducing 0.5 readings when the clinical signs seemingly fell between two consecutive integer grades. Thus, in order to avoid inconsistencies, any grading scale aiming at collecting clinical data should strive to provide well-defined categories to the physician.

Assessments are expected to be less confusing following controlled bioinstrumentation. Indeed, the different procedures are commonly more accurate, sensitive, specific, and reproducible. The power of most biometrology methods surpasses any subjective clinical grading. As a result, multiparametric dermometrology has gained popularity in the assessment of a number of skin conditions. Clear, well-designed, objective methods show increased positive predictive values. Some subclinical effects are possibly discernible, predicting the onset of overt skin reactions [11, 15, 16]. Any multipronged testing bypasses limitations linked to a single assessment. In essence, each measuring device provides information focused on a restricted range of changes about a given skin characteristic. A multipronged approach is encouraged for unraveling some complex aspects of skin biology. Typically, it aims at increasing the validity of the global assessment [15].

Patch testing is used to diagnose allergic contact dermatitis for more than a century. For that purpose, a visual scoring system is still in use, but more objective and quantitative criteria were proposed to interpret patch test results. Various dermometrology methods (colorimeter, transepidermal water loss, overall capacitance, skin capacitance mapping/imaging, laser Doppler velocimeter, reflectance spectrophotometer, and ultrasound) have been explored for the objective quantification of experimental sodium lauryl sulfate (SLS)-induced irritant dermatitis. Noninvasive techniques for evaluating skin surface contours (e.g., conventional optical and laser profilometer) and skin color are other useful tools.

2.5 Defining the Value of Skin Bioinstrumentation

Prior to performing measurements, the procedure must be validated, and the device must be adjusted and calibrated, according either to reference values or to relevant internal standards. In addition, it is essential to cope with the sensitivity, reproducibility, and range of variation of the measured parameters. It is obvious that reliable and reproducible measurements are primordial. Clearly, consistency among a set of measurements performed on the same skin condition increases confidence about the observations [17].

Method accuracy is an indication of the systemic error. It relies on the level of similarity between (1) the mean values of repeat measurements and (2) the reference value corresponding to in-house or international standards. The limit of detection refers to the lowest detectable value. By contrast, the limit of quantification is the lowest change discernible with confidence in the peculiar observational design. Linearity in value changes within a given range of data refers to the ability of the procedure to provide test data directly proportional to actual values. The range of data represents the interval between the lower and upper limits of the concerned scale of measurements.

Repeatability refers to the similarity of data collected under identical conditions, including the same operator, device, and samples, as well as a brief time interval between assessments. By contrast, reproducibility is defined by comparing data from different laboratories, operators, and samples examined at different times by different devices. The method precision refers to the scatter dispersion of measurements obtained under controlled conditions from the same homogeneous sample.

The method ruggedness refers to the effects of small changes in the test procedure on measuring performance. The method sensitivity refers to the capacity to record small variations or differences within the defined range of measurements.

2.6 Drawbacks in Skin Bioinstrumentation

The specificity and sensitivity of well-designed bioinstrumentations are typically optimized by the manufacturer, but they occasionally suffer from a series of bias. The interpretation of data is flawed when a beginner conceptually oversimplifies the aspects of the skin physiopathology under consideration. In addition, the measuring devices offer nearly unlimited possibilities that are not supported by guidelines and technical standardization. Indeed, only few recognized quality-control procedures are available for ensuring uniformity of data collection and sound interpretation. Certainly, any measurement without appropriate control introduces inherent bias and inconsistencies.

Some environmental factors notoriously affect a number of measurements. Data interpretation needs adequate expertise in the understanding of both the technical aspects and the physiopathology and microanatomy of variables under consideration. The outcome-measured parameter must support the study purpose and be objectively defined. When multiple parameters are used, the critical ones must be identified and justified by reference to publications, guidelines, or recommendations by scientific groups or regulatory authorities.

2.7 Stratum Corneum Barrier Function and Transepidermal Water Loss

The SC permeability barrier function is rapidly altered during the initial steps of both allergic and irritant contact dermatitis [18, 19]. Both the SC water content and water flux through the SC are disturbed in these conditions. They represent two distinct variables related by Fick's law. TEWL is part of the insensible perspiration contributed by both the body water diffusion through the SC and water vapor issued from the acrosyringia below the thermal sweating threshold [1, 20]. In non-emotionally sweating areas, a careful control of experimental conditions allows the contribution of sweat evaporation to remain minimal.

Sources of interferences with TEWL determinations belong to individual factors, environmental conditions, and instrumental errors. The physiologic subject-linked parameters include ethnicity, age, gender, anatomical site, skin surface temperature, SC integrity, and possibly circadian chronobiology. The relevant environmental variables encompass the probe temperature, any air flow near the test site, as well as environmental temperature and relative humidity. Some specific limitations differ according to the open or closed measurement methods.

The open-chamber diffusion technique (Tewameter, C+K Electronic, Cologne, Germany) provides continuous measurements in ambient air, with minimal alterations of the microenvironment overlying the skin surface. Another portable device (VapoMeter, Delfin Technologies Ltd., Kuopio, Finland) uses a humidity sensor in a closed chamber [21].

TEWL is one of the most relevant parameters assessing the SC permeability barrier function and its alteration in hand dermatoses. Both the open- and closed-chamber methods for TEWL determination detect the discrete to severe alterations of the SC. On the dorsum of the hands, a low TEWL ($\leq$5 g m^2/h) suggests an intact skin barrier function. By contrast, irritant xenobiotics compromising the hand barrier increase TEWL, whose value is frequently above 10 g m^2/h. TEWL on the palms is typically higher than on the dorsum of the hands. The efficacy of skin-protective creams for the hand is possibly assessed using TEWL determinations [22].

2.8 Electrometric Assessments of Stratum Corneum Moisture

The SC water content affects both skin barrier permeability and SC flexibility. It regulates the activity of hydrolytic enzymes involved in corneocyte desquamation. Failure of the SC to retain water promotes xerosis and skin harshness, which is usually misinterpreted as SC dryness. This condition frequently impairs the barrier permeability function on the hands. Thus, any reduction in the SC water-holding capacity increases the susceptibility to develop irritant and/or contact dermatitis [20]. Of note, this SC feature is difficult to maintain when exposed to a relatively dry and cold environment (low dew point). This basic SC characteristic depends on the amount and composition of the natural moisturizing factor (NMF) stored inside corneocytes and on the integrity of the SC barrier function as well.

In routine clinical settings, the SC hydration is conveniently assessed using electrometric devices [23, 24]. The determination of any of the electric conductance, capacitance, and impedance provides indirect information about the SC hydration [25]. Clearly, a series of individual-, instrument-, and environment-related variables influence the electrometric methods. Indeed, electric properties of skin are modulated by its surface texture and microrelief, as well as by the SC water and electrolyte content and the sweat production.

The capacitance method is rooted on the water permittivity ($e=81$), which is above most other molecules. Hence, the SC dielectric characteristics mainly depend on its water content [24]. According to the location of the measurement site, sources of error or variations in the data collections are possible. The main interfering factors include sweat production and vellus hair density, as well as the SC electrolyte content and some artifacts from applied xenobiotics. One of the most popular capacitance devices is the Corneometer CM 825 (C+K Electronic, Cologne, Germany). It measures the relative SC capacitance down to a depth of approximately 10–20 μm. The sensor probe consists of two closely juxtaposed finger-type metal plates. The SC water content regulates the local dielectric constant and thus a proportional capacitance change expressed in Corneometer average capacitance (CMAC). A spring present in the measuring probe guarantees a constant application pressure onto the skin.

Any regular device devoted to skin capacitance measurements provides average electrometric value of the global skin area covered by the sensor probe. By contrast, real-time skin capacitance mapping/imaging (SCM) is a nonoptical method measuring capacitance every 50 μm, providing information about the possible heterogeneity in the measured physical parameter over the test area. The sensor probe provides computer recordings of both the skin surface hydration and microrelief. The SkinChip device (L'Oréal, Paris, France) contains a network of 92,160 microcapacitors orderly dispersed on an 18×12.8 mm plate protected by a thin silicon oxide layer. The probe must be closely applied to the skin surface for approximately 5 s in order to collect relevant information without interfering with both the water flux through the SC and the water collection inside the SC. SCM is displayed on a computer screen as pixels in a range of 256 grey levels [26, 27]. SCM data correlate with corneosurfametry (CSM) assessments [28]. SCM provides information about the kinetics of surfactant-related irritation, including the successive corneocyte swelling and desiccation steps [29].

Other methods were described for assessing the SC moisture. The most sophisticated ones correspond to the microwave, thermal, and spectroscopic methods, including nuclear magnetic resonance spectroscopy, infrared spectroscopy, and Raman spectroscopy [30–33]. The near-infrared imaging and the confocal Raman microspectroscopy help determine the water gradient across the whole SC thickness [30, 33]. The Raman method is based on the inelastic light scattering of different molecules. The proportion of the intensities of the Raman bands at certain shifts determines the water-to-protein ratio. The water content is expressed in weight proportion of wet tissue.

2.9 Assessment of the Stratum Corneum Structure

Two semiquantitative noninvasive methods shed some light on the SC structure, which is particularly affected by allergic and irritant contact dermatoses. These time-honored methods correspond to the cyanoacrylate skin surface stripping (CSSS) and the self-adhesive coated disc (SACD) sampling.

2.9.1 Cyanoacrylate Skin Surface Stripping

The CSSS method entails harvesting the upper layers of the SC looking for focal corneocyte clumpiness, parakeratosis, serosity deposits, and inflammatory cells. The CSSS method consists of depositing a droplet of cyanoacrylate adhesive onto a supple transparent sheet of terephthalate polyethylene. The material (3S-biokit, C+K Electronic, Cologne, Germany) is pressed firmly onto the lesion to be sampled. After 10–20 s, a continuous SC sheet is conveniently harvested. As the adhesion mechanism of cyanoacrylate relies on a chemical reaction, the depth of the removed SC is determined by the depth of penetration of the adhesive before hardening. The cleavage level is exclusively located inside the SC. Oozing and eroded lesions, as encountered in acute eczema, are not adequately explored using CSSS. CSSS samples are conveniently harvested from any part of the body, with two main provisos [34]. First, sampling from hairy areas such as on the dorsum of the hand is painful, because of hair being pulled out. Therefore, it is advisable to shave such an area before CSSS sampling. Second, intercorneocyte cohesion on the palms is frequently stronger than the cyanoacrylate bond, thus impairing the collection of an unbroken sheet of corneocytes. However, CSSS sampling from such a site is possible in certain physiopathologic conditions associated with a compromised cohesion between corneocytes.

Disease severity and therapeutic effects are possibly assessed noninvasively on CSSS collected from the hands. For instance, xerosis corresponding to various forms of predominantly orthokeratotic hyperkeratosis [10] is found in various degrees of severity in inflammatory hand dermatoses [10, 34]. Several grades of orthokeratotic hyperkeratosis were identified on CSSS [10]. Grade 0 corresponds to the absence of hyperkeratosis, except for some discrete focal accumulation of corneocytes in the primary order lines of the skin. Grade 1 corresponds to a continuous linear hyperkeratosis of the primary lines or to focal hyperkeratosis predominant at the site of adnexal openings at hair follicle openings and acrosyringia. Grade 2 corresponds to focal hyperkeratosis of the skin surface plateaus covering one-third of the sampling at the most. Grade 3 resembles grade 2, but with a xerotic area extending over one-third of the CSSS. Grade 4 is defined by a homogeneous and diffuse hyperkeratosis with persistence of primary order lines. Grade 5 is similar to grade 4, but without recognizable tracks of primary order lines or to the most heterogeneous and diffuse hyperkeratosis vanishing the primary line network.

Corneodynamics relies on SC staining in vivo by dansyl chloride or dihydroxyacetone. Sampling CSSS 10 days later allows one to measure under the microscope any loss of dye related to the SC renewal [35, 36]. These aspects are particularly altered by contact allergic/irritant dermatitis.

2.9.2 Self-Adhesive Coated Disc Sampling

Reproducible harvesting of the stratum disjunctum, which corresponds to the loose topmost layers of the SC, is possible using SACD [37–43]. The sampling material corresponds to a transparent polyester support disc coated with a pressure-sensitive clear adhesive (Corneodisc, C+K Electronic, Cologne, Germany; D-squame, Cuderm Corp, Dallas, TX, USA). In this minimally invasive method, insufficient or inconsistent application pressure of SACD results in samples that are difficult to compare. Skillful handling by firm finger pressure provides more reliable samples after tearing off the SACD with a single continuous motion. Precision is increased when using a dynamometer delivering a calibrated application pressure in the range 100–250 g/cm^2. A clean and dry SC surface provides maximal adhesion. Conversely, presence of lipids, including greasy topical formulations, prevents accurate samplings. Delipidization of the skin surface is a convenient way to reveal discrete scaliness that is not clinically obvious. Sampling is then more uniform and reproducible.

Common SACD brands differ in composition and adhesive properties. The amount of SC removed by a single SACD strip is influenced by a series of parameters. Differences in adhesive properties between SACD brands result in different amounts of SC removed per surface area. Pressure, time elapsed between application and removal, as well as velocity of the removal process further influence corneocyte harvesting. Additionally, intrinsic skin properties related to age, gender, and ethnicity are further supposed to change SC removal. The body site and the skin condition after chemical exposure affect the corneocyte removal. Moreover, SC amount removed by SACD varies according to depth of sampling inside the SC.

The application time of SACD onto the skin influences the amount of harvested corneocytes. The maximum regular contact time is about 5 s. When it is increased up to 1 h, SACD causes occlusion. The resulting overhydration of the corneocytes loosens the intercorneocyte cohesion. As a result, the amount of SACD-harvested corneocytes is usually increased. This procedure is tentatively used for assessing the skin barrier function in combination with TEWL measurements [44, 45].

After appropriate staining in the laboratory, clumps of SACD-harvested corneocytes appear as colored objects that are adequate for the squamometry procedure. The material is gently stained for 1 min with a solution of toluidine blue and basic fuchsin. This step should not tear away corneocytes from SACD. After air drying, the stained samples are placed over a hole cut out of a plastic slide, and the sample is placed onto a white reference tile. In the reflectance colorimetry, Chroma C* is the most convenient colorimetric parameter. It combines the values of red and blue chromaticities following $(a^{*2} + b^{*2})^{1/2}$. A linear correlation exists between the amount of orthokeratotic SC and the Chroma C* of the SACD samples. Data are influenced by the presence of parakeratotic cells and serum as found in irritant and allergic contact dermatitis.

The squamometry method is applicable for qualitative and quantitative assessments of scaliness and inflammatory reactions [37, 42]. It is a convenient method for evaluating the effect of drugs in alleviating a range of skin alterations in chronic eczema. However, when the intercorneocyte cohesion is tidy with formation of adherent large scales, the squamometry-based information becomes irrelevant regarding the clinical presentation. Indeed, under these conditions, SACD only collects minute amounts of corneocytes.

Other methods for SACD examination rely on photography under polarized light [46] and the ultraviolet (UV) light reflectance using a UV-emitting camera (Visiopor, C+K Electronic, Cologne, Germany). SACD is placed on a black reference tile, and the picture is submitted to computerized image analysis [43]. Weight difference of SACD before and after SC sampling is a direct means for assessing the amount of collected SC. Another quantification relies on the determination of the total amount of proteins collected by the SACD procedure [47]. The reduction in light transmission through SACD is a procedure that exhibits a poor sensibility, and its reliability appears limited.

2.10 Skin Roughness

The skin roughness observation benefits from the in vivo ULEV method [48]. Due to the specular reflectance of the incident UV light, the contrasts are enhanced in the scaly areas. Various other noninvasive methods were designed to quantify the skin microrelief which is particularly altered in hand dermatoses. Skin roughness is conveniently assessed in vivo using standardized profilometric parameters. Diverse methods and devices have been designed [49].

The skin Visiometer SV400 and the Visioline VL650 (C+K Electronic, Cologne, Germany) share a cost-performance ratio, allowing their application in routine clinical settings. The basic principle relies on light transmission through a thin, dyed silicone replica of the skin surface. Light is absorbed according to the thickness of the silicone material. The replica reproduces a negative cast of the heights and depths of the skin. The visualization of the light absorption on a computer screen, using a black-and-white CCD camera, shows the heights and depths of the replica by a corresponding classification on a 256-grey-level pixel scale. The RT, RM, RA, RZ, and RP parameters described in the DIN-standard 4762–4768 turned out to be useful.

2.11 Vasodilation, Blood Flow Changes, and Skin Color

In the severity evaluation of skin signs, such as inflammation, a visual scoring system is widely used as a subjective method. However, it is acknowledged that interobserver variations are frequent, even among experienced dermatologists. Conversely, bioinstrumentation helps resolve these inconsistencies. Indeed, it is important to achieve objective evaluation of color distribution noninvasively. Reflectance spectrophotometry measures the intensity of light reflection from the skin in the wavelength spectrum of visible light. A conventional spectrophotometer analyzes the average value of the wavelength portion of interest without assessing the color distribution.

Some skin color variations combine the influences of scaling and vasodilation. Compared to uninvolved skin, the L*a*b* assessment of contact dermatitis commonly indicates a lower L* value, an increased a* value, and a decreased b* value [50]. The combination of these three evaluations following the ratio $(L^* \times b^*)a^{*-1}$ magnifies color changes seen in contact dermatitis. In Caucasians the ratio value reaches about 30 for lesional skin, compared to about 120 for healthy skin.

Several techniques, including laser Doppler flowmetry (LDV), laser Doppler imaging (LDI), photoplethysmography, thermal conductance, thermography, and xenon wash-out techniques, can be used in the investigation of the skin blood flow [51, 52]. The skin blood flow assessed by LDV has to show a three- to fourfold increase before the naked eye detects changes [53]. Of note, the area with increased blood perfusion extends beyond the area showing a clinically perceptible erythematous reaction. In the time course of an irritant reaction, the microcirculation assessed by LDV decreases while a* value remains increased [54].

2.12 Ultrasound Shear Wave Propagation

The propagation speed of ultrasound shear waves as assessed by the Reviscometer (C + K Electronic, Cologne, Germany) is under the influence of age, body site, and gender [55, 56] and is possibly altered in irritant dermatitis [57, 58]. Such a method has not yet been widely applied in hand dermatoses.

2.13 Noninvasive Optical Microscopy

Optical coherence tomography and in vivo confocal reflectance microscopy are applied in the scope of skin irritation [59, 60]. Structural changes in skin exposed to irritants are revealed by confocal reflectance microscopy [61]. SC cracks, as well as epidermal alterations and hyperproliferation, represent some hallmarks of irritant contact dermatitis. In addition, spongiosis, vesicle formation, and vasodilation are observed in the course of contact allergic reaction [60].

2.14 Skin Surface pH

SC pH regulates permeability, hydration, and corneocyte cohesion [62, 63]. The SC pH controls the permeability barrier homeostasis. Indeed, worsening of barrier function occurs when intact skin is exposed to an alkaline pH. Indeed, the SC pH influences the barrier function through its effects on the membrane bilayer organization and through the regulation of the extracellular lipid processing. Lipid processing refers to the post-secretory conversion of secreted lamellar body-derived polar lipid precursors into their nonpolar lipid products, a sequence that generates the extracellular lamellar membrane structures mediating barrier function.

In the field of dermometrology, the flat glass electrode method is the most commonly used for SC pH determinations. Such assessments correlate with the fluorescent dye method [64]. Various endogenous (ethnicity, anatomical site, gender, age, circadian chronobiology, and any concomitant disorder) and exogenous factors (seasons, skin-care products) alter the surface pH.

In short-term experiments, exposure of intact skin to neutral pH does not affect the epidermal barrier permeability. However, similar sustained repetitive conditions lead to an increase in both the SC pH and TEWL, without altering the SC hydration. These conditions resemble prolonged occupational contacts with mild-alkaline compounds.

2.15 Prediction of Product-Induced Irritation

In the field of hand dermatology, measuring the skin biophysical properties could help (1) predict the risk of irritant contact dermatitis, (2) detect subclinical dermatitis, and (3) monitor therapy [65]. The development of irritant contact dermatitis might thus be reduced by preventive counselling and more intensive protective measures. There are, however, some legal limitations to such screening procedures. In addition to baseline measurements, skin irritancy tests using different irritant compounds, including surfactants and other chemically aggressive xenobiotics, are commonly used to assess individual irritant reactivity [66]. The evaluations are typically performed in vivo after a single or repeat application of low-irritancy compounds [67, 68]. TEWL determination appears as an appropriate parameter in assessing irritant susceptibility testing.

Interindividual variations in skin reactivities are typically present and may be prominent. Of note, on an individual basis, skin reactivity depends on the body site and on previous skin preconditioning. In addition, the irritancy susceptibility is unstable over time in a given individual for specific products.

The dansyl chloride test was introduced for documenting effects of irritant surfactants on the epidermal and SC cell renewal. It was later demonstrated that the SC fluorescence fading was rather due to the extraction of the fluorescent dye by the surfactant and was not due to any biologic effect on the living epidermis [69].

Of note, the intraindividual reproducibility of any single in vivo test is not guaranteed over an extended period of time [70]. Hence, it is important to use a set of tests for predicting hand contact dermatitis. However, some correlations are expected between data gained by different methods [71, 72]. In the multipronged exploratory approach, the ex vivo CSM and corneoxenometry (CXM) bioassays appear to be reasonably reproducible tools.

The combination of surfactants and physical trauma induces cumulative effects on SC permeability barrier impairment. Tandem repeated irritation tests (TRITs) demonstrated that combined mechanical trauma, surfactants, and occlusion were responsible for increased effects on the epidermal barrier disruption. The TRITs procedure resembles conditions of daily life and hand exposures better than single-irritant exposure models [73].

Different mechanisms of barrier impairment are involved in various noxious stimuli. Organic solvents extract SC lipids and thus disrupt the integrity of the SC barrier. By contrast, anionic surfactants damage proteins, thus exposing new xenobiotic-binding sites, and disorganize the lipid bilayers. The process causes SC overhydration. Regardless of the nature of the noxious agent, acute permeability barrier disruption initiates the restoration processes of the SC homeostasis [74]. The triggering factor in the repair process is that the increased TEWL induces lamellar body secretion and lipid restoration.

In case of potential hazardous reaction, the ex vivo CSM and CXM bioassays on CSSS samples are possibly performed prior to any in vivo testing [30]. CSM refers to the effects of surfactants and wash solutions. The bioassay relies on CSSS samples harvested from healthy volunteers or from specific subjects. A diluted solution of the test product is sprayed over the CSSS specimens. The samples are placed in covered plastic trays.

After a predetermined incubation time at a controlled temperature, the samples are thoroughly rinsed in tap water and dried. They are stained for 3 min in a toluidine blue-basic fuchsin solution before being copiously rinsed with water and dried prior to color quantification using reflectance colorimetry. Indeed, surfactants remove lipids and denature corneocyte proteins, thus revealing sites available for stain deposition. A combined dotted and rimmed pattern is visible at the microscopic examination.

Using quantitative reflectance colorimetry, the mean luminance (L*) and Chroma C* are derived from the mean of measurements made at three distinct sites on each sample placed on a white colorimetric reference tile. Mild surfactants and other discretely irritant xenobiotics exert little effect on corneocytes, and they exhibit high L* values and low Chroma C* values. With increasing irritancy potential of the products, the L* value decreases while Chroma C* increases. The differences between L* and Chroma C* values of each sample give the colorimetric indices of mildness (CIM). The CSM index (CSMI) of the test product, corresponds to the color difference between water-treated control samples and those exposed to the test product. It is conveniently calculated according to:

$$CSMI = \left[\left(\Delta(delta)\mathrm{L}* \right)^2 + \left(\Delta(delta)\mathrm{C}* \right)^2 \right]^{0.5}$$

Microwave CSM is a rapid procedure [75]. CSSS samples are immersed in a flask containing the test surfactant solution. Samples are then placed in a microwave oven with a 500 mL water load. Microwave CSM is commonly run at 750 W for 30 s. The next steps of the method are identical to the standard CSM procedure.

Responsive CSM is a variant method where skin is preconditioned in vivo before CSSS sampling [70]. The method relies on repeat subclinical SC injuries by surfactants monitored in a controlled forearm immersion test. At completion of the in vivo procedure, CSSS specimens are harvested for the regular or microwave CSM bioassay using the same surfactant as in the preliminary in vivo procedure. Such skin preconditioning increases the CSM sensitivity for discriminating mild surfactants [76].

Shielded CSM is used for predicting the effect of skin-protective products [77, 78] that claim to provide a shielding effect against noxious agents [79]. In shielded CSM, the CSSS specimens are initially covered by the putative protective product before performing regular CSM using a reference surfactant. Comparative screenings of such formulations are conveniently performed using shielded CSM without exposing volunteers to hazardous in vivo testing.

Animal CSM is performed similarly to human CSM. The method was designed for safety testing and for determining potential interspecies differences in reactivity to irritant xenobiotics [80].

The CXM bioassay is used for testing the adverse effects of any chemical xenobiotic other than surfactants on the SC [78, 81]. The basic procedure is similar to CSM and its variants. One main indication is found in the exploration of skin irritation without risking in vivo hazards of irritant and toxic compounds [81]. Another indication deals with the comparative assessment of penetration enhancers commonly used in topical formulations [81]. Still another use concerns the ex vivo predictive assessment of skin barrier products commonly promoted for prevention of hand contact dermatitis [77].

Conclusion

Measure when you can. If there is no measurement, invent one. This adage is up-to-date because skin biometrology usually shows more sensitivity in detecting occupational dermatoses than the clinical observation alone. The methods represent important tools in skin-care management of occupational hand dermatoses. They improve the prevention strategy of skin disorders, and they presumably help establishing the predictive risk of contact dermatitis. In addition, they deliver objective and quantitative data, allowing statistical analysis that reduces the sample size in any clinical study. The rapidly emerging body of knowledge in this field paves the way for more rational developments of forthcoming therapies.

The current descriptive aspects of occupational dermatology should benefit from increased precision in the knowledge of functional alterations found in hand dermatoses. Some advances should be expected in more targeted therapies for a better control of the principal functions of the epidermis and the inflammatory reaction.

References

1. Noël F, Piérard-Franchimont C, Piérard GE, Quatresooz P. Sweaty skin, background and assessments. Int J Dermatol. 2012;51:647–55.
2. Diepgen TL. Occupational skin diseases. J Dtsch Dermatol Ges. 2012;10:297–313.
3. Vester L, Thyssen JP, Menné T, Johansen JD. Occupational food-related hand dermatoses seen over a 10-year period. Contact Dermatitis. 2012;66:264–70.
4. Bazin R, Laquièze S, Rosillo A, Lévêque JL. Photoaging of the chest analyzed by capacitance imaging. Skin Res Technol. 2010;16:23–9.
5. German GK, Engl WC, Pashkovski E, Banerjee S, Xu Y, Mertz AF, et al. Heterogeneous drying stresses in stratum corneum. Biophys J. 2012;102:424–32.
6. Piérard GE, Preud'Homme L, Quatresooz P. Predictive methods exploring sensory irritation to surfactant-based products. Househ Pers Care. 2011;7:22–4.
7. Hirao T, Denda M, Takahashi M. Identification of immature cornified envelopes in the barrier-impaired epidermis by characterization of their hydrophobicity and antigenicities of the components. Exp Dermatol. 2001;10:35–44.
8. Diridollou S, de Rigal J, Querleux B, Leroy F, Lolloway Barbosa V. Comparative study of the hydration of the stratum corneum between four ethnic groups: influence of age. Int J Dermatol. 2007;46:S11–4.
9. Uter W, Gefeller O, Schwanitz HJ. An epidemiological study of the influence of season (cold and dry air) on the occurrence of irritant skin changes of the hands. Br J Dermatol. 1998;138:266–72.
10. Piérard GE. EEMCO guidance for the assessment of dry skin (xerosis) and ichthyosis: evaluation by stratum corneum strippings. Skin Res Technol. 1996;2:3–11.
11. Zhai H, Fautz R, Fuchs A, et al. Assessment of the subclinical irritation of surfactants: a screening open assay model. Exog Dermatol. 2002;1:238–41.
12. Quatresooz P, Piérard-Franchimont C, Szepetiuk G, Devillers C, Piérard GE. Fungal chitin-glucan scaffold for managing diabetic xerosis of the feet in menopausal women. Exp Opin Pharmacother. 2009;10:2221–9.
13. Astner S, Gonzalez E, Cheung AC, Rius-Diaz F, Doukas AG, William F, et al. Non-invasive evaluation of the kinetics of allergic and irritant contact dermatitis. J Invest Dermatol. 2005;124:351–9.
14. Devillers C, Piérard GE, Quatresooz P, Piérard S. Environmental dew point and skin and lip weathering. J Eur Acad Dermatol Venereol. 2010;24:513–7.
15. John SM, Uter W, Schwanitz HJ. Relevance of multiparametric skin bioengineering in a prospectively-followed cohort of junior hairdressers. Contact Dermatitis. 2000;43:161–8.
16. Korinth G, Göen T, Koch HM, Merz T, Uter W. Visible and subclinical skin changes in male and female dispatch department workers of newspaper printing plants. Skin Res Technol. 2005;11:132–9.
17. Fluhr JW, Kuss O, Diepgen T, Lazzerini S, Pelosi A, Gloor M, et al. Testing for irritation with a multifactorial approach: comparison of eight non-invasive measuring techniques on five different irritation types. Br J Dermatol. 2001;145:696–703.
18. Schmid K, Broding HC, Uter W, Drexler H. Transepidermal water loss and incidence of hand dermatitis in a prospectively followed cohort of apprentice nurses. Contact Dermatitis. 2005;52:247–53.
19. Proksch E, Brasch J. Abnormal epidermal barrier in the pathogenesis of contact dermatitis. Clin Dermatol. 2012;30:335–44.
20. Xhauflaire-Uhoda E, Mayeux G, Quatresooz P, Scheen A, Piérard GE. Facing up to the imperceptible perspiration. Modulation influences by diabetic neuropathy, physical exercise and antiperspirant. Skin Res Technol. 2011;17:487–93.
21. Steiner M, Aikman-Green S, Prescott GJ, Dick FD. Side-by-side comparison of an open-chamber (Tewameter TM 300) and a closed-chamber (Vapometer™) transepidermal water loss meter. Skin Res Technol. 2011;17:366–72.
22. Zhai H, Brachman F, Pelosi A, Anigbogu A, Ramos MB, Torralba MC, et al. A bioengineering study on the efficacy of a skin protectant lotion in preventing SLS-induced dermatitis. Skin Res Technol. 2000;6:77–80.
23. Kuzmina N, Duval C, Johnsson S, Boman A, Lindberg M, Emtestam L. Assessment of irritant skin reactions using electrical impedance- a comparison between 2 laboratories. Contact Dermatitis. 2003;49:26–31.
24. Mayrovitz HN. Local tissue water assessed by measuring forearm skin dielectric constant: dependence on measurement depth, age and body mass index. Skin Res Technol. 2010;16:16–22.
25. Ferreira DM, Silva CS, Souza MN. Electrical impedance model for evaluation of skin irritation in rabbits and humans. Skin Res Technol. 2007;13:259–67.
26. Lévêque JL, Querleux B. SkinChip®, a new tool for investigating the skin surface in vivo. Skin Res Technol. 2003;9:343–7.
27. Xhauflaire-Uhoda E, Piérard GE, Quatresooz P. The skin landscape following nonoptical capacitance imaging. Am J Clin Dermatol. 2010;11:89–94.
28. Xhauflaire-Uhoda E, Loussouarn G, Haubrechts C, Léger DS, Piérard GE. Skin capacitance imaging and corneosurfametry. A comparative assessment of the impact of surfactants on stratum corneum. Contact Dermatitis. 2006;54:249–53.
29. Uhoda E, Lévêque JL, Piérard GE. Silicon image sensor technology for in vivo detection of surfactant-induced corneocyte swelling and drying. Dermatology. 2005;210:184–8.

30. Chrit L, Bastien P, Sockalingum GD, Batisse D, Leroy F, Manfait M, et al. An in vivo randomized study of human skin moisturization by a new confocal Raman fiber-optic microprobe: assessment of a glycerol-based hydration cream. Skin Pharmacol Physiol. 2006;19:207–15.
31. Johnsen GK, Haugsnes AB, Martinsen OG, Grimnes S. A new approach for an estimation of the equilibrium stratum corneum water content. Skin Res Technol. 2010;16:142–5.
32. Gonzalez FJ, Alda J, Moreno-Cruz B, Martinez-Escanamé M, Ramirez-Elias MG, Torres-Alvarez B, et al. Use of Raman spectroscopy for the early detection of filaggrin-related atopic dermatitis. Skin Res Technol. 2011;17:45–50.
33. Nishino K, Fujiyama T, Hashizume H, Nakauchi S. Detection and visualization of intracutaneous allergic type-specific elements using long-wavelength near-infrared hyperspectral imaging. Skin Res Technol. 2013;19:157–66.
34. Piérard-Franchimont C, Arrese Estrada J, Quatresooz P, Piérard GE. Cyanoacrylate skin surface strippings. In: Farage M, Miller KW, Maibach H, editors. Textbook of aging skin. Berlin: Springer; 2010. p. 393–9.
35. Piérard GE. Microscopic evaluation of the dansyl chloride test. Dermatology. 1992;185:37–40.
36. Piérard GE, Piérard-Franchimont C. Dihydroxyacetone test as a substitute for the dansyl chloride test. Dermatology. 1993;186:133–7.
37. Piérard GE, Piérard-Franchimont C, Saint Léger D, Kligman AM. Squamometry: the assessment of xerosis by colorimetry of D-squame adhesive discs. J Soc Cosmet Chem. 1992;47:297–305.
38. Piérard GE, Piérard-Franchimont C. Squamometry as an aid for rating severity of target lesions in atopic dermatitis. Giorn Int Dermatol Pediatr. 1994;6:125–8.
39. Piérard GE, Goffin V, Piérard-Franchimont C. Squamometry and corneosurfametry in rating interactions of cleansing products with stratum corneum. J Soc Cosmet Chem. 1994;45:269–77.
40. Piérard GE, Piérard-Franchmiont C. Squamometry in acute photodamage. Skin Res Technol. 1995;1:137–9.
41. Dreher F, Arens A, Hostynek JJ, Mudumba S, Ademola J, Maibach HI. Colorimetric method for quantifying human stratum corneum removed by adhesive-tape stripping. Acta Derm Venereol. 1998;78:186–9.
42. Piérard-Franchimont C, Henry F, Piérard GE. The SACD method and the XLRS squamometry tests revisited. Int J Cosmet Sci. 2000;22:437–46.
43. Piérard-Franchimont C, Quatresooz P, Piérard GE. Specular light reflectance of flakes in seborrheic dermatitis of the scalp. A pilot study. Clin Exp Dermatol. 2011;36:793–6.
44. Uhoda E, Piérard-Franchimont C, Debatisse B, Wang X, Piérard GE. Repair kinetics of stratum corneum under repeated insults. Exog Dermatol. 2004;3:7–11.
45. Breternitz M, Flach M, Prassler J, Elsner P, Fluhr JW. Acute barrier disruption by adhesive tapes is influenced by pressure, time and anatomical location: integrity and cohesion assessed by sequential tape stripping. A randomized, controlled study. Br J Dermatol. 2007;156:231–40.
46. Bae EJ, Seo SH, Kye YC, Ahn HH. A quantitative assessment of the human skin surface using polarized light digital photography and its dermatologic significance. Skin Res Technol. 2010;16:270–4.
47. Dreher F, Modjtahedi BS, Modjtahedi SP, Maibach HI. Quantification of stratum corneum removal by adhesive tape stripping by total protein assay in 96-well microplates. Skin Res Technol. 2005;11:97–101.
48. Szepetiuk G, Piérard S, Piérard-Franchimont C, Caucanas M, Quatresooz P, Piérard GE. Recent trends in specular light reflectance beyond clinical fluorescence diagnosis. Eur J Dermatol. 2011;21:157–61.
49. Lee E, An S, Im MS, Kim HK, Lee TR. An improved method for measurement of change in skin roughness caused by cleansing products under mild application conditions. Skin Res Technol. 2011;17:320–5.
50. Piérard GE. EEMCO guidance for the assessment of skin colour. J Eur Acad Dermatol Venereol. 1998;10:1–11.
51. Fullerton A, Rode B, Serup J. Skin irritation typing and grading based on laser Doppler perfusion imaging. Skin Res Technol. 2002;8:23–31.
52. Fullerton A, Stucker M, Wilhelm KP, Wardell K, Anderson C, Fischer T, et al. Guidelines for visualization of cutaneous blood flow by laser Doppler perfusion imaging. A report from the standardization group of the European society of contact dermatitis based upon the HIRELADO European community project. Contact Dermatitis. 2002;46:129–40.
53. Berardesca E, Lévêque JL, Masson P. EEMCO guidance for the measurement of skin microcirculation. Skin Pharmacol Appl Skin Physiol. 2002;15:442–56.
54. Zuang V, Rona C, Archer G, Berardesca E. Detection of skin irritation potential of cosmetics by non-invasive measurements. Skin Pharmacol Appl Skin Physiol. 2000;13:358–71.
55. Nizet JL, Piérard-Franchimont C, Piérard GE. Influence of body posture and gravitational forces on shear wave propagation in the skin. Dermatology. 2001;202:177–80.
56. Xin S, Man W, Fluhr JW, Song S, Elias PM, Man MQ. Cutaneous resonance running time varies with age, body site and gender in a normal Chinese population. Skin Res Technol. 2010;16:413–21.
57. Uhoda E, Piérard GE. Skin irritation and propagation speed of ultrasounds. Int J Cosmet Sci. 2003;25:31–5.
58. Paye M, Mac-Mary S, Elkhyat A, Tarrit C, Mermet P, Humbert PH. Use of the Reviscometer for measuring cosmetic-induced skin surface effects. Skin Res Technol. 2007;13:343–9.
59. Welzel J, Bruhns M, Wolff HH. Optical coherence tomography in contact dermatitis and psoriasis. Arch Dermatol Res. 2003;295:50–5.
60. Astner S, Gonzalez S, Gonzalez E. Noninvasive evaluation of allergic and irritant contact dermatitis by in vivo reflectance confocal microscopy. Contact Dermatitis. 2006;17:182–91.

61. Hicks SP, Swindells KJ, Middelkamp-Hup MA, Sifakis MA, Gonzalez E, Gonzalez S. Confocal histopathology of irritant contact dermatitis in vivo and the impact of skin color (black vs white). J Am Acad Dermatol. 2003;48:727–34.
62. Schmid-Wendtner MH, Korting HC. The pH of the skin surface and its impact on the barrier function. Skin Pharmacol Physiol. 2006;19:296–302.
63. Gunathilake R, Schurer NY, Shoo BA, Celli A, Hachem JP, Crumrine D, et al. pH-regulated mechanism account for pigment-type differences in epidermal barrier function. J Invest Dermatol. 2009;129: 1719–29.
64. Wagner H, Kostka KH, Lehr CM, Schaefer UF. pH profiles in human skin: influence of two in vitro test systems for drug delivery testing. Eur J Pharm Biopharm. 2003;55:57–65.
65. Tupker RA. Prediction of irritancy in the human skin irritancy model and occupational setting. Contact Dermatitis. 2003;49:61–9.
66. Aramaki J, Effendy I, Happle R, Kawana S, Löffler C, Löffler H. Which bioengineering assay is appropriate for irritant patch testing with sodium lauryl sulfate? Contact Dermatitis. 2001;45:286–90.
67. Goffin V, Piérard-Franchimont C, Piérard GE. Passive sustainable hydration of the stratum corneum following surfactant challenge. Clin Exp Dermatol. 1999; 24:308–11.
68. Branco N, Lee I, Zhai H, Maibach HI. Long-term repetitive sodium lauryl sulfate-induced irritation of the skin: an in vivo study. Contact Dermatitis. 2005; 53:278–84.
69. Paye M, Simion FA, Pierard GE. Dansyl chloride labelling of stratum corneum: its rapid extraction from skin can predict skin irritation due to surfactants and cleansing products. Contact Dermatitis. 1994;30: 91–6.
70. Iliev D, Hinnen U, Elsner P. Skin bioengineering methods in occupational dermatology. Curr Probl Dermatol. 1998;26:145–50.
71. Goffin V, Paye M, Piérard GE. Comparison of in vivo predictive tests for irritation induced b anionic surfactants. Contact Dermatitis. 1995;3:38–41.
72. Gabard B, Chatelain E, Bieli E, Haas S. Surfactant irritation: in vitro corneosurfametry and in vivo bioengineering. Skin Res Technol. 2001;7:49–55.
73. Wigger-Alberti W, Spoo J, Schliemann-Willers S, Klotz A, Elsner P. The tandem repeated irritation test: a new method to assess prevention of irritant combination damage to the skin. Acta Derm Venereol. 2002;82:94–7.
74. Feingold KR, Schmuth M, Elias PM. The regulation of permeability barrier homeostasis. J Invest Dermatol. 2007;127:1574–6.
75. Goffin V, Piérard GE. Microwave corneosurfametry and the short-duration dansyl chloride extraction test for rating concentrated irritant surfactants. Dermatology. 2001;202:46–8.
76. Uhoda E, Goffin V, Piérard GE. Responsive corneosurfametry following in vivo preconditioning. Contact Dermatitis. 2003;49:292–6.
77. Goffin V, Piérard-Franchimont C, Piérard GE. Shielded corneosurfametry and corneoxenometry: novel bioassays for the assessment of skin barrier products. Dermatology. 1998;196:434–7.
78. Xhauflaire-Uhoda E, Macarenko E, Denooz R, Charlier C, Piérard GE. Skin protection creams in medical settings: successful or evil? J Occup Med Toxicol. 2008;3:15–20.
79. Berndt U, Wigger-Alberti W, Gabard B, Elsner P. Efficacy of a barrier cream and its vehicle as protective measures against occupational irritant contact dermatitis. Contact Dermatitis. 2000;42:77–80.
80. Goffin V, Fontaine J, Piérard GE. Comparative surfactant reactivity of canine and human stratum corneum. A plea for the use of the corneosurfametry bioassay. Altern Lab Anim. 1999;27:103–9.
81. Goffin V, Henry F, Piérard-Franchimont C, Piérard GE. Penetration enhancers assessed by corneoxenometry. Skin Pharmacol Appl Skin Physiol. 2000;13:280–4.

3 Clinical Subtypes and Categorization of Hand Eczema: An Overview

Jean-Marie Lachapelle

Contents

J.-M. Lachapelle, M.D., Ph.D.
Department of Dermatology,
Catholic University of Louvain,
10, Avenue Hippocrate, Brussels 1200, Belgium
e-mail: jean.marie.lachapelle@uclouvain.be

3.1 Introduction

As stated by Berth-Jones [1], "no single classification of hand eczema is completely satisfactory." As with eczematous dermatoses in general, classification is based partly on etiology and partly on morphology. Several different morphological forms are seen clinically, as fairly consistent entities, but some of these entities can have several different causes. Conversely, a single cause can sometimes produce several different morphological patterns.

The classification that has been adopted is based upon morphological and etiological criteria, taking into consideration the intersection between exogenous and endogenous factors in the pathogenesis of the disease in each individual case (Table 3.1).

This important approach was pointed out by Fregert [2] many years ago, and it is still valid.

Table 3.1 Proposal for a classification of hand eczema

A. Exogenous	Irritant contact dermatitis (ICD): frictional, chemical Allergic contact dermatitis (ACD) Protein contact dermatitis (PCD)
B. Endogenous	Nummular eczema Pompholyx and/or dyshidrotic eczema Palmar hyperkeratotic eczema
C. Exogenous and/or endogenous	Atopic eczema (atopic dermatitis) Fingertip dermatitis

A. Alikhan et al. (eds.), *Textbook of Hand Eczema*,
DOI 10.1007/978-3-642-39546-8_3, © Springer-Verlag Berlin Heidelberg 2014

3.2 Irritant Contact Dermatitis

The main clinical characteristics of irritant contact dermatitis (ICD) are listed in Table 3.2.

ICD is fully described in Chap. 11. Differential diagnosis between ICD and allergic contact dermatitis (ACD) is a major clinical problem. There are some trails to guide the dermatologist, but there is no definite "clue," as both conditions partly share similar signs and symptoms. Histopathological examination is of no real interest. Therefore, patch testing and other tests are of prime importance. When the patch tests are positive, it is still possible that the clinical condition is mixed – that is, having both symptoms of ICD and ACD, with or without an atopic background.

As far as hands are concerned, keep in mind the following:

- On the back of the hand, ICD is acute and erythematous (Fig. 3.1), sometimes vesicular, almost exclusively due to chemical irritants.
- On the palm, both physical (mechanical) agents and chemicals can be incriminated. Frictional ICD is therefore common; clinical signs and symptoms include painful, dry, erythematous, and scaly lesions, with fissuring.

3.3 Allergic Contact Dermatitis

The clinical signs and symptoms of ACD, which is eczematous in most cases, vary depending on their localization and duration. This is particularly relevant for hand ACD. In most instances, acute eruptions are characterized by erythema and papules, vesicles (often coalescent), or bullae, depending on the intensity of the allergic response (Fig. 3.2). In severe cases, this can lead to abundant oozing. On the backs of the hands, edema may be prominent.

In contrast, chronic ACD presents as a thickened, scaling, occasionally fissured dermatitis,

Table 3.2 Clinical characteristics of ICD and ACD: some criteria of differential diagnosis[a]

	ICD	ACD
Clinical course	Acute ICD may appear after first exposure (at least with strong irritants)	Sensitizing exposure(s) is required
	In acute ICD, lesions appear rapidly, usually minutes to a few hours after exposure, but delayed reactions can be seen	Clinical lesions appear after subsequent challenges with re-presentation of the antigen to already primed (memory) T cells
		Lesions usually appear 24–72 h after the last exposure to the causative agent, but they may develop as early as 5 h or as late as 7 days after exposure
	Irritant reactions are characterized by the "decrescendo phenomenon." The reaction reaches its peak quickly and then starts to heal	Allergic reactions are characterized by the "crescendo phenomenon," and the kinetics of resolution may be slower
Morphology	Acute ICD includes erythema and edema and sometimes vesicles or bullae, oozing, and pustules. Necrosis and ulceration may also be seen with corrosive materials	Pustules, necrosis, or ulceration are rarely seen
	Subacute or chronic ICD is characterized by hyperkeratosis, fissuring, glazed, or scalded appearance of the skin	Intense vesiculation increases the suspicion of ACD, but it may not be present in chronic ACD
	Lesions are characteristically sharply circumscribed to the contact area (see Fig. 3.1)	Clinical lesions are stronger in the contact area, but their limits are usually ill defined
	Usually there is absence of distant lesions, but sometimes dermatitis may be generalized, depending on the nature of the exposure	Dissemination of the dermatitis with distant lesions may occur (see Fig. 3.2)
Symptoms	Symptoms of acute ICD are burning, stinging, pain, and soreness of the skin	Pruritus is the main symptom of ACD
	Pruritus may be present in chronic ICD	

[a]Adapted from [3]

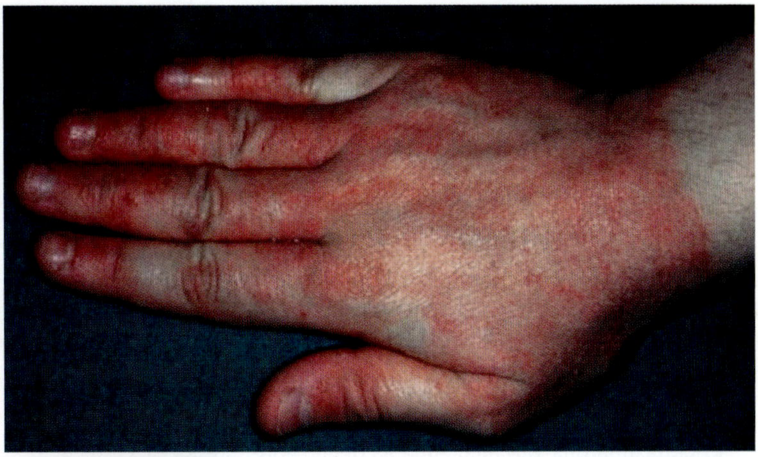

Fig. 3.1 Irritant contact dermatitis due to repeated contact with household detergents

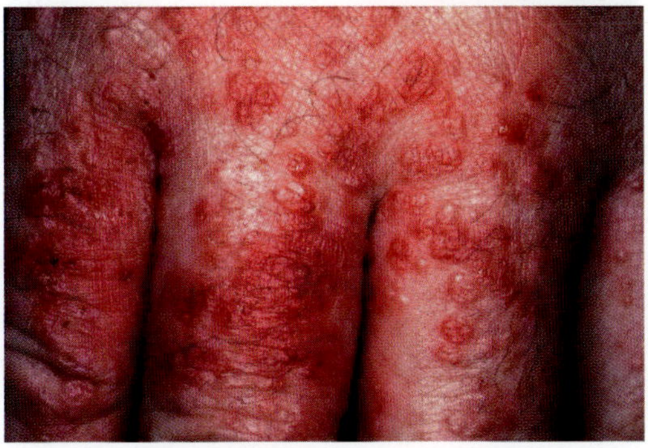

Fig. 3.2 Acute erythemato-vesicular contact dermatitis to cement chromate in a bricklayer

with or without accompanying vesiculation. The margins of the eczematous plaques, either vesicular or dry and scaly, are usually ill defined, extending beyond the site of application of the allergen(s). This has to be differentiated from the lesions of ICD, which are usually sharply demarcated.

Differential diagnosis of ICD and ACD is detailed in Table 3.2 [3].

As fully explained in Chap. 6, all these criteria must now be reexamined in light of new immunological approaches. Patch testing still remains the gold standard for differentiating ICD and ACD, but it has to be used with caution, and the evaluation procedure must include other complementary tests, such as open test, semi-open test, and ROAT test. One must keep in mind that the relevance of results to the clinical situation is of utmost importance.

3.4 Protein Contact Dermatitis

Protein contact dermatitis (PCD) is a complex immune entity, first described by Hjörth and Niels-Petersen [4] and accepted as a well-defined syndrome [5].

It results from skin contact with molecules of high molecular weight (MW > 1000), mainly proteins (vegetables, meat, fish, and other foods), but also, for instance, enzymes such as α(alpha)-amylase (wheat), xylanase (rye), protease (oat), papain (cornstarch), and cellulase (barley). An atopic background has been evoked in some cases.

The most classical clinical presentation is hand eczema (described first among food handlers) that may resemble chronic irritant or allergic contact dermatitis. However, redness, wheals, and sometimes microvesicles appear as symptoms of contact urticaria, usually within an hour after skin contact with the causative agent.

The following are some clinical variants:

- Fingertip dermatitis, mainly, but not exclusively, of the "gripping type."
- Chronic paronychia (Fig. 3.3). This is a common variant, mainly observed in patients who have chronically wet hands. Bacterial and/or *Candida albicans* infection may be associated in some cases [6].
- The nails are usually involved. Changes consist of irregular striae of the plate associated with yellowish onycholysis.

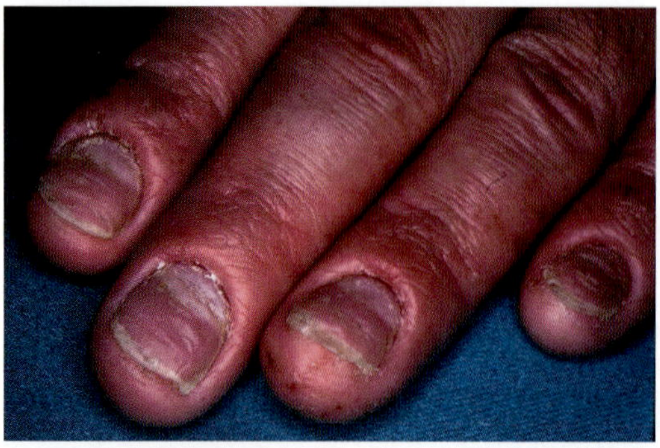

Fig. 3.3 Protein contact dermatitis to monkfish in a cook

Prick test and its variants, such as open (non-prick) test, prick-by-prick test, scratch test, and scratch-chamber test, are the key tools in the etiological diagnosis of PCD. This approach has to be linked with conventional patch testing, in order to be meaningful for complete evaluation of each individual case.

3.5 Nummular (Discoid) Eczema

Nummular (discoid) eczema is a specific form of hand eczema. The term "nummular" is based on the "coin" shape of the lesions (from the Latin *nummulum*). On the backs of the hands, it is characterized by single or multiple round or oval erythematous plaques, which may be vesicular and oozing or dry and scaly. In the latter, the plaque margins are often slightly elevated, with tiny vesicles (Fig. 3.4).

There is a particular form of dry and scaly nummular eczema on the palms. It has a distinctive topography, involving the flexor aspects of the fingers and fanning in a semicircle over the metacarpophalangeal joints, in a pattern resembling an apron; therefore, it is called "apron eczema" [7].

Nummular eczema is, in many cases, of obscure origin. It has been proposed that an atopic background could be the cause in some cases.

Finally, it can be stressed that nummular eczema is a good example of the "annularity" of some lesions in dermatology.

An algorithmic approach to the various etiologies of nummular eczema is presented in Fig. 3.5.

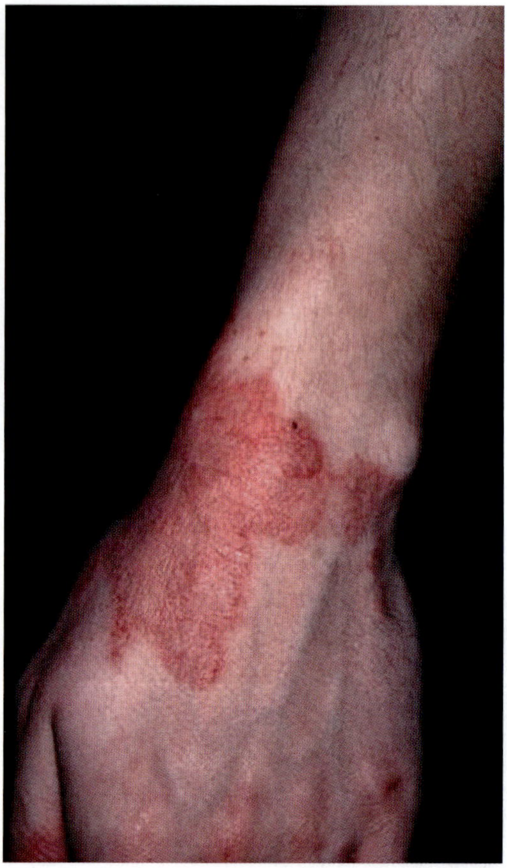

Fig. 3.4 Nummular (discoid) eczema

3.6 Pompholyx (and Dyshidrotic Eczema)

The term pompholyx has been coined by Hutchinson and is classically used in the English and American literature (cheiropompholyx from the Greek χειρ = hand and πομφολυξ = bulla and podopompholyx from the Greek ποδοσ = feet). It is synonymous with dyshidrosis, used earlier in the nineteenth century by Tilbury-Fox. Dyshidrotic eczema refers to the palmar localization of pompholyx [8]. All facets of pompholyx of the hands are summarized in this section [9]:

- The pompholyx vesicles are bunched on the lateral aspects of the fingers (Fig. 3.6). They are hard to the touch, embedded in epidermis, and translucent. They are associated with intense pruritus. They burst when scratched, leaving small ulcerations.

Fig. 3.5 An algorithmic approach to nummular eczema

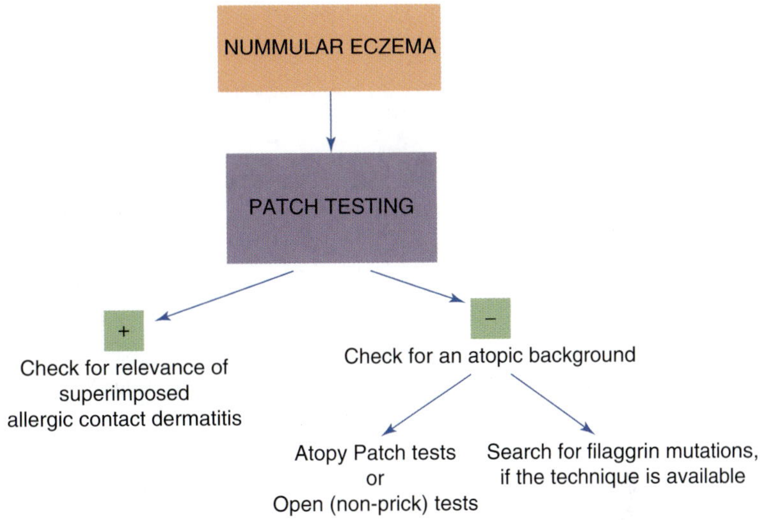

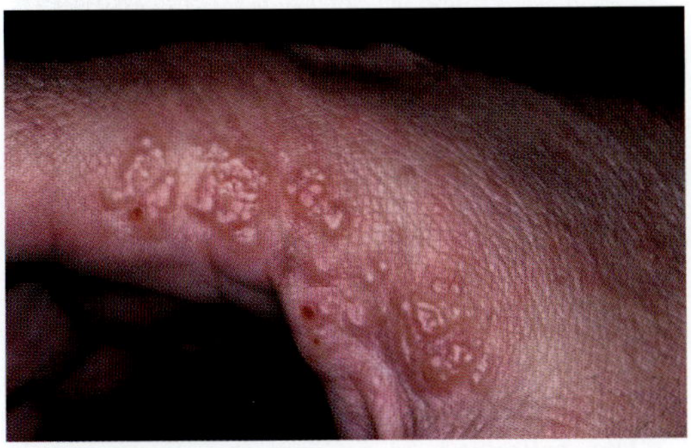

Fig. 3.6 Vesicular pompholyx of the lateral aspects of the fingers

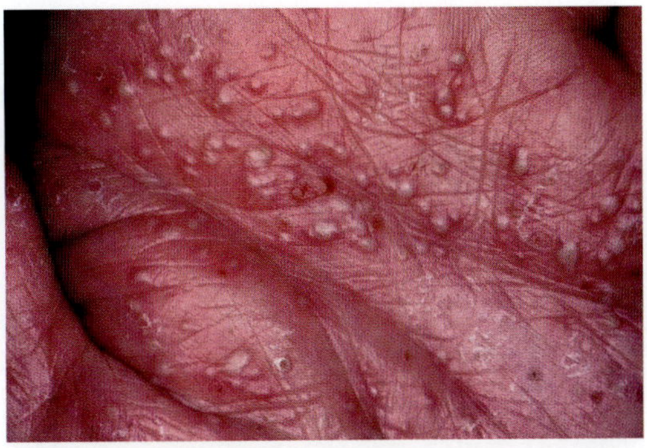

Fig. 3.7 Vesicular palmar pompholyx (dyshidrotic eczema)

- Palmar pompholyx is often characterized by large, painful bullae (Fig. 3.7). Pompholyx vesiculobullae may transform into prominent pustules scattered over the entire palm and palmar aspect of the fingers.
- After some days of acute evolution, the lesions regress gradually over several days. The receding lesions are eczematous and erythematosquamous.

An algorithmic approach related to the various etiologies of pompholyx is presented in Fig. 3.8.

3.7 Palmar Hyperkeratotic Eczema

Palmar hyperkeratotic eczema is extensively described in Chap. 14. The main features of the disease are summarized in this section.

The condition is characterized by the outbreak on the palms of hyperkeratotic, sharply demarcated plaques (Fig. 3.9). Deep, painful, sometimes bleeding crevices are common. Erythema is usually very pronounced, with well-defined margins extending around hyperkeratotic plaques, but, in some cases, it is totally absent. Itching, if present, is usually moderate. Mechanical factors can sometimes be implicated (hyperkeratotic variant of frictional dermatitis), but in most cases, environmental factors cannot be traced; therefore, palmar hyperkeratotic eczema is considered endogenous [10]. In some cases, the differential diagnosis with palmar psoriasis can be difficult. The presence of psoriasis elsewhere on the body may help to clarify the situation (see Chap. 14).

An algorithmic approach to the various potential etiologies of palmar hyperkeratotic eczema is presented in Fig. 3.10.

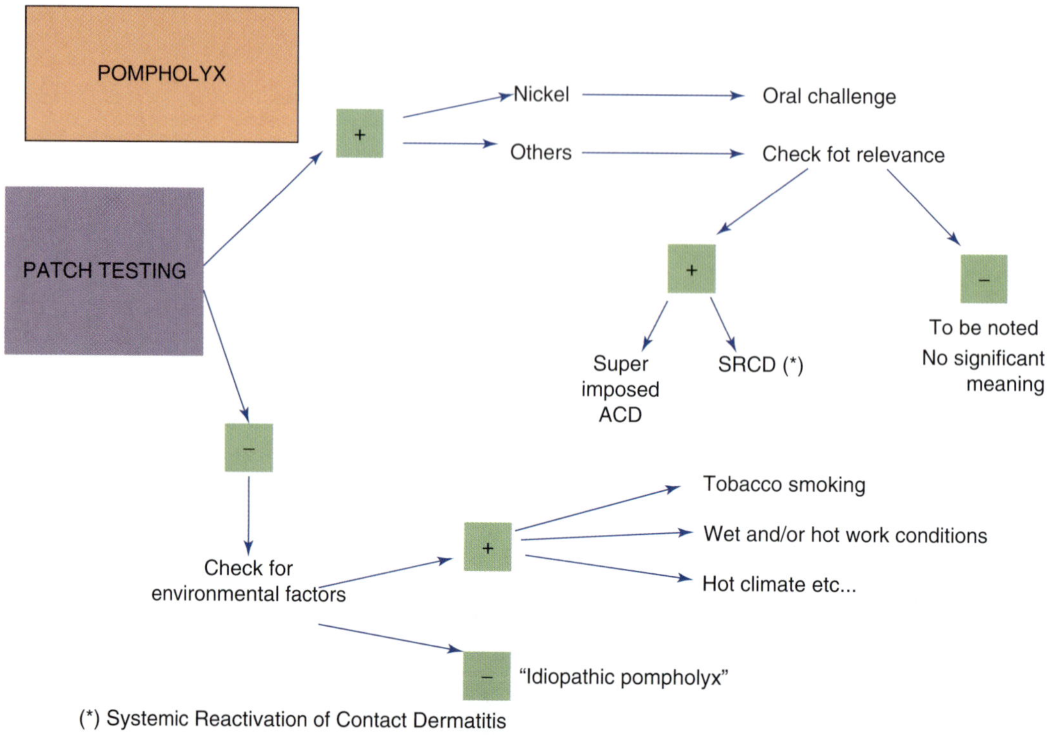

Fig. 3.8 An algorithmic approach of pompholyx

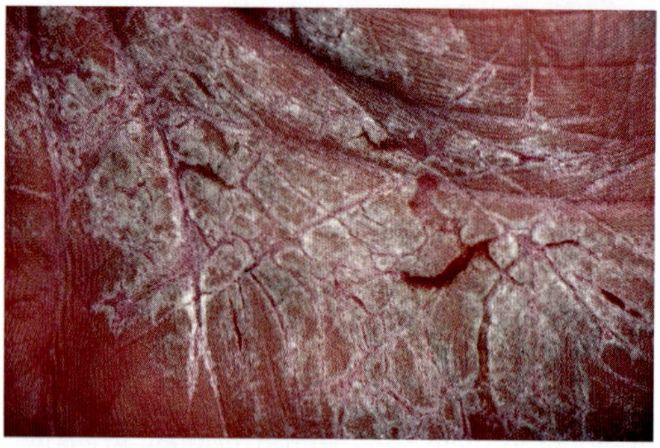

Fig. 3.9 Palmar hyperkeratotic eczema

3.8 Atopic Eczema (Atopic Dermatitis)

Atopic subjects with or without evidence of atopic dermatitis in other body areas may develop hand eczema from contact irritants. The cardinal features (fully described in Chap. 12) are intense pruritus, a predilection for the dorsum of the hands and fingers, and a random distribution [11] (i.e., avoiding some areas but in a manner that differs from patient to patient) [12].

The following variations are illustrated in Figs. 3.11, 3.12, and 3.13:

- Acute exudative eczema with yellowish crusts and scratch marks. There is a massive staphylococcal colonization. Note the involvement of the dorsum of the index finger; absolutely no other fingers are involved (Fig. 3.11).
- Chronic crusting, deeply fissured eczema. The backs of the hand, thumb, index, and middle fingers are entirely covered in eczema, while the ring and little finger are unaffected (Fig. 3.12).
- In the last case, there is chronic erythematosquamous eczema with erosions and fissures, spreading symmetrically to the dorsa of all the fingers and distal dorsa of the hands while leaving the proximal parts intact. The topography is highly characteristic of atopic eczema (Fig. 3.13).

An important paper has been published recently by Danish authors [13]. They have studied

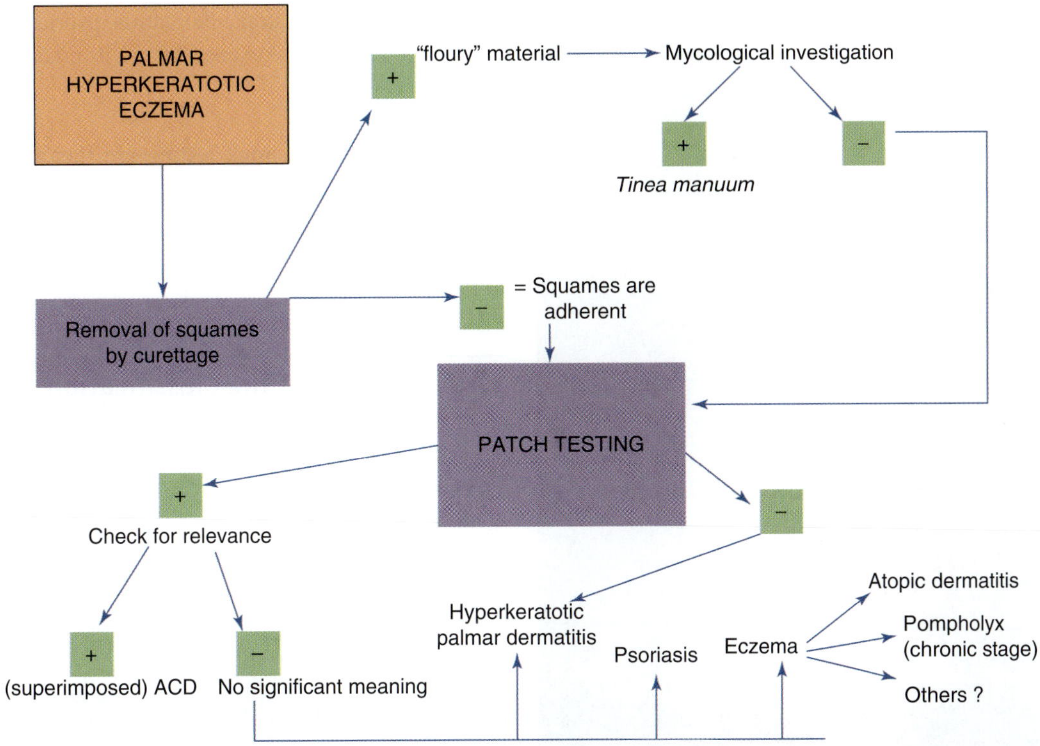

Fig. 3.10 An algorithmic approach to palmar hyperkeratotic eczema

healthy and diseased hands from individuals with filaggrin gene (FLG) mutations to describe the clinical entity of hand eczema. Xerosis and hyperkeratosis of the dorsal aspects of the hands should alert the clinician about a possible inherited barrier abnormality of the skin resulting from FLG mutations, with the improvement of our knowledge about atopic dermatitis and the etiopathogenic pathways leading to the onset of lesions (particularly filaggrin genetic defects). It can be considered that atopic hand eczema is partly exogenous (extrinsic atopic eczema) and partly endogenous (intrinsic atopic eczema).

Refer to Chap. 12 for more complete information on this topic.

3.9 Fingertip Dermatitis

Fingertip dermatitis is synonymous with chapping. It is very common and extends from the distal crease to ventral aspects of the fingertip (Fig. 3.14). The term used in French textbooks is "pulpite" (pulpitis), in reference to the digital pulpa. Subjective symptoms include itching, stinging, burning of the fingertips, tingling, or slight numbness. Painful crevices develop on an eczematous background, and bleeding may occur in severe cases. We would like to emphasize that fingertip dermatitis limited to the thumb and index (and eventually medius) finger of one or both hands frequently implies irritant (frictional and/or chemical) or allergenic factors. In those cases, fingertip dermatitis may be typical of (1) ICD, (2) ACD, or (3) PCD. We call this the "gripping form" of fingertip dermatitis [14]. These topographical features are only indicative of an exogenous (exclusively environmental) origin, but they may offer useful guidelines.

When some fingers are randomly involved and others are spared, or in case of complete involvement of all fingers of both hands, resolving the etiological factors may be quite difficult, even for well-trained dermatologists.

Three options must be considered:

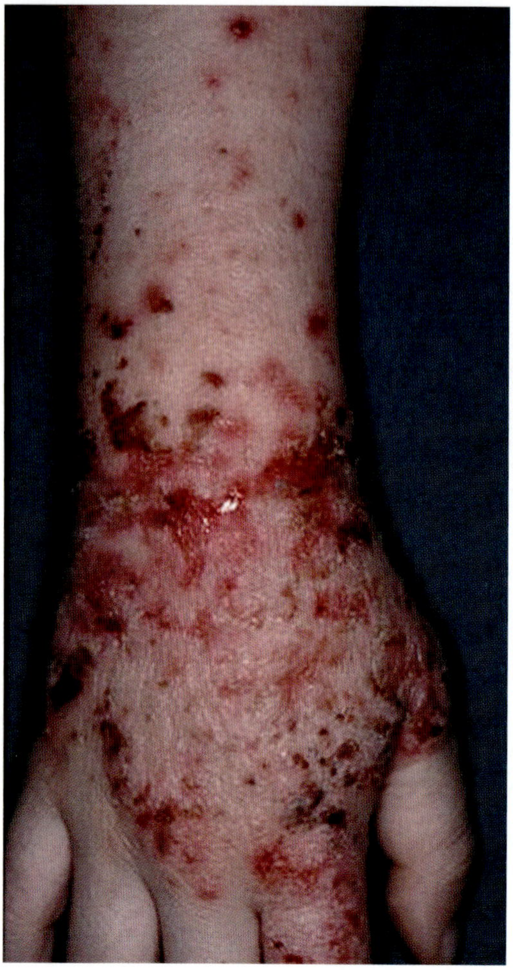

Fig. 3.11 Atopic eczema. Acute exudative eczema with crusts and scratch marks

- Endogenous (i.e., atopic dermatitis, psoriasis)
- Endogenous, but worsened by environmental factors
- Exogenous

Patch testing and prick testing are therefore highly recommended in each individual case.

An algorithmic approach to the various potential etiologies of fingertip dermatitis is presented in Fig. 3.15.

3.10 Failures of the Classification: Overlapping Diseases

The classification of the different categories of hand eczema, as reported above, seems to be very adequate for clinical and educational purposes. But it has to be moderated when exploring each individual patient. Indeed, overlapping of diseases does occur frequently (Fig. 3.16).

The scrutiny of the dermatologist is therefore highly recommended in the following cases:

- ICD and ACD can be superimposed, either simultaneously or subsequently.
- ICD is a classical component of atopic eczema. In 1980, Cronin [15] proposed the term "irritant contact dermatitis on an atopic background" instead of "atopic dermatitis of the hands." Recent research in the field of filaggrin mutations in atopic dermatitis has reevaluated this classical view [13].

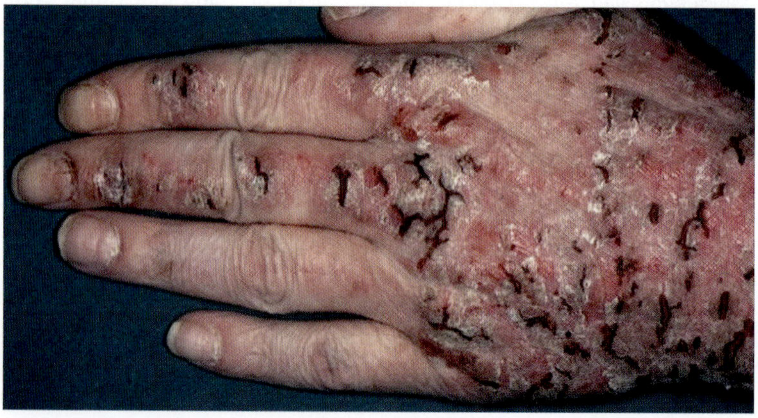

Fig. 3.12 Atopic eczema. Chronic crusting, deeply fissured eczema

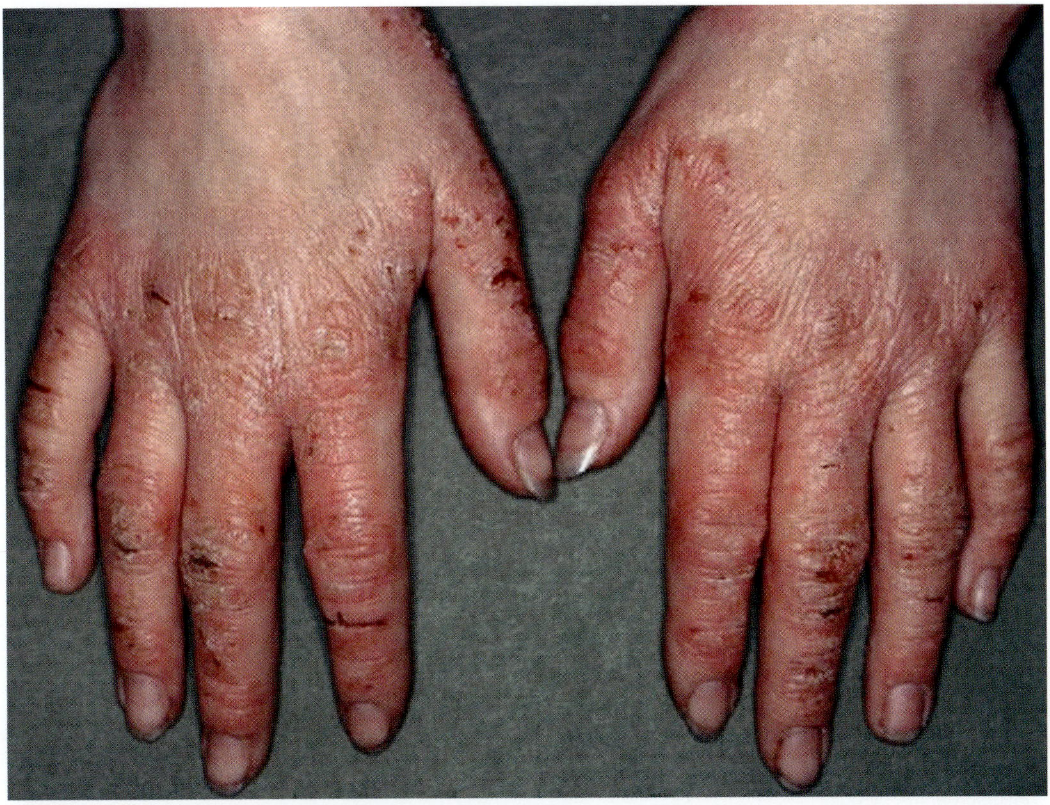

Fig. 3.13 Atopic eczema. Chronic erythematosquamous lesions

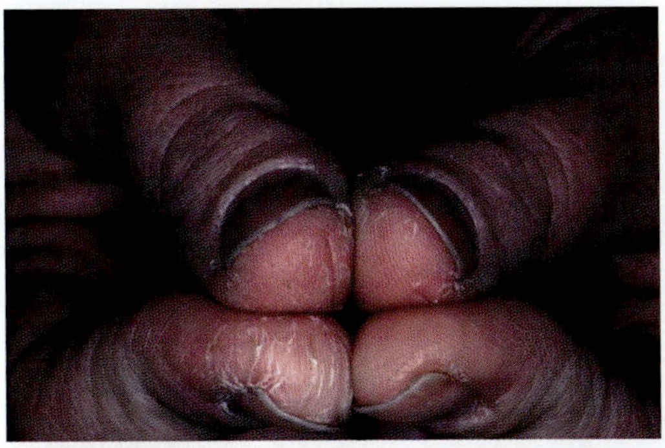

Fig. 3.14 Fingertip dermatitis

- Practically, for all other diseases (i.e., pompholyx, nummular eczema, palmar hyperkeratotic eczema, atopic eczema, fingertip dermatitis), it is very important to mention that they can be aggravated by ACD. It is essential to conduct a complete investigation in order to include (or exclude) all environmental factors suspected to worsen the clinical condition (Table 3.3).

3.11 Recent New Trends in the Classification of Hand Eczema

Many papers have been published in the recent years that focus on a reevaluation of the classification of hand eczema.

The general trend is to consider hand eczema as a "specific condition," including all morphological, topographical, and etiological facets of the disease. It also takes into account the overlap that frequently exists between the clinical variants.

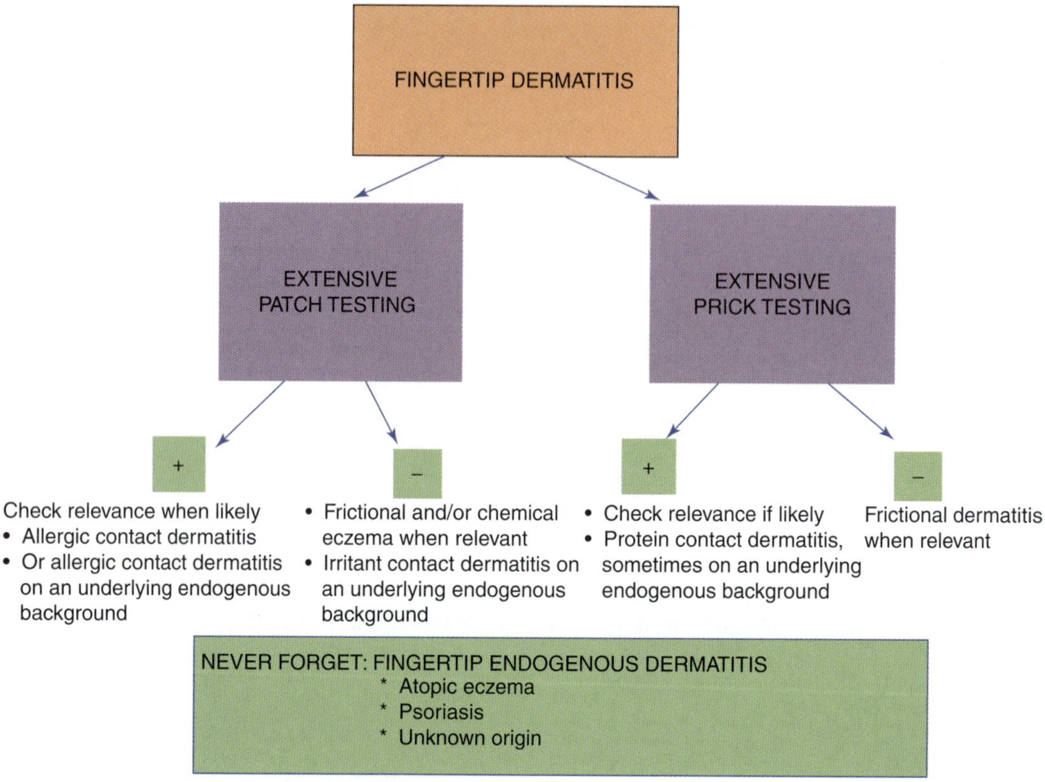

Fig. 3.15 An algorithmic approach to fingertip dermatitis

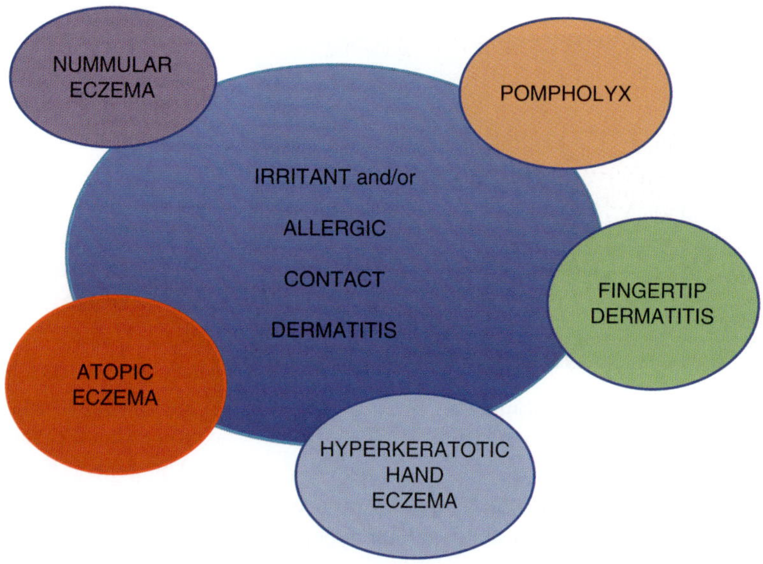

Fig. 3.16 Overlapping of diseases in hand eczema

Table 3.3 Tools of investigation available when hand eczema is suspected

Patch test	Prick-by-prick test
Strip patch test	Scratch test
Open test	Scratch-chamber test
Semi-open test	Intradermal test
ROAT test	Mycologic investigation (to exclude *tinea manuum*)
Spot tests	Skin biopsy (in rare instances)
Atopy patch test	Biological checkup (referring, for instance, to IgE-specific antigens)
Open (non-prick) test	
Prick test	

Diepgen [16], who developed this new approach, found it very useful, particularly in the field of occupational dermatology, in terms of management of each individual patient, not only for clinical assessment but also for elaborating educational programs, preventive measures, and modalities of treatment. The Danish Contact Dermatitis Group has also proposed a slightly modified classification (defined as "guideline") based on clinical and etiological criteria [17, 18].

3.12 The Hand Eczema Severity Indexes

Scoring the severity of hand eczema is not a usual practice among dermatologists, but it needs to be mentioned in this overview.

Several indexes have been proposed in the recent literature:

- The Hand Eczema Severity Index (HECSI) [19]
- The Osnabrueck Hand Eczema Severity Index (OHSI) [20]
- The Occupational Contact Dermatitis Disease Severity Index (ODDI) [21]

We refer the reader to the papers that explain the criteria for evaluating each patient individually. Their validity and reliability have been demonstrated [22, 23].

Nevertheless, some discrepancies can be observed between patient- and physician-rated scores [24].

In my view, scoring the severity of hand eczema may be of great interest when treatment results are concerned.

3.13 Algorithmic Approach for Differential Diagnosis: Key Role of Patch Testing and/or Prick Testing

Each patient presenting with clinical signs and symptoms suggestive of hand eczema requires a complete investigation built on grounds of evidence-based dermatology. An algorithmic approach to problems is an efficient way to reach a good evaluation in terms of diagnosis and management ("holistic approach"). It represents a major taxonomic challenge. The procedure is extremely useful, particularly when dealing with the multiple variants of "hand dermatitis." From this perspective, patch testing is, of course, one of the pieces of the puzzle [3]. Other algorithms have also been proposed in the recent literature [25].

The different tools of investigation are presented in Table 3.3.

A few algorithms were presented as examples in Figs. 3.5, 3.8, 3.10, and 3.15. It is recommended that dermatologists hang them up in the patch test clinic.

Conclusion

A classification of clinical subsets of hand eczema was proposed. Although it has some failures, it is a useful guide for the clinician in search of a precise etiology.

References

1. Berth-Jones J. Hand eczema. In: Burns T et al., editors. Rook's textbook of dermatology. 8th ed. Oxford: Wiley-Blackwell; 2010. p. 23.13–23.
2. Fregert S. Manual of contact dermatitis. 2nd ed. Copenhagen: Munksgaard; 1981. 138 pages.
3. Lachapelle J-M. Diseases for which patch testing is recommended: patients who should be investigated. In: Lachapelle J-M, Maibach HI, editors. Patch testing and prick testing. A practical guide. 3rd ed. Berlin: Springer; 2012. p. 11–33. Ch.2.

4. Hjorth N, Roed-Petersen J. Occupational protein contact dermatitis in food handlers. Contact Dermatitis. 1976;2:28–42.
5. Janssens V, Morren M, Dooms-Goossens A, Degreef H. Protein contact dermatitis: myth or reality? Br J Dermatol. 1995;132:1–6.
6. Lachapelle J-M. Protein contact dermatitis. In: Lachapelle J-M, Maibach HI, editors. Patch testing and prick testing. A practical guide. 3rd ed. Berlin: Springer; 2012. p. 153–6. Ch.10.
7. Wilkinson DS. Introduction, definition and classification. In: Menné T, Maibach HI, editors. Hand eczema. 2nd ed. Boca Raton: CRC Press; 2000. p. 1–13. Ch.1.
8. Lachapelle J-M. Dysidrose et eczéma dysidrosique. In: Saurat J-H, Lachapelle J-M, Lipsker D, Thomas L, editors. Dermatologie et infections sexuellement transmissibles. 5th ed. Paris: Masson; 2009. p. 83–5. Ch.2.
9. Pompholyx WU. A review of clinical features, differential diagnosis and managements. Am J Clin Dermatol. 2010;11:305–14.
10. Lachapelle J-M. Hyperkeratotic palmar dermatitis. In: Lachapelle J-M, Maibach HI, editors. Patch testing and prick testing. A practical guide. 3rd ed. Berlin: Springer; 2012. p. 29–30. Ch.2.
11. Lachapelle J-M, Tennstedt D, Marot L. Atlas of environmental dermatology. Braine l'Alleud: UCB Pharma Sector; 1997. p. 214.
12. Veien NK, Hattel T, Laurberg G. Hand eczema: causes, course and prognosis. Contact Dermatitis. 2008;58:330–4.
13. Kaae J, Menné T, Carlsen BC, Zachariae C, Thyssen JP. The hands in health and disease of individuals with filaggrin loss-of-function mutations: clinical reflections on the hand eczema phenotype. Contact Dermatitis. 2012;67:119–24.
14. Lachapelle J-M. Fingertip dermatitis. In: Lachapelle J-M, Maibach HI, editors. Patch testing and prick testing. A practical guide. 3rd ed. Berlin: Springer; 2012. p. 30. Ch.2.
15. Cronin E. Contact dermatitis. Edinburgh: Churchill Livingstone; 1980. 915 pages.
16. Diepgen TL, Andersen KE, Brandao FM, Bruze M, Bruynzeel DP, Frosch P, Gonçalo M, et al. Hand eczema classification: a cross-sectional, multicentre study of the actiology and morphology of hand eczema. Br J Dermatol. 2009;160:353–8.
17. Menné T, Johansen JD, Sommerlund M, Veien NK. Hand eczema guidelines based on the Danish guidelines for the diagnosis and treatment of hand eczema. Contact Dermatitis. 2011;65:3–12.
18. Johansen JD, Hald M, Andersen BL, Laurberg G, Danielsen A, Avnstorp C, et al. Classification of hand eczema: clinical and aetiological types. Based on the guidelines of the Danish Contact Dermatitis Group. Contact Dermatitis. 2011;65:13–21.
19. Held E, Skoet R, Johansen JD, Agner T. The hand eczema severity index (HECSI): scoring system for clinical assessment of hand eczema. A study of inter- and intraobserver reliability. Br J Dermatol. 2005;152: 302–7.
20. Skudlik C, Dulon M, Pohrt U, Appl KC, John SM, Nienhaus A. Osnabrueck hand eczema severity index – a study of the interobserver reliability of a scoring system assessing skin diseases of the hands. Contact Dermatitis. 2006;55:42–7.
21. Dulon M, Skudlik C, Nübling M, John SM, Nienhaus A. Validity and responsiveness of the Osnabrück Hand Eczema Severity Index (OHSI): a methodological study. Br J Dermatol. 2009;160:137–42.
22. Curr N, Dharmage S, Keegel T, Lee A, Saunders H, Nixon R. The validity and reliability of the occupational contact dermatitis disease severity index. Contact Dermatitis. 2008;59:157–64.
23. Coenrads PJ. Hand eczema. N Engl J Med. 2012;367: 1829–37.
24. van Coevorden AM, van Sonderen E, Bouma J, Coenraads PJ. Assessment of severity of hand eczema: discrepancies between patient – and physician – rated scores. Br J Dermatol. 2006;155:1217–22.
25. Molin S, Diepgen TL, Ruzicka T, Prinz JC. Diagnosing chronic hand eczema by an algorithm: a tool for classification in clinical practice. Clin Exp Dermatol. 2011;36:595–601.

Nail Alterations in Hand Eczema

4

Robert Baran

Contents

R. Baran, M.D.
Nail Disease Center,
Rue des Serbes, Cannes 06400, France
e-mail: baran.r@wanadoo.fr

4.1 Anatomy of the Nail Apparatus

The nail plate is the permanent product of the nail matrix. Its normal appearance and growth depend on the integrity of the perionychium and the bony phalanx [1, 2] (Fig. 4.1). The nail is a semi-hard, horny plate covering the dorsal aspect of the tip of the digit. The nail is inserted proximally in an invagination that is practically parallel to the upper surface of the skin and laterally in the lateral nail grooves. This pocket-like invagination has a roof, the proximal nail fold, and a floor, the matrix from which the nail is derived. The matrix extends approximately 5 mm under the proximal nail fold, and its distal portion is only visible as the white semicircular lunula. Injury to the nail matrix will manifest in the nail plate several weeks later. The general shape of the matrix is a crescent, concave in its posteroinferior portion. The lateral horns of this crescent are more developed in the great toe and are located at the coronal plane of the bone. The ventral aspect of the proximal nail fold encompasses both a lower portion, which the matrix continues, and an upper portion (roughly three-quarters of its length), called the *eponychium*. The germinal matrix forms the bulk of the nail plate. The proximal element forms the superficial third of the nail plate, whereas the distal element provides its inferior two-thirds. The ventral surface of the proximal nail fold adheres closely to the nail for a short distance and forms a gradually desquamating tissue, the cuticle, made of the stratum

A. Alikhan et al. (eds.), *Textbook of Hand Eczema*,
DOI 10.1007/978-3-642-39546-8_4, © Springer-Verlag Berlin Heidelberg 2014

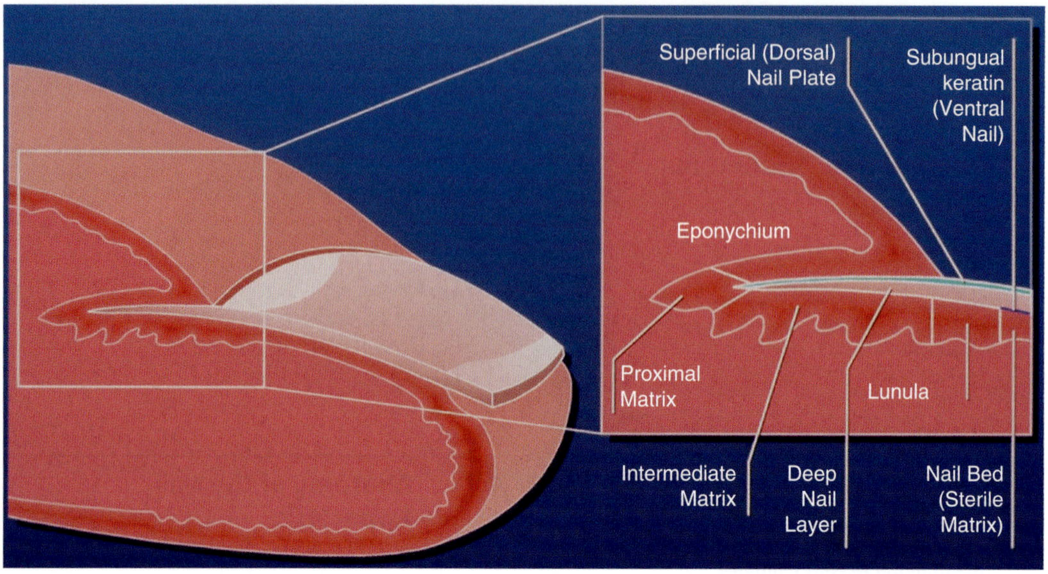

Fig. 4.1 Anatomy of the nail apparatus

corneum of both the dorsal and the ventral sides of the proximal nail fold. The cuticle seals and protects the nail cul-de-sac.

The nail plate is bordered by the proximal nail fold, which is a modified extension of the digit and is an actual fold of skin containing both epidermis and dermis but no subcutaneous tissue. Enthesitis may modify the appearance of the posterior fold [3]. This nail fold is continuous with the similarly structured lateral nail fold on each side. The nail bed extends from the lunula to the hyponychium.

In contrast to the matrix, the nail bed has a firm attachment to the nail plate, and avulsion of the overlying nail plate denudes the nail bed. The nail bed is composed of parallel longitudinal grooves and ridges consisting of an epithelium and a dermal connective tissue. Colorless but translucent, this highly vascular connective tissue, containing glomus organs, transmits a pink color through the nail.

Distally, adjacent to the nail bed, lays the hyponychium, an extension of the volar epidermis under the nail plate, which marks the point at which the nail separates from the underlying tissue. The distal nail groove, which is convex anteriorly, separates the hyponychium from the fingertip. The circulation of the nail apparatus is supplied by two digital arteries that course along the digits and give off branches to the distal and proximal arches. The sensory nerves to the distal phalanx of the three middle fingers are derived from fine, oblique, dorsal branches of the volar collateral nerves. Longitudinal branches of the dorsal collateral nerves supply the terminal phalanx of the fifth digit and also the thumb.

Among its multiple functions, the nail provides counterpressure to the pulp, which is essential to the tactile sensation involving the fingers and to the prevention of hypertrophy of the nail bed and the distal pulp.

4.2 Introduction to Nail Changes in Dermatitis

The worker's health, as well as that of any citizen, is an entitlement. Thus, the investment for health care has grown, because occupational diseases often cause irreversible damage. Skin diseases are among these important diseases, including allergic disorders of the nail unit in occupational diseases. However, to acknowledge their prevalence is complex, because many of them do not come to the attention of specialists and are not even noted.

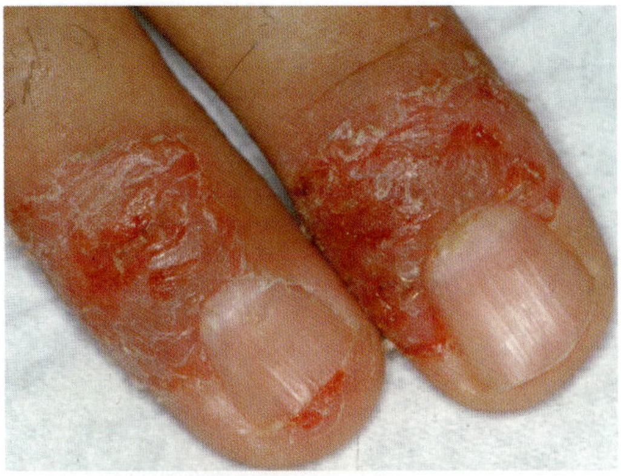

Fig. 4.2 Periungual eczema

The nail apparatus is particularly vulnerable to eczematous involvement irrespective of the nature of the allergen or the route by which it reaches the nail apparatus.

The mechanism of nail changes is obvious when the eczema is periungual (Fig. 4.2). However, the cause must be sought elsewhere if, as is frequently the case, the nail disorder is not associated with periungual eczema. General examination may reveal a specific type of eczema (e.g., atopic dermatitis, discoid eczema, pompholyx). Modifications of the nail plate result mainly from disturbances of the matrix (Table 4.1). These may present as thickening with discoloration, trachyonychia (roughness), pitting (Fig. 4.3), onychomadesis, and sometimes irregular, transverse furrows in the nails. These abnormalities may accompany a vesicular eruption of the periungual area and the nail matrix. Careful inspection of the nails may alert the dermatologist to the previous occurrence of eruptions. Nails may sometimes be shed. Fingernails continuously grow on average 0.1 mm per day. Toenails form over a period of 12–18 months.

A variety of different diagnoses unified by their pathology may present a similar clinical picture in the nail apparatus. The differential diagnosis of the disease actually causing the nail changes may vary from atopic dermatitis to irritant contact dermatitis and many others. The diagnosis may be established from a good history and physical examination of the configuration and distribution of the rash of the cutaneous surface.

Table 4.1 Clinical reaction patterns may originate from the different structures of the nail unit

1	Proximal matrix	
	1.1	Pitting (small depressions on the dorsum of the plate)
	1.2	Beau's lines and transverse grooving
	1.3	Trachyonychia (rough nails due to excessive ridging)
	1.4	Onychomadesis (detachment of the nail in its proximal portion)
	1.5	Nail shedding (loss of fingernail due to persistent contact dermatitis in an artificial gel nail designer is rarely reported) [12, 32]
2	Distal matrix	Leukonychia
3	Nail bed and hyponychium	Onycholysis (distal and/or lateral detachment of the nail plate)
4	Paronychium	
	4.1	Paronychial involvement (LE-like erythema and periungual telangiectasia among coffee plantation workers)
	4.2	When eczema occurs on the proximal and lateral nail folds, erythema, edema, and loss of the cuticle can result, characteristic of a chronic paronychia. The potential space between the proximal nail fold and the nail plate harbors moisture and *Candida* yeast Eczema will affect the most proximal part of the matrix if it involves the proximal nail fold
5	Surrounding tissue	Changes in the surrounding tissue (pulpitis, fissures)
6	Surrounding contour	Changes in the texture and contour of the nail plate, onychauxis, worn-down nail plate (usure des ongles), brittle nails, koilonychias (seasonal koilonychias in Ladakh after exposure to cold, wet mud) [33]
7	Underlying bone	Distal bony phalanx anomalies (they are mainly responsible for shape of the nail [pseudo-acro-osteolysis])

Eczema of the nail bed is no longer associated with cosmetic products such as base coats or hair-setting lotions; nevertheless, artificial nails remain the exception. The nail changes resulting from allergic contact sensitivity at this site appear

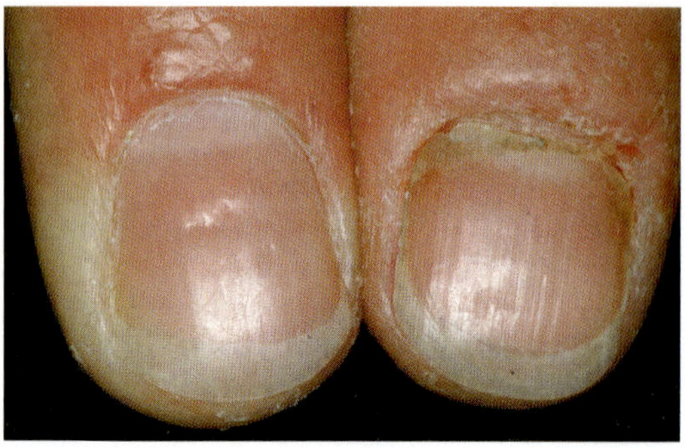

Fig. 4.3 On the left digit: pitting and vesicles on the proximal nail fold. On the right digit, onychomadesis

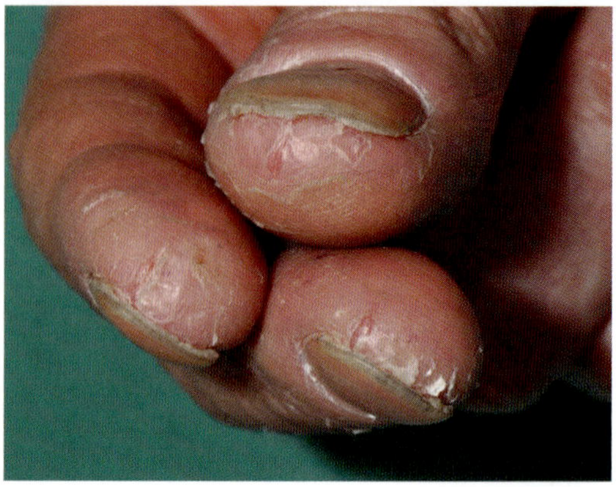

Fig. 4.4 Fissures of the first three fingers (Courtesy of Claire Bernier, MD, France)

hours, days, or even weeks later as splinter hemorrhages, soon followed by the development of subungual hyperkeratosis and, occasionally, koilonychia; onycholysis and paronychia may also be seen, often as a result of formaldehyde application. Color changes vary from a bluish-red appearance, initially, to "rust" and finally yellow. The affected areas may be intensely painful.

Occupational nail disorders and periungual changes may be produced, maintained, or exacerbated by agents present in the professional environment. These agents can attack the nail plate and surrounding skin. Occupational contact dermatitis (OCD) represents 80 % of cases of work-related dermatoses. Certain factors predispose individuals to the development of the OCD, such as age, sex, and color of the individual, as well as the temperature and humidity levels in their professional environment. Added to these, there is the possibility of exposure to irritants and factors inherent to the worker, such as hygiene care and use of personal protective equipment.

The potential space between the proximal nail fold and nail plate often harbors moisture and *Candida* yeast. The subungual space is important because it can potentially provide infection spread by scratching [4].

From a practical point of view, nail alterations in hand eczema may be divided into acute and chronic eczema. The latter is currently defined as an anatomic and a clinical syndrome that often has a multifactorial origin. The factors involved in both the development of the lesions and that of the flares are multiple and not always clearly identified. Their severity is variable, depending on the patients and the flares, which explain the diversity of the clinical appearances of chronic eczema in the same subject.

Common sensitizers in OCD may induce a wide range of clinical patterns in the nail area. Minimal damage may simply produce onycholysis. Subungual hyperkeratosis is frequent and may be accompanied by erythema, scaling, and fissuring (Fig. 4.4).

The main changes of the nail unit by sensitizing agents are as follows: modification of the color of the nail (yellow chromonychia), loss of coloration, onychoschizia and granulation surface of the nail plate, brittle nails, onycholysis, paronychia, transverse furrows, onychomadesis, subungual hyperkeratosis, periungual fissures, and alterations to the formation of the cuticle.

Irritant contact dermatitis is observed mainly in the hands, in the region around the fingernails, with abnormal formation of the cuticle, onycholysis, and thin subungual hyperkeratosis. There is often a secondary infection. The diagnosis is made through a detailed history, characterization of the disease, and identification of causative agents.

In patients with atopic dermatitis (intrinsic), in addition to personal and family history of atopy in patients (atopic dermatitis found in 41 % of the patients in infancy) [5], an open (non-prick) or prick test may be carried out by which means it is possible to detect sensitivity to allergens of the environment. Another possibility, though less reliable, is that one examine the immunoglobulin E (IgE) levels in serum specific for certain antigens. Careful examination of nails is also essential for diagnosis of OCD. In cases of suspected lesions by contact, patch tests can be performed and read later.

Standardized batteries are used, and each substance is placed in aluminum disks (Finn Chambers), which are preferably placed on the back of the patient. They are reinforced with tape, and reading takes place in 48 and 72 h, according to the International Contact Dermatitis Research Group, or in 48 and 96 h, as recommended by the Brazilian Group Study in Contact Dermatitis. The diagnosis of occupational allergic contact dermatitis will be confirmed if there is consistency between the test results, the location of lesions, and history of occupational exposure to those agents. When dermatitis is caused by a primary irritant, the patch test will be negative. Other important tests to evaluate possible differential diagnosis are biopsy, as well as bacteriological and mycological direct and indirect testing.

4.3 Causes of Contact Dermatitis that Can Affect the Nail

A list of main causes and their reactions is presented in this section [6].

Plants and flowers:

- Alstroemeria dermatitis: onycholysis of thumb and index fingers.
- Hydrangea dermatitis: clinical picture of paronychia and nail dystrophy.
- Nasturtium (common plant used in salads): fingertip dermatitis.
- Rhus dermatitis: onycholysis and xanthonychia.
- Wooden orange stick (cuticle remover): responsible for persistent eczema of the right hand of a manicurist.
- Tabernaemontana coronaria: fingertip dermatitis of the first three fingers of both hands.
- Tulip fingers: painful, dry, fissured, hyperkeratotic eczema. It starts under the free margin of the nails and extends to the fingertips and periungual regions (Fig. 4.5).
- Turpentine: in craft workers, it can cause eczema of the fingers and periungual tissues with subungual hyperkeratosis.

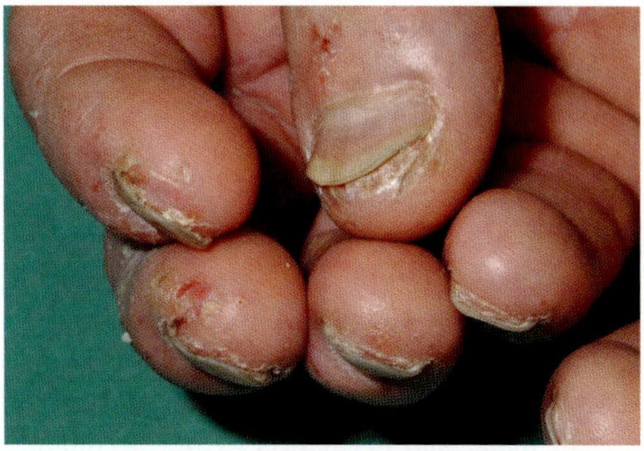

Fig. 4.5 Distal subungual hyperkeratosis with onycholysis (Courtesy of Claire Bernier, MD, France)

Among common sensitizers, nail cosmetics are a special type of allergen of the nail region [7]. After a few months of applications of nail cosmetics, patients may begin to show an allergic contact dermatitis, usually of the dorsal aspects of some of the fingers and paronychial tissue, the face, and the eyelids [8]. Pain and persistent paresthesia have been reported with sculptured nails and gels, but this may occur without an allergic reaction [9].

Manicurists who apply these artificial nails to clients may become sensitized. The thumb and index [10] or middle fingers of the left hand are constantly exposed as the manicurist holds the client's finger during the building-up process of the sculptured nails.

Today, acrylates have a broad area of application in various products (see Chap. 17 for more details). Repeated contact with acrylic materials, especially the sensitizing liquid monomers, has long been known to be responsible for contact dermatitis in dental staff and orthopedic surgeons. More recently, a wider public has been affected by the practice of wearing sculptured artificial nails [11, 12].

Dimethacrylates used in industrial sealants mainly affect the pulp of the fingers and can extend as scaly eczema under the free margin of the nails [10]:

- Epoxy resin dermatitis especially involves the first two right fingertips of nail technicians, producing erosion and crusting or necrotic-appearing lesions. The resin oligomer may collect under the free edge of the nail and polymerize slowly as it dries [13, 14].
- p-Tertiary-butyl phenol formaldehyde resin, an adhesive to attach a brand of plastic artificial nail, was responsible for onycholysis, subungual hyperkeratosis, atrophy of the nail plate, and dermatitis of the periungual skin [15].

Other sensitizers in different fields have been reported. Among them are the following:

- Printing workers sensitized to photopolymerizable acrylic resin may show eczematous lesions on the fingertips and around the nail plate, extending to the distal subungual area.
- Current dermatitis may be allergic due to dichromate content or may result from alkaline irritation and burns.
- In dermatitis of the dorsum of the proximal nail fold, koilonychia is frequent. It is usually accompanied by distolateral subungual hyperkeratosis, lifting the lateral edges of the nail. Painful fissures in the same area are common [16].
- Codeine sensitization in pharmaceutical workers has been associated with subungual hyperkeratosis, onycholysis, and nail atrophy [17].
- Beside these examples, we can also quote "caine" local anesthetics, glutaraldehyde, hydroxolamine, 1-methylquinoxalinium, p-toluene sulfonate, propacetamol, quaternium-15, etc. The same lesions, previously described, may be observed.

Food allergy (onions, garlic, tomatoes, etc.) may develop finger pulp dermatitis with hyperkeratosis and fissuring, paronychia (Fig. 4.6), and onycholysis. The nails may also present with several transverse depressions. Food handlers who have contact with uncooked food may develop immediate-type hypersensitivity in the form of protein contact dermatitis, a variant of contact urticaria.

When eczema involves the posterior nail fold, it will often also affect the proximal tip of the matrix. This results in surface irregularities such as ridges, furrows, and pits. The nail bed, and particularly the hyponychium, may be involved with consequent subungual hyperkeratosis and loss of nail adhesion to the nail bed. Histopathology reveals spongiosis, spongiotic vesicles, variable parakeratosis, and granular layer with intermittent orthokeratotic foci. The dermis shows a predominantly superficial perivascular lymphocytic infiltrate. Giemsa stain usually exhibits severe alterations in the stain ability of the nail plate, which may become disorderly and wavy. The pits do not usually contain parakeratotic onychocytes. PAS stain may show pronounced staining of the intercellular spaces, probably due to trapping of serum glycoproteins in between the cells of the nail plate.

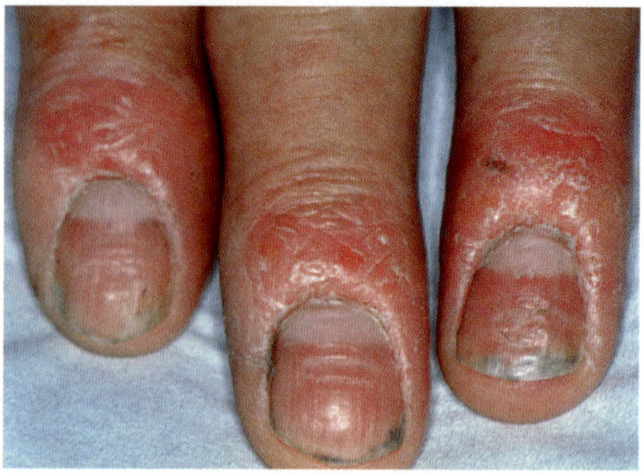

Fig. 4.6 Paronychial dermatitis and transverse grooves of the nail plate

4.4 Chemical Irritants and Cumulative Primary Irritants

Contact dermatitis by primary irritant (CDPI), or irritant contact dermatitis, is the most common and can occur in anyone and is subject to the concentration of the irritant and the frequency and duration or contact. Acids, alkalis, solvents, soaps, detergents, abrasives, oils, and oxidizing and reducing agents are examples of irritants (Fig. 4.7). No immune mechanism is involved, while allergic contact dermatitis (ACD) results from hypersensitivity reactions of type IV Gell and Coombs, more specifically, type IVa.

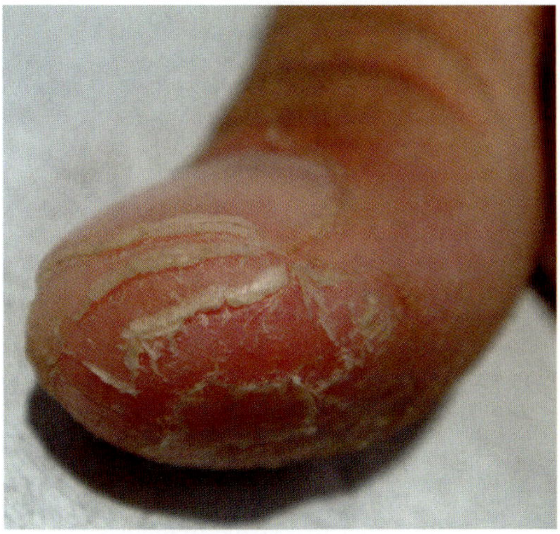

Fig. 4.7 Distal desquamation due to irritants

The time required for a patient to become sensitized is around 14–21 days. Once sensitized, whenever there is new contact with the substance, the ACD reaction occurs, and this will be faster, growing at 24–48 h. An irritant patch test reaction appears as sharply demarcated erythema with minimal infiltration and small pustules [18].

Below are nail changes appreciated in irritant contact dermatitis due to various chemicals:

- The nails can be softened and gradually destroyed by prolonged immersion in water containing high concentrations of alkalis, alkaline chlorine-containing compounds, solvents, soap, or powerful detergents. Abrasives, oils, and oxidizing and reducing agents are examples of irritants.
- Permanent wave chemicals (ammonium thioglycolate) may cause koilonychias in hairdressers in conjunction with soreness of the distal nail beds. Thioglycolates in depilatories (chemical hair removers) are a further domestic cause of acute chemical onycholysis. Several fingernails are involved at the same time [19].
- Weed killers diquat and paraquat can soften and discolor the nail plate, leading to nail loss [20]. Similar changes have been described in a man using 5 % dinitro-ortho-cresol, without further recommended dilution, for spraying fruit trees [21]. Dinobuton handlers may present with yellow hair and nails [22].
- Hydrofluoric acid especially damages the subungual tissues, which are a common portal of entry for this highly destructive chemical. The acid readily diffuses through minute holes in rubber gloves. Frequently, the burn is unrecognized until up to 24 h later, when excruciating pain begins. The subungual tissues are especially susceptible to its destructive effect. Specific treatment with a topical 2 % calcium gluconate preparation is indicated or, even better, intra-arterial injection with a bolus of calcium (14 mg/kg) followed by prophylactic nail avulsion and continuous topical calcium gluconate therapy for 4–6 days [23]. Hydrofluoric acid is widely used in the semiconductor industry but can be a component of rust-removing agents. It is also used in the manufacture of plastics, germicides, dye tanning solutions, solvents, and fire-proofing materials; the glazing of pottery; cleaning brick, stone, iron, and steel; and the brewing of beer to control fermentation and to cleanse rubber pipes.
- Formaldehyde is responsible for sensitization in many occupational groups, including hospital staff, where eczema of the fingers with nail dystrophy may result [24]. Prolonged occupational contact with formaldehyde solutions can cause softening and brown discoloration of the nail. Formalin (37–50 % solution of formaldehyde in water) is widely used industrially, as a preservative, as a tanning agent, and to augment the water resistance of paper. Formalin is a generic name for a substance that contains 59 % methylene glycol and 0.0466 % formaldehyde, mixed in water with a small amount of methanol to prevent the methylene glycol (which is a liquid) from converting into a solid polymer. Products containing 5 % formalin (or less) contain less than 0.0025 % formaldehyde. The test methods used actually measure both methylene glycol and formaldehyde together as though they were only one chemical (D. Schoon, personal communication).

Other chemical irritants that warrant mention include gold potassium cyanide (purplish-brown discoloration and onycholysis), organic solvents and motor oils that soften the nail plate, and oxalic acid used in bleaching animal and vegetable materials (swelling and redness of the fingertips presents with a bluish discoloration and brittleness of the nails).

Nails and fingertips are often involved in cumulative irritant contact dermatitis.

The nails may show onycholysis, subungual hyperkeratosis, and textural irregularities of the nail plate with pitting and transverse depressions. Painful fissures and cracks occur at the transition of nail plate to fingertip. Wear and tear and chemical exposure may damage the fingertips with painful cracks, lamellar sealing, and abrasion of the epidermis.

4.5 Allergic and Irritant Contact Dermatitis: The Same Disease?

Many irritants and sensitizing agents are responsible for OCD; consequently, many professionals are exposed to them. Some examples are construction workers (who are exposed to chromium cement), chefs, service staff (responsible for general maintenance and cleaning), mechanics, painters, health professionals, gardeners, farmers, and others. Plants can cause changes at the nail and periungual regions, ranging from change of color to important dystrophies. Acrylates have been widely cited in the literature in terms of their use in adhesives, textures, orthopedic prostheses, dental materials, nail polish, artificial nails, and paint, among other products. Formaldehyde used as a nail hardener can cause throbbing pain, onycholysis, subungual hematoma, and yellowish chromonychia.

The only discriminative test between irritant and allergic contact dermatitis would be revealing specific T lymphocytes to the incriminated allergen in allergic contact dermatitis.

Unfortunately, this is not possible in daily practice, and the diagnosis is based on a combination of data (obtained in history) with clinical investigation and, of course, patch testing. However, in general, there is no single characteristic in

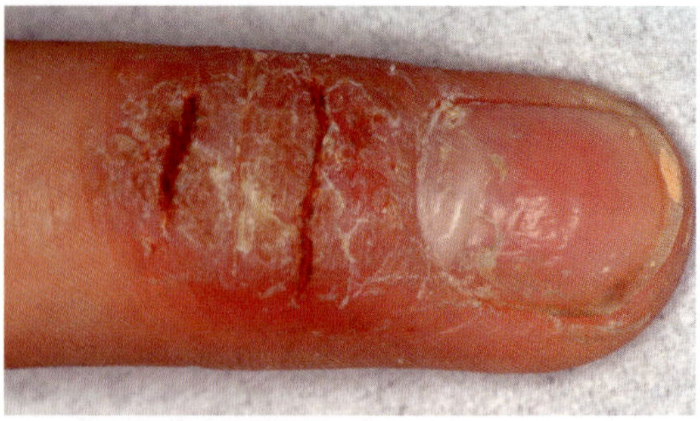

Fig. 4.8 Distal dorsal digit involvement in atopic dermatitis

the clinical picture of cumulative irritant contact dermatitis that makes the diagnosis certain. This is particularly true for the hands that are in contact with such a large range of various occupational products, household chores, and topical drugs usually bought by the patient for various reasons.

Nail changes may occur in any type of dermatitis involving the hands and in particular the skin adjacent to the nail, but atopic dermatitis more frequently affects the nails than do other types (Fig. 4.8). In atopic dermatitis and in pompholyx, the nail changes sometimes predominate. One must assume in these cases that the eczematous process is most marked on the undersurface of the dorsal nail fold.

The usual change is an atrophic process that consists of the development of irregular ridges across the nail. In addition, coarse pitting may affect one or more nails. The ridges occur independently on one or several nails, and the overall change is a very ugly nail. If the grooves are deep enough (Fig. 4.9), they may result in temporary shedding of part of the nail. In the early stages, only the proximal part of the nails will be involved. Subungual hemorrhages, either petechial or more extensive, may complicate the picture, as may chronic paronychia. The ridges must be distinguished from ridges formed by other causes and in particular the traumatic nail dystrophy produced by a habit tic.

The sudden onset of generalized dermatitis may be accompanied by the formation of a depression on all nails similar to Beau's lines, but

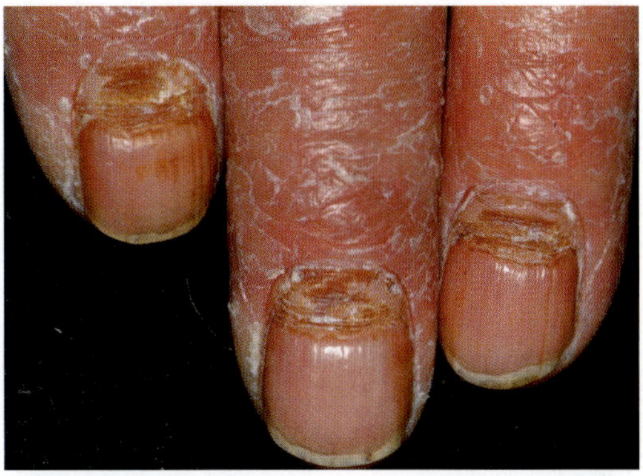

Fig. 4.9 Deep transverse grooves leading to temporary nail shedding

in dermatitis the nail behind the depression is likely to be deformed. In exfoliative dermatitis, the nails may be shed.

Although the usual nail change in dermatitis is an atrophic process, occasionally gross hypertrophy occurs. These cases are associated with inflammation of the nail fold, and the nail becomes very thick and irregular.

Onycholysis is not infrequently seen in association with dermatitis of the fingertips, presumably as a result of irritant material being trapped under the free edge of the nail and then penetrating further proximally. Occasionally, the irritant material may pass through the nail plate to reach the nail bed [25]. Shelley [26] has noted onycholysis from the topical application of 5 % 5-fluorouracil to the fingertips under occlusion. The condition was reversible and was not produced by a 2 % preparation.

Koilonychia may be associated with the use of organic solvents and motor oils [27]. Both irritant and allergic contact reactions may result from the use of nail cosmetics, causing a variety of nail abnormalities. Highly polished nails are sometimes seen in patients with generalized eczema or erythroderma. This is, of course, an indirect effect of the patients rubbing their hands on their skin to obtain relief from itching, preferring this to actual scratching because it does less damage. Another change sometimes encountered is the so-called usure des ongles, a wearing away of the nails due to scratching.

4.6 Hand Eczema in Atopics

In a study of 777 consecutive patients with atopic eczema by Simpson et al. [28], hand involvement was observed in 58.9 % and nail dystrophy was seen in 16 %.

Nail changes were noted to be relatively common. Like other eczemas, atopic palmar eczema can lead to impairments of the matrix and/or nail bed. There are slight changes (e.g., pits or transverse grooves) but also more marked changes (e.g., trachyonychia). As seen before, constant rubbing and scratching of the skin, as in atopic dermatitis or erythroderma, causes the nails to be buffed; the surface of the nails becomes "polished" and shiny, and the free edge may be worn down. The prevalence of *Staphylococcus* beneath the nails of atopics has been described as ten times greater than that of normal controls. This illustrates the importance of nail care and careful cleaning when there is eczema.

In atopic hand eczema (dorsal type), lichenification and fissuring, particularly over the knuckles, are observed; the nails are polished from extensive scratching. In atopic hand eczema (ventral type), symmetric nummular infiltrates, both chronic (lichenified) and acute (vesicular, crusted) in nature, may be seen.

It has been suggested that parakeratosis pustulosa, probably the juvenile type of nail psoriasis, may be a variant of atopic eczema. Interestingly, trachyonychia, which may result from psoriasis, lichen planus, or alopecia areata, presents with histopathologic features of eczema in the latter. This may be a problem when diagnosing isolated nail involvement in alopecia areata. Allergic contact dermatitis may also be a precipitant in some instances.

Atopic antecedents are also considered risk factors. In atopic skin, which is chronically inflamed, xerotica with several structural changes in the skin barrier are more vulnerable when exposed to chemicals, whether they are primary irritants or sensitizing. Thus, depending on the type of exposure that the atopic patient suffers in his/her work environment, there will be a greater predisposition to development of ACD, which may be responsible, among other injuries, for important changes at the nail unit.

Dermatitis can play havoc with the nails, and in most cases the cause of the nail damage is obvious. At times, however, the dermatitis is under control before the patient complains of the nail changes; in these cases, one has to rely on the history for confirmatory diagnosis. Such patients are usually referred to as having suspected fungal infection of the nails; this is generally easily excluded with lab tests [25].

4.7 Treatment

Treatment of the nail folds with topical corticosteroids or tacrolimus [29] is often helpful, in association with the hand-care measures that are employed in psoriatic nail disease. An additional antimicrobial ingredient may be required (e.g., mupirocin). If a potent steroid is used long term, there may be a risk of premature closure of the underlying epiphyses in children and acroatrophy [30]. It could be argued that steroid use would increase the risk of secondary infection, such as osteomyelitis of the distal phalanges, as reported in three children [31]; however, untreated eczema is likely to represent a risk of, at least, similar proportions.

Many things have changed during the last few years concerning "eczemas."

From an etiopathogenic point of view, irritant contact dermatitis and allergic contact dermatitis have moved closer. At present, irritant contact dermatitis, which stems from innate immunity, and allergic contact dermatitis, which stems from adaptative immunity, share commonalities in some reactional mechanisms and in implicated cells, such as intervention of numerous cytokines.

Treatment should be primarily preventive in nature. It has three objectives: (1) the promotion of worker's health through guidance, training, proper nutrition, hygiene, and other standards; (2) secondary prevention, which includes outpatient care at the company, inspection of places of work, and periodic examinations; and (3) tertiary prevention in the patients with active lesions. Appropriate therapeutic measures are adopted (topical medications and/or systemic), potential occupational allergens are detected and removed, and, where appropriate, the patient may be rehabilitated for another activity. Wearing adapted gloves is essential for protection.

Conclusion

In conclusion, the purpose of this chapter was to emphasize the vulnerability of the nail apparatus in the different types of hand dermatitis, even in the absence of cutaneous hand lesions.

References

1. Baran R. Nail surgery. In: Goldsmith LA, Katz SI, Gelderest BA, Puller AS, Leffell DJ, Wolff K, editors. Fitzpatrick's dermatology in general medicine. New York: McGraw Hill; 2012.
2. Morgan AM, Baran R, Haneke E. Anatomy of the nail unit in relation to the distal digit. In: Krull E, Zook E, Baran R, Haneke E, editors. Nail surgery – a text and atlas. Philadelphia: Lippincott William & Wilkins; 2001.
3. McGonagle D. Enthesitis: an autoinflammatory lesion linking nail and joint involvement in psoriatic disease. J Eur Acad Dermatol Venereol. 2009;23 suppl 1:9–13.
4. Halioua B, Richard MA. Mise au point sur l'eczéma chronique des mains. Ann Dermatol Venereol. 2010;173:315–27.
5. Nishijima S, Namura S, Higashi T, Kawai S. Staphylococcus aureus in the anterior pares and subungual spaces of the hands in atopic eczema. J Int Med Res. 1997;25:155–8.
6. Baran R, Rycroft RJG. Occupational abnormalities and contact dermatitis. In: Baran R, De Berker DAR, Holzberg M, Thomas L, editors. Diseases of the nails and their management. 4th ed. Oxford: Wiley-Blackwell; 2012.
7. Schoon D, Baran R. Cosmetics: the care and adornment of the nail. In: Baran R, De Berker DAR, Holzberg M, Thomas L, editors. Diseases of the nails and their management. 4th ed. Oxford: Wiley-Blackwell; 2012.
8. Hemmer W, Focke M, Wantke F, Götz M, Jarisch R. Allergic contact dermatitis to artificial finger nails prepared from UV light-cured acrylates. J Am Acad Dermatol. 1996;35:377–80.
9. Baran RL, Schibli H. Permanent paresthesia to sculptured nails. A distressing problem. Dermatol Clin. 1990;8:139–41.
10. Condé-Salazar L, Guimaraens D, Romero LV. Occupational allergic dermatitis from anaerobic acrylic sealants. Contact Dermatitis. 1986;18:129–32.

11. Freeman S, Lee MS, Gudmundsen K. Adverse contact reactions to sculptured acrylic nails: four case reports and literature review. Contact Dermatitis. 1995;33:381–5.
12. Cruz MJ, Baudrier T, Curha AP, Ferreira O, Azevedo F. Severe onychodystrophy caused by allergic contact dermatitis to acrylates in artificial nails. Cutan Ocul Toxicol. 2011;30:323–4.
13. Guin JD, Bass K, Nelson-Adesokan P. Contact sensitization to cyanoacrylate adhesive as a cause of severe onychodystrophy. Int J Dermatol. 1998;37:31–6.
14. Lazarov A. Sensitization to acrylates in a common adverse reaction to artificial nails. J Eur Acad Dermatol Venereol. 2007;21:169–74.
15. Rycroft RJG, Wilkinson JD, Holmes R, Hay RJ. Contact sensitization to p-tertiary butylphenol (PTBP) resin in plastic nail adhesive. Clin Exp Dermatol. 1980; 5:441–5.
16. Calnan CD. Cement dermatitis. J Occup Med. 1960; 2:15–22.
17. Romaguera C, Grimalt F. Dermatitis de contacto profesional por codeina. Bol Inform GEIDC. 1983;5:21–3.
18. Militello G. Contact and primary irritant dermatitis of the nail unit: diagnosis and treatment. Dermatol Therap. 2007;20:47–53.
19. Baran R. Acute onycholysis from rust-removing agents. Arch Dermatol. 1980;116:382–3.
20. Botella R, Sastre A, Castello A. Contact dermatitis to paraquat. Contact Dermatitis. 1985;13:123–4.
21. Baran R. Nail damage caused by weed killers and insecticides. Arch Dermatol. 1974;10:46–7.
22. Wahlberg JE. Yellow nail staining of hair and nails and contact sensitivity to dinobuton. Contact Dermatitis Newsl. 1974;16:481.
23. Sebastian G. General practice-relevant therapeutic recommendations in hydrofluoric acid burns. Hautarzt. 1994;45:453–9.
24. Cronin E. Contact dermatitis. Edinburgh: Churchill-Livingston; 1980. p. 586.
25. Samman PD, Fenton DA. Nail disorders associated with other dermatological conditions. In: Samman PD, Fenton DA, editors. Samman's the nails in disease. 5th ed. Oxford: Butterworth–Heinemann; 1995. p. 72–6.
26. Shelley WB. Onycholysis due to topical 5 fluorouracil. Acta Derm Venereol. 1972;52:320.
27. Dawber R. Occupational koilonychia. Clin Exp Dermatol. 1977;2:115–6.
28. Simpson EL, Thompson MM, Hanifin JM. Prevalence and morphology of hand eczema in patients with atopic dermatitis. Contact Dermatitis. 2006;17:153–7.
29. Lee DY, Kim WS, Lee KJ, Kim JA, Park JH, Cho HJ, et al. Tacrolimus ointment in onychodystrophy associated with eczema. J Eur Acad Dermatol Venereol. 2007;21:1137–8.
30. Requena L, Zamora E, Martin L. Acropathy secondary to long standing applications of topical steroids. Arch Dermatol. 1990;126:1013–4.
31. Boiko S, Kaufman RA, Lucky AW. Osteomyelitis of the distal phalanx in 3 children with severe atopic dermatitis. Arch Dermatol. 1988;124:418–23.
32. Haglmüller T, Hemmer W, Kusa I, et al. Loss of fingernails due to persistent allergic contact dermatitis in an artificial nail designer. J Allergy Clin Immun. 1995;95:250.
33. Anan IS, Harris P. Koilonychia in Ladakhis. Br J Dermatol. 1988;119:267–8.

Other Dermatoses Affecting the Hand: Differential Diagnosis

5

Jean-Marie Lachapelle and Dominique Tennstedt

Contents

J.-M. Lachapelle, M.D., Ph.D. (✉)
D. Tennstedt, M.D.
Department of Dermatology, Catholic University of Louvain, 10, Avenue Hippocrate, Brussels 1200, Belgium
e-mail: jean.marie.lachapelle@uclouvain.be; dominique@tennstedt.be

5.1 Introduction

Various skin diseases, unrelated to eczema, may affect the hands. For most (but not all) of those, the typical lesions can be observed on other body

A. Alikhan et al. (eds.), *Textbook of Hand Eczema*,
DOI 10.1007/978-3-642-39546-8_5, © Springer-Verlag Berlin Heidelberg 2014

parts and facilitate the diagnosis. However, in certain cases, the diseases may in an early stage of their evolution be exclusively located on the hands. As several variants of hand eczema could be relevant, differential diagnosis is sometimes problematic (Table 5.1).

Table 5.1 Other dermatoses affecting the hands: differential diagnosis with hand eczema

Hand dermatoses	Differential diagnosis
Acrokeratosis paraneoplastica	Palmar hyperkeratotic eczema Psoriasis Fingertip dermatitis
Antisynthetase antibodies syndrome "mechanic's hands"	Chronic irritant contact dermatitis "Wear and tear" dermatitis Palmar hyperkeratotic eczema
Bullous pemphigoid	Vesiculobullous pompholyx or dyshidrotic eczema
Candidiasis	Protein contact dermatitis
Contact urticaria	Protein contact dermatitis Acute allergic contact dermatitis on the backs of the hands
Crusted scabies	Palmar hyperkeratotic eczema Hyperkeratotic irritant and/or allergic contact dermatitis (chronic stage) Atopic dermatitis Psoriasis
Cutaneous T-cell lymphoma	Allergic contact dermatitis Atopic dermatitis Psoriasis Palmar *tinea manuum*
Darier's disease	Palmar hyperkeratotic eczema
Dermatitis artefacta	Irritant contact dermatitis Allergic contact dermatitis Protein contact dermatitis
Dermatomyositis	No real problem of differential diagnosis. Be alert
Lichen planus	Lichenoid allergic contact dermatitis Lichenoid drug eruption Lichenification
Linear IgA bullous dermatosis	Vesiculobullous pompholyx or dyshidrotic eczema
Palmoplantar keratodermas	Palmar hyperkeratotic eczema Palmoplantar psoriasis
Palmoplantar pustulosis	Acute vesicular *tinea manuum* or *tinea pedis* Chronic allergic contact dermatitis Linear IgA bullous dermatitis
Porphyria cutanea tarda	Phototoxic contact dermatitis Photoallergic contact dermatitis
Psoriasis	Palmar hyperkeratotic eczema
Recurrent palmar peeling	Desquamation stage of pompholyx
Syphilis	Palmar psoriasis Palmar hyperkeratotic eczema
Tinea manuum	Chronic hand eczema

Some patients, suffering from a skin disease unrelated to hand eczema, are referred erroneously to a patch and/or prick test clinic.

Infections and tumoral diseases of the hand have been excluded in this review.

The purpose of the chapter is to describe the most important dermatoses of the hands, related (or not) to those variants of hand eczema.

5.2 Acrokeratosis Paraneoplastica (Bazex Syndrome)

The condition described at first by Bazex in France is a rare, but classical, paraneoplastic syndrome, much commoner in males than in females, associated particularly with squamous cell carcinoma of the upper respiratory or gastrointestinal tracts. The presence of an underlying malignancy is required for the diagnosis [1, 2]. The skin lesions (Fig. 5.1a, b) are characterized by violaceous erythema and scaling and are mainly acral – that is, helices of the ears, tip of the nose, hands, and feet (especially the distal portion of the digits).

Symptoms on hands can include the following:

- At a very early stage, lesions can be limited to pulpar fingertips, and differential diagnosis with "common" fingertip dermatitis is needed.
- Erythematous, keratotic, and fissural lesions of periungual areas and pulpar fingertips. These are constantly described as "psoriasiform."
- On the palms, keratoderma may appear progressively, during the course of the disease.
- Nail dystrophy is often present.

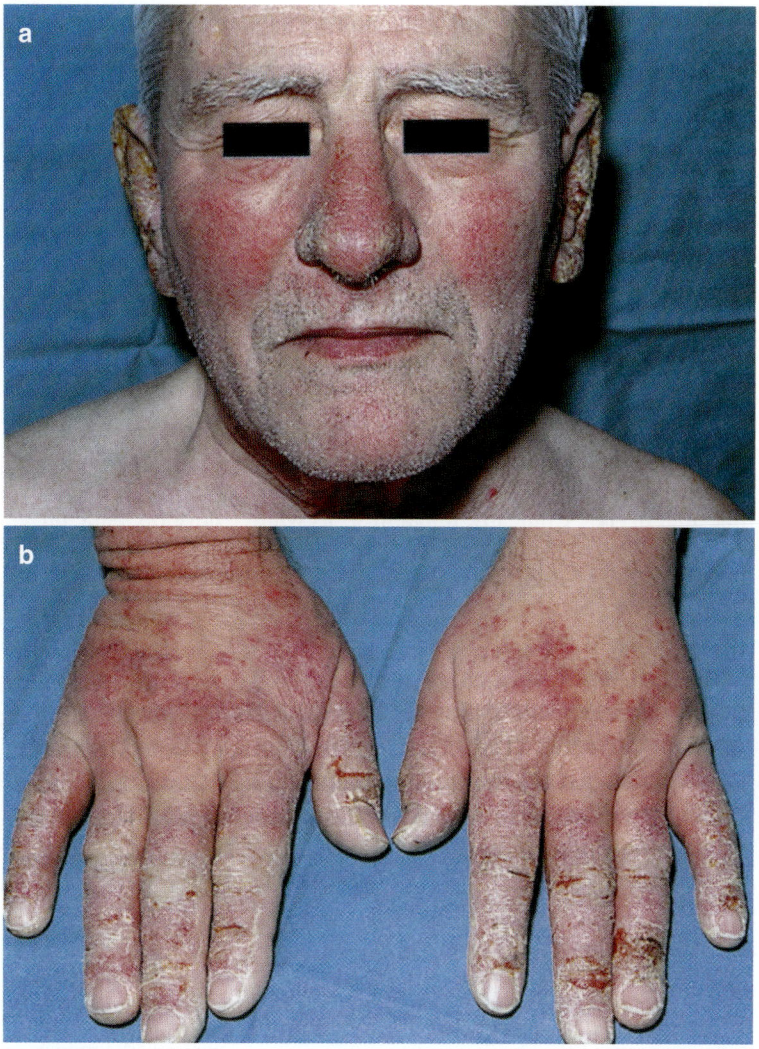

Fig. 5.1 Acrokeratosis paraneoplastica (Bazex syndrome). Skin lesions are characterized by violaceous plaques and scaling. They are mainly acral. (**a**) Lesions of the face. (**b**) Lesions of the hands

It can be concluded that the most difficult differential diagnosis is related to psoriasis [3], particularly when the underlying carcinoma has not yet been suspected. However, chronic hyperkeratotic eczema must also be taken into consideration.

5.3 Antisynthetase Antibodies Syndrome ("Mechanic's Hands")

In the antisynthetase antibodies syndrome, finger lesions mimic irritative and/or "wear and tear" dermatitis. The lesions, which are painful and keratotic with fissures, are present on the fingertips. The periungual and lateral aspects of the fingers are mainly involved, with a predominance on those that are submitted to hard, manual work. Therefore, the lesions have been described as "mechanic's hands" or "machinist's hands." The patients are frequently suffering from polymyositis, fibrosing interstitial pneumopathy, polyarthritis, and Raynaud's syndrome. In exceptional cases, the lesions can become necrotic (see Chap. 10, Fig. 10.1) [4].

Histology shows hyperkeratosis, acanthosis, a mononuclear dermal infiltrate, and liquefaction necrosis of the basal layer. The antibody anti-Jo-1 is the most characteristic among the anti-aminoacryl-ARNE synthetases in those patients.

Differential diagnosis is primordial with chronic irritant dermatitis, "wear and tear" dermatitis, and palmar hyperkeratotic dermatitis.

5.4 Aquagenic Syringeal Acrokeratoderma

This is a rare condition that has only been described in the last 10 years. Basically, it is an acquired disorder that predominantly develops in young women. It is clinically characterized by a burning sensation and whitish discoloration on the hands, and rarely on the soles, after brief immersion in water that resolves within a short time after drying. Clinically, it manifests as whitish or yellowish flattened, translucent papules and whitish microvesicles, located in areas of pressure or trauma on the palms and/or soles (Fig. 5.2). Involvement is usually bilateral [5].

Histopathological examination suggests that an aberration in the sweat gland apparatus may be the underlying cause of the condition [6]. Some patients arrive in their physician's office with their hand in a bucket of water to more readily demonstrate their lesion; this is known as the "hand-in-the-bucket sign." This cooperation with the patient is of great help to the clinician. It has also been described recently as "idiopathic aquagenic wrinkling of the palms," in such a common presentation that it almost can be regarded as pathognomonic [7].

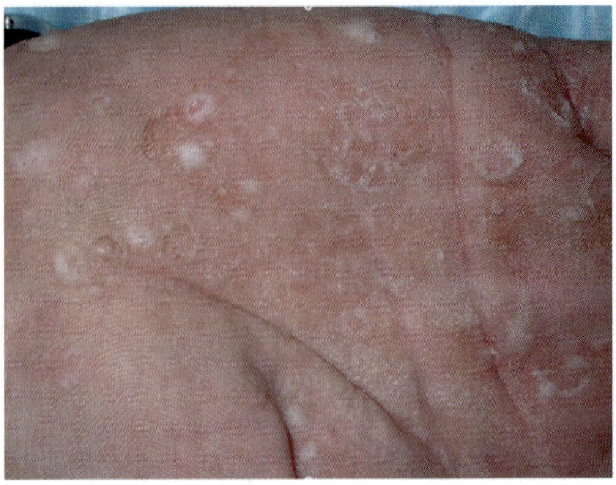

Fig. 5.2 Aquagenic syringeal acrokeratoderma

5.5 Bullous Dermatoses

Some bullous dermatoses may be a challenge for dermatologists, particularly when the early stage of the disease is limited to the hands. The differential diagnosis of vesiculobullous hand dermatitis can pose a conundrum.

5.5.1 Bullous Pemphigoid

Bullous pemphigoid (BP) is defined as a blistering disease that occurs mainly in elderly people. It often starts with pruritus and urticated and erythematous lesions. Later, large, tense blisters develop both on erythematous and on normal skin, and there may be mucosal involvement with blisters and erosions. In some cases, some selective drugs can boost the onset of the disease. Characteristics of BP from pathogenesis to treatment are fully explained in textbooks of dermatology [8].

On the backs of the hands, clinical diagnosis is clear-cut: tense, hemorrhagic bullae and erosions surrounded by a slightly erythematous and pruritic skin are the hallmark of BP, usually associated with lesions on other parts of the body.

Special attention has to be paid to palmar BP. When widespread BP is undiagnosed and nevertheless treated symptomatically by systemic corticosteroids, it is commonly observed that the lesions disappear on most body areas, except, for some obscure reasons, on the palms of the hands [9–11].

Palmar BP is characterized by tense vesicles and bullae of different sizes. They are almost always whitish, opalescent (Fig. 5.3) as compared to pompholyx, exceptionally hemorrhagic, and usually very pruritic and/or painful. In these circumstances, differential diagnosis with vesicular bullous pompholyx or dyshidrotic eczema is of concern. We have coined the terms "pseudo-pompholyx" or "pseudo-dyshidrosis" to emphasize the existence of this particular situation. Skin biopsy is diagnostic, based on histopathological and immunohistopathological criteria.

When the corticosteroids are tapered, BP lesions reappear on different sites (face, trunk, back, inferior limbs, etc.).

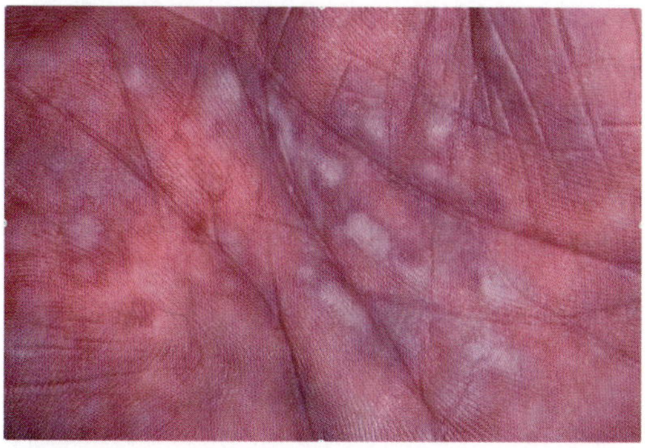

Fig. 5.3 Palmar bullous pemphigoid is characterized by tense vesicles and bullae of different size, almost always whitish and opalescent ("pseudo-dyshidrosis" or "pseudo-pompholyx")

5.5.2 Linear IgA Bullous Dermatosis (Linear IgA Disease)

Linear IgA bullous dermatosis is a chronic, acquired, subepidermal disease of children and adults, with cutaneous and mucosal involvement, characterized by IgA basement membrane antibodies. In children and in adults (two distinct varieties), the onset may be insidious. Symptoms vary from mild pruritus to severe pruritus and burning. The trunk is involved most of the time, and the limbs, face and scalp, and hands and feet are commonly affected. The lesions comprise urticarial plaques, papules, vesicles, and bullae.

In practice, due to the widespread localization of lesions on various sites of the skin, it cannot be confused with vesiculobullous hand eczema. Nevertheless, in some cases, lesions can be limited to palms (particularly when corticosteroids have been prescribed systemically). The vesicles and/or bullae are whitish and opalescent. The only potential differential diagnoses of concern are pemphigoid and pompholyx [12].

5.5.3 Dermatitis Herpetiformis

Dermatitis herpetiformis is not a matter of differential diagnosis with hand dermatitis. Indeed, lesions very rarely involve hands. The sites of predilection of vesicles and/or bullae, often excoriated, are the extensor aspects of the limbs, buttocks, axillary folds, shoulders, face, and scalp [13].

5.5.4 Epidermolysis Bullosa Acquisita (Acquired Epidermolysis Bullosa)

This very rare condition can mimic either pemphigoid or linear IgA bullous dermatosis. Comments relative to the disease are therefore similar to those presented in the preceding paragraphs. A striking clinical feature is the presence of milia (similar to those observed in porphyria cutanea tarda).

5.6 Candidiasis

5.6.1 *Candida* Intertrigo of the Interdigital Folds

An erythematous, glazed, "velvety" macerated area of one or more folds is the usual clinical picture. There is often a collarette of desquamation at the periphery (Fig. 5.4). Similar lesions can also develop under rings. It is worthwhile to mention erosio interdigitalis blastomycetica, which is caused by *Candida* and most often occurs in the third interdigital web space. In those cases, it is often considered that candidiasis is triggered by a previous skin irritation, mainly linked with detergents and/or with sugar; this could explain the occurrence of the disease in bakeries, confectioner's shops, chocolate factories, fruit-packing trade, and so forth. Minor trauma (such as superficial abrasions) could initiate the infection. A steady decline in this condition recently is likely due, in part, to the introduction of automation in most factories.

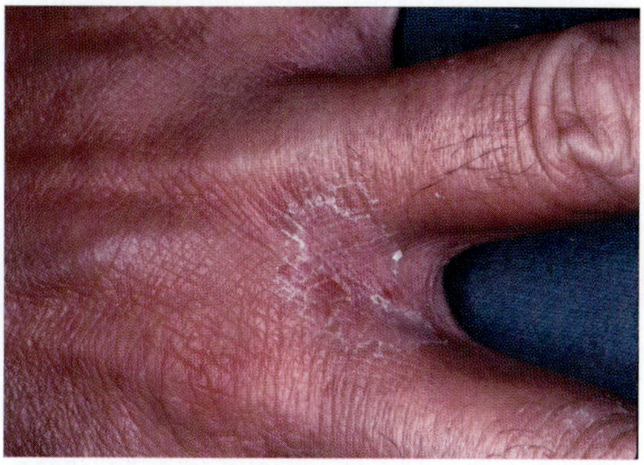

Fig. 5.4 *Candida* intertrigo

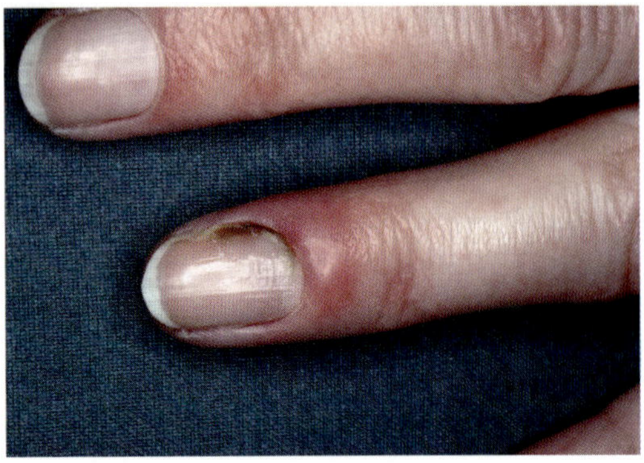

Fig. 5.5 *Candida* paronychia

5.6.2 *Candida* Paronychia

Candida albicans can be isolated in some cases of chronic paronychia (Fig. 5.5). The yeast has traditionally been considered to play an etiological role in the condition, but bacteria and irritant or allergic contact dermatitis also play a role, although the contribution of each varies from patient to patient. A more recent approach is to envisage the primary role of a repeated contact with various kinds of foods. Proteins of foods could induce a protein contact dermatitis [14, 15] and eventually, later on, an infection by *Candida albicans*. When considering this new concept, the primary role of the yeast is therefore minimized. Professions at risk apart from those already quoted as prone to develop *Candida intertrigo* of the interdigital folds include all categories of workers handling food, including cooks and housewives. Clinical symptoms are obvious. Several fingers are usually infected, but one or all may be involved, and lesions are painful. The nail fold is red and swollen; there is loss of the cuticle and detachment of the nail fold from the dorsal surface of the nail plate, leading to pocketing. Occasionally, thick, white pus may discharge – often force is needed to express it. In more advanced cases, nail dystrophy and onycholysis do occur.

5.7 Circumscribed Palmar Hypokeratosis

This very rare condition, recently described, has to be quoted but does not interfere with hand eczema. It is characterized by a well-circumscribed area of erythematous skin and slightly depressed area of erythema. Any history of trauma or contributory incident has been identified.

Histologically, lesions show a well demarcated, abrupt decrease in the thickness of the stratum corneum with a central area of thinning and hypogranulosis. The borderline of the lesion between the areas of the thick and thin layers is somewhat shaggy but relatively well demarcated [16, 17].

5.8 Contact Urticaria

The contact urticaria syndrome (CUS) is a well-known entity, first described by Maibach and Johnson [18], and updated in a recent review [19]. CUS is classified in four stages, according to morphology and severity. Contact urticaria (CU) can be immunological or non-immunological.

We are focusing on CU limited to the hands (stage 1). The signs and symptoms can be described as follows [15]:

- In mildest cases, there are only subjective symptoms (invisible contact urticaria). These are reported as itching, tingling, or burning sensations, without any objective change, or just a discrete erythema occurs.
- Urticarial lesions of CU do not differ clinically from those observed in common urticaria. Itchy, erythematous macules develop (at the site of contact) into wheals consisting of pale-pink, edematous, raised skin, often with a surrounding flare. They appear in various numbers and sizes, ranging from a few millimeters to lesions that cover a large area, corresponding to the site of contact.
- When contact has ceased, excoriations may be the only clinical symptom.
- These clinical variants are well illustrated in CU to rubber latex (Fig. 5.6), a clinical entity that has exploded (in terms of numbers of cases) during the two last decades [15]; mainly the backs and, more rarely, the palms of the hands may be involved.

In the vast majority of cases, diagnosis of CU is clear-cut, but in some there may be an overlap between CU and protein contact dermatitis, and symptoms of both conditions are superimposed

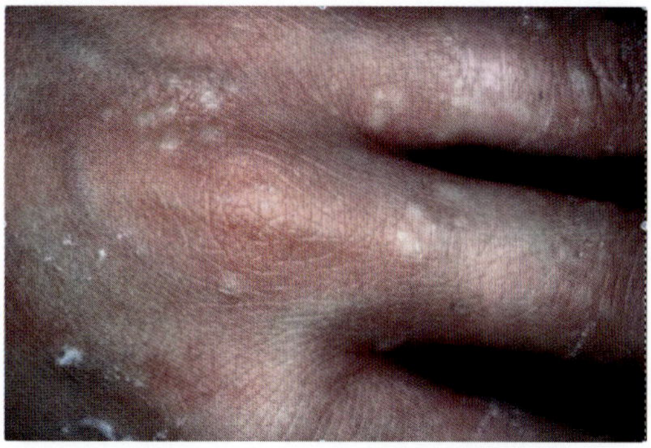

Fig. 5.6 Immunological contact urticaria of the dorsum of the hand from internally powdered latex gloves

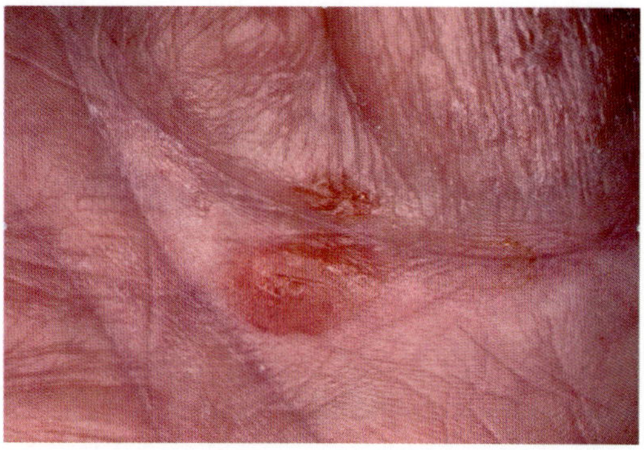

Fig. 5.7 Cutaneous T-cell lymphoma of the palm of the hand

(see Chap. 3). Differential diagnosis with acute hand eczema (mainly on the backs of the hands) has to be considered.

Open (non-prick) testing and prick testing are of great help for an accurate diagnosis [15].

5.9 Cutaneous T-Cell Lymphoma (Mycosis Fungoides)

Mycosis fungoides (MF) is the most common primary cutaneous T-cell lymphoma (CTCL), but other subsets with clearly identifiable clinicopathological features and varying prognoses have also been described [20]. Lesions of MF appear on different parts of the body, consisting of patches or plaques. Most often, subtle, fine, scaly, and often slightly atrophic erythematous plaques are observed on the trunk and may also involve the limb girdle areas, breast, and particularly the buttocks. The differential diagnosis includes pityriasis rosea, dermatophytosis, mild eczematous dermatitis, or even a rather atypical form of psoriasis. Later on, tumoral lesions do occur, but these may appear at an early stage of the disease ("tumeur d'emblée"). Erythroderma is also reported [21].

Our interest is focused on a particular variety of MF – one that is localized exclusively on the palms of the hands, in a very early stage. The lesions appear as erythematous, scaly, sometimes slightly hyperkeratotic plaques (Fig. 5.7). They are sharply demarcated and may be pruritic or not. Among the differential diagnoses, the following have to be considered:

- Allergic contact dermatitis
- Atopic dermatitis
- Psoriasis
- Palmar *tinea manuum*

Skin biopsy is helpful but may not be conclusive. Multiple biopsies are sometimes needed to confirm a clinical suspicion of MF, including a very complete immunopathological investigation [22].

5.10 Darier's Disease

Darier's disease (keratosis follicularis) is an autosomal dominant condition, characterized by a persistent eruption of hyperkeratotic papules.

The distinctive lesion is a firm, red papule that is skin-colored, yellow brown, or brown. Seborrheic areas of the trunk and face, particularly the scalp margins, temples, ears, and scalp, are most often involved. The hands are also a site of predilection [23].

The lesions can be described as follows:

- On the backs of the hands (and feet), discrete papules are clinically indistinguishable from acrokeratosis verruciformis of Hopf. These may be the earliest manifestations of the disease. Nail changes are very characteristic (Fig. 5.8). They include red or white longitudinal bands of various width and also "coin-shaped" alterations, linked with terminal notching of the nail (nail dystrophy).
- Palmar lesions may be very varied. They show minute pits or punctate and filiform keratoses in severe cases; palmoplantar hyperkeratosis may occur; palm prints show focal interruption

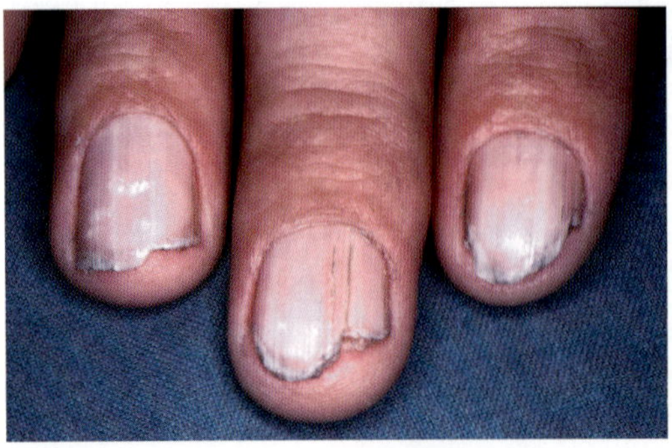

Fig. 5.8 Darier's disease. Typical lesions of the nails

of dermatoglyphics, best visualized by dermoscopy [24].

- Hemorrhage into palmoplantar lesions is found with specific *ATP2 A2* mutations [25].

Since many areas of the body are usually involved, there is (in most cases) no problem of differentiating between Darier's disease and other dermatoses of the hand, including hand eczema, except potentially palmar hyperkeratotic eczema.

5.11 Dermatitis Artefacta (Dermatitis Factitia) and Dermatitis Simulata

Dermatitis artefacta is a well-known skin disease caused entirely by the actions of the fully aware (i.e., consciously or not consciously) impaired patient on the skin.

The backs of the hands are a quite common site of involvement, and our comments are limited to this specific location.

Some lesions are characterized by erosions and/or ulcerations, symmetrical or asymmetrical, mainly located on the nondominant hand, and predominantly monomorphic. The margins of the lesions may be angular and may or may not be surrounded by an erythematous area. They are claimed by the patient to occur very rapidly at night or on the way from work to home. A biopsy is often diagnostic [26]. In some other cases, patients voluntarily reproduce previous lesions (Figs. 5.9 and 5.10), particularly in occupational medicine, to obtain, perpetuate, or increase compensation linked with their work [26]. It may be difficult to reach a correct diagnosis.

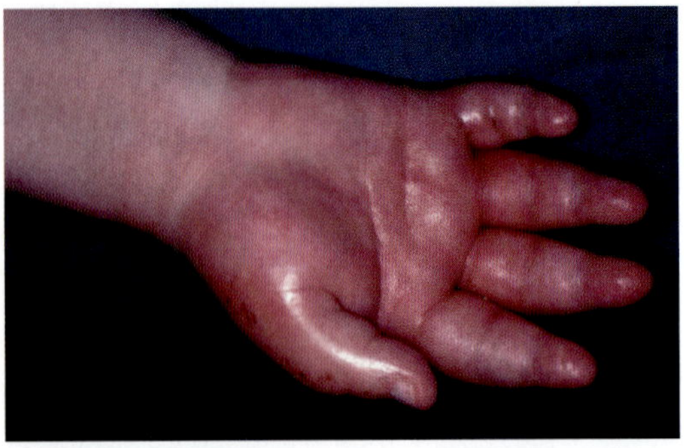

Fig. 5.9 A variant of dermatitis artefacta (Secrétan syndrome), characterized by lymphedema of one hand, caused by wearing a constricting band around the arm

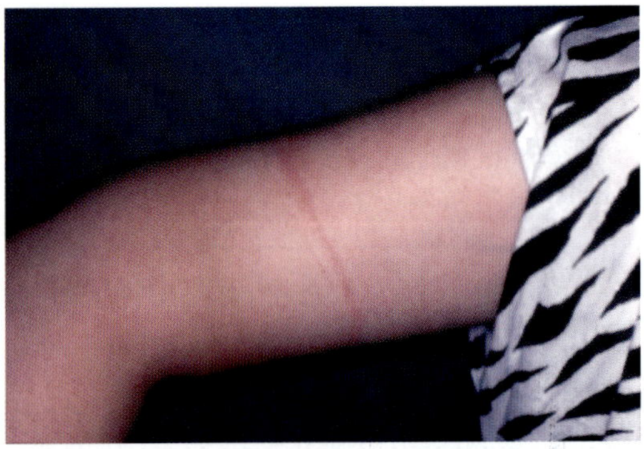

Fig. 5.10 The clue to diagnosis of dermatitis artefacta is an erythematous and perfectly horizontal ring around the limb proximal to the edema

The following example is very illustrative in this respect. A worker developed allergic contact dermatitis after repeated contact with humid cement. The diagnosis was confirmed by a positive patch test to chromates. He obtained compensation rights, and later on, when he visited the occupational physician, he worked with cement, privately, in order to maintain his status [26].

Differential diagnosis includes irritant contact dermatitis, allergic contact dermatitis, and protein contact dermatitis.

It should be noted that palms of the hands are not usually concerned, because they are rarely involved.

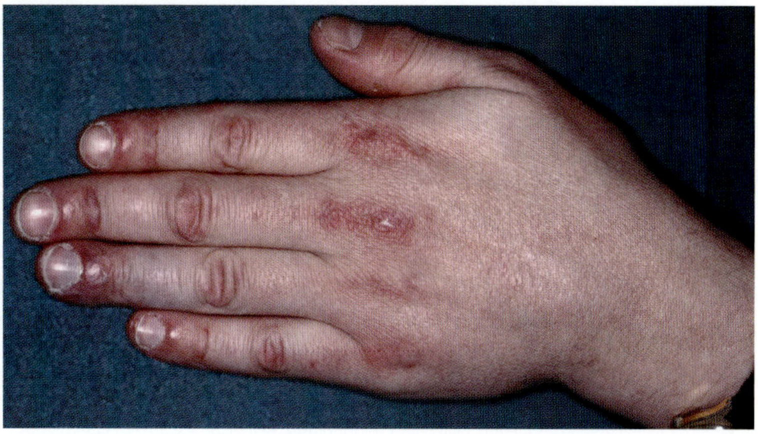

Fig. 5.11 Dermatomyositis of the dorsum of the hand

5.12 Dermatomyositis

Dermatomyositis is a multisystemic disorder mainly affecting skin, muscle, and blood vessels. We refer the reader to textbooks of dermatology for a full description of the disease. Characteristic erythematous and edematous skin lesions are predominant on the face. There is purplish-red or heliotrope erythema, especially involving the eyelids, the upper cheeks, forehead, and temples. Edema of the eyelids and periorbital tissues is not uncommon. Edema of the hands and arms, and sometimes of much of the body, may also occur, and this is usually associated with erythema of the backs of the forearms, the upper back, and, sometimes, elsewhere. The dorsal aspects of the hands are a site of predilection (Fig. 5.11).

The lesions can be described as follows:

- Linear erythematous streaking over the extensor tendon sheaths.
- Diffuse redness and shininess of the nail folds.
- The capillary loops of the nail folds may be dilated, irregular, and tortuous, easily visible with or without a lens or by dermoscopy and/or capillaroscopy.
- A quite specific sign is the presence of erythematous or violaceous flat papules (Gottron's papules) and small plaques on the dorsa of the finger joints and around the nail folds (Fig. 5.12).

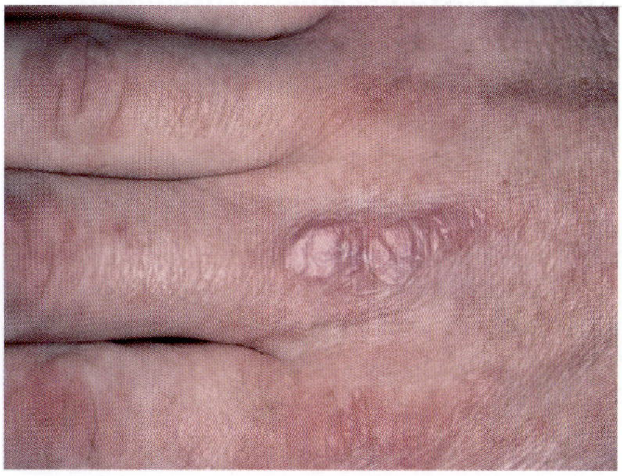

Fig. 5.12 Dermatomyositis: Gottron's papules

- Thickening, roughness, hyperkeratosis, and irregularity of the cuticles, with minimal or no redness.

All these symptoms can also be observed in other types of connective tissue disorders.

5.13 Human Scabies

5.13.1 Common Human Scabies

Human scabies is a parasitic disease caused by *Sarcoptes scabiei*. Blackish burrows, from 5 to 15 mm in length, end in a vesicle at one end ("mite hill"). The fingers (particularly web spaces) and the volar surface of the wrist are sites of predilection. Numerous marks of excoriation, sometimes accompanied by fine, more or less translucent vesicles spread all over the skin. These excoriations are mainly the sign of severe itching in the evening and at night.

Dermoscopy is a very useful tool to detect burrows on the lateral aspects of the fingers, in most cases (i.e., when these are not easily visualized at clinical examination).

Surprisingly, scabies is often misdiagnosed, even by skilled practitioners. The occurrence of confluent excoriations is too often interpreted as chronic hand eczema.

5.13.2 Crusted Scabies (Norwegian Scabies)

Crusted scabies is an infection with *Sarcoptes scabiei* var. *hominis* in which the mite population is enormous and may number millions. The grossly thickened, horny layer is honeycombed with cavities that contain large numbers of mites, and these are shed into the environment of the patient. An undiagnosed case of crusted scabies may be the source of an outbreak (mainly institutional) of common scabies. Immunosuppressed and elderly patients are particularly at risk.

Large, warty crusts form on the backs of the hands and feet. In the meantime, the palms and soles may be irregularly thickened and fissured. Flexures of the palms are characteristically white and hyperkeratotic (Fig. 5.13). Erythema and scaling occur on the face, scalp, neck, trunk, and genitals. Pruritus is mild to severe. Diagnosis is

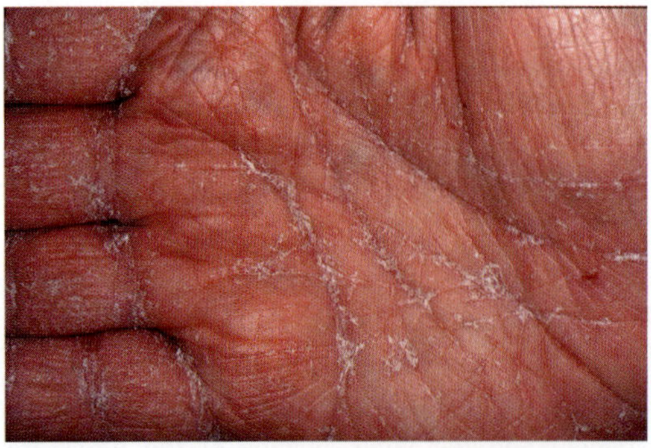

Fig. 5.13 Crusted scabies of the palm of the hand

crucial, to avoid epidemics of common human scabies in the neighborhood. Dermoscopy is illustrative: a typical “triangular” shape of the lesions is seen. Scraping or curettage is diagnostic; microscopic examination with mineral oil reveals large numbers of mites.

Differential diagnosis is of prime importance; it refers to several diseases:

- Palmar hyperkeratotic eczema
- Hyperkeratotic irritant and/or allergic contact dermatitis (chronic stage [27])
- Atopic dermatitis
- Psoriasis
- Darier’s disease

It is the authors clinical experience that many cases are misdiagnosed, sometimes over several visits, despite the fact that there are self-evident clues to reach a correct diagnosis.

5.14 Lichen Planus

The basic lesion of this immune disease is a firm, reddish-violet polygon that shines in oblique light and shows whitish or grayish striae caused by keratotic thickening (termed Wickham’s striae). One of the preferred sites is the flexor aspect of the forearm. The lesions are highly pruriginous, and papules may appear along the excoriations caused by scratching (Koebner’s phenomenon).

Lesions of the backs of the hands are quite similar to those observed on other sites of the body.

On the contrary, lesions of the palms and soles are quite different (Fig. 5.14). This is a remarkable illustration related to the interaction between the different anatomoclinical structures and the pathological (immunological) process inducing lichen planus. There are usually no papules, but erythematosquamous plaques, either circumscribed or widespread, are present. They tend to be firm and rough, with a yellowish hue. Pruritus is usually absent [28, 29]. The concomitant presence of typical papules on the flexural aspect of the forearms is diagnostic. Biopsy is confirmatory. The involvement of nails is also a very important clue to the diagnosis.

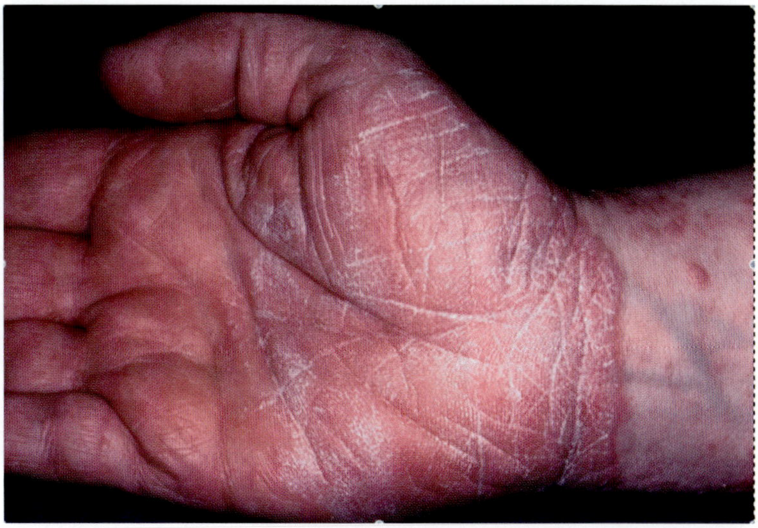

Fig. 5.14 Lichen planus: typical papules are present on the volar aspect of the forearm. On the contrary, lesions of the palms are erythematosquamous plaques that are often misdiagnosed and confused with hyperkeratotic hand eczema

The main nail findings are as follows:

- There is exaggeration of the longitudinal lines and linear depressions, due to slight thinning of the nail plate.
- Adhesion between the epidermis of the dorsal nail fold and the nail bed may cause partial destruction of the nail (*pterygium unguis*).
- Rarely, the nail is completely shed [30].

Lichen planus of the backs of the hands has to be differentiated from lichenoid allergic contact dermatitis (see Chap. 3) and lichenoid drug eruption, but, in the latter, lesions are not limited to the hands. Lichenification (lichen simplex) and/or lichenified hand eczema must also be considered.

Lichen planus of the palms, due to its particular manifestations, has to be differentiated from psoriasis, keratoderma, syphilis, and even callosities and warts, when such changes occur in isolation [31].

5.15 Lupus Erythematosus

Lupus erythematosus (LE) is an autoimmune disease of unknown origin, implicating genetic, immunological, and environmental factors. It is characterized by a kaleidoscope of systemic and skin symptoms, which are very important to recognize, as early diagnosis is important. We refer the reader to textbooks of dermatology for a complete overview of the disease [32].

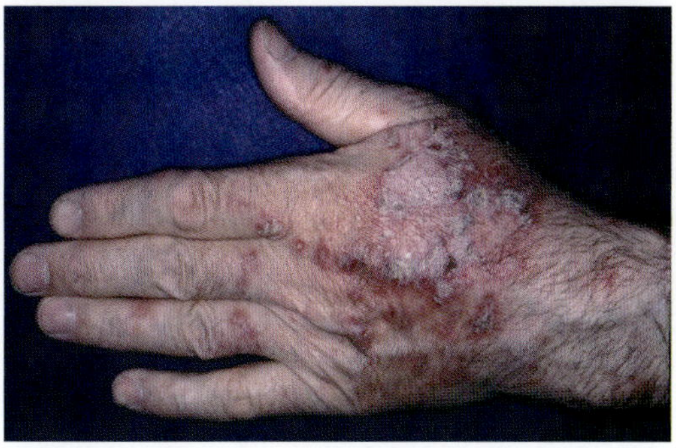

Fig. 5.15 Lupus erythematosus of the dorsum of the hand

Lesions of the hands are multifaceted [32]:

- Typical erythematosquamous, adherent, sharply demarcated plaques, sometimes surrounded by an erythematous, slightly raised edge. In some cases, the plaques may show prominent flattening in the center, giving rise to annular lesions (Fig. 5.15).
- On the palms, hyperkeratotic lesions may become papulonodular, mimicking hypertrophic lichen planus or even nodular prurigo (Fig. 5.16).
- Unusual spindling of the fingers and hyperextension of the distal phalanges.
- Raynaud's phenomenon.

Practically, differential diagnosis of LE is not a problem. Typical lesions are present on other skin sites, such as the face, neck, ears, and trunk,

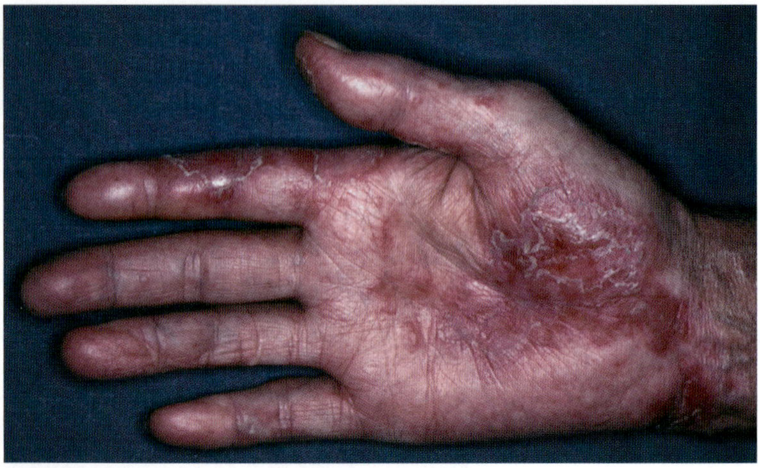

Fig. 5.16 Lupus erythematosus of the palm of the hand

and are diagnostic. LE and psoriasis of the hands share similar clinical features, but LE is not typically confused with hand eczema.

5.16 Palmoplantar Keratodermas

Palmoplantar keratodermas are a diverse group of hereditary and acquired disorders defined by epidermal thickening of palms and soles.

Most keratoderma syndromes are restricted to palms and soles (mainly the variety Thost-Unna), but marked palmoplantar hyperkeratosis may also be seen in generalized disorders of keratinization, such as ichthyosis vulgaris or epidermolysis bullosa, for instance. As so many types of keratodermas are described in textbooks, the role of the clinician is to precisely identify the type in each individual patient. In principle, there is no problem of diagnosis, when using the various tools of investigation now available.

The only differential diagnosis that can be evoked is palmar hyperkeratotic eczema (see Chap. 14) and/or palmoplantar psoriasis, but the onset of keratoderma is, nevertheless, quite different.

5.17 Palmoplantar Pustulosis

Palmoplantar pustulosis is a common condition in which erythematous and scaly plaques are studded with sterile pustules persisting on the palms or soles. The disease is chronic and very resistant to treatment. At the present time, there is still some controversy about the relationship with psoriasis [33].

The current classification of the various types of palmoplantar pustuloses is described in the following sections.

5.17.1 Palmoplantar Pustular Psoriasis and Palmoplantar Pustulosis

There is a debate about this entity. Is it one or two diseases? There is no real answer so far. The clinical features are very similar; hence, they are described together. The disease presents with one or more well-defined plaques. Pustules are either yellow or greenish (Fig. 5.17). On the hands, the thenar eminence is the most common site. Less commonly, the hypothenar eminence, the central palm, or the distal palm are involved. On the feet, the instep, the medial or lateral border of the foot (at the level of the instep), or the back of the heels are involved. The lesions are usually chronic. The classical histopathological distinction between unilocular or multilocular pustules is now outdated. Differential diagnosis is of prime importance. Tinea and/or eczema are the most common alternatives. Acute vesiculopustular *tinea manuum* or *pedis* is more common in hot weather. Chronic allergic contact dermatitis also has to be taken into consideration.

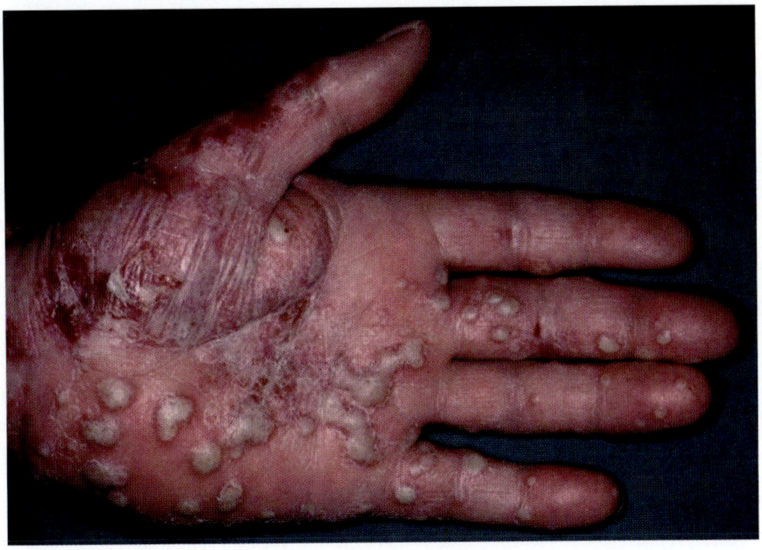

Fig. 5.17 Palmoplantar pustulosis

The term "bacterid of Andrews" to define palmoplantar pustulosis is now outdated.

Some systemic symptoms can be associated with palmoplantar pustulosis. The most common are synovitis, acne, hyperostosis, and osteitis. The occurrence of such associations has been described under the name "SAPHO syndrome" [34, 35].

5.17.2 Acrodermatitis Perstans (Hallopeau)

This is a very particular disease, characterized by a chronic, sterile, pustular eruption affecting initially the tips of the fingers or (rarely or exceptionally) toes, that slowly tends to extend locally. The first lesion starts on a finger. Onset is often related by the patient to minor trauma or infection at the tip of the digit. The skin over the distal phalanx becomes red and scaly, and pustules develop. The nail folds and nail bed may be involved, leading to nail dystrophy. Eventually, other digits may be involved. Acrodermatitis perstans may evolve into generalized pustular psoriasis. In terms of differential diagnosis, the following diseases are considered: *tinea manuum*, irritant and/or allergic contact dermatitis, and candidiasis [36].

5.18 Pityriasis Rubra Pilaris

Pityriasis rubra pilaris is a skin disease of unknown origin, described extensively in all textbooks of dermatology. It is most often widespread all over the body. It appears either in children or in adults and is, therefore, classified in different subtypes. The eruption usually starts as an erythematous, slightly scaly macula. Further macules appear within a few weeks. Then a profusion of perifollicular papules, with central keratotic acuminate plugs, is classic. Follicular lesions appear singly at first and then coalesce to form groups of two, three, or more. Interfollicular erythema appears, and the follicular lesions are gradually submerged in sheets of erythema, with a slight orange color, which typically spread from head to feet.

As far as hands are concerned, a few remarks are needed:

- The palms and soles become hyperkeratotic and orange and are described as "PRP sandal" (Fig. 5.18).
- The nails are thickened and discolored distally, showing splinter hemorrhages, but unlike psoriasis, there is no dystrophy of the nail plate and pitting is minimal.

Practically, it would be difficult to confuse PRP with chronic hand eczema, but the condition deserves mention as it can be quite severe.

5.19 Porphyria Cutanea Tarda

Porphyria cutanea tarda (PCT) is the commonest of all the porphyrias. Almost all patients notice increased fragility on light-exposed skin, particularly the backs of the hands and forearms. Minor trauma can shear the skin away to leave sharply marginated erosions (Fig. 5.19). Most patients suffer from bullae, which can be over 1 cm in diameter and may be painful. They are worsened by sun exposure. They crust and resolve over a few weeks, leaving atrophic scars, milia (Fig. 5.20), and mottled hyper – or hypopigmentation [37]. Other major symptoms include scarring alopecia of the scalp and hypertrichosis of the face, particularly of the temples and ears. Palms of the hands are consistently spared. The clinical symptoms are so obvious that the disease cannot be confused with others. Nevertheless, the condition can be missed by inexperienced practitioners. Two differential diagnoses we can mention are phototoxic or photoallergic contact dermatitis on the backs of the hands and forearms, although these share quite different symptoms, and linear IgA bullous dermatosis, which is also characterized by milia. Another consideration is pseudoporphyria, though it requires negative porphyria laboratory tests and an appropriate clinical scenario [38].

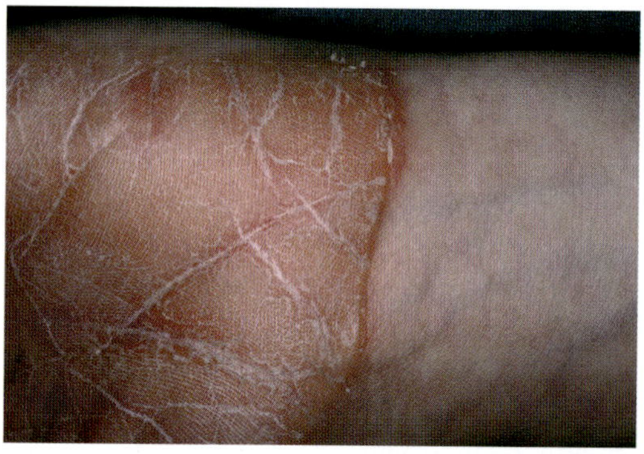

Fig. 5.18 Pityriasis rubra pilaris

5.20 Psoriasis

Our knowledge of psoriasis has exploded in recent years. Our new perspective of the disease as an inflammatory disorder with several genetic and environmental risk factors is revealing the multifaceted nature of psoriasis and its associated diseases. The perception of disease pathophysiology from a hyperkeratotic disorder of keratinocytes to a deregulation of the immune system (a "T-cell mediated disease") is now unanimously recognized. T-helper (Th-1, Th-17, and Th-22)

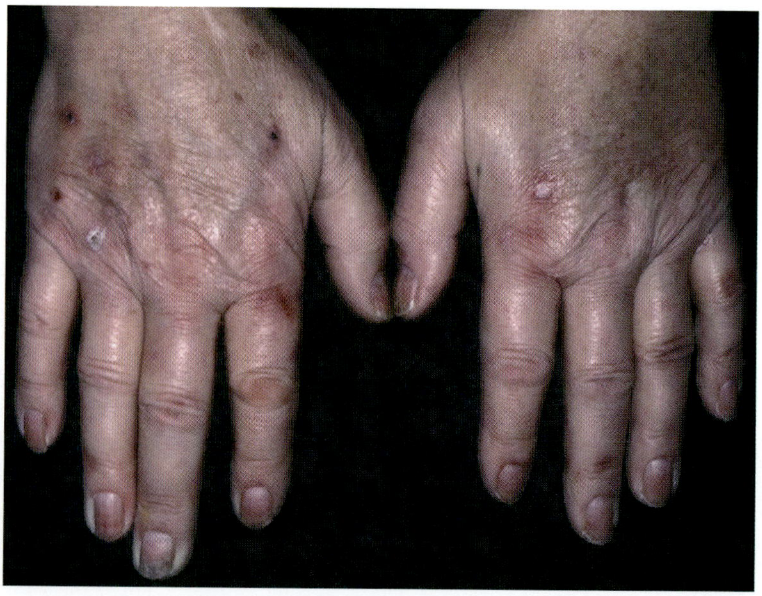

Fig. 5.19 Porphyria cutanea tarda of the dorsum of the hands. Skin fragility, skin erosions, and scars

cell populations are expanded and stimulated to release inflammatory cytokines [39–41]. Innate and adaptive immunity are most likely implicated. Histopathological characteristics are not always diagnostic. Nevertheless, there is no clue to a specific immunological marker, so far. On the backs of the hands, the psoriatic lesions are similar to those observed on other parts of the body – either erythematous, sharply demarcated plaques, covered by fine scales, or more keratotic, presenting as thick, adherent, micaceous plaques with a thin border of erythema at the edge of the lesion.

There may be relationship to trauma or occupational irritants (Koebner's sign). When present, nail alterations are characteristic and therefore of great help for the clinician.

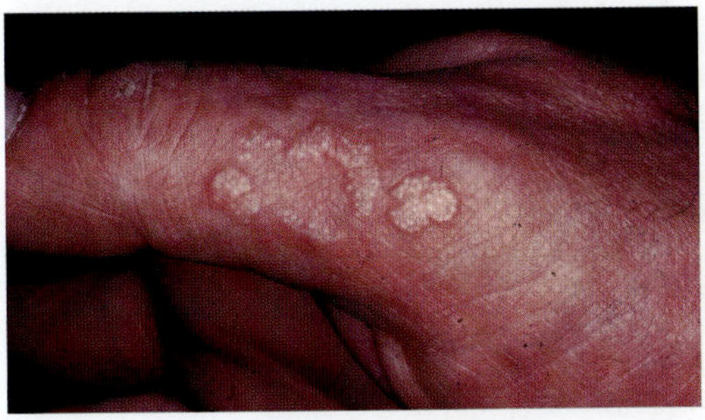

Fig. 5.20 Milia of the lateral aspects of the fingers. Very characteristic but also encountered in some varieties of epidermolysis bullosa, but never in hand eczema

They can be described as follows [42]:

- Pits
- Discoloration of the nail
- Onycholysis ("oil drop sign")
- Subungual hyperkeratosis
- Nail plate abnormalities
- Splinter hemorrhages
- Proximal destruction of the nail

When located exclusively on the palms (or soles), psoriasis may be difficult to diagnose [43]. Erythematous and scaly plaques are present, usually with well-defined margins (Fig. 5.21). It may sometimes be extremely difficult to distinguish psoriasis from palmar hyperkeratotic hand eczema (dermatitis) (Fig. 5.22). There is still some controversy about whether they represent one or two distinct entities, as explained in Chap. 14. It is claimed that a sharply defined edge at the wrist or forearm and absence of vesiculation are helpful signs in diagnosing palmar psoriasis.

5.21 Puffy Hand Syndrome

The puffy hand syndrome is observed in drug addicts who inject themselves with various drugs in the dorsal veins of the hands. Edema of the backs of both hands (mainly the "nondominant" hand) is typically the presenting sign. The lesions

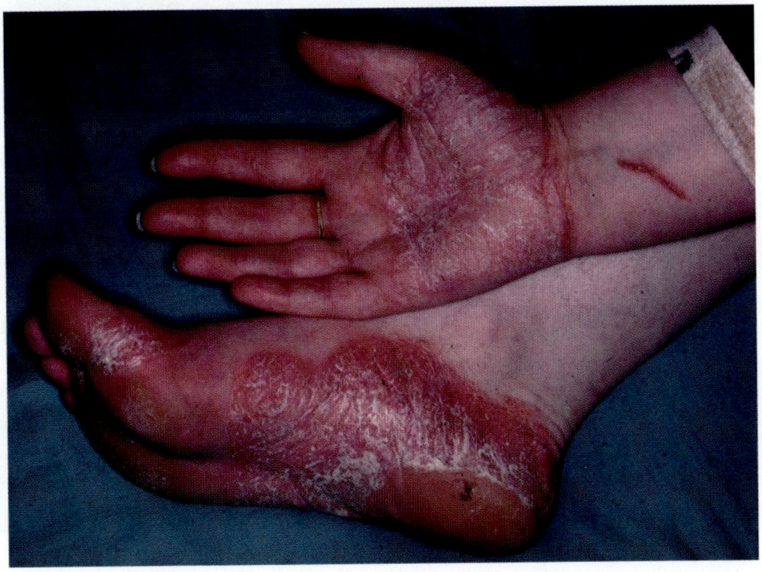

Fig. 5.21 Palmoplantar psoriasis

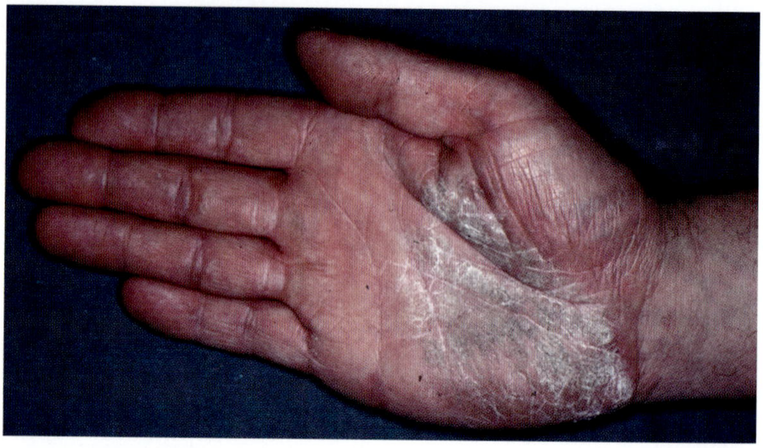

Fig. 5.22 Isolated palmar psoriasis

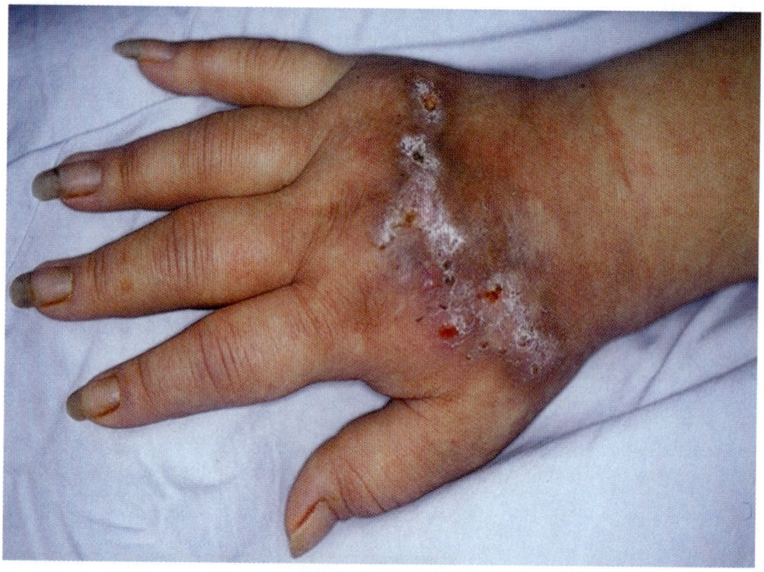

Fig. 5.23 Puffy hand syndrome

are impressive, painful or not. It is a well-defined entity [44–46], and sometimes patients are referred to the patch test clinic (Fig. 5.23).

5.22 Recurrent Palmar Peeling ("Desquamation Estivale en Aires des Mains")

This highly distinctive condition occurs mainly in summertime, disappearing (sometimes incompletely) in winter. It is unrelated to external irritation. It affects the palmar aspect of the hands and fingers and simply consists of dry and extremely superficial detachment of the epidermis. Initially, and in mild cases, the lesion is the size of a small pinhead. It then broadens slightly with a small, circular but soon incomplete border. Peeling often spreads centrifugally, and the various circles may converge in wavy lines (Fig. 5.24).

The etiology of the disease is unknown. It has been proposed that it could be related to the desquamation stage of pompholyx but without any real proof. In very rare cases, it could represent a part of the generalized peeling skin syndromes. It must also be differentiated from aquagenic syringeal acrokeratoderma.

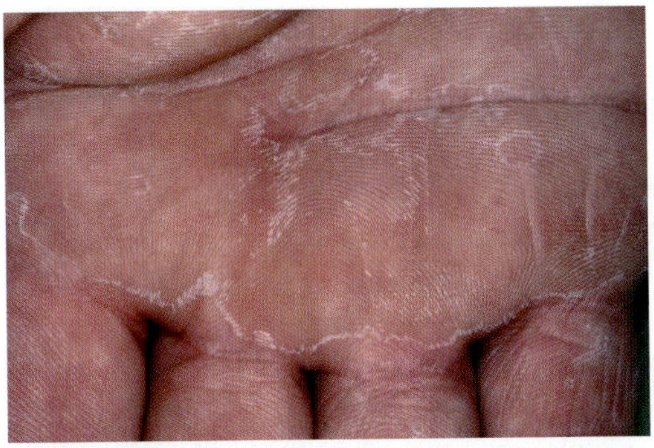

Fig. 5.24 Recurrent palmar peeling of the hands ("Desquamation estivale en aires des mains")

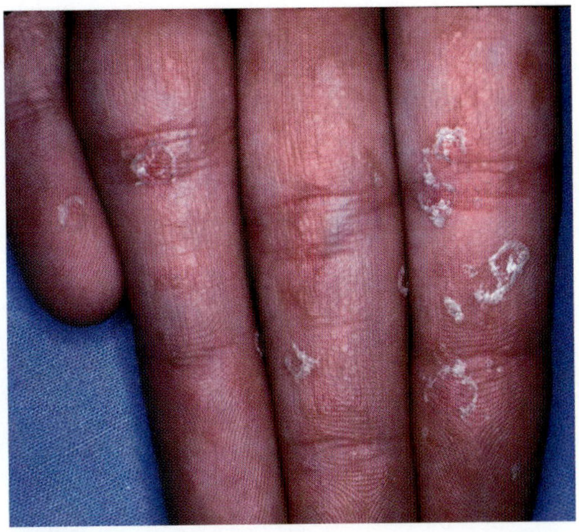

Fig. 5.25 Secondary stage of syphilis. Palmar syphilides

5.23 Syphilis

During the secondary stage of syphilis, palmar and plantar skin lesions are quite common ("papulosquamous syphilides"). At first, they consist of typical firm papules, round to oval in shape. Early papules tend to be shiny, but gradually a thin layer of scale forms and is quickly shed. In the late stages of papular syphilis, nummular lesions, less than 1 cm in diameter, are covered by massive layer of scales which are easily removed by curettage. They are psoriasiform and are more commonly, but not exclusively, formed in black populations. These hyperkeratotic lesions of the palms and soles may flake, peel, and fissure (Fig. 5.25).

Differential diagnosis is practically limited to palmar psoriasis (mainly when atypical), pompholyx, and *tinea manuum*, i.e., three conditions characterized by peeling of abundant scales, when lesions are scraped.

On the other hand, syphilis may not be confused with palmar hyperkeratotic eczema, which is clinically different.

5.24 *Tinea Manuum*

Tinea manuum is synonymous with fungal infection of the hands by dermatophytes. It may or may not be associated with other dermatophyte infections: *tinea pedis* (very commonly) and/or *tinea cruris*. It can be isolated and may be precipitated by gardening or other activities involving contact with contaminated soil (geophilic dermatophytes, such as *M. gypseum*; zoophilic dermatophytes, such as *M. canis*, *M. mentagrophytes*; but also anthropophilic dermatophytes such as *T. rubrum*).

The clinical picture on the backs of the hands is similar to that observed on other parts of the body (i.e., round or annular erythematosquamous lesions, with an elevated margin, either scaly or vesicular). The condition is often misdiagnosed by general practitioners and even well-trained dermatologists. The use of topical corticosteroids (sometimes for months or years) modifies the clinical characteristic of the lesions (Fig. 5.26); there is a reduction of the inflammatory component, and the appearance of small pustules along the lesion edges [47].

The clinical picture on the palms and palmar aspect of the fingers is entirely different. There is dusty desquamation on an erythematous background with pearl-white accentuation of the palmar flexor folds. A very particular feature is the fact that the disease is clinically unilateral (Fig. 5.27), and, so far, there is no explanation for this. When toe webs are also affected (both feet), a specific syndrome has been described ("one hand, two feet") [48].

Onychomycosis may or may not be present. *Tinea manuum* is a diagnostic trap with regard to chronic hand eczema, in particular when palms or interdigital webs are concerned, because it can be easily confused with hyperkeratotic palmar dermatitis (or eczema) and chronic pompholyx.

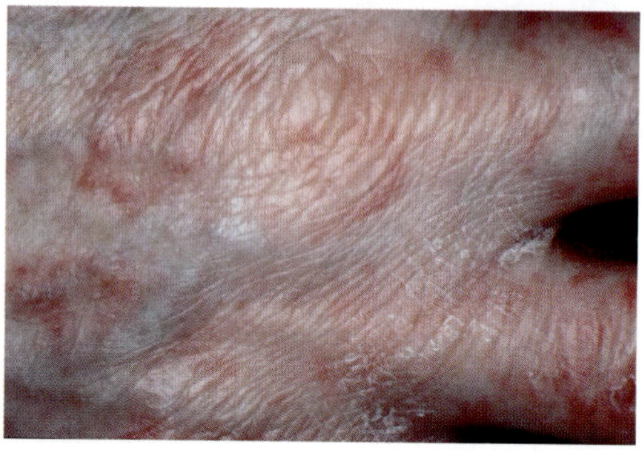

Fig. 5.26 *Tinea manuum* of the dorsum of the hand. Small, round, well-delineated erythematosquamous lesions, modified by applications of corticosteroid creams

Nevertheless, several clues are available to differentiate both conditions:

- Unilateral localization of lesions (Fig. 5.27), particularly in the case of palmar *tinea manuum*.
- The frequent association with other dermatophyte lesions, such as *tinea pedis* or *tinea cruris*.
- Floury desquamation on an erythematous background. Scraping (curettage) yields a flurry of disintegrated scales (Fig. 5.28). In contrast, in hyperkeratotic palmar dermatitis, scales are most often quite adherent and are not easily peeled off by curettage.
- Microscopic examination, after clearing with potassium hydroxide (with or without Parker blue ink), is diagnostic and usually reveals a network of concentrated dermatophyte filaments. Culture identifies the incriminated dermatophyte.
- Skin surface biopsy (cyanoacrylate stripping) can also be used as an alternative to sampling, but only on the backs of the hands, and not on the palms, because the procedure is too painful.

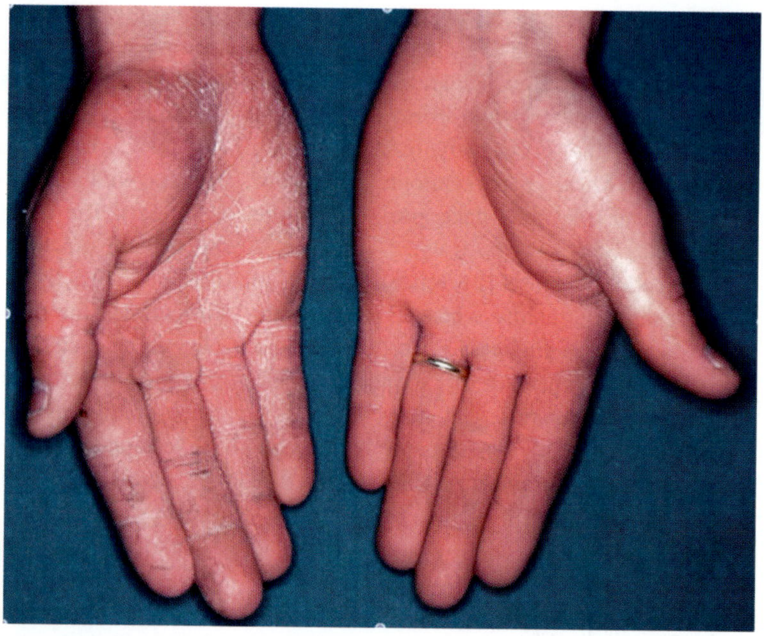

Fig. 5.27 Palmar *tinea manuum*. It can be mistaken for chronic palmar eczema. In most cases, it is strictly unilateral, which provides a first clue to the diagnosis

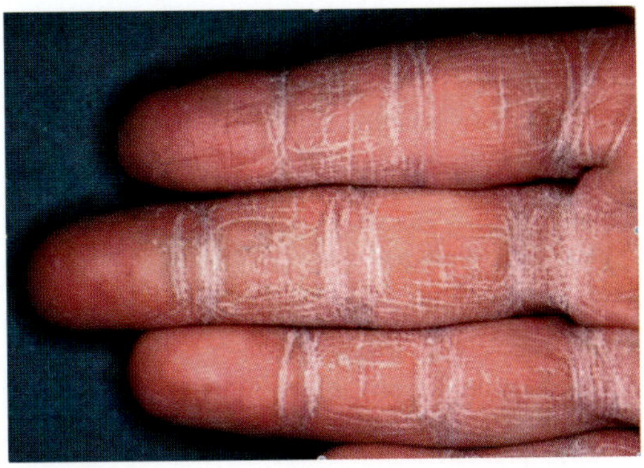

Fig. 5.28 *Tinea manuum* of the palmar aspect of the fingers

When scraping is negative (not a rare event) but clinical symptoms seem obvious, a trial treatment with an antimycotic systemic drug is advised.

Conclusion

When chronic hand eczema is suspected, the alert dermatologist must always keep in mind the potential differential diagnosis with *tinea manuum*. A mycologic investigation is strongly advised when there is any suspicion.

References

1. Ramos-E-Silva M, Carvalho JC, Carneiro SC. Cutaneous paraneoplasia. Clin Dermatol. 2011;29:541–7.
2. Zarzour JG, Singh S, Ander A, Cafardi JA. Acrokeratosis paraneoplastica (Bazex syndrome): report of a case associated with small cell lung carcinoma and review of the literature. J Radiol Case Rep. 2011;5:1–6.
3. Koh WL, Ang CC, Lim SP. Psoriasiform dermatitis in a case of newly diagnosed locally advanced pyriform sinus tumour: Bazex syndrome revisited. Singapore Med J. 2012;53:12–4.
4. Disdier P, Bolla G, Harle JR, Pache X, Weiller-Merli C, San Marco M, et al. Nécroses digitales révélatrices d'un syndrome des antisynthétases. Ann Dermatol Venereol. 1994;121:493–5.
5. Luo DQ, Li Y, Huang YB, Wu LC, He DY. Aquagenic syringeal acrokeratoderma in an adult man: case report and review of the literature. Clin Exp Dermatol. 2009;34:907–9.
6. Baldwin BT, Prakash A, Fenske NA, Messina JL. Aquagenic syringeal acrokeratoderma; report of a case with histological findings. J Am Acad Dermatol. 2006;54:899–902.
7. Vale R, Adam DN. Idiopathic aquagenic wrinkling of the palms in sisters. J Dermatol. 2011;38:472–3.
8. Wojnarowska F, Venning VA. Bullous pemphigoid. In: Burns T et al., editors. Rook's textbook of dermatology. 8th ed. Oxford: Wiley-Blackwell; 2010. p. 40.26–35.
9. Veien NK. Bullous pemphigoid masquerading as recurrent vesicular hand eczema. Acta Derm Venereol. 2010;90:4–5.
10. Lupi F, Masini C, Ruffelli M, Puddu P, Cianchini G. Dysidrosiform palmoplantar pemphigoid in a young man: response to dapsone. Acta Derm Venereol. 2010;90:80–1.
11. Yamada Y, Sugita K, Izu K, Nakamura M, Hashimoto T, Tokura Y. A case of dyshidrosiform pemphigoid. J UOEH. 2011;33:183–7.
12. Wojnarowska F, Venning VA. Linear IgA disease. In: Burns T et al., editors. Rook's textbook of dermatology. 8th ed. Oxford: Wiley-Blackwell; 2010. p. 40.45–51.
13. Wojnarowska F, Venning VA. Dermatitis herpetiformis. In: Burns T et al., editors. Rook's textbook of dermatology. 8th ed. Oxford: Wiley-Blackwell; 2010. p. 40.58–62.
14. Tosti A, Buerra L, Mozelli R. Role of food in the pathogenesis of chronic paronychia. J Am Acad Dermatol. 1992;27:706–10.
15. Lachapelle J-M, Maibach HI. Spectrum of diseases for which prick testing and open (non-prick) testing are recommended: patients who should be investigated. In: Lachapelle J-M, Maibach HI, editors. Patch testing and prick testing. A practical guide. 3rd ed. Berlin: Springer; 2012. p. 147–57.
16. Tanioka M, Miyagawa-Hayashino A, Manabe T. Circumscribed palmo-plantar hypokeratosis: a disease with two subtypes. J Invest Dermatol. 2009;129:1045–7.
17. Akasaka K, Maesawa C, Takahashi K, Masuda T, Akasaka T. Circumscribed palmar or plantar hyperkeratosis: two cases and a review of published work. J Dermatol. 2011;38:314–6.
18. Maibach HI, Johnson HL. Contact urticaria syndrome. Contact urticaria to diethyltoluamide (immediate type hypersensitivity). Arch Dermatol. 1975;111:726–30.

19. Basketter D, Lahti A. Immediate contact reactions. In: Johansen JD, Frosch PJ, Lepoittevin J-P, editors. Contact dermatitis. 5th ed. Berlin: Springer; 2011. p. 137–53.
20. Whittaker S. Biological insights into the pathogenesis of cutaneous T-cell lymphomas (CTCL). Semin Oncol. 2006;33:S3–6.
21. Kashani-Sabet M, Mc Millan A, Zackheim H. A modified staging classification for cutaneous T-cell lymphoma. J Am Acad Dermatol. 2001;45:700–6.
22. Grubb B, Henderson DB, Pandya AG. Adult T-cell lymphoma/leukemia presenting as pagetoid reticulosis of the palms and soles. J Am Acad Dermatol. 2011;65:1063–4.
23. Judge MR, Mc Lean WHI, Munro CS. Dariers' disease. In: Burns T et al., editors. Rook's textbook of dermatology. 8th ed. Oxford: Wiley-Blackwell; 2010. p. 19.81–6.
24. Grim KD, Maroon ML, Metry DW. Congenital wart-like papules on hands and feet. Pediatr Dermatol. 2010;27:93–4.
25. Ruiz-Perez VL, Carter SA, Healey E. ATP2 A2 mutations in Darier's disease: variant cutaneous phenotypes are associated with missense mutations, but neuropsychiatric features are independent of mutation class. Hum Mol Genet. 1999;8:1621–30.
26. Lachapelle J-M. Dermatoses simulées en médecine du travail. In: Lachapelle JM, Frimat P, Tennstedt D, Ducombs G, editors. Dermatologie Professionnelle et de l'Environnement. Paris: Masson; 1992. p. 263–6.
27. Wolf R, Wolf D, Viskoper RJ. Norwegian-type scabies mimicking contact dermatitis. Postgrad Med. 1985;78:228–30.
28. Mugoni MG, Monteso MA, Cottoni F. Lichen planus on the palms and soles. J Eur Acad Dermatol Venereol. 1994;3:535–40.
29. Sanchez-Pérez J, Rios-Buceta L, Fraga J, Garcia-Diez A. Lichen planus with lesions on the palms and/or soles. Prevalence and clinicopathological study of 36 patients. Br J Dermatol. 2000;142:310–4.
30. Nishizawa A, Satoh T, Yokozeki H. Close association between metal allergy and nail lichen planus: detection of causative metals in nail lesions. J Eur Acad Dermatol Venereol. 2012. doi:10.1111/j.1468-3083.2012.04561.
31. Zeng YP, Sun QN, Liu YH, Fang K. Lichen planus with palmoplantar involvement: rapid therapeutic response to acitretin. Eur J Dermatol. 2011;21:632–3.
32. Goodfield MJD, Jones SK, Veale DJ. Lupus erythematosus. In: Burns T et al., editors. Rook's textbook of dermatology. 8th ed. Oxford: Wiley-Blackwell; 2010. 51.2-51.1-51.62.
33. Reitamo S, Erkko P, Remitz A. Palmoplantar pustulosis. Eur J Dermatol. 1992;2:311–4.
34. Benhamou CL, Bardet M, Luthier F, Caplan F, Brigant S. Chronic arthritis in palmo-plantar pustulosis. Bacterid of Andrews. Rev Rhum Mal Osteoartic. 1985;52:487–90.
35. Zhao Z, Li Y, Zhao H, Li H. Synovitis, acne, pustulosis, hyperostosis and osteitis (SAPHO) syndrome with review of the relevant published work. J Dermatol. 2011;38:155–9.
36. Griffiths CEM, Barker JNWN. Localized pustular psoriasis. In: Burns T et al., editors. Rook's textbook of dermatology. 8th ed. Oxford: Wiley-Blackwell; 2010. p. 20.44–8.
37. Sarkany RPE, Breathnach SM, Morris AAM, Weismann K, Flynn PD. Porphyria cutanea tarda. In: Burns T et al., editors. Rook's textbook of dermatology. 8th ed. Oxford: Wiley-Blackwell; 2010. p. 59.12–6.
38. Green JJ, Manders SM. Pseudoporphyria. J Am Acad Dermatol. 2001;44(1):100–8.
39. Griffiths CEM, Barker INWN. Pathogenesis and clinical features of psoriasis. Lancet. 2007;370:263–71.
40. Torti DC, Feldman SR. Interleukin-12, interleukin-23 and psoriasis: current prospects. J Am Acad Dermatol. 2007;57:1059–68.
41. Reich K. The concept of psoriasis as a systemic inflammation: implications for disease management. J Eur Acad Dermatol Venereol. 2012;26(Suppl2):3–11.
42. Baran R, Dawber RPK, editors. Diseases of the nails and their management. 2nd ed. London: Blackwell Scientific Publications; 1994. p. 135–47.
43. Samitz MH, Albom JJ. Palmar psoriasis. Arch Dermatol Syphilol. 1951;64:199–204.
44. Neviaser RJ, Butterfield WC, Wieche DR. The puffy hand of drug addiction: study of the pathogenesis. J Bone Joint Surg Am. 1972;54:629–33.
45. Del Giudice P, Durant J, Dellamonica P. Hand edema and acrocyanosis: "puffy hand syndrome". Arch Dermatol. 2006;142:1084–5.
46. Tennstedt D, Bulinckx A, Del Giudice P. Drogues "dures" et peau. In: Raison-Peyron N, editor. Progrès en Dermato-Allergologie. Montpellier 2011. Montrouge: John Libbey Eurotext; 2011. p. 1–28.
47. Kiraz N, Metintas S, Oz Y, Koc F, Koku Aksu EA, Kalyoncu C, et al. The prevalence of tinea pedis and tinea manuum in adults in rural areas of Turkey. Int J Environ Health Res. 2010;20:379–86.
48. Zhan P, Ge YP, Lu XL, She XD, Li ZH, Liu WD. A case-control analysis and laboratory study of the two feet-one hand syndrome in two dermatology hospitals in China. Clin Exp Dermatol. 2010;35:468–72.

Irritant Versus Allergic Contact Dermatitis: An Etiopathological Approach

6

Audrey Nosbaum and Jean-François Nicolas

Contents

A. Nosbaum, M.D. (✉) • J.-F. Nicolas, M.D., Ph.D.
Department of Allergology and Immunology, Centre Hospitalier Lyon-Sud, Hospices Civils de Lyon, 395 Chemin du Grand Revoyet, Pierre-Bénite 69495, France
e-mail: nosbaumaudrey@yahoo.fr; jean-francois.nicolas@chu-lyon.fr

6.1 Introduction

Contact dermatitis comprises two main groups, irritant (ICD) and allergic (ACD) contact dermatitis. It presents as acute, subacute, or chronic eczema. Although it is possible to differentiate ICD from ACD on clinical grounds, both diseases can have very similar clinical, histological, and molecular presentations. They can be considered as a xenoinflammation, induced by the skin penetration of low-molecular-weight xenobiotic chemicals [1].

The mechanisms at the origin of the eczema are different in the two types of dermatitis, at least as far as the initiation stages of the skin inflammation are concerned (Fig. 6.1). ICD is a nonspecific inflammatory dermatosis, mainly due to the toxicity of chemicals on the skin cells, which triggers inflammation by activation of the skin innate immune system. ACD, on the other hand, corresponds to a delayed-type hypersensitivity response, and the skin inflammation is mediated by antigen-specific T cells. Thus, ICD and ACD can be differentiated on the basis of the presence (ACD) or absence (ICD) of antigen-specific effector T cells in the eczema lesions [2]. The new classification of allergic diseases proposes that dermatitis should be classed as a delayed hypersensitivity reaction (DHS) (as it develops several hours after contact with the hapten) and further as allergic (mediated by antigen-specific T cells, ACD) or nonallergic (mediated by the intrinsic proinflammatory properties of chemicals, ICD) [3].

A. Alikhan et al. (eds.), *Textbook of Hand Eczema*,
DOI 10.1007/978-3-642-39546-8_6, © Springer-Verlag Berlin Heidelberg 2014

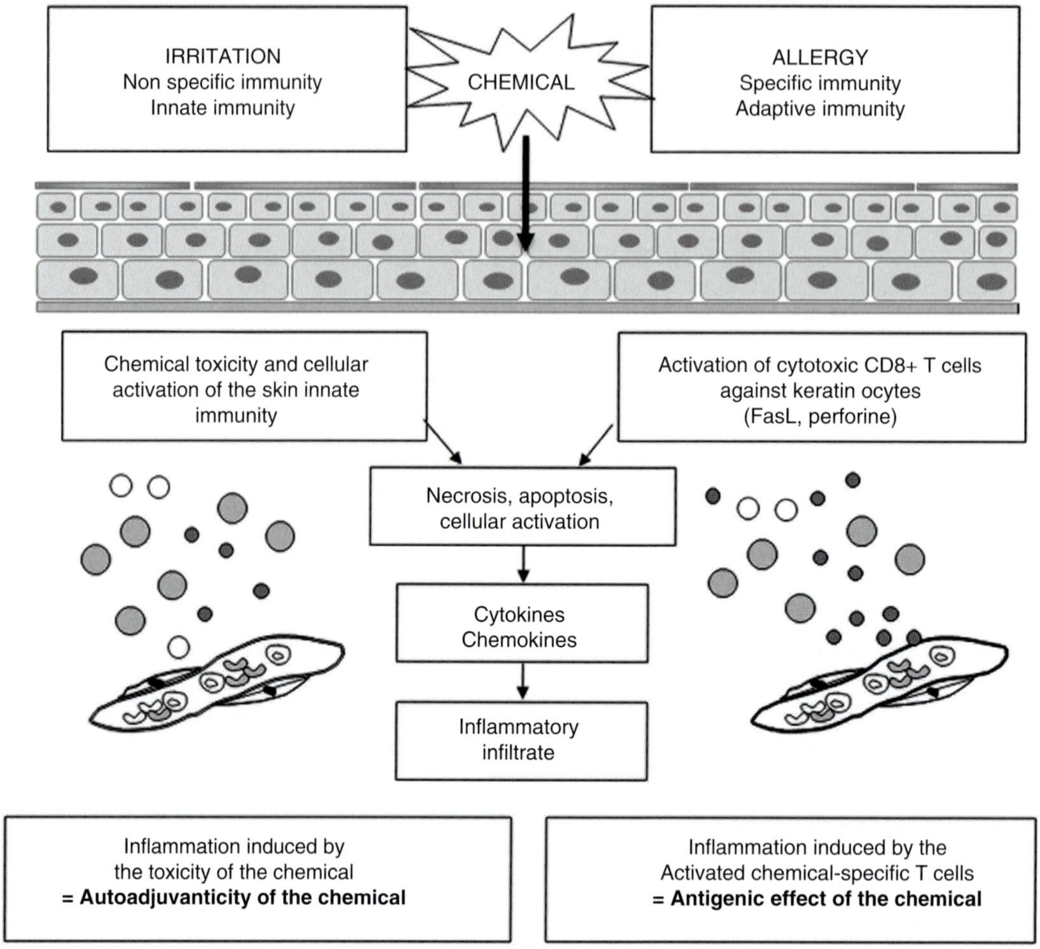

Fig. 6.1 Mechanisms of irritant and allergic contact dermatitis. ICD and ACD are induced by skin contact with chemicals. The early stages are different, as the chemical is proinflammatory by its direct "toxicity" on the skin cells in ICD, while the active chemical triggers an inflammatory reaction mediated by specific T cells in ACD. The later stages giving rise to an eczema lesion are, on the other hand, very similar and involve cytokines, chemokines, phenomena of apoptosis and cellular necrosis, and the recruitment of a polymorphic inflammatory infiltrate. This explains why ACD and ICD lesions can be confused clinically and histologically

6.2 Pathophysiology of Irritant and Allergic Skin Inflammation

ICD has long been considered a non-immunological inflammation, and ACD, an immunological inflammation. In fact, both types of eczema implicate the immune cells, but ICD follows the activation of innate immunity, while ACD is the result of acquired immunity and the induction of specific proinflammatory T-cell effectors [4, 5]. It should be noted that the development of ACD initially requires the activation of innate immune cells, which permit maturation of the cutaneous dendritic cells. The dendritic cells are then required for the presentation of allergens to T cells in the lymph nodes, and thus to the induction of an acquired immune response.

6.2.1 Dual Effects of Chemicals

All chemicals, whether they are responsible for ICD or ACD, can be considered as irritants with very important differences in the concentrations necessary to induce irritation [6, 7]. For example,

DNFB is an irritant at 0.05 %, while geraniol is an irritant at 50 %. On the other hand, only those chemicals that behave as haptens are allergens. Indeed, they interact in a covalent manner or not, with amino acids, and thus are able to modify the proteins giving rise to neoantigens. Contact allergens are, thus, only a minority of chemicals.

Skin contact with an irritant may only induce an ICD. However, contact with a hapten can induce ICD or ACD, the latter occurring only if the individual has been immunized during the previous skin exposures to the same chemical. Thus, contact allergens exhibit dual effects. They can simultaneously activate the innate and adaptive immune system. Both their built-in adjuvant effect (also known as autoadjuvanticity), which induces nonspecific inflammation, and their antigenic effect (formation of T-cell epitopes), which leads to a contact allergen-specific inflammation, depend on their chemical reactivity [8].

6.2.2 Skin Irritation: Activation of Innate Immunity

6.2.2.1 Innate Immunity

Innate immunity refers to all the cells and molecules capable of distinguishing "danger signals" of an infectious, physical, or chemical nature and of inducing an inflammatory reaction. The inflammation enables the individual to eliminate the infection and repair the damage caused by the physical and/or chemical agents (wound healing). Innate immunity is, therefore, synonymous with inflammation. In the blood, the innate immune cells are the hematopoietic cells, with the exception of T and B lymphocytes, which form the acquired arm of the immune response. In the skin, the totality of the epidermal and dermal cells participates in the skin's innate immunity. The recognition of chemicals as sterile, dangerous molecules for the body (i.e., xenobiotics) is very similar to that of microorganisms that deliver danger signals [9]. Through a poorly described process, chemicals induce the production of reactive oxygen species (ROS), which lead to the release of ATP and possibly other damage-associated molecular patterns (DAMPs), as well as to the generation of low-molecular-weight hyaluronic acid. Low-molecular-weight hyaluronic acid is sensed by neighboring cells via toll-like receptor 2 (TLR2) and TLR4, resulting in increased expression of inactive pro-IL-1β (beta) and pro-IL-18, through the NF-κ(kappa)B pathway [10]. ATP is sensed through the purinergic receptor P2X7 and activates the inflammasome, resulting in caspase 1 activity and the generation of active IL-1β and IL-18 [11]. Nickel has a unique adjuvant property and can directly bind histidine residues in the extracellular domain of TLR4, triggering the activation of this receptor [12]. This leads to the production of inflammatory cytokines and chemokines, especially IL-1β, IL-6, IL-8, IL-18, and TNF-α (alpha). Molecules of innate immunity also include complements, the plasmatic enzyme systems of coagulation and fibrinolysis, and interferons.

6.2.2.2 Skin Irritation: Mechanisms of Action

The penetration of a chemical through the different layers of the skin, notably the epidermis and the dermis, is responsible for the release of a large number of cytokines and chemokines by different cell types whose respective roles in the induction of inflammation are not yet well understood [11]. Keratinocytes represent 95 % of epidermal cells and are the principal and first cells to secrete cytokines after an epicutaneous stimulus, thus giving them an essential role in the initiation and development of ICD [13]. Other cell types are activated by the chemicals and contribute to the induction of inflammation. Current studies with transgenic mice, deficient in certain types of cells, should bring a better understanding of the respective contributions of mast cells, macrophages/dendritic cells (DC), endothelial cells, γ(gamma)δ(delta) T cells, and NK cells in the development of ICD lesions [14–16].

The profile of cytokine expression during ICD varies over time and also depends on the nature, environment, and dose of the chemical. The most frequently found mediators of ICD are IL-1α(alpha), IL-1β(beta), IL-6, IL-8, TNF-α(alpha), GM-CSF (granulocyte/macrophage-colony stimulating factor), and IL-10, which is an anti-inflammatory cytokine [11]. However, initiation of the inflammation seems to be mainly linked to IL-1α, TNF-α, and derivatives of arachidonic acid. Indeed, IL-1α and TNF-α are two primary cytokines capable of inducing secondary mediators (including numerous cytokines, chemokines, adhesion molecules, growth factors) that are essential for the recruitment of leukocytes to the altered skin site. Thus, a multistep cascade in the production of inflammatory mediators takes place, finally inducing histological modifications followed by the clinical expression of eczema.

6.2.2.3 Direct Responsibility of the Chemical in ICD

In ICD, the chemical is directly responsible for the cutaneous inflammation by its autoadjuvanticity, linked to its "toxic" physicochemical properties, which are proinflammatory. The analysis of the inflammation of the ICD finds all the characteristics of a nonspecific inflammatory reaction (i.e., a hyperproduction of cytokines and chemokines, the presence of a polymorphic inflammatory infiltrate and lesions of apoptosis/necrosis of the epidermal cells with a compensatory proliferation of keratinocytes). There is no argument for an involvement of T cells.

6.2.3 Skin Allergy: The Role of Specific Immunity

6.2.3.1 Antigen-Specific Immunity

Specific immunity involves B cells (humoral immunity) and T cells (cellular immunity). Specific immunity takes care of the immune memory, which protects us from reinfection but which is also responsible for the chronicity of eczema in allergic patients.

6.2.3.2 Skin Allergy: Mechanisms of Action

ACD lesions are secondary to the activation, at the site of contact with the hapten, of specific T cells that have been induced during previous contacts [4] (see Fig. 6.1). First the chemical activates skin inflammation, which is responsible for the recruitment of blood leukocytes. The specific T cells are recruited in the skin and activated by skin cells, which present the hapten to them on MHC class I and II molecules. The activated T cells produce type 1 cytokines (IFN-γ(gamma), IL-2, IL-17) and are cytotoxic, inducing keratinocyte apoptosis. This series of events allows the recruitment of new cells in the skin, resulting in eczema lesions. Knowledge of the mechanisms of ACD comes mainly from preclinical mouse models that illustrate the cytotoxic proinflammatory effector role of CD8+ T cells, while CD4+ T cells comprise anti-inflammatory regulatory populations known as Treg cells [17, 18].

6.2.3.3 Indirect Responsibility of Chemicals in Skin Irritation

In the case of ACD, the chemical is indirectly responsible for the skin inflammation. The hapten needs to react with a protein to form epitopes which will be recognized by T cells. It is the T cells which induce specific inflammation to a skin haptenized protein. The hapten itself is not sufficiently toxic to create an inflammatory reaction, either because its concentration is not high enough or because, at the concentration used, the patient is not sensitive to the irritant potential of the chemical.

6.3 Irritant and Allergic Inflammation: The Connection Between Innate and Acquired Immunity

As previously discussed, the induction of an efficient specific immunity requires the activation of innate immunity, necessary for the maturation of immature dendritic cells into potent antigen-presenting cells.

In the case of eczema, it is known that ICD creates the conditions for the development of ACD, on the basis of observations that patients who have ICD are more easily sensitized to the products they handle than patients who do not present any cutaneous irritation [19]. This hypothesis has been recently confirmed by experimental results showing that the intensity of an ACD response to a hapten is proportional to the cutaneous irritation induced by contact with this

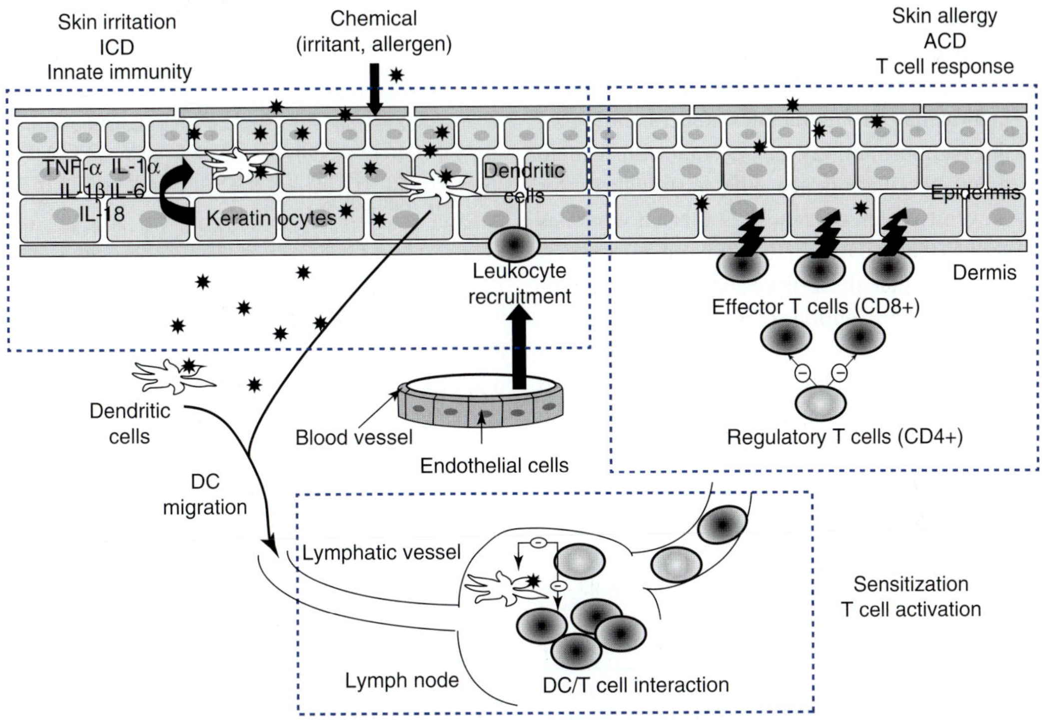

Fig. 6.2 Pathophysiology of allergic contact dermatitis. Activation of innate immunity is necessary to the development of ACD. Sensitization phase: The chemicals, in contact with the skin and capable of crossing the corneal layer, activate innate immunity and induce inflammation/irritation, which may or may not be visible but which is necessary to the recruitment of leukocytes and the activation of resident and recruited DCs. Cutaneous haptens are taken up by dendritic cells, which migrate to the draining lymph nodes, where they present the antigenic peptides to specific CD8+ and CD4+ T cells, which have, respectively, effector and regulatory functions. Activated specific T-cell clones leave the lymph nodes and circulate in the blood, tissues, and secondary lymphatic organs. Expression of eczema phase: During subsequent contact with the same hapten, its penetration induces cutaneous irritation, which permits the recruitment of effector T cells, which are activated by presentation of peptides of MHC class I and II molecules in skin cells. Experimental work has shown that effector T cells in eczema are CD8+ Tc1 cells producing IFN-γ and are responsible for apoptosis of keratinocytes though direct cytotoxicity. The CD4+ T cells control the expansion of CD8+ T cells in the lymphatic organs and their activation in the skin

hapten during sensitization [20]. In this example, the chemical tested was dinitrofluorobenzene (DNFB), which has both irritant and allergic properties. At low doses of DNFB during sensitization, there is no skin irritation on day 1 and no eczema on day 5. At higher doses, the intensity of the allergic reaction on day 5 is directly correlated to the intensity of the irritation on day 1 and is proportional to the concentration of DNFB.

Figure 6.2 summarizes the above discussion and shows the different steps of the ACD reaction. The reaction starts with inflammation, clinically visible (ICD) or totally unseen, induced by application of the chemical to the skin. This innate inflammatory reaction has several important consequences for the later development of ACD: (1) activation of skin dendritic cells (DC); (2) recruitment to the skin of DC precursors, which are blood monocytes; and (3) maturation and migration of skin DC to the lymph nodes draining the site of exposure to the chemical. In the lymph nodes, the immunogenic DCs activate specific T-cell effectors, which proliferate and migrate to the site of the contact with the chemical. In fact, in the absence of activation of innate immunity, the maturation of skin DC is incomplete, and proinflammatory T-cell effectors are not able to be activated. On the other hand, immature DCs are capable of activating anti-inflammatory regulatory T cells [21].

Conclusion

In conclusion, progress in the knowledge of the mechanisms at the origin of skin inflammation has brought better understanding of the pathophysiology of eczema with a main practical consequence: the justification for preventive measures in ACD. Recent work has shown that ICD and ACD are closely associated and that the prevention of ACD implicates the prevention of ICD. This can be achieved by protecting consumers from the most irritating chemicals, using gloves to reduce the risk of hand dermatitis or simply by using chemicals at low, nonirritating doses. The prevention of eczema also requires the maintenance of a good quality barrier function of the skin, which limits the penetration of chemicals and thus the appearance of ICD.

References

1. Martin SF. Allergic contact dermatitis: xenoinflammation of the skin. Curr Opin Immunol. 2012;24(6): 720–9.
2. Nosbaum A, Vocanson M, Rozieres A, Hennino A, Nicolas J-F. Allergic and irritant contact dermatitis. Eur J Dermatol. 2009;19(4):325–32.
3. Johansson SGO, Bieber T, Dahl R, Friedmann PS, Lanier BQ, Lockey RF, et al. Revised nomenclature for allergy for global use: report of the nomenclature review committee of the world allergy organization, October 2003. J Allergy Clin Immunol. 2004;113(5):832–6.
4. Vocanson M, Hennino A, Rozières A, Poyet G, Nicolas J-F. Effector and regulatory mechanisms in allergic contact dermatitis. Allergy. 2009;64(12): 1699–714.
5. Fyhrquist-Vanni N, Alenius H, Lauerma A. Contact dermatitis. Dermatol Clin. 2007;25(4):613–23.
6. Lepoittevin J-P, Leblond I. Hapten determinants for T cells. Eur J Dermatol. 1997;7(3):151–4.
7. Basketter DA, Kan-King-Yu D, Dierkes P, Jowsey IR. Does irritation potency contribute to the skin sensitization potency of contact allergens? Cutan Ocul Toxicol. 2007;26(4):279–86.
8. Martin SF. Contact dermatitis: from pathomechanisms to immunotoxicology. Exp Dermatol. 2012;21(5):382–9.
9. Martin SF, Esser PR, Weber FC, Jakob T, Freudenberg MA, Schmidt M, et al. Mechanisms of chemical-induced innate immunity in allergic contact dermatitis. Allergy. 2011;66(9):1152–63.
10. Martin SF, Dudda JC, Bachtanian E, Lembo A, Liller S, Dürr C, et al. Toll-like receptor and IL-12 signaling control susceptibility to contact hypersensitivity. J Exp Med. 2008;205(9):2151–62.
11. Kaplan DH, Igyártó BZ, Gaspari AA. Early immune events in the induction of allergic contact dermatitis. Nat Rev Immunol. 2012;12(2):114–24.
12. Schmidt M, Raghavan B, Müller V, Vogl T, Fejer G, Tchaptchet S, et al. Crucial role for human toll-like receptor 4 in the development of contact allergy to nickel. Nat Immunol. 2010;11(9):814–9.
13. de Jongh CM, Lutter R, Verberk MM, Kezic S. Differential cytokine expression in skin after single and repeated irritation by sodium lauryl sulphate. Exp Dermatol. 2007;16(12):1032–40.
14. Dudeck A, Dudeck J, Scholten J, Petzold A, Surianarayanan S, Köhler A, et al. Mast cells are key promoters of contact allergy that mediate the adjuvant effects of haptens. Immunity. 2011;34(6):973–84.
15. Macleod AS, Havran WL. Functions of skin-resident γδ T cells. Cell Mol Life Sci. 2011;68(14):2399–408.
16. Rouzaire P, Luci C, Blasco E, Bienvenu J, Walzer T, Nicolas J-F, et al. Natural killer cells and T cells induce different types of skin reactions during recall responses to haptens. Eur J Immunol. 2012;42(1): 80–8.
17. Vocanson M, Hennino A, Chavagnac C, Saint-Mezard P, Dubois B, Kaiserlian D, et al. Contribution of CD4(+) and CD8(+) T-cells in contact hypersensitivity and allergic contact dermatitis. Expert Rev Clin Immunol. 2005;1(1):75–86.
18. Cavani A, De Luca A. Allergic contact dermatitis: novel mechanisms and therapeutic perspectives. Curr Drug Metab. 2010;11(3):228–33.
19. Basketter D, Darlenski R, Fluhr JW. Skin irritation and sensitization: mechanisms and new approaches for risk assessment. Skin Pharmacol Physiol. 2008;21(4):191–202.
20. Bonneville M, Chavagnac C, Vocanson M, Rozieres A, Benetiere J, Pernet I, et al. Skin contact irritation conditions the development and severity of allergic contact dermatitis. J Invest Dermatol. 2007;127(6): 1430–5.
21. Vocanson M, Rozieres A, Hennino A, Poyet G, Gaillard V, Renaudineau S, et al. Inducible costimulator (ICOS) is a marker for highly suppressive antigen-specific T cells sharing features of TH17/TH1 and regulatory T cells. J Allergy Clin Immunol. 2010;126(2): 280–9.

7 Scope of the Problem: Epidemiology of Hand Eczema

Birgitta Meding and Karin Wrangsjö

Contents

B. Meding, M.D., Ph.D. (✉) • K. Wrangsjö, M.D., Ph.D.
Unit of Occupational and Environmental Dermatology, Institute of Environmental Medicine, Karolinska Institute, 210, Stockholm 17177, Sweden
e-mail: birgitta.meding@ki.se; karin.wrangsjo@ki.se

7.1 Introduction

Hand eczema is a common disease and is regarded as a public health problem. Hand eczema is also the most common occupational skin disease. The long-term prognosis is poor, with a tendency for the disease to become chronic. As with other chronic diseases, optimal treatment and preventive measures are demanded. The concept "scope of hand eczema" also includes an estimation of the economic impact of the disease, on society and on the individual. Consequences on the individual level such as sick leave, occupational changes, unemployment, and influence on the quality of life are of importance. In the last decades, the interest in these issues has grown, something that is reflected by an increasing number of publications.

7.2 Occurrence

The 1-year prevalence of self-reported hand eczema has been investigated in population-based studies. In 1983, a questionnaire was mailed to 20,000 randomly selected individuals of working age (18–65 years) in Gothenburg, Sweden, with a response rate of 83 % [1]. The individuals who reported hand eczema were later invited to a clinical examination and patch testing. The 1-year prevalence was found to be 11.8 % (females 14.5 % and males 8.9 %). In order to study the occurrence of hand eczema over time, a similar questionnaire was sent, 13 years later, to a random

A. Alikhan et al. (eds.), *Textbook of Hand Eczema*,
DOI 10.1007/978-3-642-39546-8_7, © Springer-Verlag Berlin Heidelberg 2014

sample of 3,000 individuals in the same age, in Gothenburg [2]. The response rate in the second study was 74 %, and the 1-year prevalence of hand eczema was somewhat lower, in total 9.7 % (females 12.3 % and males 7.0 %). The suggested reason for the lower prevalence was a different situation on the labor market with higher unemployment, as occupational skin exposure is considered to be an important cause of hand eczema. Other population-based studies including older people have found a 1-year prevalence of 6.5–8.0 % [3–5]. In a Danish study with limited response rate [44 %], the 1-year prevalence of hand eczema was 11.7 % [6].

In Sweden there is a long tradition of epidemiologic surveillance of the population with public health surveys being performed in different parts of the country or nationwide [7]. A validated question on 1-year prevalence of hand eczema has been included in many of these surveys [8]. Data from public health surveys are thus available regarding large numbers of individuals. The self-reported 1-year prevalence of hand eczema was found in these surveys to be in the range of 9–10 % [9–13]. For Sweden, this means that about 600,000 individuals of working age have hand eczema in a year – a number to consider when allocating resources for medical care and when assessing costs in terms of production loss due to hand eczema.

To estimate the occurrence of hand eczema in cross-sectional studies, the *1-year prevalence* is usually the preferred measure. The reason for this is that hand eczema often has a varying, relapsing course with seasonal variation. The question used in many of the Swedish hand eczema studies is "Have you had hand eczema on any occasion during the past 12 months?" This question has been validated, and the sensitivity was found to be 53–59 % and the specificity 96–99 % [8]. It was found that the question gives some underestimation of the true 1-year prevalence. The *point prevalence* gives the prevalence at a certain point in time. Considering the relapsing course of the disease, with repeated free intervals in many individuals, the point prevalence of hand eczema gives a considerable underestimation of the problem overall. In the Gothenburg hand eczema study, the point prevalence was 5.4 %, thus about half of the 1-year prevalence [1]. A point prevalence of 2–3 % was found in a population-based hand eczema study in Sweden performed by Agrup in 1964–1965 in a mainly rural population [14]. *Lifetime prevalence* (cumulative prevalence) of hand eczema is sometimes presented. This measure is, of course, dependent on the age of the responders, and recall bias may be a problem. "Ever hand eczema" has been reported by 9.2 % of Danish schoolchildren [15] and by 11.0–17.4 % of adults in Swedish population-based studies [4, 16].

One measure that gives valuable information is the *incidence rate*. This measure gives the number of new cases per person-year. In the second population-based study of hand eczema in Gothenburg, a question about the year for onset of hand eczema was included in the questionnaire [16]. That information made calculation of incidence rate possible using a retrospective design. The incidence rate was found to be in total 5.5 cases per 1,000 person-years (females 7.1 and males 4.0) among individuals of working age (18–65 years). In a Dutch study, the incidence rate of hand eczema in the general population was 7.9 cases per 1,000 person-years [17], and in a Danish twin study, the crude incidence rate was 8.8 cases per 1,000 person-years in individuals of 19–52 years of age [18]. High incidence rates are found in some occupational groups with extensive skin exposure (e.g., hairdressing apprentices, nurses' apprentices, car industry apprentices, nurses, bakers, and hairdressers) [19–24].

7.3 Age and Sex Distribution

The occurrence of hand eczema is usually found to be higher in females than in males. The female/male ratio of 1-year prevalence was in the range of 1.6–1.8 in various studies [2, 4, 5, 9]. There are also age differences, with a tendency for higher prevalence in young individuals, particularly young females. Results from the Swedish national environmental health survey in 2007 illustrate the distribution of 1-year prevalence of hand eczema in relation to sex and age (Fig. 7.1) [12, 13, 25].

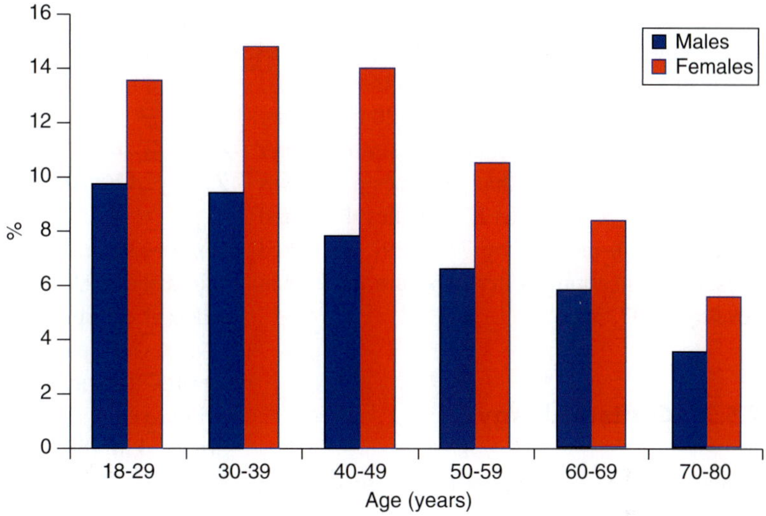

Fig. 7.1 Self-reported 1-year prevalence of hand eczema in relation to sex and age ($n=25778$). Results from the national Swedish environmental health survey 2007 (Reprinted with permission from Meding et al. [25]. © 2010 The Authors. BJD © 2010 British Association of Dermatologists)

A difference in incidence rate between the sexes was found only in individuals younger than 30 years in a Swedish study [16]. The highest incidence rate was found in females aged 20–29 years (11.4 cases per 1,000 person-years).

An interesting observation is the tendency for early onset of hand eczema; 35 % of female cases and 27 % of male cases reported onset before 20 years of age [16]. In epidemiological studies in Sweden and Denmark, the 1-year prevalence of hand eczema in schoolchildren was between 5 % and 10 % [15, 26, 27]. The reason for the early onset of hand eczema is not fully known, although atopic eczema constitutes the background in many cases.

There are no differences between males and females regarding susceptibility to skin irritants [28]. The reason for the sex differences observed in the occurrence of hand eczema is considered to be due mainly to differences in exposure, particularly wet exposure. In population-based studies in Sweden, water exposure was reported more frequently in females than in males and more frequently in younger adults than in older [29, 30].

7.4 Genetic Factors

Genetic factors are shown to be of importance for the development of hand eczema. Atopic eczema is a well-known risk factor entailing skin barrier defects [31]. An increased risk of hand eczema in individuals with a history of atopic eczema has been shown in many studies [2, 9, 14, 32, 33]. In questionnaire-based epidemiological studies in Sweden, the validated question "Have you had childhood eczema?" has often been used for self-reporting of atopic eczema [34]. In various studies, odds ratios (OR) in the range of 3.2–5.7 were found for hand eczema in relation to childhood eczema [2, 9, 33, 35]. The influence of atopic eczema on incidence of hand eczema seems to be of importance mainly at ages lower than 30 years [16]. Danish twin studies indicate that there exist genetic factors independent of atopy that are of importance for the development of hand eczema [35, 36]. When controlling for age and atopic dermatitis, the effect of genetic factors was estimated to explain 41 % of the variance in liability to develop hand eczema, leaving 59 % of the variance to be explained by environmental factors [36].

7.5 Environmental Factors

7.5.1 Skin Irritation

Environmental factors of importance for the development of hand eczema are typically those causing skin irritation. Occupational, as well as nonoccupational, exposure should be considered.

Knowledge about the extent of wet exposure in the general population is limited. In a population-based survey, 22 % (females 30 %, males 12 %) reported water exposure more than 20 times *during the entire day* [30]. In another survey, water exposure *at work* more than 20 times a day was reported by 6 % (females 8 %, males 4 %) and more than 2 h per day by 7 % [29]. Validated questions concerning water exposure have been developed [37, 38].

7.5.2 Contact Allergy

Contact allergy is an important cause of hand eczema. The presence of contact allergy is a common finding in clinical cases, and there is abundant literature on contact allergy in hand eczema patients. Contact allergy has been shown to be a risk factor for increased severity of hand eczema [39, 40] and to relate to persisting symptoms [41]. Nickel is the most common contact allergen, and its relevance as a cause and maintaining factor for hand eczema is under debate. In several occupations, exposure to contact allergens, such as chromium, rubber chemicals, epoxy, and permanent hair dyes, entails a risk for hand eczema. Little is known about the role of contact allergy for hand eczema in the general population. Few population-based patch test studies have been performed [6, 42, 43], probably due to costliness and logistical complexity.

7.5.3 Lifestyle Factors

A possible relation between lifestyle factors and hand eczema has been investigated in a few studies. In a cross-sectional public health study in Sweden, it was found that hand eczema was more common in individuals who reported stress, obesity, and smoking and less common in those who reported high physical exercise levels [44]. A positive relation between smoking and hand eczema has also been seen in other studies [6, 25], and a positive dose relation was revealed [25]. In a study on upper secondary schoolchildren, neither tattoos nor a vegetarian diet were found to be related to hand eczema [27]. No relation has been found between alcohol consumption and hand eczema [6, 18, 44].

7.6 Occupational Hand Eczema

Hand eczema is the most frequent occupational skin disease. Data published regarding the occurrence of occupational skin disease are compiled in a review paper from 2009 [45]. In several reports, the incidence was 6–8 cases per 10,000 person-years. In a number of reports, occupational skin disease constituted a considerable proportion of all cases of occupational disease – in Germany, 34 %, in Finland, 16 %, and in the United Kingdom, 22 %. In the United States, it was estimated that 10–15 % of occupational disease was skin disease [46]. Reports to occupational disease registers are to be regarded as uncertain sources of data that do not represent the true occurrence of occupational disease. Different insurance systems are in use in different countries, and the incentive to report is not the same in all countries. Examples of heavy underreporting to occupational disease registers have been demonstrated in several countries [24, 46–48]. Many factors in the work environment may contribute to hand eczema. Wet exposure occurs in many occupations, particularly in health care and service, and conveys an increased risk of hand eczema [49, 50]; in some occupations, there is skin exposure to contact allergens.

Incidence rate, which identifies new cases, is the preferred measure when occurrence of hand eczema in different occupations is addressed. When comparing data on occurrence of hand eczema from different studies and in different occupational subpopulations, it is necessary to perform adjustments for age and sex. Hand eczema has a protracted course, which implies that prevalence is a less suitable measure. The prevalence is also probably modified by the healthy worker effect in many occupations [51]. The limited information obtained regarding differences in hand eczema occurrence in different occupations is illustrated in a paper from the Gothenburg hand eczema study [52]. The results were based on 1-year prevalence in a large cross-sectional study where questionnaires were mailed to 20,000 individuals. When adjusting for age and sex, the only statistically significant difference identified was a higher 1-year prevalence of hand eczema among cleaners (21.3 %). In the analysis, 46 different occupations were compared.

7.7 Course and Severity of Hand Eczema

Hand eczema is a disease that often has a long duration and a tendency to become chronic. In one population-based study, the mean reported duration from onset of the disease to the time of examination was 11.6 years [1]. The disease has a relapsing course in many individuals. In the same study, 23 % reported continuous symptoms from the onset of the disease to the time of examination [1]. There are also seasonal variations – low temperature and low humidity are found to increase skin irritation [53]. Bacterial infection with *Staphylococcus aureus* on the hands is suggested to be a cofactor for persistence of hand eczema [54].

The prognosis of hand eczema is considered to be poor. In a follow-up of a population-based hand eczema cohort, almost half of the individuals had ongoing hand eczema after 15 years [55]. In selected groups, like occupational hand eczema cases or patients at dermatology clinics, the long-term prognosis was found to be even worse [56–59]. Negative factors for the prognosis are shown to be extent of involvement of the eczema, history of childhood eczema, and young age at disease onset [41]. A worse prognosis of hand eczema was found to be associated with longer delay before medical attention [60].

The ability to assess the severity of the disease is of importance for evaluation of effects of treatments and different preventive interventions. There is no generally accepted method for estimating the severity of hand eczema. In a review article published in 2009, a systematic search of the literature identified 45 different methods for quantifying hand eczema [61]. Most of the scoring systems are based on recordings of morphology and affected area, and in some scores subjective complaints are included. The Osnabrück hand eczema severity index (OHSI) [62] and the hand eczema severity index (HECSI) [63] have been validated. Physician Global Assessment (PGA) has been used for evaluating treatment of hand eczema [64]. The occupational contact dermatitis disease severity index (ODDI) is an instrument designed to also include functional disability [65]. A photo guide has been developed and validated [66], and this has also been used by patients [67]. In a follow-up study, it was found that morphology data did not significantly add information regarding long-term prognosis of hand eczema [68]. A simple scoring system based merely on the extent of the hand eczema has been developed, and a good correlation between the scores set by dermatologists, nurses, and the patients themselves is shown [69]. To evaluate the impact of the hand eczema, severity scoring should preferably be supplemented with an instrument to assess health-related quality of life.

7.8 Cost of Hand Eczema

The cost of illness is measured in two categories: direct and indirect costs. Direct costs are related to expenses for medical care and include additional costs in daily life for the patient. Indirect costs include the cost of loss of productivity. Hand eczema constitutes the main form of occupational dermatitis, has a poor long-term prognosis, and may cause sick leave, especially in health care and food-handling professions, where leave can be mandatory. All these factors may have an economic impact.

Few studies on the costs related to hand eczema have been published, and in a systematic review on the effectiveness of hand eczema prevention, no cost study following Cochrane criteria was found [70]. However, some studies have explored the economic burden of hand eczema on society and the individual. The results indicate that the diagnosis has considerable economic consequences even if the individual is not "seriously ill," since many individuals are affected. In a 12-year follow-up study in Sweden of individuals who had reported their skin disease to the Social Insurance Office,

32 % declared their private economic situation was worse due to occupational skin disease [56]. In a similar study from Finland, 23 % reported during follow-up that their economic situation was worse due to the hand eczema [71].

The economic burden of dermatitis was measured on individuals working in seven US industry sectors. The total cost (direct and indirect) was estimated to be around USD $1.2 billion and USD $570 per individual with dermatitis in 2004 [72]. In another population-based study in the United States, published in 2006, the direct cost per month was estimated to USD $70 for every patient with chronic hand eczema [73]. In an analysis of workers' compensation claims in Oregon in the United States during 1990–1997, the average cost was USD $3,552 per claim of occupational dermatitis (of which hand eczema constituted 38 %) [74].

In the Netherlands (with 15 million inhabitants), the direct medical costs in 1995 for occupational skin diseases were estimated to about EUR 42 million [75]. In a detailed study on hand eczema prevention, direct and indirect costs will be measured, with results expected in 2014 [76]. The cost of 1 day lost at work in Germany was estimated to be EUR 400–700, and in a survey from 2006, the annual indirect costs for occupational dermatitis were estimated to exceed EUR 1.5 billion [75]. In Great Britain, approximately four million working days are estimated to be lost every year due to work-related skin diseases [77].

In a German study from 2011 that included patients with severe chronic hand eczema refractory to topical steroids, the total annual cost per patient was estimated to EUR 2128 (direct costs EUR 1742, indirect costs EUR 386). The costs correlated to clinical severity of the eczema [78]. The major cost drivers in the direct costs were hospital care and drugs.

7.9 Sick Leave and Occupational Changes

In hand eczema treatment, sick leave is prescribed to facilitate medical treatment and to minimize skin irritation from wet work or other manual work. In patient care and food handling, the risk of transmitting infection from wounded skin must also be considered.

Several studies report figures on sick leave and occupational changes caused by hand eczema and occupational dermatitis [55–57, 60, 71, 79, 80]. Fear of unemployment has also been clearly expressed in a German semi-structured-guided interview study of patients with occupational skin disease [81]. Several factors influence the extent to which sick leave will be prescribed and utilized and occupational changes will be performed. Besides the severity of the disease, several surrounding factors play an important role: type of occupation and education, form of employment, possibility to get temporary job relief, actual labor market, and the models of the national social insurance systems. When interpreting the figures in studies on sick leave and occupational changes, it is important to have all these circumstances in mind and also to pay special attention to the study design, including populations and time intervals studied.

In a Swedish population-based study published in 1990, 21 % of individuals with hand eczema reported sick leave, with a median total time of 8 weeks, and 8 % reported change of occupation due to the eczema [79]. At follow-up 15 years later, 6 % reported sick leave periods of more than a week during the follow-up period, and 3 % reported change to another occupation [55].

Hand eczema patients (of which 26 % were occupational) from dermatological clinics in Denmark were followed up after 6 months. Sick leave during the last year was reported by 9 % [60]. Patients with occupational hand eczema diagnosed at the Finnish Institute of National Health were followed up after 7–14 years [71]. Sick leave was reported by 23 %, change of occupation by 34 %, and loss of job (unemployment or retirement) by 25 %.

Study populations can be recruited from national insurance registers on occupational diseases. In a detailed survey of the individuals who had reported their hand eczema to the Danish National Board of Industrial Injuries Registry, it was found that patients with low economic status had a high risk of prolonged sick leave, occupational changes, and loss of job [57]. In a 1-year follow-up, 57 % reported sick leave during the last year, and 23 % reported that they had lost their job at least once during the last year [80]. Working in food-related occupations has been documented to imply an enhanced risk to lose jobs [71, 80].

In a Swedish 12-year follow-up of individuals who reported occupational skin disease to the Social Insurance Office, 48 % reported sick leave for at least 1 week during follow-up, and 44 % reported a change of occupation [56]. Fifteen percent were excluded from the labor market through unemployment or retirement.

7.10 Hand Eczema and Quality of Life

Besides the medical and socioeconomic impacts of hand eczema, the disease also has effects on daily activities and may entail an emotional stress factor. Indications from questionnaire studies and clinical work have drawn attention to the importance of the issue, and during the last decades, abundant studies with a focus on quality of life (QoL) and hand eczema have been published [5, 39, 82–91]. Review articles are also accessible [92–96]. Impaired health-related quality of life (HRQoL) of the same magnitude as in asthma and psoriasis is reported by individuals in a population-based study [88]. Patients with severe occupational hand eczema got "impairment scores" similar to those found with atopic dermatitis and psoriasis [86].

Measuring QoL is complex. Definitions and concepts are developing together with a huge number of abbreviations. Structured instruments are often used to measure HRQoL. The validation of these presents difficulties, as does interpretation of the results. Cultural and other differences in study populations may also give less generally applicable results. In addition to the use of HRQoL instruments, further research has focused on the patients' subjective illness perceptions, using qualitative methods [81].

Three different types of instruments to study HRQoL are used: generic, dermatology specific, and disease specific.

1. Generic instruments permit comparison between different diseases and may include healthy controls. Examples are EQ-5D, developed by the EuroQol Group [97], and SF-36, Short Form Health Survey [98, 99].
2. Dermatology-specific instruments have been developed to measure HRQoL in skin diseases in general. Dominating instruments are DLQI (Dermatology Life Quality Index) [100] and different versions of Skindex [101].
3. Disease-specific instruments for hand eczema have hitherto, to the best of our knowledge, not been presented.

It has been shown in population-based studies [5, 88, 90], as well as in studies on clinical patients [39, 82–87, 89, 91], that HRQoL is negatively affected in individuals with hand eczema. Hitherto, DLQI has often been used [39, 57, 82, 83, 85–87, 89–91]. In some studies, both generic and dermatology-specific instruments are used [82, 85, 90, 91]. Correlation between HRQoL and severity of the hand eczema has been shown [57, 87, 91].

References

1. Meding B. Epidemiology of hand eczema in an industrial city. Acta Derm Venereol Suppl. 1990;153: 1–43.
2. Meding B, Järvholm B. Hand eczema in Swedish adults – changes in prevalence between 1983 and 1996. J Invest Dermatol. 2002;118:719–23.
3. Meding B, Lidén C, Berglind N. Self-diagnosed dermatitis in adults. Results from a population survey in Stockholm. Contact Dermatitis. 2001;45:341–5.
4. Montnémery P, Nihlén U, Löfdahl CG, Nyberg P, Svensson Å. Prevalence of hand eczema in an adult population and the relationship to risk occupation and smoking. Acta Derm Venereol. 2005;85:429–32.
5. Bingefors K, Lindberg M, Isacson D. Quality of life, use of topical medications and socio-economic data in hand eczema: a Swedish nationwide survey. Acta Derm Venereol. 2011;91:452–8.
6. Thyssen JP, Linneberg A, Menné T, Nielsen NH, Johansen JD. The effect of tobacco smoking and alcohol consumption on the prevalence of self-reported hand eczema: a cross-sectional population-based study. Br J Dermatol. 2010;162:619–26.
7. Erikssson CG, Granvik M, Kindblad I, Lindgren G, Nyström L, Rosén M, et al. Health problems in a Swedish county – what can we learn from official sources? Soc Sci Med C. 1981;15:143–51.

8. Meding B, Barregård L. Validity of self-reports of hand eczema. Contact Dermatitis. 2001;45:99–103.
9. Stenberg B, Meding B, Svensson Å. Dermatology in public health – a model for surveillance of common skin diseases. Scand J Public Health. 2010;38: 368–74.
10. Stockholms läns landsting, Sweden. Folkhälsorapport 2007. Stockholm: Centrum för folkhälsa; 2007.
11. Stockholm County Council, Sweden. Public Health Report 2007, Summary. Stockholm Centre for Public Health. 2007. Available: http://www.folkhalsoguiden.se/Informationsmaterial.aspx?id=2998 Accessed on 21 Oct 2013.
12. Socialstyrelsen, Sweden. Miljöhälsorapport 2009. Stockholm: Socialstyrelsen; 2009.
13. National Board of Health and Welfare, Sweden. Environmental Health Report 2009. Extended Summary. Stockholm: National Board of Health and Welfare; 2009.
14. Agrup G. Hand eczema and other hand dermatoses in South Sweden. Acta Derm Venereol (Stockh). 1969;49 Suppl 61:28–37.
15. Mortz CG, Lauritsen JM, Bindslev-Jensen C, Andersen KE. Prevalence of atopic dermatitis, asthma, allergic rhinitis, and hand and contact dermatitis in adolescents. The Odense adolescence cohort study on atopic diseases and dermatitis. Br J Dermatol. 2001;144:523–32.
16. Meding B, Järvholm B. Incidence of hand eczema – a population-based retrospective study. J Invest Dermatol. 2004;122:873–7.
17. Lantinga H, Nater JP, Coenraads PJ. Prevalence, incidence and course of eczema on the hands and forearms in a sample of the general population. Contact Dermatitis. 1984;10:135–9.
18. Lerbaek A, Kyvik KO, Ravn H, Menné T, Agner T. Incidence of hand eczema in a population-based twin cohort: genetic and environmental risk factors. Br J Dermatol. 2007;157:552–7.
19. Smit HA, van Rijssen A, Vandenbroucke JP, Coenraads PJ. Susceptibility to and incidence of hand dermatitis in a cohort of apprentice hairdressers and nurses. Scand J Work Environ Health. 1994;20: 113–21.
20. Smit HA, Coenraads PJ. A retrospective cohort study on the incidence of hand dermatitis in nurses. Int Arch Occup Environ Health. 1993;64:541–4.
21. Uter W, Pfahlberg A, Gefeller O, Schwanitz HJ. Prevalence and incidence of hand dermatitis in hairdressing apprentices: results of the POSH study. Int Arch Occup Environ Health. 1998;71:487–92.
22. Funke U, Fartasch M, Diepgen TL. Incidence of work-related hand eczema during apprenticeship: first results of a prospective cohort study in the car industry. Contact Dermatitis. 2001;44:166–72.
23. Brisman J, Meding B, Järvholm B. Occurrence of self-reported hand eczema in Swedish bakers. Occup Environ Med. 1998;55:750–4.
24. Lind M-L, Albin M, Brisman J, Kronholm Diab K, Lillienberg L, Mikoczy Z, et al. Incidence of hand eczema in female hairdressers. Occup Environ Med. 2007;64:191–5.
25. Meding B, Alderling M, Wrangsjö K. Tobacco smoking and hand eczema: a population-based study. Br J Dermatol. 2010;163:752–6.
26. Yngveson M, Svensson Å, Isacsson A. Prevalence of self-reported hand dermatosis in upper secondary school pupils. Acta Derm Venereol. 1998;78: 371–4.
27. Röhrl K, Stenberg B. Lifestyle factors and hand eczema in a Swedish adolescent population. Contact Dermatitis. 2010;62:170–6.
28. Agner T. Noninvasive measuring methods for the investigation of irritant patch test reactions. Acta Derm Venereol. 1992; Suppl. 173:14.
29. Anveden Berglind I, Alderling M, Järvholm B, Lidén C, Meding B. Occupational skin exposure to water: a population-based study. Br J Dermatol. 2009;160:616–21.
30. Meding B, Lindahl G, Alderling M, Wrangsjö K, Anveden Berglind I. Is skin exposure to water mainly occupational or non-occupational? A population-based study. Br J Dermatol. 2013;168:1281–6.
31. Cork MJ, Robinson DA, Vasilopoulus Y, Ferguson A, Moustafa M, MacGowan A, et al. New perspectives on epidermal barrier dysfunction in atopic dermatitis: gene-environment interactions. J Allergy Clin Immunol. 2006;118:3–21.
32. Rystedt I. Long term follow-up in atopic dermatitis. Acta Derm Venereol Suppl (Stockh). 1985;114:117–20.
33. Bingefors K, Svensson Å, Isacson D, Lindberg M. Self-reported lifetime prevalence of atopic dermatitis and comorbidity with asthma and eczema in adulthood: a population-based cross-sectional survey. Acta Derm Venereol. 2013;93:438–41.
34. Stenberg B, Lindberg M, Meding B, Svensson Å. Is the question "Have you had childhood eczema?" useful for assessing childhood atopic eczema in adult population surveys? Contact Dermatitis. 2006;54:334–7.
35. Bryld LE, Hindsberger C, Kyvik KO, Agner T, Menné T. Risk factors influencing the development of hand eczema in a population-based twin sample. Br J Dermatol. 2003;149:1214–20.
36. Lerbaeck A, Kyvik KO, Mortensen J, Bryld LE, Menné T, Agner T. Heritability of hand eczema is not explained by comorbidity with atopic dermatitis. J Invest Dermatol. 2007;127:1632–40.
37. Anveden I, Lidén C, Alderling M, Meding B. Self-reported skin exposure – validation of questions by observation. Contact Dermatitis. 2006;55:186–91.
38. Anveden I, Meding B. Skin exposure in geriatric care – a comparison between observation and self-assessment of exposure. Contact Dermatitis. 2007;57: 253–8.
39. Agner T, Anderson KE, Brandao FM, Bruynzeel DP, Bruze M, Frosch P, et al. Contact sensitisation in hand eczema patients-relation to subdiagnosis, severity and quality of life: a multi-center study. Contact Dermatitis. 2009;61:291–6.

40. Hald M, Agner T, Blands J, Ravn H, Johansen JD. Allergen associated with severe symptoms of hand eczema and a poor prognosis. Contact Dermatitis. 2009;61:101–8.
41. Meding B, Wrangsjö K, Järvholm B. Fifteen-year follow-up of hand eczema: predictive factors. J Invest Dermatol. 2005;124:893–7.
42. Nielsen NH, Linneberg A, Menné T, Madsen F, Frølund L, Dirksen A, et al. The association between contact allergy and hand eczema in 2 cross-sectional surveys 8 years apart. The Copenhagen allergy study. Contact Dermatitis. 2002;46:71–7.
43. Dotterud LK, Smith-Sivertsen T. Allergic contact sensitization in the general adult population: a population-based study from Northern Norway. Contact Dermatitis. 2007;56:10–5.
44. Anveden Berglind I, Alderling M, Meding B. Life-style factors and hand eczema. Br J Dermatol. 2011; 165:568–75.
45. Keegel T, Moyle M, Dharmage S, Frowen K, Nixon R. The epidemiology of occupational contact dermatitis (1990–2007): a systematic review. Int J Dermatol. 2009;48:571–8.
46. Lushniak BD. Occupational contact dermatitis. Dermatol Ther. 2004;17:272–7.
47. Hansen HS, Søstedt H. Hand eczema in Copenhagen hairdressers – prevalence and under-reporting to occupational registers. Contact Dermatitis. 2009;61:361–3.
48. Lyons G, Keegel T, Palmer A, Nixon R. Occupational dermatitis in hairdressers: do they claim workers' compensation? Contact Dermatitis. 2013;68:163–8.
49. Keegel TG, Nixon RL, LaMontagne AD. Exposure to wet work in working Australians. Contact Dermatitis. 2011;66:87–94.
50. Ibler KS, Jemec GBE, Agner T. Exposures related to hand eczema: a study of healthcare workers. Contact Dermatitis. 2012;66:247–53.
51. Rothman KJ. Epidemiology. An introduction. New York: Oxford University Press; 2002. p. 97–8.
52. Meding B, Swanbeck G. Occupational hand eczema in an industrial city. Contact Dermatitis. 1990;22:13–23.
53. Uter W, Gefeller O, Schwanitz HJ. An epidemiological study of the influence of season (cold and dry air) on the occurrence of irritant skin changes of the hands. Br J Dermatol. 1998;138:266–72.
54. Haslund P, Bangsgaard N, Jarløv JO, Skov L, Skov R, Agner T. *Staphylococcus aureus* and hand eczema severity. Br J Dermatol. 2009;161:772–7.
55. Meding B, Wrangsjö K, Järvholm B. Fifteen-year follow-up of hand eczema: persistence and consequences. Br J Dermatol. 2005;152:975–80.
56. Meding B, Lantto R, Lindahl G, Wrangsjö K, Bengtsson B. Occupational skin disease in Sweden – a 12-year follow-up. Contact Dermatitis. 2005;53:308–13.
57. Cvetkovski RS, Zachariae R, Jensen H, Olsen J, Johansen JD, Agner T. Prognosis of occupational hand eczema. Arch Dermatol. 2006;142:305–11.
58. Veien NK, Hattel T, Laurberg G. Hand eczema: causes, course, and prognosis I. Contact Dermatitis. 2008;58:330–4.
59. Veien NK, Hattel T, Laurberg G. Hand eczema: causes, course, and prognosis II. Contact Dermatitis. 2008;58:335–9.
60. Hald M, Agner T, Blands J, Johansen JD. Delay in medical attention to hand eczema: a follow-up study. Br J Dermatol. 2009;161:1294–300.
61. Weistenhöfer W, Baumeister T, Drexler H, Kütting B. An overview of skin scores used for quantifying hand eczema: a critical update according to the criteria of evidence-based medicine. Br J Dermatol. 2010;162:239–50.
62. Skudlik C, Dulon M, Pohrt U, Appl KC, John SM, Nienhaus A. Osnabrueck hand eczema severity index – a study of the interobserver reliability of a scoring system assessing skin diseases of the hands. Contact Dermatitis. 2006;55:42–7.
63. Held E, Skoet R, Johansen JD, Agner T. The hand eczema severity index (HECSI): a scoring system for clinical assessment of hand eczema. A study of inter- and intraobserver reliability. Br J Dermatol. 2005;152:302–7.
64. Ruzicka T, Lynde CW, Jemec GBE, Diepgen T, Berth-Jones J, Coenraads PJ, et al. Efficacy and safety of oral alitretinoin (9-*cis* retinoic acid) in patients with severe chronic hand eczema refractory to topical corticosteroids: results of a randomized, double-blind, placebo-controlled, multicenter trial. Br J Dermatol. 2008;158:808–17.
65. Curr N, Dharmage S, Keegel T, Lee A, Saunders H, Nixon R. The validity and reliability of the occupational contact dermatitis disease severity index. Contact Dermatitis. 2008;59:157–64.
66. Coenraads PJ, van der Walle H, Thestrup-Pedersen K, Ruzicka T, Dreno B, de la Loge C, et al. Construction and validation of a photographic guide for assessing severity of chronic hand dermatitis. Br J Dermatol. 2005;152:296–301.
67. Hald M, Veien NK, Laurberg G, Johansen JD. Severity of hand eczema assessed by patients and dermatologist using a photographic guide. Br J Dermatol. 2007;156:77–80.
68. Meding B, Wrangsjö K, Järvholm B. Hand eczema extent and morphology – association and influence on long-term prognosis. J Invest Dermatol. 2007;127: 2147–51.
69. Carlsson A, Gånemo A, Anderson CD, Meding B, Stenberg B, Svensson Å. Scoring of hand eczema: good agreement between patients and dermatological staff. Br J Dermatol. 2011;165:123–8.
70. Van Gils RF, Boot CRL, van Gils PF, Bruynzeel D, Coenraads PJ, van Mechelen W, et al. Effectiveness of prevention programmes for hand dermatitis: a systematic review of the literature. Contact Dermatitis. 2011;64:63–72.
71. Mälkönen T, Alanko K, Jolanki R, Luukkonen R, Aalto-Korte K, Lauerma A, et al. Long-term follow-up study of occupational hand eczema. Br J Dermatol. 2010;163:999–1006.
72. Blanciforti LA. Economic burden of dermatitis in US workers. J Occup Environ Med. 2010;52:1045–54.

73. Fowler JF, Ghosh A, Sung J, Emani S, Chang J, Den E, et al. Impact of chronic hand dermatitis on quality of life, work productivity, activity impairment, and medical costs. J Am Acad Dermatol. 2006;54:448–57.
74. McCall BP, Horwitz IB, Feldman SR, Balkrishnan R. Incidence rates, costs, severity, and work-related factors of occupational dermatitis. A workers' compensation analysis of Oregon, 1990–1997. Arch Dermatol. 2005;141:713–8.
75. Diepgen TL. The cost of skin disease. In EDF White Book. Eur J Dermatol. 2006;16:456–61.
76. Van der Meer EWC, Boot CRL, Jungbauer FHW, van der Klink JJL, Rustemeyer T, Coenraads PJ, et al. Hands4U: A multifaceted strategy to implement guideline-based recommendations to prevent hand eczema in health care workers: design of a randomized controlled trial and (cost) effectiveness evaluation. BMC Public Health. 2011;11:669.
77. English JSC. Current concepts of irritant contact dermatitis. Occup Environ Med. 2004;61:722–6.
78. Augustin M, Kuessner D, Purwins S, Hieke K, Posthumus J, Diepgen TL. Cost-of-illness of patients with chronic hand eczema in routine care: results from a multicentre study in Germany. Br J Dermatol. 2011;165:845–51.
79. Meding B, Swanbeck G. Consequences of having hand eczema. Contact Dermatitis. 1990;23:6–14.
80. Cvetkovski RS, Rothman KJ, Olsen J, Mathiesen B, Iversen L, Johansen JD, et al. Relation between diagnoses on severity, sick leave and loss of job among patients with occupational hand eczema. Br J Dermatol. 2005;152:93–8.
81. Bathe A, Diepgen TL, Matterne U. Subjective illness perceptions in individuals with occupational skin disease: a qualitative investigation. Work. 2012;43:159–69.
82. Hutchings CV, Shum KW, Gawkrodger DJ. Occupational contact dermatitis has an appreciable impact on quality of life. Contact Dermatitis. 2001;45:17–20.
83. Holness DL. Results of quality of life questionnaire in a patch test clinic population. Contact Dermatitis. 2001;44:80–4.
84. Kadyk DL, McCarter K, Achen F, Belsito DV. Quality of life in patients with allergic contact dermatitis. J Am Acad Dermatol. 2003;49:1037–48.
85. Wallenhammar L-M, Nyfjäll M, Lindberg M, Meding B. Health-related quality of life and hand eczema – a comparison of two instruments, including factor analysis. J Invest Dermatol. 2004;122:1381–9.
86. Cvetkovski RS, Zachariae R, Jensen H, Olsen J, Johansen DJ, Agner T. Quality of life and depression in a population of occupational hand eczema patients. Contact Dermatitis. 2006;54:106–11.
87. Agner T, Andersen KE, Brandao FM, Bruynzeel DP, Bruze M, Frosch P, et al. Hand eczema severity and quality of life: a cross-sectional, multicentre study of hand eczema patients. Contact Dermatitis. 2008;59:43–7.
88. Moberg C, Alderling M, Meding B. Hand eczema and quality of life: a population-based study. Br J Dermatol. 2009;161:397–403.
89. Hald M, Agner T, Blands J, Johansen JD. Quality of life in a population of patients with hand eczema: a six-month follow-up study. Acta Derm Venerol. 2011;91:484–6.
90. Lindberg M, Bingefors K, Meding B, Berg M. Hand eczema and health-related quality of life; a comparison of EQ-5D and the Dermatology Life Quality Index (DLQI) in relation to the Hand Eczema Extent Score (HEES). Contact Dermatitis. 2013;69:138–43.
91. Boehm D, Schmid-Ott G, Finkeldey F, John SM, Dwinger C, Werfel T, et al. Anxiety, depression and impaired health-related quality of life in patients with occupational hand eczema. Contact Dermatitis. 2012;67:184–92.
92. Skoet R, Zachariae R, Agner T. Contact dermatitis and quality of life: a structured review of the literature. Br J Dermatol. 2003;149:452–6.
93. Both H, Essink-Bot M-L, Busschbach J, Nijsten T. Critical review of generic and dermatology-specific health-related quality of life instruments. J Invest Dermatol. 2007;127:2726–39.
94. Basra MKA, Fenech R, Gatt RM, Salek MS, Finlay AY. The dermatology life quality index 1994–2007: a comprehensive review for validation data and clinical results. Br J Dermatol. 2008;159:997–1035.
95. Basra MKA, Shahrukh M. Burden of skin diseases. Expert Rev Pharmacoecon Outcomes Res. 2009;9:271–83.
96. Basra MKA, Chowdhury MMU, Smith EV, Freemantle N, Piguet V. A review of the use of the dermatology life quality index as criterion in clinical guidelines and health technology assessments in psoriasis and chronic hand eczema. Dermatol Clin. 2012;30:237–44.
97. Rabin R, de Charro F. EQ-5D: a measure of health status from the EuroQol group. Ann Med. 2001;33: 337–43.
98. Sullivan M, Karlsson J. SF-36 Hälsoenkät. Svensk manual och tolkningsguide (Swedish manual and interpretation guide). Göteborg: Sahlgrenska University Hospital; 1994.
99. Sullivan M, Karlsson J, Ware JE. The Swedish SF-36 Health Survey I. Evaluation of data quality, scaling assumptions, reliability and construct validity across general populations in Sweden. Soc Sci Med. 1995;41:1349–58.
100. Finlay AY, Khan GK. Dermatology life quality index (DLQI) – a simple practical measure for routine clinical use. Clin Exp Dermatol. 1994;19:210–6.
101. Chren MM, Lasek RJ, Quinn LM, Mostow EN, Zyzanski SJ. Skindex, a quality-of-life measure for patients with skin disease: reliability, validity, and responsiveness. J Invest Dermatol. 1996;107:707–13.

Risk Factors in Hand Eczema

8

Thomas L. Diepgen and Elke Weisshaar

Contents

T.L. Diepgen, M.D., Ph.D. (✉)
Department of Social Medicine,
University Hospital Heidelberg, Thibautstrasse 3,
Heidelberg, Baden-Württemberg 69115, Germany
e-mail: thomas.diepgen@med.uni-heidelberg.de

E. Weisshaar, M.D., Ph.D.
Department of Clinical Social Medicine,
Occupational and Environmental Medicine,
Heidelberg University Hospital,
Thibautstr 3, Heidelberg 69115, Germany
e-mail: elke.weisshaar@med.uni-heidelberg.de

8.1 Introduction

Although eczema of the hand is one of the most common skin diseases, a clear and worldwide accepted definition of what is included as "hand eczema" does not exist, and even dermatologists differ in their interpretation. After having excluded disorders of known etiology (e.g., tinea manuum, scabies), well-defined noneczematous morphology (e.g., psoriasis, lichen planus, granuloma annulare, porphyria cutanea tarda, keratosis palmoplantaris, fixed drug eruption), and neoplastic disorders from the category of hand eczema (HE) and if hands are not involved as part of an extensive skin disorder, the diagnosis of characteristic and established cases of HE usually presents little difficulty. But opinions differ on the validity of including mild and transient cases or those in which dryness, cracking, and superficial fissuring are the only features. It is also difficult to subclassify HE according to morphologic-etiologic or pathogenetic classifications used in dermatology.

Hand eczema and *hand dermatitis* are used interchangeably to describe a particular type of inflammatory disorder of the skin that mainly targets the epidermis. Clinically, it is a polymorphic eruption. Among the primary lesions that may be observed are macules, papules, and vesicles. Among the secondary lesions are oozing, crusting, scaling, lichenification, and fissuring. Pruritus is common in all types of hand eczema/dermatitis.

Acute and subacute HE can be defined as eczema, localized to the hands, that lasts for less

A. Alikhan et al. (eds.), *Textbook of Hand Eczema*,
DOI 10.1007/978-3-642-39546-8_8, © Springer-Verlag Berlin Heidelberg 2014

than 3 months and does not occur more than once per year [1, 2]. In the acute stage, vesicles will be present in most cases, although not always in irritant HE. Erythema, representing inflammation, is pronounced in acute HE as is edema. A subjective sensation of burning and itching is present in most cases.

Chronic HE refers to an eczematous process that lasts for more than 3 months or relapses twice or more per year [1, 2]. Scaling and fissures are found in most cases of chronic HE. Hyperkeratosis is present in chronic irritant HE but is also found in the endogenous hyperkeratotic HE and in other chronic cases.

HE is a multifactorial disease in which both exogenous and endogenous factors play a role. General aspects of those risk factors in hand eczema will be considered in this chapter. Besides the fact that HE is not a single entity but an affliction with multiple causes, an attempt to discuss the general role of risk factors using the literature poses additional problems: some studies are based on selected samples like patch test patients or special occupational groups (e.g., hairdressers, nurses), while other population-based studies are based on questionnaires and often "control" groups were not included. Finally, there is no clear agreement on the definition of endogenous risk factors like an atopic diathesis, which is believed to be often related to HE.

In this chapter, demographic and clinical characteristics of patients with hand eczema will be introduced, and general aspects of exogenous and endogenous risk factors in hand eczema are discussed.

8.2 Demographic and Clinical Characteristics of Hand Eczema

In Germany, a registry of chronic HE was established under the auspices of the German Dermatological Society (Deutsche Dermatologische Gesellschaft: DDG). Detailed information on the project is available at http://carpe.dermis.net. The aim of this carpe registry (German acronym *carpe*: Chronisches Handekzem-Register zum Patienten-Langzeitmanagement, equivalent to chronic hand eczema registry on long-term patient management) is to investigate characteristics and medical care in patients affected by chronic hand eczema (chronic HE defined as disease duration > 3 months or > two flares within the previous 12 months).

The sociodemographic and some clinical characteristics of 1,163 chronic HE patients of the *carpe* registry are as follows [3]: In total 54.6 % of all patients were female. Mean age was 47.0 years (SD, 13.7 years; min, 17.1 years; max: 84.3 years; median: 48.9 years). Average duration of HE was 7.6 years (SD 9.1 years, median 3.8 years). Mean body mass index (BMI) was 26.7 (SD, 4.6; median, 26.0) kg/m^2. Of the included patients, 32.2 % had received in-patient treatment (hospital treatment or rehabilitation measure) prior to inclusion in the registry; 81.7 % were currently gainfully employed. Of these, 24.2 % were currently unable to work, and 36.1 % had been on sick leave due to HE in the past 12 months. Overall, 5.1 % had lost or changed their occupation due to HE.

The localization of chronic HE on the hands is illustrated in Fig. 8.1. The most frequently reported localization was on the palm of the hand, while the least frequently reported localization was the wrist.

In Table 8.1 clinical characteristics of irritant, allergic, and atopic HE are presented. HE includes several clinical subtypes such as pompholyx, vesicular, atopic, endogenous, discoid, acral, irritant, allergic, tylotic, and hyperkeratotic eczema [4]. There is no single universally accepted classification for HE. Most published classifications invoke a combination of etiological factors (irritant, allergic, atopic disease) and morphological features (pompholyx, vesicular, hyperkeratotic eczema). No existing system completely avoids the existence of hybrids and combination of the various morphological categories or overcomes the inability to determine etiology in a substantial fraction of cases.

Diagnoses of chronic HE according to the carpe registry are presented in Fig. 8.2. Irritant contact dermatitis was the most frequently occurring diagnosis (45.1 %), followed by hyperkeratotic rhagadiform (34.0 %), atopic hand eczema (34.0 %), and allergic contact dermatitis (22.3 %). In 47.8 % a contact sensitization had been previously

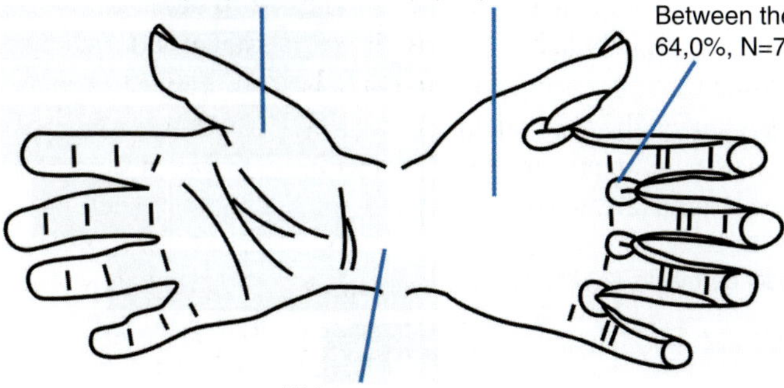

Fig. 8.1 Localization of chronic HE on the hands (Adapted from [3])

Table 8.1 Characteristics of irritant, allergic, and atopic hand eczema[a]

1. **Irritant (subtoxic cumulative) hand eczema**
Pathogenesis:
Result of repeated effects on the skin of irritating toxic substances over a longer period of time in minor concentrations
In occupational disease, gradual development with work, little improvement over the weekend, healing only after a prolonged leave of absence
Constitutional factors facilitate the development: atopic skin diathesis, sebostasis, hyperhidrosis
Localization:
Mainly on the backs of the hands and fingers as well on exposed areas of the forearms, only later on the palms of the hands
Skin symptoms limited to the hands, no spread, relatively sharply bordered
Morphology:
Initially raw, dry, scaly skin
Later redness, infiltration, and rhagades
Finally, hyperkeratotic rhagadiform appearance
Pruritus generally not as severe as in allergic contact dermatitis
Painful rhagades (common)
2. **Allergic hand eczema**
Pathogenesis:
Due to type IV hypersensitivity (patch test verification)
Rarely protein contact dermatitis
Close temporal relationship between exposure and disease, for occupational disease: development and exacerbation when working, improvement on the weekends, healing during vacation, recurs within a few days of returning to work
Localization:
Location on the skin related to allergen exposure
Exposure sites affected (airborne sensitization also possible)
Spread to surrounding areas (differentiate from irritant hand dermatitis)
Irregular border at exposure sites
Morphology:
In acute stages: redness, small blisters, severe itching
In chronic stages: hyperkeratosis, rhagades
3. **Atopic hand eczema**
Pathogenesis:
Result of atopic eczema or atopic skin diathesis
Rarely also protein contact dermatitis
Course often independent of working pattern
Initial manifestation, possibly transitory disease or exacerbation due to toxic substances at the workplace
Localization:
Often involves the back of the hands as in irritant dermatitis
Nail involvement common, fingertip eczema (pulpite sèche)
Often involves flexural surfaces of the wrist, lichenification
Involvement of the anatomical "snuff box" with poorly bordered lichenified lesions
Involvement of other regions of the body (neck, joint flexures, dorsum of the foot)
Morphology:
Palmar and interdigital blistering (vesicular morphology) are common
Lichenification (backs of the hands, flexural surfaces of the wrist)
Scaling, rhagades (fingertips)
Nummular lesions (backs of the hands, usually poorly bordered) possible

[a]Adapted from [1]

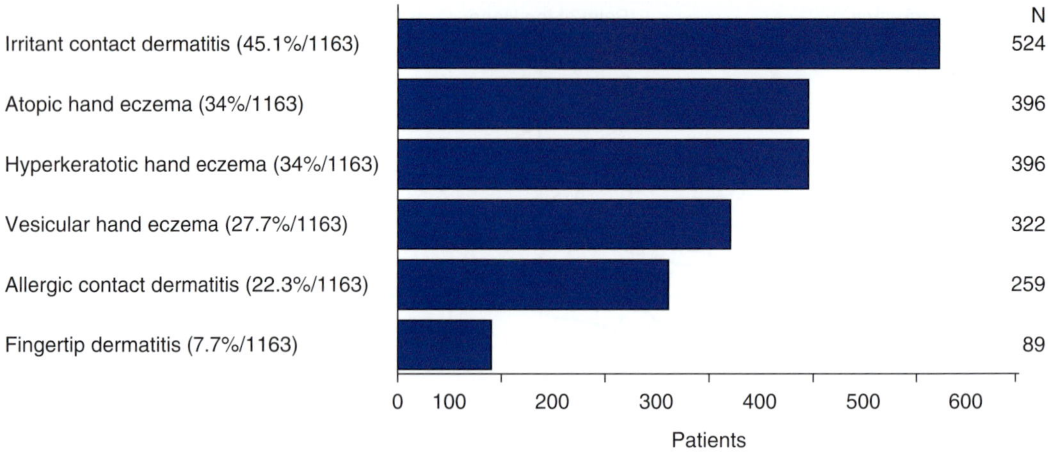

Fig. 8.2 Diagnoses of chronic HE (multiple answers possible) (Adapted from [3])

Fig. 8.3 The seven most frequently used sub-diagnoses or combinations of sub-diagnoses for HE in males and females. *ACD* allergic contact dermatitis, *ICD* irritant contact dermatitis, *AHE* atopic hand eczema (Reprinted from Diepgen et al. [5], with permission from John Wiley and Sons. © 2008 The Authors. © Journal Compilation British Association of dermatologists)

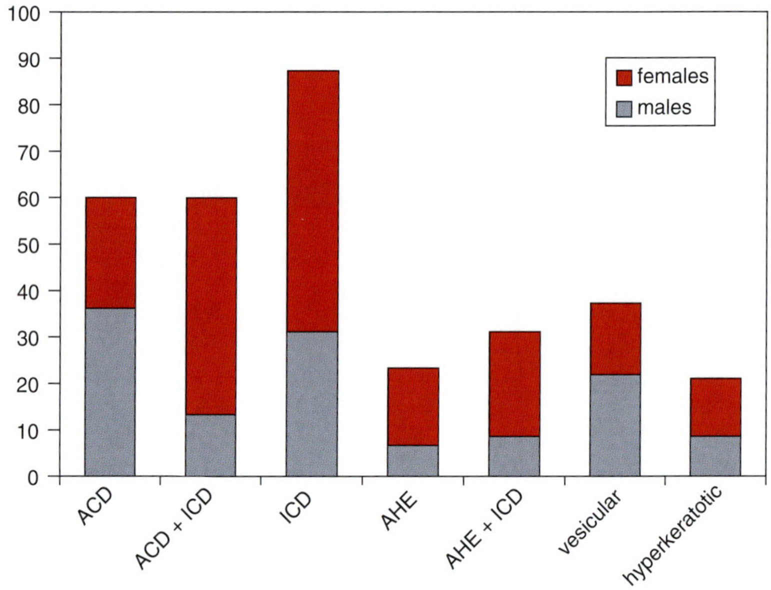

diagnosed by patch testing. Of the 1163 patients, 572 had a monodiagnosis (49.2 %). Hyperkeratotic rhagadiform hand eczema was the most frequent monodiagnosis ($n = 198$).

In a European study, 416 consecutive HE patients from 10 participating European clinics were included [5]. The seven most frequently used sub-diagnoses or combinations of sub-diagnoses for HE were allergic contact dermatitis (ACD), allergic plus irritant contact dermatitis (ACD+ICD), irritant contact dermatitis (ICD), atopic hand eczema (AHE), atopic hand eczema plus irritant contact dermatitis (AHE+ICD), vesicular hand eczema, and hyperkeratotic hand eczema, and these diagnoses comprised 319 patients (80.6 %) [5]. The distribution of these sub-diagnoses of HE in relation to gender is presented in Fig. 8.3. Different diagnoses in relation to age groups are shown in Fig. 8.4, with statistically significant variation in age distribution between the sub-diagnostic groups (Kruskal-Wallis test $p < 0.0001$). Patients with AHE were

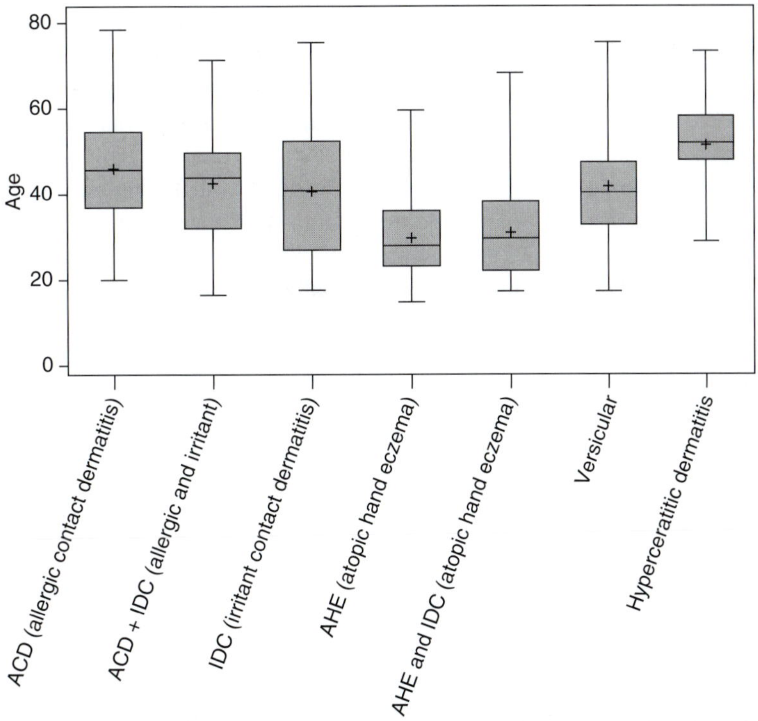

Fig. 8.4 Age in relation to sub-diagnoses (n=319 patients). A statistical significant difference was found in age distribution between the diagnostic subgroups (p<0.0001). Youngest age was found for patients with AHE and highest for patients with hyperkeratotic eczema (Diepgen et al. [5], with permission from John Wiley and Sons. © 2008 The Authors. © Journal Compilation British Association of dermatologists)

the youngest on average (median age 28), while those with hyperkeratotic eczema were the oldest on average (median age 52).

8.3 Exogenous Risk Factors

Chronic HE often has its origins in irritant or allergic contact dermatitis. Irritant contact dermatitis (ICD) may be caused by exposure to agents such as wet work, food, gloves, and oils [6]. Exposure to water can be a contact irritant and thereby an external causal or contributing factor. Allergic contact dermatitis (ACD) is caused by exposure to allergens, such as chromate, nickel, biocides, and rubber chemicals. Ingested allergens (e.g., nickel) may also provoke HE [7].

Often, a combination of irritant, allergic, and endogenous factors are acting in concert [1, 5]. It has been suggested that the multifactorial origin of HE is responsible for the chronic course of the condition and for its poor response to treatment [8].

In many chronic HE patients, a clear etiology cannot be identified or no longer contributes to the clinical features and the activity of the disease. In particular, patients with multifactorial etiology may develop chronic disease that is not related to any single identifiable causative factor.

8.3.1 Irritants and Irritant Hand Eczema

The first signs of irritant contact dermatitis are raw, dry, and slightly scaly skin with increasing redness and infiltration after prolonged or repeated exposure to an irritant. This is followed by formation of rhagades, and with continued exposure there are hyperkeratotic plaques interspersed with rhagades. Itching is generally not as severe as in allergic contact dermatitis. Irritant HE primarily affects the backs of the hands and fingers as well as exposed portions of the forearms (e.g., contact surfaces). Over the course of disease, the inner surfaces of the hands can also be affected. The eczematous lesions remain normally limited to exposure sites and there is normally no secondary spread.

The onset of irritant contact dermatitis is promoted by atopic skin diathesis, which often causes barrier damage as a result of genetically related changes. The development is highly dependent on the duration and intensity of exposure. In two-phase dermatitis, allergic contact dermatitis can arise from underlying irritant contact dermatitis. Allergic contact dermatitis should be excluded and the presence of atopic diathesis should be assessed.

8.3.1.1 Irritants

One of the most frequent and important irritants is wet work. The harmful effects of wet work can be seen in occupations that require frequent hand washing (e.g., healthcare workers) and in those that require the wearing of gloves for a long period of time. Sweat becomes trapped in close contact to the skin, leading to as significant a risk as direct water contact. Other common irritants include soaps, detergents, solvents, food, and oils. Intensive or frequent washing can also induce irritant contact dermatitis. According to the German regulation of hazardous substances at the work place, "wet work" is defined as individuals having their skin exposed to liquids longer than 2 h per day, or using occlusive gloves longer than 2 h per day, or cleaning the hands very often (e.g., 20 times per day or less if the cleaning procedure is more aggressive).

Irritant contact dermatitis frequently occurs in occupations with damp conditions.

The role of low humidity and strong winds is often overlooked, but can cause the stratum corneum to become dry and brittle. Repetitive mild friction to the skin, such as continually working with paper, may also worsen dermatitis.

8.3.2 Allergens and Allergic Hand Eczema

Allergic HE is caused by exposure to allergens, usually direct skin contact with chromate, nickel, preservatives, rubber, and so on in already sensitized individuals. A distinction has to be made between induction (sensitization) and effector (elicitation) phase.

The development of allergic HE is frequently triggered by a combination of domestic and occupational exposures. Environmental factors such as low humidity, high temperatures, occlusion, and frequent contact with water or other liquids (including sweating) may also adversely impact the epidermal barrier and, at identical levels of exposure, enhance the effects of irritants and/or allergens.

The clinical presentation varies greatly, making allergic and irritant HE difficult to distinguish clinically and histologically. Allergic HE is generally more acute, however. Morphological signs can include redness, scaling, blistering, papules, pustules, exudation, and excoriation. In chronic disease, rhagades can form and there may be lichenification and hyperkeratosis. Patients usually have itching and burning.

The first signs are evident at contact sites. Unlike irritant contact dermatitis, the borders of the lesions are poorly defined. In allergic contact dermatitis, additional lesions can appear on other parts of the body that have not come into contact with the allergen (secondary spread).

Allergic HE should be presumed if the patient history suggests occupational-related causes (onset and worsening during work, improvement on the weekend, healing on vacation, recurrence upon returning to work) and there is an association between the affected site and occupational contact. Unlike irritant HE, the borders around the exposed sites are poor and there is an almost pathognomic secondary spread to other areas of the body. When there is primarily involvement of the dorsal aspects of the hands, differential diagnosis should include photoallergic contact eczema.

8.3.3 Relevant Allergens and Irritants in Occupational Hand Eczema

Table 8.2 gives an overview of common sources of occupational eczematous diseases in higher-risk occupational groups. The table includes important allergens and chemical irritants.

Known irritants include water and working in wet or moist conditions, as well as detergents,

Table 8.2 Allergens and/or irritants (selection) in occupations with a significantly higher risk of work-related contact dermatitis. Most of these types of jobs involve working in wet conditions (definition in Table 8.3)[a]

Activities	Effects	Selection of important allergens and chemical irritants
Hairdressers	Perming agents, hair dyes, bleaches, shampoos, rubber gloves	Esters and salts of thioglycolic acid, p-phenylenediamine, p-toluenediamine, dyes, resorcinol, parabens, persulfates, preservatives, fragrances, plant extracts, cocamidopropyl betaine, emulsifiers, accelerators[b], natural latex
Bakers, pastry makers	Dough, fragrances and spices, preservatives, antioxidants	Wheat, rye, soy flour, amylase, vanilla, bitter almonds, anise, orange peel extract, cinnamon, benzoic acid, sorbic acid, octyl, propyl, and dodecyl gallates
Galvanization workers	Galvanic baths, protective rubber gloves	Nickel and chromate ions, cobalt compounds, acids, alkaline substances, accelerators[b], natural latex
Gardeners, florists	Ornamental plants, pesticides	Primrose, chrysanthemums, Asteraceae, Alstroemeria, tulip bulbs, carbamate, thiuram, pyrethrum
Construction workers, brick layers tile layers	Cement, freshly mixed concrete, plastics	Chromate ion, cobalt compounds, uncured epoxy resins and hardeners, isocyanate, thiuram
Metal workers	Solid cooling lubricants (especially water soluble), metals, metal glue	Preservatives (formaldehyde splitters, triazine, isothiazolinones), emulsifiers, anti-corrosive agents, ethanolamine, tall oil, mineral oil, nickel or cobalt or chromate ions, epoxy resins, acrylate, hardeners
Plastics workers	Uncured synthetic resins	Epoxy resins and hardeners, acrylates, cobalt, accelerators[b], peroxides, melamine/urea/phenol formaldehyde resins, isocyanates, phthalates, solvents
Cooks, kitchen workers	Foodstuffs	Flour, enzymes, meat, fish, crustaceans, vegetables, spices, preservatives, dyes
	Cleaning agents, rubber gloves	Preservatives (isothiazolinones, formaldehyde, parabens), fragrances, accelerators[b], natural latex
Hospital and nursing care employees	Disinfectants, medications, rubber gloves	Formaldehyde, glutaraldehyde, mercury compounds, chlorocresol, phenols, antibiotics, local anesthetics, phenothiazine (photo allergens), essential oils, accelerators[b], natural latex
Dental technicians	Dental chemicals	Uncured acrylates, eugenol, nickel, cobalt, palladium, amalgam, acids
Textile manufacturers and processors	Textile dyes, glaze, special equipment, rubber thread, clothing parts	Azo dyes, anthraquinone dyes, chromate compounds, formaldehyde resins, acrylate, polyurethane, accelerators[b], natural latex, nickel, cobalt ions
Leather and fur industry workers	Tanning agents, adhesives, waterproofing agents	Chromate ions, tannin, acids, lye, rosin, p-tert-butylphenol formaldehyde resin
Woodworkers, cabinet makers, carpenters	Lumbers, adhesives, stains, wood preservatives	Rosewood (various types), teak, cherry mahogany, mahogany, coniferous woods, formaldehyde resins, rosin, epoxy resins, acrylate, chromate ions, azo dyes, insecticides, fungicides

(continued)

Table 8.2 (continued)

Activities	Effects	Selection of important allergens and chemical irritants
Painters, work with varnish, house painters, flooring technicians	Dyes, synthetic resins, adhesives, diluting agents	Chromate ions, turpentine and substitutes, dye pigments, formaldehyde resins, rosin, epoxies, acrylate, isocyanate, solvents
Soldering, electronics engineer	Soldering agents, metal adhesives, metals	Rosin, metal chloride, acids, epoxy resins, acrylate, hardeners, nickel/cobalt/chromate ions
Cleaning industry workers	Detergents, disinfectants, floor cleansing/preserving products, rubber gloves	Tensides and cleaning agents, formaldehyde, glutaraldehyde, phenols, fragrances, accelerators, natural latex
Photo lab workers	Color developer, photo chemicals, rubber gloves	p-phenylenediamine, hydroquinone, Metol, chromate ions, formaldehyde, accelerators[b], natural latex
Rubber manufacturers and processors	Rubber, rubber additives	Natural latex, thiuram, thiocarbamates, mercaptobenzothiazole, p-substituted amines
Agricultural occupations	Animal feed dust, animal hair, rubber ingredients, disinfectants, pesticides	Grains, medications, etc., additives to animal feed

[a]Reprinted from Diepgen [9], with permission from John Wiley and Sons
[b]Thiuram, thiocarbamates, mercaptobenzothiazole; preservatives, etc.

cleansers, solid cooling lubricants, preservatives, and hand cleansers [9]. A few of these substances are not only responsible for triggering irritant HE but also for allergic HE. The "risk to the skin from working in wet (moist) conditions" is highly relevant given that it is the most significant risk to the skin in terms of numbers. The definition of working in wet conditions is found in the technical regulations for hazardous materials (TRGS) 401 "risk related to skin contact – identification, evaluation, measures" (http://www.baua.de/de/Themen-von-A-Z/Gefahrstoffe/TRGS/TRGS-401_content.html). According to this, "wet conditions" include "activities in which workers spend a significant portion of their time, i.e., regularly more than 2 h a day with their hands in a moist environment or must often or intensively wash their hands or must wear protective gloves for a certain period of time resulting in occlusion (preventing escape of heat and moisture). Impermeable protective gloves prevent the evaporation of sweat. Wearing gloves for a prolonged period of time can thus cause maceration of the skin and impair its barrier effect. The resulting damage makes it easier for irritants, potentially allergenic (sensitizing) substances, and pathogens to penetrate the skin."

The amount of time spent working in wet conditions and the amount of time spent wearing impermeable gloves should be added if no effective measures are taken for regeneration of the skin [9].

Hairdressers are especially at risk as they often work many hours a day in wet conditions (e.g., hair washing) and, in addition, are exposed to hairdressing chemicals that have strong irritant properties and contain potent allergens [9]. It is easy to imagine that against the backdrop of irritant damage (subtoxic cumulative HE), delayed hypersensitivity could develop to occupational substances and that allergic contact dermatitis may arise as two-phase eczema.

Other occupational groups that are at risk include cleaners as well as medical care personnel and caregivers. Among medical personnel, there is a risk due to prolonged wearing of impermeable gloves and working with cleansers and disinfectants (especially in hospital employees). In healthcare and other caregiving professions, there is the added factor of frequent hand washing and disinfecting [9].

Constant exposure to moist or wet conditions is also present in the food industry (e.g., bakers, pastry chefs, cooks, and butchers) [9]. Due to contact with foodstuffs, the hands are constantly moist and also must often be washed. There is also a risk of type I hypersensitivity (protein contact dermatitis). Workers generally do not adequately protect their hands. In addition, these occupations often involve cleaning activities.

In the metalworking industry, metal grinders are exposed to greater moisture due to work with water-soluble solid cooling lubricants. Solid cooling lubricants also contain many additives such as anti-foaming agents, anti-corrosive agents, and antibacterial substances. The irritants are usually highly potent, and there is also the risk of delayed hypersensitivity [9]. When solid cooling lubricants dry on the skin, it is often more damaging than constant wetting of the skin because the harmful substances of cooling lubricants are in direct contact with the skin for a longer period of time. Other polishing jobs that also use solid cooling lubricants or lubricants are also associated with an increased risk of skin disease (e.g., glass and stone polishing).

Frequent and aggressive hand washing also poses an increased risk of skin disease. Thus, all occupations that involve hand cleansing must be considered hazardous to the skin [9]. In addition to working in wet conditions, alkaline solutions are also skin irritants. Given their alkaline properties, cement and plaster can cause severe chemical burns ("cement necrosis"). This affects all employees in the building trade.

Occupational skin contact with organic solvents always poses a risk to the skin. This applies to workers in paint and varnish manufacturing and processing (printers, painters, and craftsmen who work with varnish) [9]. Solvents are also used in the metal industry, for instance, to remove grease from metal parts and machinery. Given additional exposure to solid cooling lubricants, there is an especially high risk of contact dermatitis.

Physical factors, such as excessive warmth or cold, facilitate the development of irritant HE. Workers in outdoor occupations thus require special protection against the cold. However, dry agents and materials that create dust, such as textile fibers, wood, plastic, or construction materials, can irritate the skin due to their hydroscopic effects. Glass and mineral fibers are a particular problem as they can penetrate the skin and cause microtrauma. This usually occurs at areas of the body that are covered (due to friction with the clothing, especially on flexural surfaces). This applies especially to occupations in which fibers are manufactured and processed. Metal cuttings can also cause microtrauma, if for instance, the same cloth is used to clean the machine and the hands. Even if the cloth is cleaned in between uses, cuttings can remain in the textile fibers [9].

All occupations that involve the wearing of waterproof gloves over an extended period of time must be considered hazardous to the skin. Gloves act as a moist chamber, and their occlusive effect enhances the irritant and/or allergenic effects of harmful substances [9].

Occupational skin diseases often develop gradually, and an attempt must be made as soon as possible to counteract the possible development of occupational disease through optimized prevention, targeted diagnosis, and specific treatment [9].

8.4 Endogenous Risk Factors

8.4.1 The Relationship Between Hand Eczema and Atopic Eczema

According to the studies of Lammintausta and Kalimo [10] and Rystedt [11], atopic disease and especially atopic eczema in childhood are risk factors for HE in adults. Today, it is generally agreed that the atopic skin has a disturbed barrier function and a reduced resistance to irritants, and that consequently individuals with a history of or with current atopic eczema (AE) have a tendency to develop an irritant contact dermatitis located mainly on the hands [12]. The clinical pattern is dry, scaly, and fissuring skin at the dorsum of the hand with a tendency of lichenification. In chronic cases, even a short direct skin contact to mild irritants such as water or wet work will induce a relapse of the inflammatory skin disease. It is usually impossible to distinguish between irritant contact dermatitis on an atopic base caused by work-related exogenous factors and an atopic HE mainly elicited by endogenous factors. A typical pattern for atopic HE is the involvement of eczematous lesions at the wrist, in contrast to an irritant contact dermatitis, where this location is unusual.

In severe chronic cases, the palms can be involved and the morphology of the skin lesions is characterized by hyperkeratosis and tylotic rhagadiform eczema [12]. Another variant is the tylotic, rhagadiform, fingerpad eczema, so-called *pulpite sèche*. Concomitant pain leads to impairment of functions in the involved hand. In chronic cases, the nails are also involved.

In over 50 % of patients, atopic HE shows vesicular volar eruption, sometimes with extension from the distal part of the palm to proximal fingers (apron sign) [12]. Very often the vesicular eruptions begin with intense pruritus at the lateral sides of the fingers. It can be difficult to clinically distinguish this vesicular type of atopic hand eczema from other hand eczema (pompholyx, e.g., induced by allergens) (see also Table 8.1).

In many cases of HE, the diagnosis must rest on clinical features while an absolute marker for AE awaits recognition. Therefore, it is important to examine the whole body carefully for minimal eczematous lesions at typical locations such as the neck, the flexural area of the elbow and knee, dorsa of the feet, and ear rhagades.

In adults, the most common location of atopic eczema is the hands [13–15], and atopic eczema is a well-known factor influencing the course and prognosis of hand eczema [10, 11].

8.4.2 Atopic Skin Diathesis and Hand Eczema

Lammintausta [16] introduced the term atopic skin diathesis (ASD) as a useful definition of the skin condition that might be involved in the development of HE. This condition was defined as:

- Dry skin
- A history of low pruritus threshold for two of three nonspecific irritants (sweat, dust, rough material)
- White dermographism
- Facial pallor/infraorbital darkening

This atopic skin diathesis was found in 35 % of subjects with respiratory atopy and in 18 % of the nonatopics and significantly increased the risk of HE among employees engaged in wet work. In her careful follow-up studies of atopic children, Rystedt [11] found a four to ten times higher frequency of HE in subjects who had atopic eczema in childhood than in those who had not. Patients with a history of respiratory allergy without associated AE ($n = 222$; 14 % HE) showed no increased frequency of HE compared to controls without personal or family atopy ($n = 199$; 11 % HE). Therefore, it seems to be necessary to subclassify the atopic state of possible skin involvement for occupational risk assessment.

In order to establish a diagnostic score for atopic skin diathesis (ASD), basic and minor features of atopic eczema were evaluated systematically in established cases of atopic eczema and in subjects randomly collected from the Caucasian population of young adults in a prospective study [17, 18]. Anamnestic and clinical atopic basic and minor features were investigated in all test subjects by two investigators to obtain a good interobserver agreement. Based on statistical modeling methods, a diagnostic scoring system was constructed based on anamnestic and clinical features without laboratory investigations (Table 8.3). The presence of an itching flexural dermatitis was not included since this was the selection base. For practical use, every atopic feature obtained a value between 1 and 3 points according to its statistical significance. Based on this scoring system, patients with more than 10 points should be considered to have ASD; patients with more than 6 points are suspected of having ASD.

8.5 Hand Eczema and Occupational Skin Diseases

HE has a substantial health economic and sociomedical impact, and occupational skin disease has been the most commonly reported occupational disease for years. Occupations at particularly high risk include hairdressers, bakers, butchers, florists, cashiers, electroplaters, dental technicians,

Table 8.3 Criteria of atopic skin diathesis (ASD). Individuals with at least 10 points have an ASD; between 7 and 9 points, ASD is suspected[a]

	Points
Family history of atopy (1st degree relatives)	
Eczema	2
Respiratory atopy	1
Personal history of atopy	
Flexural eczema	
Allergic rhinitis	1
Allergic asthma	1
Cradle cap	1
Itch when sweating	3
Intolerance to wool	3
Intolerance to metal	1
Photophobia	1
Minor manifestations of AE	
Xerosis	3
Ear rhagades	2
Dyshidrosis	2
Pityriasis alba	2
Atopic foot/pulpitis sicca	2
Nipple eczema	2
Perlèche	1
Atopic stigmata	
Atopic palms	2
Hertoghe sign	2
Dirty neck	2
Keratosis pilaris	1
White dermographism	3
Acrocyanosis	1

[a]Adapted from [18, 23]

machine operators, workers in metal surface processing, and healthcare workers [6, 19]. The annual incidence of new reports of occupational skin diseases is 0.7–0.8 per 1,000 employees [20, 21], yet the number of occupational skin conditions that go unreported is many times greater [22]. In a study conducted at 10 European centers, 28 % of HE patients were unfit for work, and disability persisted for longer than 12 weeks in 12 % of cases [5]. In this study, the etiology was considered occupational in 52 % of the HE patients.

Occupations associated with an increased risk of HE are listed in Table 8.4. Most risks are related to irritants and/or allergy-inducing materials present at the workplace. Common risks, and thus particularly relevant ones to occupational dermatology, are not necessarily strong irritants or allergens. Important irritants include water, for instance, in employees working in wet conditions [1].

Table 8.4 Professional fields with an increased risk of occupational hand eczema[a]

I. Risk to the skin due to working in wet conditions[b] (moist environment) – wet working conditions are defined as jobs in which:
Employees routinely spend a considerable amount of time, i.e., more than ¼ of each shift (or roughly 2 h), with their hands in a moist environment
Must wear waterproof gloves for the same amount of time
Must wash their hands often or intensely (about 20 times or less often but with more aggressive hand washing with the same effect)
II. Occupations involving considerable stress to the skin (highly problematic for patients with atopic eczema): hairdressers, bakers, florists, pastry makers, massage therapists, tilers, metal polishers, cutters, dental technicians, employees in photo laboratories, cooks, painters, craftsmen working with varnish, tanners, hospital and nursing care workers
III. Occupations involving stress to the skin (problematic for patients with atopic eczema): ceramic and glass painters, drilling jobs, plasterers, certain food industry jobs (butcher, vegetable processing), bricklayers and concrete workers, laboratory workers, printers, housekeeping, cleaning services, and gastronomy

[a]Adapted from [9]

[b]See also TRGS 401 Risk related to skin contact – identification, evaluation, measures (Internet link: http://www.baua.de/de/Themen-von-A-Z/Gefahrstoffe/TRGS/TRGS-401_content.html)

In some occupations, such as hairdressing, the responsible allergens are relatively well known, while in others (e.g., metalworkers) the allergens are often unknown or are based on isolated case reports. This may mean that for patch testing, comprehensive testing with less standardized substances is needed.

Environmental factors (low humidity, high temperatures, occlusion, sweating) can be very detrimental to the epidermal barrier and given the same level exposure may enhance the effect of irritants and/or allergens. Contact dermatitis often initially manifests as a result of the combination of occupational exposure and individual predisposition to disease given constitutional factors (e.g., atopic skin diathesis).

Table 8.5 A practical guide for occupational pre-employment counseling in persons with atopic eczema (AE)[a]

Step 1: Defining the occupational risk category	Step 2: Occupational counseling for each risk category
First risk category Moderate to severe AE with hand involvement Chronic hand eczema Change of work due to irritant contact dermatitis	For the first risk category: Occupations with wet work or other exposure to irritants not advisable Pre-employment medical-occupational counseling and medical advice is required
Second risk category AE without involvement of the hands Dyshidrosis (history of pompholyx) Allergic rhinitis or asthma in occupations with increased risk for type I allergies (e.g., bakers)	For the second risk category: Technical and organizational protection measures Personal protection measures Repeated follow-up examinations every 3 months in the first year and every 6 months in the second year
Third risk category Evidence for low threshold to nonspecific irritants: Wool intolerance Itch due to sweating Unusually dry skin	For the third risk category: Technical and organizational protection measures Follow-up examinations after 6, 12, and 24 months

[a]Adapted from [24]

8.6 Occupational Guidelines for Patients with a Personal History of AE

Summarizing the evidence thus far, it is clear that AE patients run a certain risk of developing HE, and that this risk is dependent on the severity of their AE. Thus, in evaluating AE patients, a history of hand involvement or a present involvement of the hands plays a central role. Proper advice at a pre-employment examination is essential, and regular follow-up and counseling of persons with an increased risk will help them to keep functioning in their jobs. Recently, the German occupational organizations (which also administer the occupational insurance funds) have reached consensus on a series of guidelines for pre-employment advice to employees opting for occupations that carry increased skin risk. As an analogy, this chapter can be concluded with Table 8.5, which presents guidelines for preventive advice to individuals with a personal history of AE. As a first step, the risk category is defined, and as a second step the corresponding advice is formulated.

Although the guidelines are restricted to occupational aspects, it is clear that domestic exposure, such as household wet work or handicraft work, should not be neglected and that this should be an important component of occupational counseling.

References

1. Diepgen TL, Elsner P, Schliemann S, Fartasch M, Köllner A, Skudlik C, John SM, Worm M. Guidelines on the management of hand eczema. J Dtsch Dermatol Ges. 2009;7 Suppl 3:S1–16.
2. Diepgen TL, Andersen KE, Chosidow O, Pieter Jan Coenraads PJ, Elsner P, English J, et al. Guidelines for diagnosis, treatment and prevention of hand eczema. 2013 (submitted).
3. Apfelbacher CJ, Akst W, Molin S, Schmitt J, Bauer A, Weisshaar E, et al. Characteristics and provision of care in patients with chronic hand eczema: updated data from the carpe registry. 2013 (in press).
4. McFadden JP. Hand eczema. In: Rycroft RJG, Menne T, Frosch PJ, Lepoittevin JP, editors. Textbook of contact dermatitis. Berlin: Springer; 2001. p. 403–11.
5. Diepgen TL, Andersen KE, Brandao FM, Bruze M, Bruynzeel DP, Frosch P, et al. Hand eczema classification: a cross-sectional, multicentre study of the aetiology and morphology of hand eczema. Br J Dermatol. 2009;160:353–8.
6. Skoet R, Olsen J, Mathiesen B, Iversen L, Johansen JD, Agner T. A survey of occupational hand eczema in Denmark. Contact Dermatitis. 2004; 51:159–66.
7. Jensen CS, Menne T, Lisby S, Kristiansen J, Veien NK. Experimental systemic contact dermatitis from nickel: a dose-response study. Contact Dermatitis. 2003;49:124–32.
8. Hogan DJ, Dannaker CJ, Maibach HI. The prognosis of contact dermatitis. J Am Acad Dermatol. 1990;23:300–7.
9. Diepgen TL. Occupational skin diseases. J Dtsch Dermatol Ges. 2012;10:297–313.
10. Lammintausta K, Kalimo K. Atopy and hand dermatitis in hospital wet work. Contact Dermatitis. 1981;7:301–8.

11. Rystedt I. Hand eczema and long term prognosis in atopic dermatitis (thesis). Acta Derm Venereol. 1985; 117(suppl):1–59.
12. Diepgen TL. Occupational aspects of atopic eczema with emphasis on atopic hand eczema. In: Ring J, Przybilla B, Ruzicka T, editors. Handbook of atopic eczema. Berlin: Springer; 2006. p. 166–77.
13. Breit R, Leutgeb C, Bandmann HJ. Zum neurodermitischen Handekzem. Arch Dermatol Forsch. 1972;244: 353.
14. Forsbeck M, Skog E, Asbrink E. Atopic hand dermatitis: a comparison with atopic dermatitis without hand involvement, especially with respect to influence of work and development of contact sensitization. Acta Derm Venereol (Stockh). 1983;63:9.
15. Rystedt I. Factors influencing the occurrence of hand eczema in adults with a history of atopic dermatitis in childhood. Contact Dermatitis. 1985;12:185–91.
16. Lammintausta K. Risk factors for hand dermatitis in wet work. Turku: Academic dissertation. 1982.
17. Diepgen TL, Fartasch M, Hornstein OP. Evaluation and relevance of atopic basic and minor features in patients with atopic dermatitis and in the general population. Acta Derm Venereol Suppl. 1989;144:50–4.
18. Diepgen TL, Sauerbrei W, Fartasch M. Development and validation of diagnostic scores for atopic dermatitis incorporating criteria of data quality and practical usefulness. J Clin Epidemiol. 1996;49:1031–8.
19. Diepgen TL. Occupational skin-disease data in Europe. Int Arch Occup Environ Health. 2003;76:331–8.
20. Dickel H, Bruckner T, Berhard-Klimt C, Koch T, Scheidt R, Diepgen TL. Surveillance scheme for occupational skin disease in the Saarland, FRG: first report from BKH-S. Contact Dermatitis. 2002;46:197–206.
21. Lerbaek A, Kyvik KO, Ravn H, Menne T, Agner T. Incidence of hand eczema in a population-based twin cohort: genetic and environmental risk factors. Br J Dermatol. 2007;157:552–7.
22. Diepgen TL, Schmidt A. Werden Inzidenz und Prävalenz berufsbedingter Hauterkrankungen unterschätzt? Arbeitsmed Sozialmed Umweltmed. 2002;37: 477–80.
23. Diepgen TL, Fartasch M, Hornstein OP. Kriterien zur Beurteilung der atopischen Hautdiathese. Dermatosen. 1991;39:79–83.
24. Coenraads PJ, Diepgen TL. Risk for hand eczema in employees with past or present atopic dermatitis. Int Arch Occup Environ Health. 1998;71:7–13.

Chemical Skin Burns and Hand Eczema

9

Magnus Bruze and Malin Engfeldt

Contents

M. Bruze, M.D., Ph.D. • M. Engfeldt, M.Sc. (Chem Eng), Ph.D. (✉)
Department of Occupational and Environmental Dermatology, Skåne University Hospital, Lund University, Jan Waldenströmsgata 18, Malmö 205 02, Sweden
e-mail: magnus.bruze@med.lu.se; malin.engfeldt@med.lu.se

9.1 Introduction

Chemical skin burns are particularly common in industry, but also occur in the non-working environment. Corrosive chemicals used in hobbies are an increasing cause of skin burns. Disinfectants and cleansers are examples of household products that can cause chemical burns. In most cases, the cause of a chemical burn is obvious to the affected persons, and the damage is minimal and heals without medical care. Sometimes, the chemical burns are severe and extensive, with risk of complications and long-term disability. In the acute stage, there is a varying risk of systemic effects, including a fatal outcome, depending on exposure conditions and incriminating agent.

9.2 Definition

- A chemical burn is an acute, severe irritant reaction in which the cells have been damaged to a point where there is no return to viability.
- The corrosive action of chemicals depends on chemical properties as well as body region, previous skin damage, and possibly individual resistance capacity.

This chapter is based upon Bruze M, Fregert S, Gruvberger B. Chemical skin burns. In: L. Kanerva L, Elsner P, Wahlberg JE, Maibach HI, eds. Handbook of occupational dermatology. Berlin: Springer; 2000; with permission from Springer Science+Business Media.

A. Alikhan et al. (eds.), *Textbook of Hand Eczema*,
DOI 10.1007/978-3-642-39546-8_9, © Springer-Verlag Berlin Heidelberg 2014

- Products that, under ordinary exposure, cause weak irritant reactions can, under occlusion, cause chemical burns.

A chemical burn is an acute, severe irritant reaction in which the cells have been damaged to a point where there is no return to viability (i.e., a necrosis develops) [1–3]. A single skin exposure to certain chemicals can result in a chemical burn. These chemicals react with intra- and intercellular components in the skin. The action of toxic chemicals varies, giving partly different reactions morphologically. They can damage the horny layer, cell membranes, lysosomes, mast cells, leukocytes, DNA synthesis, blood vessels, enzyme systems, and metabolism. The corrosive action of chemicals depends on properties such as concentration, pH, alkalinity, acidity, temperature, solubility, interaction with other substances, and duration of contact. It also depends on the body region, previous skin damage, and possibly on individual resistance capacity.

Many substances cause chemical burns only when applied under occlusion from, for example, gloves, boots, clothes, face masks, adhesive plasters, rings, or from skin folds (e.g., under breasts and in the axillae). Products that, under ordinary exposure, cause weak irritant reactions can, under occlusion, cause chemical burns (e.g., detergents, solvents, plants, topical medicaments, toiletries, pesticides, preservatives, plastic monomers, and Portland cement).

Chemical and thermal burns differ. Chemical agents cause progressive damage until either no more chemical remains unreacted in the tissue or the agent is inactivated by treatment. Thermal damaging effects cease shortly after removal of the heat source.

The most commonly reported chemicals that can cause chemical burns are listed in Table 9.1.

9.3 Diagnosis

It is usually easy to diagnose a chemical skin burn, as the symptoms are easily recognized and the exposure to a corrosive agent obvious. However, sometimes the exposure is concealed, at least initially. For example, hospital personnel may be exposed to ethylene oxide remaining in gowns and straps after sterilization [4], and cleaners may occasionally be exposed to a corrosive agent contaminating nonhazardous objects in a laboratory. Corrosive substances under occlusion may also confuse and delay the diagnosis. Occasionally, a chemical burn can mimic other dermatoses (e.g., ethylene oxide can mimic bullous impetigo).

9.4 Clinical Features

- Morphologically, chemical burns are characterized by erythema, blisters, erosions, ulcers, and necrosis with surrounding erythema.
- Alkalis, with the exception of hydrofluoric acid, often give more severe damage than acids.

Not only the skin but also the eyes, lips, mouth, esophagus, nasal septum, glottis, and lungs can be directly affected. As a result of resorption, the blood, bone marrow, liver, kidneys, nerves, brain, and other organs can be damaged. The most common locations of chemical burns on the skin are the hands and face/neck, but the whole body can be affected. The major symptoms are burning and smarting. Morphologically, chemical burns are characterized by erythema, blisters, erosions, ulcers, and necrosis with surrounding erythema. Usually, the symptoms develop immediately or in close connection to exposure, but certain chemicals, such as phenols, diluted hydrofluoric acid, and sulfur mustard gas can give delayed reactions that first appear several hours, or even a day, after exposure.

9.4.1 Strong Acids

Strong acids coagulate skin proteins, and further penetration is diminished by the barrier formed. Principally, all strong acids give the same symptoms and major features, including erythema, blisters, and necrosis. Some acids discolor the skin (e.g., nitric acid gives a yellow color). The action of hydrofluoric acid in the skin differs from that of strong acids [5, 6]. It is a weak acid that exists predominantly in the undissociated

Table 9.1 Agents causing chemical burns[a]

Acids	Bases	Miscellaneous
Acetic acid	Amines	Acetyl chloride
Acrylic acid	Ammonia	Acrolein
Benzoic acid	Barium hydroxide	Acrylates
Boric acid	Calcium carbonate	Acrylonitril
Bromoacetic acid	Calcium hydroxide	Alkali ethoxides
Chloroacetic acids	Calcium oxide	Alkali methoxides
Chlorosulfuric acid	Hydrazine	Allyl diiodine
Fluorophosphoric acid	Lithium hydroxide	Aluminum bromide
Fluorosilicic acid	Potassium hydroxide	Aluminum chloride
Fluorosulfonic acid	Sodium carbonate	Aluminum trichloride
Formic acid	Sodium hydroxide	Ammonium difluoride
Fumaric acid	Sodium metasilicate	Ammonium persulfate
Hydrobromic acid		Ammonium sulfide
Hydrochloric acid		Antimone trioxide
Hydrofluoric acid		Aromatic hydrocarbons
Lactic acid		Arsenic oxides
Nitric acid		Benzene
Perchloric acid		Benzoyl chloride
Peroxyacetic acid		Benzoyl chlorodimethylhydantoin
Phosphonic acids		Benzoyl chloroformiate
Phosphoric acids		Borax
Phthalic acids		Boron tribromide
Picric acid		Bromine
Propionic acid		Bromotrifluoride
Salicylic acid		Calcium carbide
Sulfonic acids		Cantharides
Sulfuric acid		Carbon disulfide
Tartaric acid		Carbon tetrachloride
Toluenesulfonic acid		Chlorobenzene
Trifluoroacetic acid		Chlorhexidine gluconate
		Chlorinated acetophenons (tear gas)
		Chlorinated solvents
		Chlorocresols
		Chloroform
		Chlorophenols
		Chromates
		Chromium oxychloride
		Chromium trioxide
		Creosote
		Cresolic compounds
		Crotonaldehyde
		Peroxides
		Benzoyl
		Cumene
		Cyclohexanone
		Hydrogen
		Methyl ethyl ketone
		Potassium

(continued)

Table 9.1 (continued)

Acids	Bases	Miscellaneous
		Sodium
		Phenolic compounds
		Phosphorus
		Phosphorus bromides
		Phosphorus chlorides
		Phosphorus oxychloride
		Phosphorus oxides
		Piperazine
		Potassium
		Potassium cyanide
		Potassium difluoride
		Potassium hypochlorite
		Potassium permanganate
		Povidone-iodine
		Propionic oxide
		Propylene oxide
		Quaternary ammonium compounds
		Reactive diluents
		Sodium
		Sodium borohydride
		Sodium difluoride
		Sodium hypochlorite
		Sodium sulfite
		Sodium thiosulfate
		Styrene
		Sulfur dichloride
		Sulfur dioxide
		Sulfur mustard
		Tetramethylammonium hydroxide
		Thioglycollates
		Thionyl chloride
		Tributyltin oxide
		Trichloroethylene
		Trifluoroacetic anhydride
		Turpentine
		Vinyl pyridine
		White spirit
		Zinc chloride

[a]The chemicals listed are the most common reported to cause chemical burns in industries, hobbies, and households. Acids and alkalis have been grouped separately, as the corrosive effect within the respective group is exerted through the same mechanism. The other compounds are listed together, although their corrosive effects are mediated through different mechanisms. The list contains strong corrosive substances and also less irritating compounds that require special conditions (e.g., occlusion) to give chemical burns

state, which permits it to penetrate deep into the skin, where the fluoride ion is liberated and causes necrosis and electrolyte abnormalities by binding the cations Ca^{2+} and Mg^{2+} [7]. Penetration may continue for days. When an area above 1 % of the total body surface is affected, systemic effects can arise. Hydrofluoric acid causes much more intense pain than other acids. The intense pain is presumably due to electrolyte shifts at nerve endings caused by the fluoride ion, which is a metabolic poison that inhibits the Na-K ATPase, allowing efflux of potassium [7]. Hydrofluoric acid can penetrate to the bone and cause decalcification. Also, fluorides and fluorosilicic acid can give the same type of symptoms. However, not all substances containing fluorine have the capability to produce fluoride. Trifluoroacetic acid used industrially in the production of peptides, for example, does not release fluoride ions, but it is a strong acid and should be treated accordingly [8].

9.4.2 Alkalis

Alkalis often give more severe damage than acids, with the exception of hydrofluoric acid [9–11]. The necrotic skin first appears dark brown, then changes to black. Later, the skin becomes hard, dry, and cracked. Generally, no blisters appear in the skin. Alkalis split proteins and lipids, and there is saponification of the released fatty acids. The emulsifying effect of the soap formed facilitates further penetration into deeper layers of the skin. Chemical burns from alkaline chemicals are generally more painful than from acids. Because of its alkalinity, cement mixed with water can cause an acute ulcerative damage [12–19]. Severe skin damage has involved the lower limbs, often after kneeling on wet concrete or when getting inside shoes. Sometimes, necrotic skin appears 8–12 h after exposure. Rarely, hands can also be affected, particularly when the insides of gloves are contaminated.

9.4.3 Phenolic Compounds

Phenolic compounds such as phenol, cresol, chlorocresol, and unhardened phenolic resins penetrate the skin easily and can damage peripheral nerves resulting in insensibility, sometimes, without a visible damage to the skin. After exposure to phenolic compounds, the local blood vessels become constricted, contributing to the development of necrosis. Shock and renal damage can appear after absorption of phenolic compounds [20–22].

9.4.4 Sulfur Mustard

Sulfur mustard, 2,2′-dichlorodiethyl sulfide, is a chemical warfare agent [23–25]. It is a liquid below and a gas above 14°C. On the skin, the liquid causes blisters and necrosis 10–12 h after skin exposure. The gas attacks mainly the eyes and respiratory organs. Sometimes the skin is affected by direct gas contact, and the chemical burn then clinically appears 3–6 h after exposure; initial redness is followed by blisters and ulcers. Tear gas can cause a bullous dermatitis [26].

9.4.5 Ethylene Oxide

Ethylene oxide gas used for sterilization of surgical materials can remain in these objects for several days, if not ventilated well enough [4, 27]. Thus, the exposure to ethylene oxide is not always obvious, and the symptoms, including erythema, edema, and large bullae, may be misdiagnosed as other skin diseases.

Accidental skin exposure to chemicals under high pressure (e.g., hydraulic oil) can result in deep penetration into the skin, where a chemical burn with necrosis can develop.

9.5 Treatment

- Chemical agents cause progressive damage until either no more chemical remains unreacted in the tissue or the agent is inactivated by treatment.
- Rinsing with water is the first-aid treatment.
- Certain types of toxic agents, such as hydrofluoric acid, phosphorous, bromine, iodine, phenol compounds, and sulfur mustard, require specific antidotes.
- Several chemicals can also give systemic effects without severe skin injury; for hydrofluoric acid or chromic acid, systemic effects can occur when more than 1 % of the total body surface is affected.

Table 9.2 Treatment for chemical skin burns caused by some specific chemicals

Chemical	Treatment
Hydrofluoric acid	Calcium gluconate gel (2.5 %)
Phosphorous	Copper (II) sulfate in water (1 %)
Bromine, iodine	Sodium thiosulfate in water (5 %)
Phenolic compounds	Polyethylene glycol 300 or 400
	Ethanol in water (10 %)
Sulfur mustard liquid	Mixture of 75 % calcium hypochlorite and 25 % magnesium sulfate

Rinsing with water, preferably tepid running tap water, is the first-aid treatment. Irrigation should not be done at high pressure, as the corrosive agent may be splashed on other parts of the body or on the persons treating the burn. Treatment should be started immediately after exposure, and copious volumes of water should be supplied, sometimes for hours. Occasionally, chemical burns are caused by substances which are insoluble in water; in such cases, a solution of water and soap should be used instead. Sometimes specific antidotes for certain types of chemical burns are required (Table 9.2). Two specific products are marketed as irrigation fluids for personal decontamination of hydrofluoric acid (Hexafluorine) and other strong acids and bases (Diphoterine) [28, 29]. Clothes, watches, rings, shoes, and so forth can be contaminated, so they should be removed.

Theoretically, neutralizing solutions could be an alternative treatment to water after exposure to acids and alkalis [30–32]. However, this is not recommended for two reasons: (1) irrigation should not be delayed while waiting for a specific antidote and (2) neutralization of the corrosive agent may produce an exothermic reaction, and the heat can cause further damage [33]. The pH of the skin can be monitored by simply holding a pH paper against the skin.

Heat is generated when strong sulfuric acid and phosphorus acid are exposed to water; hence, a thermal burn can add to the chemical burn. To prevent this, copious volumes of running water should be applied. However, water is contradicted in extinguishing burning metal fragments of sodium, potassium, and lithium because a chemical burn can be caused by hydroxides formed when water reacts with hot metals. These metals spontaneously ignite when exposed to water. To extinguish the burning metal, sand can be used. The burn should then be covered with mineral oil to isolate the metal from water. Metal pieces should be mechanically removed, and embedded pieces surgically removed. First, the area is irrigated with water to prevent an alkali burn from the hydroxides formed from the metal and water naturally present in the skin.

Skin exposed to hydrofluoric acid should be carefully irrigated with copious volumes of water and then treated with calcium gluconate gel (2.5 %) by massaging into the burned skin for at least 30 min [32, 34–36]. The gel should be applied repeatedly to the skin until the pain has disappeared. Necrotic tissue should be excised, blisters debrided, and the underlying tissue treated with the calcium preparation. Nails should be removed if the acid penetrates to the nail bed and causes pain there. If the topical treatment does not have an effect within 2 h, 10 % calcium gluconate (0.5 ml/cm^2) should be injected into and under the lesions. No anesthetics should be given since the disappearance of pain is a sign of successful treatment. Without treatment, the burn can continue in depth for several weeks.

Superficial chemical burns from chromic acid over more than 1 % of the total body surface may cause systemic damage to many organs [37]. Therefore, immediate irrigation with copious volumes of water is necessary. Thereafter, and within 2 h after the exposure, all burned tissue must be excised. To remove the circulating chromium, peritoneal dialysis has to be carried out in the first 24 h. Solid particles of, for example, lime and cement tend to fix to the skin and should be mechanically removed before or during irrigation.

Phosphorus is oxidized by air and can ignite spontaneously, causing a thermal burn [38–41]. In water, oxidized phosphorus forms phosphoric acid, which can cause a chemical burn; therefore, particles should be mechanically removed before washing with soap and water. The skin is treated with 1 % copper (II) sulfate in water, which reacts with phosphorus and forms black copper phosphide, making any remaining phosphorus visible and easily removable. Wet dressings of copper sulfate should never be applied on wounds because of the risk of systemic copper poisoning. To minimize the copper absorption, a water solution of 5 % sodium bicarbonate and 3 % copper sulfate suspended in 1 % hydroxyethyl cellulose can be used for irrigation instead. It should be stressed that copper is toxic. Copper sulfate must, therefore, be used only for a few minutes to visualize phosphorous, and after mechanical removal of the phosphide, the skin should be irrigated with water.

Skin contaminated with bromine or iodine should be washed with soap and water and then treated with 5 % sodium thiosulfate, which reacts with the agents, forming ions less hazardous to the skin [42, 43].

Skin contaminated with phenolic compounds can initially be washed with soap and water and as early as possible treated with undiluted polyethylene glycol 300 or 400, or with 10 % ethanol, which all dissolve phenolic compounds [20–22]. Tissue with deep damage from phenolic compounds should be excised immediately.

Skin contaminated with sulfur mustard liquid should be treated with a mixture of 75 % calcium hypochlorite and 25 % magnesium sulfate for some minutes before washing with soap and water. Contaminated objects should also be treated with this mixture [23–25].

Hot tar, pitch, and asphalt mainly cause thermal burns. They stick to the skin and should not be removed mechanically, as the skin can be further damaged, which increases the risk of secondary infection. The material will fall off spontaneously in due time.

Generally, an antibacterial cream should be applied to chemical skin burns to protect the surface and prevent secondary infection. If there is a significant element of inflammation in non-necrotic areas, a mild topical corticosteroid preparation can be used. Frequent examinations of primarily superficial and limited burns are advisable as they can become deeper in a few days.

Surgical treatments, such as excision, debridement of blisters, transplantation, and removal of nails, can be of great value. When a limb is affected circumferentially, there is a risk of blood vessel compression. The best method for treating the black, adherent necrotic tissue caused by cement and other toxic compounds is excision. Excision of necrotic tissue can diminish the healing time of cement burns from 8–10 weeks to 3 weeks.

Several chemicals can also give systemic effects without severe skin injury (e.g., phenolic compounds, hydrofluoric acid, chromic acid, sulfur mustard, and gasoline) [44, 45]. When there is a risk of systemic damage, an analysis including hematological screening and liver and kidney function should be performed, both at the first examination and then later in the course of treatment. These analyses are performed mainly to enable necessary precautions and measures to prevent and diminish damage on internal organs, but also partly for legal reasons.

Patients with severe and extensive skin damage and/or with systemic symptoms should be treated in intensive care units. Hospitalization is also recommended for persons having concurrent illnesses, implying that they are high-risk patients, as well as for persons with chemical burns on the hands, feet, and perineum [44, 45].

9.6 Complications

When a potential sensitizer has caused a chemical burn, the patient should be patch tested with the sensitizer after healing of the burn.

Chemical skin burns can cause hyper- or hypopigmentation. Chemical burns involving deeper parts of the skin heal with scarring. Tumors of both malignant and benign types may rarely develop in scars. In the acute stage of chemical burns from phenolic compounds and hydrofluoric acid/fluorides, the sensory nerve system is frequently affected.

Many contact sensitizers also have irritant properties. Patch testing with such sensitizers at high concentrations can cause an irritant reaction or a chemical burn, which seems to facilitate active sensitization. However, only a few sensitizers can cause chemical burns without occlusion (e.g., formaldehyde, chromic acid, amines, chloroacetophenone, some plastic monomers, and methylisothiazolinones). Even a single contact with these chemicals can cause a chemical burn and induce sensitization, with a subsequent risk of allergic contact dermatitis [46–48]. Therefore, when a potential sensitizer has caused a chemical burn, the patient should be patch tested with the sensitizer after healing of the burn, independent of the subsequent development of eczema.

Another type of eczematous dermatitis that can follow after a chemical burn is "post-traumatic eczema" [49]. It can present as discoid eczema and is a poorly understood complication of skin injuries [50]. It can appear after both physical and chemical skin injuries, including chemical burns, and is always unrelated to infection and topical treatment.

Conclusion

Thousands of chemicals and products can cause chemical skin burns, some only under special circumstances (e.g., occlusion). Clinically, a chemical burn is characterized by erythema, blisters, and necrotic skin. Some corrosive chemicals, such as phenolic compounds, sulfur mustard, chromic acid, hydrofluoric acid, and gasoline, may cause systemic effects that require hospitalization. Other chemical burns, particularly those affecting hands, feet, and perineum, may also require hospitalization. To prevent and diminish the damage after exposure to corrosive agents, it is important to administer immediate treatment. Irrigation with copious volumes of water is a universal remedy, except for treatment of burning metal fragments of sodium, potassium, and lithium. First-aid treatment after exposure to water-insoluble corrosive agents consists of washing with soap and water. Sometimes, specific antidotes are needed as for chemical burns from hydrofluoric acid, phenolic compounds, phosphorous, iodine, bromine, and sulfur mustard (see Table 9.2). Surgical intervention may be required for certain chemical burns. A few corrosive compounds are potential sensitizers, and one exposure to such a compound may cause a chemical burn and induce sensitization with a subsequent allergic contact dermatitis.

References

1. Cartotto RC, Peters WJ, Neligan PC, Douglas LG, Beeston J. Chemical burns. Can J Surg. 1996;39(3):205–11.
2. Sykes RA, Mani MM, Hiebert JM. Chemical burns: retrospective review. J Burn Care Rehabil. 1986;7(4):7–343.
3. Stewart CE. Chemical skin burns. Am Fam Physician. 1985;31(6):149–57.
4. Biro L, Fisher AA, Price E. Ethylene oxide burns. A hospital outbreak involving 19 women. Arch Dermatol. 1974;110(6):924–5.
5. Kirkpatrick JJ, Enion DS, Burd DA. Hydrofluoric acid burns: a review. Burns. 1995;21(7):483–93.
6. Vance MV. Hydrofluoric acid (HF) burns. In: Adams RM, editor. Occupational skin disease. 2nd ed. Philadelphia: WB Saunders; 1990. p. 18–21.
7. Palao R, Monge I, Ruiz M, Barret JP. Chemical burns: pathophysiology and treatment. Burns. 2010;36(3):295–304.
8. Dahlin J, Engfeldt M, Svedman C, Mowitz M, Zimerson E, Isaksson M, et al. Chemical burns caused by trifluoroacetic acid. Contact Dermatitis 2013;69:176–80.
9. Gelmetti C, Cecca E. Caustic ulcers caused by calcium hydroxide in 2 adolescent football players. Contact Dermatitis. 1992;27(4):265–6.
10. Beausang E, Herbert K. Burns from a dust explosion. Burns. 1994;20(6):551–2.
11. Winemaker M, Douglas L, Peters W. Combination alkali/thermal burns caused by 'black liquor' in the pulp and paper industry. Burns. 1992;18(1):68–70.
12. Adams RM. Cement burns. In: Adams RM, editor. Occupational skin disease. 2nd ed. Philadelphia: WB Saunders; 1990. p. 15–6.
13. Fisher AA. Chromate dermatitis and cement burns. In: Fisher AA, editor. Contact dermatitis. 3rd ed. Philadelphia: Lea & Febiger; 1986. p. 762–72.
14. Lane PR, Hogan DJ. Chronic pain and scarring from cement burns. Arch Dermatol. 1985;121(3):368–9.
15. Stoermer D, Wolz G. Cement burns. Contact Dermatitis. 1983;9(5):421–2.
16. McGeown G. Cement burns of the hands. Contact Dermatitis. 1984;10(4):246.
17. Tosti A, Peluso AM, Varotti C. Skin burns due to transit-mixed Portland cement. Contact Dermatitis. 1989;21(1):58.
18. Morley SE, Humzah D, McGregor JC, Gilbert PM. Cement-related burns. Burns. 1996;22(8):646–7.
19. Onuba O, Essiet A. Cement burns of the heels. Contact Dermatitis. 1986;14(5):325.
20. Lin CH, Yang JY. Chemical burn with cresol intoxication and multiple organ failure. Burns. 1992;18(2):162–6.
21. Horch R, Spilker G, Stark GB. Phenol burns and intoxications. Burns. 1994;20(1):45–50.
22. Shibata K, Yoshita Y, Matsumoto H. Extensive chemical burns from toluene. Am J Emerg Med. 1994;12(3):353–5.

23. Newman-Taylor AJ, Morris AJ. Experience with mustard gas casualties. Lancet. 1991;337(8735):242.
24. Smith WJ, Dunn MA. Medical defense against blistering chemical warfare agents. Arch Dermatol. 1991;127(8):1207–13.
25. Ruhl CM, Park SJ, Danisa O, Morgan RF, Papirmeister B, Sidell FR, et al. A serious skin sulfur mustard burn from an artillery shell. J Emerg Med. 1994;12(2): 66–159.
26. Zekri AM, King WW, Yeung R, Taylor WR. Acute mass burns caused by o-chlorobenzylidene malononitrile (CS) tear gas. Burns. 1995;21(8):586–9.
27. Fisher AA. Ethylene oxide (EO) burns. In: Adams RM, editor. Occupational skin disease. 2nd ed. Philadelphia: WB Saunders; 1990. p. 17–8.
28. Donoghue AM. Diphoterine for alkali chemical splashes to the skin at alumina refineries. Int J Dermatol. 2010;49(8):894–900.
29. Mathieu L, Burgher F, Blomet J. Comparative evaluation of the active eye and skin chemical splash decontamination solutions Diphoterine and Hexafluorine with water and other rinsing solutions: effects on burn. J Chem Health Saf. 2007;14:32–9.
30. Erdmann D, Hussmann J, Kucan JO. Treatment of a severe alkali burn. Burns. 1996;22(2):141–6.
31. Yano K, Hata Y, Matsuka K, Ito O, Matsuda H. Effects of washing with a neutralizing agent on alkaline skin injuries in an experimental model. Burns. 1994;20(1): 36–9.
32. Dunn BJ, MacKinnon MA, Knowlden NF, Billmaier DJ, Derelanko MJ, Rusch GM, et al. Topical treatments for hydrofluoric acid dermal burns. Further assessment of efficacy using an experimental piq model. J Occup Environ Med. 1996;38(5):507–14.
33. Sawhney CP, Kaushish R. Acid and alkali burns: considerations in management. Burns. 1989;15(2): 132–4.
34. Seyb ST, Noordhoek L, Botens S, Mani MM. A study to determine the efficacy of treatments for hydrofluoric acid burns. J Burn Care Rehabil. 1995;16(3 Pt 1): 7–253.
35. Chick LR, Borah G. Calcium carbonate gel therapy for hydrofluoric acid burns of the hand. Plast Reconstr Surg. 1990;86(5):935–40.
36. Anderson WJ, Anderson JR. Hydrofluoric acid burns of the hand: mechanism of injury and treatment. J Hand Surg Am. 1988;13(1):52–7.
37. Terrill PJ, Gowar JP. Chromic acid burns; beware, be aggressive, be watchful. Br J Plast Surg. 1990;43(6): 699–701.
38. Eldad A, Wisoki M, Cohen H, Breiterman S, Chaouat M, Wexler MR, et al. Phosphorous burns: evaluation of various modalities for primary treatment. J Burn Care Rehabil. 1995;16(1):49–55.
39. Kaufman T, Ullmann Y, Har-Shai Y. Phosphorus burns: a practical approach to local treatment. J Burn Care Rehabil. 1988;9(5):5–474.
40. Eldad A, Chaouat M, Weinberg A, Neuman A, Ben Meir P, Rotem M, et al. Phosphorous pentachloride chemical burn–a slowly healing injury. Burns. 1992;18(4):340–1.
41. Eldad A, Simon GA. The phosphorous burn–a preliminary comparative experimental study of various forms of treatment. Burns. 1991;17(3):198–200.
42. White A, Joseet M. Burns from iodine. Anaesthesia. 1990;45(1):75.
43. Corazza M, Bulciolu G, Spisani L, Virgili A. Chemical burns following irritant contact with povidone-iodine. Contact Dermatitis. 1997;36(2):115–6.
44. Andersen KE. Systemic toxicity from percutaneous absorption of industrial chemicals. In: Adams RM, editor. Occupational skin disease. 2nd ed. Philadelphia: WB Saunders; 1990. p. 73–88.
45. Chan TC, Williams SR, Clark RF. Formic acid skin burns resulting in systemic toxicity. Ann Emerg Med. 1995;26(3):383–6.
46. Bruze M, DAhlquist I, Gruvberger B. Chemical burns and allergic contact dermatitis due to Kathon WT. Am J Contact Dermatitis. 1990;1:3–91.
47. Kanerva L, Tarvainen K, Pinola A, Leino T, Granlund H, Estlander T, et al. A single accidental exposure may result in a chemical burn, primary sensitization and allergic contact dermatitis. Contact Dermatitis. 1994;31(4):229–35.
48. Isaksson M, Gruvberger B, Bruze M. Occupational contact allergy and dermatitis from methylisothiazolinone after contact with wall covering glue and after a chemical burn from a biocide. Dermatitis. 2004;15(4): 201–5.
49. Mathias CG. Post-traumatic eczema. Dermatol Clin. 1988;6(1):35–42.
50. Wilkinson DS. Discoid eczema as a consequence of contact with irritants. Contact Dermatitis. 1979;5(2): 118–9.

10 Mechanical Trauma and Hand Eczema

Klaus Ejner Andersen and Flemming Andersen

Contents

K.E. Andersen, M.D., Dr., Med., Sc. (✉)
F. Andersen, M.D., Ph.D..
Department of Dermato-venerology
and the Allergy Centre,
Odense University Hospital,
Sdr. Boulevard 29, 5000 Odense C, Denmark
e-mail: klaus.ejner.andersen@rsyd.dk;
flemming.andersen@rsyd.dk

10.1 Introduction

Constant low-level mechanical trauma to an area of the skin, as encountered in handicraft jobs, may result in the development of the following:

- "Trademarks" – localized hardening of skin due to use of trade specific implements
- Friction dermatitis/mechanical dermatitis
- Koebner phenomenon in diseased skin

Occupation-specific calluses and hyperkeratoses are not viewed as skin disease, but rather as honorific "trademarks," as described by Vernois and Purdon in French and Irish workers [1 2]. With the Industrial Revolution, these trademarks have mostly faded into oblivion. As sports activities have replaced physical labor, new sports-related skin injuries due to repetitive minor trauma have been observed, such as jogger's nipples and turf toes, as well as sports-related contact dermatitis. However, these lesions are viewed as diseases, rather than as honorifics [3, 4].

Eczema patients may complain that their eczema occurred after an injury to the skin. In some cases, this appears to be coincidental, but in other cases mechanical trauma precipitates eczema, thus leading to posttraumatic eczema that persists or recurs for long periods of time [5, 6]. Further, patients with preexisting skin disease may experience localized aggravation of the disorder as a consequence of mechanical trauma to diseased skin, such as Koebner phenomenon in palmar psoriasis [7].

A. Alikhan et al. (eds.), *Textbook of Hand Eczema*,
DOI 10.1007/978-3-642-39546-8_10, © Springer-Verlag Berlin Heidelberg 2014

Table 10.1 Skin manifestations and conditions resulting from mechanical insults[a]

Lichenification	Hyperpigmentation
Hyperkeratoses/calluses	Fissuring
Blistering/friction injury	Increased susceptibility to infection
Increased susceptibility to irritants and allergens	Development of foreign body reactions
Traumatic tattoos	Pressure urticaria
Scars and keloids	Cutaneous neoplasms
Koebner's phenomenon from friction	Raynaud's phenomenon from vibration

[a]Adapted from [7]

Repetitive mechanical trauma to the skin may result in a plethora of conditions, which are presented in Table 10.1, depending on the nature of the work and individual susceptibility.

If a dynamic relationship between trauma and the development of hand eczema is probable, and no other cause can be found, then it has important medical implications when the injury is job-related. While Wilkinson has previously reviewed dermatitis from repeated trauma in a broader perspective [8], this chapter focuses on repetitive trauma in occupational skin diseases.

10.2 Individual Factors

It is likely that genetic factors play a role in the response of the skin to mechanical strain. Exacerbation of atopic dermatitis and psoriasis (both partly inheritable skin diseases) may occur after mechanical trauma. Filaggrin loss-of-function mutations appear to be disease modifiers, but only in patients with atopic dermatitis [9]. Physiological factors, such as hydration of the skin, are important [10]. Moderate sweating hydrates the corneal layer and increases the coefficient of friction, whereas dry or wet skin diminishes the friction of resistance. Neurological diseases may impair the withdrawal response to mechanical stimuli and lead to injury of the skin.

Attempts at screening for heightened susceptibility to occupational skin diseases have been part of prevention systems for several years; because the causes are multifactorial, the screening systems tend to be elaborate [11]. Nonetheless, there is still no magic bullet for picking healthy workers.

10.3 Causes and Frequency of Occupational Skin Injuries

By convention, traumatic injuries result from single and brief episodes of cutaneous exposure and a subsequently rapid onset of a skin ailment, whereas irritant cutaneous reactions require multiple low-grade and prolonged exposures and show a relatively delayed onset of the disorder. Irritative mechanical stress significantly affects the barrier properties of the skin measured by transepidermal water loss and capacitance [10].

In private industry in the United States in 2006, skin diseases constituted about 1 % of nonfatal illnesses, while cuts, lacerations, and punctures constituted about 10 % according to the US Bureau of Labor Statistics [12]. In most cases the hands are probably involved, but exact figures are lacking. The lack of a standard definition for skin diseases explains the difficulty in obtaining accurate epidemiological data. However, several studies have found trends suggesting an underestimation of, and regular increase in, the frequency and gravity of observed skin diseases [13].

Common complications of skin injuries include scar formation, infection, persistent pain, and contact dermatitis from topical drugs used for treatment. Furthermore, local eczema may also appear and is common in susceptible individuals, such as amputees [14].

10.4 Hand Eczema Following a Mechanical Injury

Posttraumatic eczema is a poorly understood complication of skin injuries caused by thermal or chemical burns, lacerations, punctures, abra-

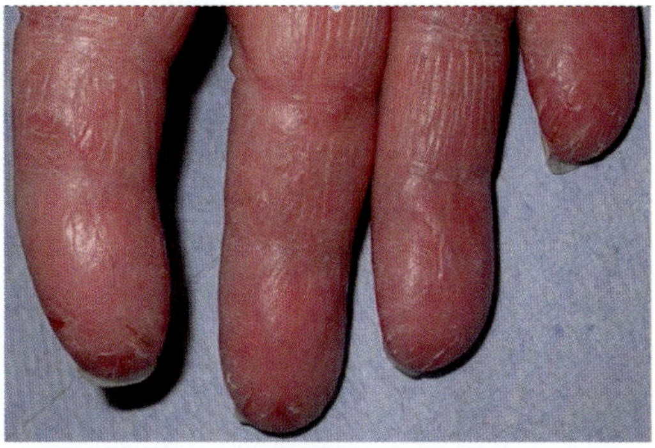

Fig. 10.1 Glossy pulpitis in a housewife who uses a mildly irritant detergent several times daily for an extended period of time. Note that the fingerprints have disappeared due to friction. Image courtesy of Prof. Jean-Marie Lachapelle, Unit for Occupational Dermatology, Louvain University, Brussels, Belgium

sions, or chemical injury. The interval between the trauma and the development of eczema is usually a few weeks. Mathias divided posttraumatic eczema into two types [15]. It may occur in association with an underlying endogenous eczema (isomorphic reaction of Koebner phenomenon) or occur as an isolated idiopathic reaction, when long-time follow-up shows that no new lesions develop on non-traumatized skin.

Continuous low-level mechanical and irritant irritation may cause a characteristic condition in which the friction ridges of the finger tips are eradicated, resulting in pulpitis with a dry glossy surface (Fig. 10.1).

In palmar hyperkeratotic hand eczema, currently regarded as an endogenous eczema, years of low-level mechanical injury to the palms may act as a disease modifier, especially in middle-aged men who engage in repetitive manual labor.

10.5 Differential Diagnoses

Friction dermatitis should be expected on a case history of repetitive low-grade trauma to a well-defined area of the skin, often the hands. Friction dermatitis may coexist with both irritant and allergic contact dermatitis, and this may obfuscate the picture. Diagnostic patch testing may be indicated to exclude aggravating allergenic exposures from working material, protective gloves, and topical remedies.

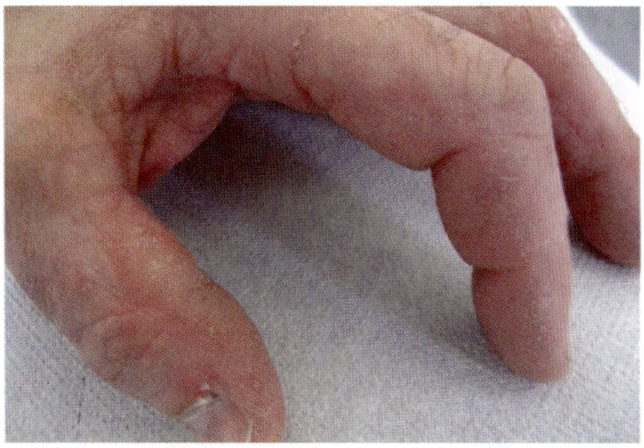

Fig. 10.2 Mechanic's hands with hyperkeratoses and fissuring in a 52-year-old man with anti-synthetase syndrome

In cases in which the patient has developed dermatitis with fissuring on the lateral aspect of the fingers without a plausible cause for the condition as well as systemic complaints, mechanic's hands should be suspected (Fig. 10.2). The patient should be interviewed with regard to fatigue, respiratory symptoms, arthralgia, and intermittent fever, and screened for anti-Jo-1 antibodies and RO/SSA antibodies, and so forth. Mechanic's hand is a marker for connective tissue diseases, especially anti-synthetase syndrome [16–18].

Conclusion

Mechanical injury and friction are still relevant as causes of dermatoses and skin conditions. Trademarks from specific repetitive trauma in specific trades are disappearing, as the trades are being industrialized. At the same time, however, there is a significant revival movement that may act as a conservatory for trademarks and friction dermatoses that would otherwise have been lost.

Careful questioning and demonstration of routines are necessary when assessing the role of friction in suspected occupational dermatoses. In cases of fissuring dermatitis on the lateral aspect of the fingers, with systemic complaints, suspect mechanic's hands as a marker of connective tissue diseases and myositis.

Mechanical dermatitis may be moving from the workplace to leisure activities, as shown in the rise of new sports-related dermatoses.

References

1. Vernois AGM. De la main des ouvriers et des artisans au point de vu de l'hygiene et de la médecine légale. Libraires de L'Académie Impériale de Médecine. Paris: J-B Bailliére et Fils; 1862. http://archive.org/details/delamaindesouvri00vern. Accessed on 28 Oct 2013.
2. Purdon HS. Trade callosities. Dublin J Med Sci. 1899;108(3):173–4.
3. Adams BB. Dermatologic disorders of the athlete. Sports Med. 2002;32(5):309–21.
4. Kockentiet B, Adams BB. Contact dermatitis in athletes. J Am Acad Dermatol. 2007;56(6):1048–55.
5. Mathias CG, Morrison JH. Occupational skin diseases, United States. Results from the bureau of labor statistics annual survey of occupational injuries and illnesses, 1973 through 1984. Arch Dermatol. 1988; 124(10):1519–24.
6. Warshaw E, Lee G, Storrs FJ. Hand dermatitis: a review of clinical features, therapeutic options, and long-term outcomes. Am J Contact Dermat. 2003; 14(3):119–37.
7. Samitz MH. Repeated mechanical trauma to the skin: occupational aspects. Am J Ind Med. 1985;8(4–5): 265–71.
8. Wilkinson DS. Dermatitis from repeated trauma to the skin. Am J Ind Med. 1985;8(4–5):307–17.
9. Landeck L, Visser M, Skudlik C, Brans R, Kezic S, John SM. Clinical course of occupational irritant contact dermatitis of the hands in relation to filaggrin genotype status and atopy. Br J Dermatol. 2012; 167(6):1302–9.
10. Pedersen L, Jemec GB. Mechanical properties and barrier function of healthy human skin. Acta Derm Venereol. 2006;86(4):308–11.
11. Weistenhöfer W, Baumeister T, Drexler H, Kütting B. How to quantify skin impairment in primary and secondary prevention? HEROS: a proposal of a hand eczema score for occupational screenings. Br J Dermatol. 2011;164(4):807–13.
12. http://www.bls.gov/iif/oshwc/osh/os/osh06_13.pdf. Accessed on 28 Oct 2013.
13. European Agency for Safety and Health at Work. Occupational skin diseases and dermal exposure in the European Union (EU-25):policy and practice overview. http://osha.europa.eu/en/publications/reports/TE7007049ENC_skin_diseases. Accessed on 28 Oct 2013.
14. Lyon CC, Kulkarni J, Zimerson E, Van Ross E, Beck MH. Skin disorders in amputees. J Am Acad Dermatol. 2000;42(3):501–7.
15. Mathias CG. Post-traumatic eczema. Dermatol Clin. 1988;6(1):35–42.
16. Stahl NI, Klippel JH, Decker JL. A cutaneous lesion associated with myositis. Ann Intern Med. 1979;91(4):577–9.
17. Bachmeyer C, Tillie-Leblond I, Lacert A, Cadranel J, Aractingi S. "Mechanic's hands": a misleading cutaneous sign of the antisynthetase syndrome. Br J Dermatol. 2007;156(1):192–4.
18. Bygum A, Velander MJ, Knudsen JB. Mechanic's hands imitating hand eczema. Dermatitis. 2010;21(6):334–5.

Irritant Contact Dermatitis

11

Gianfranco A. Frojo, Henk B. van der Walle, and Howard I. Maibach

Contents

G.A. Frojo, BS (✉)
University of Alabama at Birmingham,
1720 2nd Avenue, South Birmingham,
AL 35205, USA
e-mail: frojo@uab.edu

H.B. van der Walle, M.D., Ph.D.
Center of Occupational Dermatology, President
Kennedylaan 100, 6883AZ Velp, The Netherlands
e-mail: hvanderwalle@online.nl

H.I. Maibach, M.D.
Department of Dermatology,
University of California, San Francisco,
90 Medical Center Way, Surge 110,
San Francisco, CA 94143-0989, USA
e-mail: maibach@derm.ucsf.edu

11.1 Definition

Irritant contact dermatitis is a localized non-immunological inflammatory response to one or more external agents called irritants. Any agent that produces damage is an irritant. Damage is caused by the agent's chemical, physical, or mechanical properties. A single insult or repeated exposure to a single agent over time may cause the dermatitis, or it may result from the cumulative effect of minor damage caused by simultaneous or sequential exposure to several different agents.

11.2 Introduction

In the general population, the incidence of hand eczema varies between 2 % and 10 % [1–3]. In high-risk occupations, such as hairdressing, cleaning, agriculture, construction, and steelworking, the incidence may occasionally be as high as 40 %. Dermatological disorders are responsible for 30–40 % of all occupational diseases. Scientific reports show a gradual increase of interest in irritant contact dermatitis, but most exogenous dermatitis reports still deal with allergic contact dermatitis. In the 1970s, Malten [4, 5] stimulated the development and application of noninvasive techniques to investigate the damaging effects of irritants on human skin. With water vapor loss measurements, he demonstrated the concept of cumulative irritant contact dermatitis (Fig. 11.1).

An excess of irritant factors in relation to the defensive mechanisms and repairing capacity of

A. Alikhan et al. (eds.), *Textbook of Hand Eczema*,
DOI 10.1007/978-3-642-39546-8_11, © Springer-Verlag Berlin Heidelberg 2014

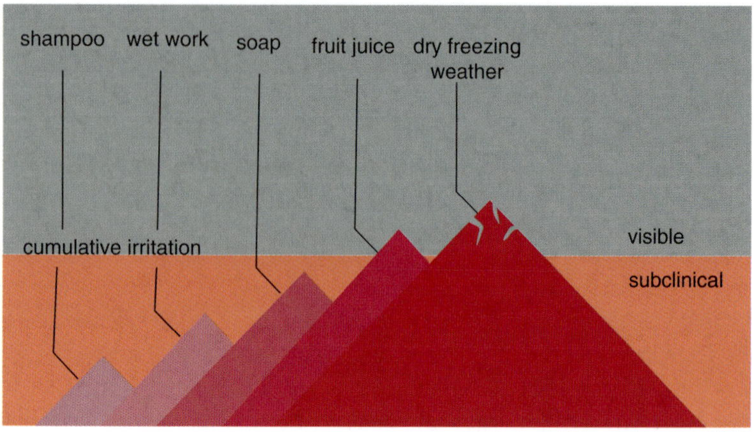

Fig. 11.1 Cumulative irritant contact dermatitis. A free interpretation of the concept as described by Malten (Adapted from [6])

the skin causes irritant contact dermatitis. The clinical picture of contact dermatitis of the hands shows a variety of expressions, ranging from the typical oligomorphic picture of dermatitis to the classic polymorphic picture of eczema. Both representations may be an expression of an irritant or allergic contact dermatitis. The final diagnosis is based on a combination of history, clinical picture, and patch test results. Diagnosis is the starting point for the management and treatment of the individual patient and, if necessary, adaptations in the work environment.

11.3 Clinical Picture

The clinical picture is the visual outcome of the dynamic interaction between the chemical, physical, and mechanical characteristics of the irritant and the biological makeup of the exposed skin. Numerous factors, belonging to either the irritant or the involved skin of the individual, are responsible for the degree of damage. The spectrum of irritant contact dermatitis varies from invisible sensation, such as stinging, burning, pain, and itching, to clinical signs, such as erythema, vesicles, blisters, necrosis, papules, scaling, and fissures. In other words, the clinical picture varies from monomorphic with one typical lesion (e.g., a blister) to a clear polymorphic picture, clinically indistinguishable from a classic eczema [5]. The clinical picture shows a variation in time, strongly influenced by the skin's repairing capacity, variation in exposure to irritants, and applied treatment.

Hand dermatitis may show a varying course with improvements and exacerbations, implying that the dermatologist is often not confronted with the dermatitis in its most active phase. In some cases, it is useful to request the patient to return when the dermatitis relapses. An allergic eczematous contact dermatitis may show an oligomorphic aspect in its healing phase when exposure to the allergen is omitted or if the reaction is suppressed by local corticosteroids.

Acute contact dermatitis develops after a single exposure to an irritant, the damaging force of which immediately overwhelms the defense capacity of the exposed skin. The skin may show a reaction with erythema, blisters, pustules, and necrosis, accompanied by a stinging, burning, or painful sensation. The lesions are sharply demarcated and often restricted to small spots or to a certain area of the hands. The most severe damage is seen at places where the concentration or intensity of the offending agent was the highest or the defense capacity of the skin the lowest. The clinical picture depends strongly on the characteristics of the involved skin and properties of the irritant. For example, a droplet of strong alkaline solution may cause necrosis when spilled on the dorsum of the hand, but the thick stratum corneum of the palmar side may limit the damage to a painful sensation with erythema or a small blister.

Chronic irritant contact dermatitis is caused by repetitive exposure to the same damaging factor or the cumulative effect of a variety of minor damaging factors. In many wet-work occupations, the clinically normal skin is damaged on a subclinical level by exposure to water, soap, and detergents. Slight erythema with fine scaling is the first visible sign of damage. A sudden change in occupational exposure or in climate conditions [7] may push the damage from the subclinical level over the threshold to a clearly visible contact dermatitis with redness, edema, scaling, chapping (fissures in the horny layer), and erythema craquelé (fissures into the epidermis) or even to hemorrhagic fissures caused by cracks into the dermis. In long-standing cases of cumulative irritant contact dermatitis, the clinical picture varies from a dry palmar dermatitis with erythema, fine scaling, chapping, and shiny fingertips (in "wear-and-tear" dermatitis, as seen in cleaning and housekeeping) to a more eczematous dermatitis with erythema, edema, itch, and lichenification.

Any part of the hand may be involved in cumulative irritant contact dermatitis, but there are general characteristics. Chapping, for example, is predominantly seen on the dorsal hand, whereas fissures and cracks are seen on the bending parts of the dorsal fingers and on the palm. Fissures and cracks at the fingertips often occur in occupations with prolonged exposure to organic solvents, as seen in painters and offset printers. Finger-web dermatitis occurs in wet-work occupations and may spread to the back of the hands, a scenario often seen in hairdressers and restaurant workers. The localization of contact dermatitis may be determined by the use of the right or left hand in certain occupations. If the dominant hand is exposed to the irritant, the dermatitis will occur on this hand, but in many occupations the dominant hand is used for handling tools or instruments, and the nondominant hand is exposed to wet work and irritants. A classic example is cumulative irritant contact dermatitis on the fingertips of the "wet hand" or "working hand" of the hairdresser, which is the nondominant hand. In occupations with wear-and-tear irritants (e.g., agriculture), the dermatitis often occurs on the first three fingers of the hands. Sometimes a contact dermatitis occurs on one or two fingers, despite equal exposure to irritants by all fingers. Obviously, the barrier function or defensive capacity of the individual fingers varies.

Nails and fingertips are often involved in cumulative irritant contact dermatitis. The nail may show onycholysis, subungual hyperkeratosis, and textural irregularities of the plate with pitting and transverse depressions. Painful fissures and cracks occur at the transition of plate to fingertip. "Wear and tear" and chemical exposure may damage the fingertips with painful cracks, lamellar scaring, and abrasion of the epidermis.

11.4 Diagnosis

Diagnosis is based on the combination of data obtained from patient history, clinical investigation, patch testing, and, if necessary, from information collected by investigation of the workplace. In general, histology via skin biopsy and monoclonal analysis of dermal infiltrates offer no typical clues to establish the diagnosis of irritant contact dermatitis [8]. The clinical picture should be carefully examined, keeping in mind that in general there is no single characteristic that makes the diagnosis certain. The examination should focus on localization, demarcation, and morphological expressions, such as redness, vesicles, blisters, necrosis, papules, scaling, fissures, or eczema. Besides the lesions on the hands, other skin parts should be examined, and special attention must be paid to the skin of the face and neck, because many occupational dermatoses occur on both the hands and face. Finally, the patient should be examined for minor and major signs of atopy, psoriasis, and active eczema.

Characteristics of the clinical picture are important facts to guide questioning. An extensive history of the patient's daily activities at work, in hobbies, and at home is essential. A thorough knowledge of various occupations is important; sometimes, it is necessary to visit the workplace or to consult the occupational hygienist to obtain an accurate impression of the occupational exposure. Cellular phone photographs are a recent addition to evaluating the workplace and often substitute for an on-site visit. Attention should be paid to the use of gloves, skin care products at work and in the home, and the use of both prescription and over-the-counter medications. The course of the dermatitis may offer important clues for the final diagnosis. The dermatologist must search for a relation between improvements and relapses of the dermatitis and activities in occupation, the home environment, within weekends, holidays, sick leave, the use of gloves, and so on. Healing time of a cumulative irritant contact dermatitis after omitting the exposure to irritants is rather slow, in contrast to an allergic contact dermatitis, in which avoidance of the allergen may lead to a rapid reduction of symptoms. Reexposure to the allergen aggravates the symptoms within several days to a week, while reexposure to minor irritants gradually aggravates the dermatitis in 1 or 2 weeks.

Patch testing is important in most cases of hand dermatitis. The testing focuses on exposure to allergens in the occupation, the home environment, and to skin care products and cosmetics. Screening series of standardized allergens related to the occupation of the patient should be, if necessary, supplemented with materials from the patient's work environment. The reliability of positive reactions to a patient's own materials should always be checked in patch testing of control persons and, if necessary, repeated with a dilution series and sometimes use tests. The information obtained in history, clinical examination, and patch testing will make the diagnosis of cumulative irritant contact dermatitis very likely, likely, or uncertain. The interpretation of positive patch test reaction should be made carefully. A negative reaction may support the diagnosis of an irritant contact dermatitis, but it may be a false-negative reaction, or an important allergen may simply be missed. In the same careful way, a positive reaction should be interpreted. The reaction may be either false-positive or have no relevance to the dermatitis on the hands. In many cases, the dermatologist deals with a combination of allergic and irritant contact dermatitis, aggravated by endogenous factors. Lachapelle provides details of the interpretation of a positive patch test result [8].

11.5 Differential Diagnosis

The differentiation of cumulative irritant contact dermatitis from another dermatitic process or an eczematous lesion of the skin is a challenge with moderate success rate. Atopic dermatitis often occurs on the hands in young adults and is provoked and aggravated in occupations with a high exposure to water and irritants, such as hairdressing, cleaning, and housekeeping [9, 10]. It is often difficult to weigh the individual role of irritants and atopic constitution. In many cases, it is the atopic disorder of the skin that is primarily responsible for the development of a cumulative irritant contact dermatitis [11]. Psoriasis of the hands can imitate eczema or an irritant contact dermatitis [12]. Careful examination of the whole skin to look for minor signs of psoriasis is important. In the follow-up of these patients, psoriasis may develop in other areas. Sometimes a combination of atopy and psoriasis occurs on the hands with itchy vesicles. Some of these patients experience a sudden aggravation of the dermatitis after exposure to water. Tinea of the hands may simulate a dry palmar dermatitis. Unilateral localization and involvement of the nails are important clues to diagnose tinea. Prolonged exposure to organic solvents may cause scaly, fissured, hyperkeratotic skin on the palmar side of the hands, which has to be differentiated from the hyperkeratotic palmar eczema (tylotic eczema). Irritants and allergens may complicate hyperkeratotic eczema, another endogenous dermatosis with features of psoriasis and eczema [13].

The differentiation between a cumulative irritant and an allergic contact dermatitis is a great challenge but not often possible (Fig. 11.2). In general, an allergic contact dermatitis is more polymorphic, with an unsharp demarcation, with a tendency for spreading, and with occasional localizations at the wrist, the forearm, and the face, especially on the eyelids. The course is often relapsing, with improvement during weekends and holidays. In the work environment, only one or a few persons are affected, and a relevant positive patch test makes the diagnosis definitive. Especially in the case of fingertip dermatitis and eczema, it is impossible to differentiate an allergic

Chronic Irritant Contact Dermatitis		Allergic Contact Dermatitis
Oligomorphic; redness, scaling, chapping	⟷ Clinical lesion	Polymorphic; redness, papules, vesicles, crusts, exudation, erosions, lichenification
Patchy, relatively unsharp	⟷ Demarcation	Unsharp, tendency to spread (wrist, underarm, face)
Fingertips, finger web, dorsum of the hand, ball of the thumb	⟷ Localization	Interdigital, fingers, palmar, and dorsal side
Chronic aggravation by climatic changes, wet work, detergents, gloves	⟷ Course	Relapsing, healing in weekends and holidays
More persons affected in same work environment	⟷ Epidemiology	One person affected in same work environment
Dry skin, atopic dermatitis, psoriasis palmaris, and exposure to irritants	⟷ Risk factors	Exposure to allergens
Negative Positive, nonrelevant	⟷ Patch testing	Positive relevant Negative, allergen missed!

Fig. 11.2 Characteristics of occupational hand dermatitis; chronic irritant versus allergic contact dermatitis (Adapted from [6])

contact dermatitis from a cumulative irritant contact dermatitis or psoriasis. Long-standing cases of allergic contact dermatitis with a lichenified character (nickel and chromate allergies) may change in character from eczematous to more psoriasis-like.

A typical type I allergy causes a contact urticaria lesion, but daily exposure to allergens in patients with type I allergies may cause a persistent dermatitis with eczematous aspects. This frequently occurs in occupations with intense exposure to biological materials (e.g., exposure to vegetables, fish, and meat in kitchen; wheat, flavors, and fruits in bakeries; and meat in slaughterhouses). Immunological contact urticaria, with or without dermatitis, is suspected on the basis of history – burn, sting, or itch – minutes after exposure and confirmed with open and/or prick testing.

Amin provides details [14]. Pompholyx (dyshidrotic eczema) may be caused by irritants, as described in metalworkers [15]. In many cases, the combination of constitutional, irritant, and allergic factors is the cause of chronic hand dermatitis. The start is often an irritant or allergic contact dermatitis, but the dermatitis may continue after avoiding irritants and allergens as a constitutional post-insult form of eczema [16].

11.6 Pathophysiology

The chemical, physical, or mechanical properties of an irritant may damage intercellular and cellular structures and molecules, which for each individual has their own characteristics. The interaction between these components of the skin and the characteristics of the irritant may lead to a disturbance in the metabolism and histological or anatomical structures of the skin. Gradually, the different mechanism of action of irritants is unraveled [17, 18]. Detergents damage the horny layer and cellular membranes and stimulate DNA synthesis and epidermal metabolism, leading to acanthosis. Others, including phorbol esters and croton oil, stimulate leukocyte activity and migration. Organic solvents quickly penetrate the epidermis and directly attack blood vessels in the dermis, causing hyperemia.

The irritant effect of water is an intriguing phenomenon. The overhydration of the skin in wet-work occupations not only enhances the penetration of many irritants but may also release inflammatory mediators and their inhibitors from the stratum corneum, the mechanism of which may lead to a gradual damage of the skin. In the first instance, irritants cause damage on a subclinical level, which is demonstrated by noninvasive methods, such as transepidermal water loss and laser Doppler flowmetry. These methods have shown that skin reacts in different ways to the exposure of irritants [19]. First, there is a strong repairing and hardening mechanism that limits the progression to a visible contact dermatitis and enables the skin to withstand the daily exposure to a great variety of low-grade irritants. If the cumulative effect of the repeated exposure to one irritant or to a variety of different irritants gradually breaches the stratum corneum skin barrier, the defense and repairing capacity of the skin is overwhelmed, and a visible cumulative irritant contact dermatitis develops. In its most classic form, there is a slight erythema with fine scales, a tendency to chapping, some itch, and ill-defined demarcation. This scenario is often seen in wet-work occupations, such as hairdressing, housekeeping, and cleaning work. In these occupations, the daily exposure to water, soap, detergents, and other irritants gradually causes an irritant contact dermatitis, which is often suddenly provoked by an increase in workload (e.g., hairdressing in the weeks before Christmas) or by a sudden change in climate, often from higher humidity with low pressure to high pressure and dry wind [7]. A fully developed cumulative contact dermatitis is often maintained by the exposure to low-grade irritants, which normally are innocuous to the skin.

Several exogenous and endogenous factors may influence the development or course of a cumulative irritant contact dermatitis. An increase in temperature, a low environmental humidity, and exposure under occlusion, which causes hyperhydration of the skin, make the skin more susceptible to irritation [20]. Atopy is the most important endogenous factor that negatively influences the response of the skin to an irritant. Individuals may have hyperirritable skin without relation to race or atopy. There seems to be an association with light skin (e.g., Fitzpatrick types I and II) and with a high baseline transepidermal water loss [21]. Increased susceptibility to some irritants occurs in eczematous patients or in patients with active skin ulceration (e.g., leg ulcer) [22].

11.7 Management and Treatment

Because cumulative irritant contact dermatitis is caused by an overbalance of irritant exogenous factors in relation to the defense and repairing capacity of the skin, which in some patients is influenced by endogenous factors such as atopy and hyperirritable skin, management and treatment should be directed to restoring this balance by the following strategy:

1. Reduction of the irritant factors
2. Skin protection
3. Enhancement of the defense and repairing capacity of the skin

This implies that for every patient a tailored treatment and management plan should be designed. If the patient is working in a profession with a high incidence of irritant contact dermatitis, initiatives should be taken to change working conditions by consultancy and cooperation with occupational hygienists, management of the factory, and producers of materials involved. The basis for action is reduction of possibilities to expose the skin to a wide variety of irritants and water. It is often necessary to change work procedures, to introduce instruments and tools, to modify the application form of products, and to supply adequate protective materials (e.g., gloves). In the meantime, the individual patient has to be treated, primarily via protection and local treatment of the skin. This can sometimes be accomplished by using the correct type of barrier protection in the appropriate location. It is important to select the adequate type of glove and to instruct the patient on how and when to use the gloves. The choice of gloves should be based on the requirements of the occupation. Some chemicals degrade the polymer of the glove or penetrate the glove material easily [23]. The elasticity, thickness, and type of polymer greatly determine the acceptability of a certain type of glove for a certain task. Damaging factors at home and with hobbies should not be overlooked. The patient must be instructed to take care with dish and hair washing and all other activities at home in which contact with water, detergents, or organic solvents may occur. In severe cases, the patient may be instructed to use a simple polyethylene glove when washing hair, purchase a dishwasher, and use gloves when doing "dirty work" to avoid the use of strong detergents to clean the skin afterwards.

Barrier creams do not really exist, but some ointments show a protective effect, especially during exposure to water and water-soluble irritants. The acceptability of this "barrier cream" depends strongly on the cosmetic acceptance of the product. Ointments that stay sticky are not typically acceptable to most people. Some glycerine-containing ointments are not sticky or greasy a few minutes after application and may be beneficial to a certain degree in the protection of skin in wet-work professions [24]. Special attention should be given to the cleaning of skin. It should be as mild as possible, and the patient should avoid the use of hard brushes or other abrasives. For details on barrier cream efficacy and toxicity, see Zhai [25, 26].

Medical treatment is based on the severity of the contact dermatitis and the occurrence of endogenous factors. No medication should be chosen that contains ingredients that irritate the skin and/or have a negative effect on the defensive capacity of the skin. This means that application of potent corticosteroids should be avoided, if possible, because they impair the thickness of the stratum corneum. Local UVB treatment may be considered to enhance the defensive capacity of the skin. In severe cases, especially in combination with allergic contact dermatitis or psoriasis, PUVA treatment of the hands should be considered [27, 28]. Furthermore, with some ingenuity and simple equipment, arrangements can be organized for home phototherapy treatment [29].

References

1. Lantinga H, Nater JP, Coenraads PJ. Prevalence, incidence and course of eczema on the hands and forearms in a sample of the general population. Contact Dermatitis. 1984;10:135.
2. Agrup G. Hand eczema and other hand dermatoses in South Sweden. Acta Derm Venereol (Stockholm). 1969;49 Suppl 61:5–91.
3. Meding B. Epidemiology of hand eczema in an industrial city. Acta Derm Venereol Suppl (Stockholm). 1990;153:1–43.
4. Malten KE, den Arend JACJ. Irritant contact dermatitis: traumiterative and cumulative impairment by cosmetics, climate, and other daily loads. Dermatosen. 1985;33:125.
5. Malten KE. Thoughts on irritant contact dermatitis. Contact Dermatitis. 1981;7:435.
6. Menne T, Maibach HI, editors. Textbook of hand eczema. 2nd ed. London: Informa Healthcare; 2000.
7. Gaul LE, Underwood GR. Relation of dew point and barometer pressure to chapping of normal skin. J Invest Dermatol. 1952;19:9.

8. Lachapelle JM, Maibach HI. Patch/prick testing. 3rd ed. Heidelberg: Springer; 2012.
9. Brasch J, Burgard J, Wolfram S. Common pathogenetic pathways in allergic and irritant contact dermatitis. J Invest Dermatol. 1992;98:166.
10. Rystedt I. Factors influencing the recurrence of hand eczema in adults with a history of atopic dermatitis in childhood. Contact Dermatitis. 1985;12:247.
11. Baurle G, Hornstein OP, Diepgen TL. Professionelle Handekzeme und Atopie. Dermatosen. 1985;33:161.
12. Maibach HI, Epstein E. Eczematous psoriasis. Semin Dermatol. 1983;2:45.
13. Feldman S. Hyperkeratotic eczema. In: Menne T, Maibach HI, editors. Hand eczema. 2nd ed. Boca Raton: CRC Press; 2000.
14. Amin S, Lahti A, Maibach HI. Contact urticaria and the contact urticaria syndrome. In: Menne T, Maibach HI, editors. Hand eczema. 2nd ed. Boca Raton: CRC Press; 2000. p. 485–504. Chapter 38.
15. de Boer EM, Bryunzeel DP, van Ketel WG. Dyshidrotic eczema as an occupational dermatitis in metal works. Contact Dermatitis. 1988;19:184.
16. Wilkinson JD, Rycroft RJG. Textbook of dermatology. 5th ed. Oxford: Blackwell Scientific; 1992. p. 611.
17. Frosch P. Hautirritation und empfindliche Haut. Berlin: Grosse Verlag; 1985.
18. Frosch PJ, Dooms-Goossens A, Lachapelle JM, Rycroft RJG, Scheper RJ. Current topics in contact dermatitis. Berlin: Springer; 1989. p. 385.
19. Marzulli FN, Maibach HI. Dermatotoxicology. 3rd ed. Washington, DC: Hemisphere; 1987.
20. Rothenberg HW, Menne T, Sjolin KE. Temperature dependent primary irritant dermatitis from lemon perfume. Contact Dermatitis. 1977;3:37.
21. Pinnagoda J, Tupker RA, Coenraads PJ, Nater JP. Prediction of susceptibility to an irritant response by transepidermal water loss. Contact Dermatitis. 1989;20:341.
22. Bjornberg A. Skin reactions to primary irritants in patients with hand eczema. Goteborg: Isacsons; 1968.
23. Mellstrom G. Protective gloves of polymeric materials. Acta Derm Venereol Suppl. 1991;163:1–54.
24. Kurte A, Zylka M, Frosch PJ. New text model for evaluating the efficacy of barrier creams, International Symposium on Irritant Contact Dermatitis, final program and abstract book, Stichting Milieu-en Arbeidsdermatologie, Groningen, Holland, October 3–5; 1991. p. 45.
25. Honbgo Z, Maibach HI. Barrier creams. In: Chew A, Maibach HI, editors. Irritant dermatitis. Berlin: Springer; 2006. p. 435–8. Chapter 46.
26. Loden M, Maibach H. Treatment of dry skin syndrome: art and science of moisturizers. Heidelberg: Springer; 2012.
27. Taube KM, Lubbe D. UV-radiation suppresses irritative and allergic skin reactions. International Symposium on Irritant Contact Dermatitis, final program and abstract book, Stichting Milieu-en Arbeidsdermatologie, Groningen, Holland, October 3–5; 1991, p. 29.
28. Rosen K, Mobacken H, Swanbeck G. Chronic eczematous dermatitis of the hands: a comparison of PUVA and UVB treatment. Acta Derm Venereol. 1987;67:48.
29. Epstein E. Home PUVA treatment for chronic hand and foot dermatoses. Cutis. 1989;44:423–7.

Atopic Hand Eczema

12

Sari Lehtimäki and Antti Lauerma

Contents

S. Lehtimäki, Ph.D.
Unit of Immunotoxicology,
Finnish Institute of Occupational Health,
Topeliuksenkatu 41 b, Helsinki 00250, Finland
e-mail: slehtim@gmail.com

A. Lauerma, M.D., Ph.D. (✉)
Department of Dermatology,
University of Helsinki, Meilahdentie,
Helsinki 00250, Finland
e-mail: antti.lauerma@hus.fi

12.1 Introduction

Atopic hand eczema represents an important entity of hand dermatitis. An increase in atopic diseases, atopic allergies, and atopic skin has made this subset of hand eczema increasingly important. Proper diagnostic procedures and treatments and avoidance of aggravating factors, however, enable successful maintenance of this skin condition, so that this disease will not likely significantly worsen quality of life and impair the patient's ability to work.

12.2 Mechanisms

The non-lesional skin of patients with atopic dermatitis (AD) differs from healthy skin. Lowered hydration, modified lipid synthesis, enhanced infiltration of CD3+ and CD11c + cells, and elevated expression of Th1, Th2, and Th22 cytokines have been reported. In the lesional skin, elevated amounts of thymic stromal lymphopoietin (TSLP), which instructs dendritic cells (DCs) to induce Th2 responses, have been detected. The acute skin lesions are dominated by Th2 cells, while chronic lesions are maintained by Th1 cells [1, 2]. IgE levels in the serum are usually upregulated.

Polymorphism in genes controlling skin barrier function has been shown to correlate with AD [3]. Filaggrin (FLG) is a structural protein of the cornified envelope of the epidermis and has been shown to be associated with AD in at least 20 different studies [4]. Loss-of-function mutation

A. Alikhan et al. (eds.), *Textbook of Hand Eczema*,
DOI 10.1007/978-3-642-39546-8_12,

of filaggrin results in the impairment of the skin barrier [5], which in turn facilitates the penetration of the allergen into the skin and might also render AD patients more susceptible to infections [4, 6]. In addition, filaggrin deficiency plays a role in decreased hydration of stratum corneum in AD patients [3, 7, 8]. Compared to AD patients without FLG mutation, FLG-deficient patients have an earlier onset and a more severe and persistent form of AD and are also more likely to develop asthma or other allergies [5, 9, 10].

Association between AD and polymorphism in other structural genes of the skin, such as hornerin and claudin-1, has also been reported [11–13]. In addition, Th2 cytokines have been shown to reduce the expression of cornified envelope proteins [14, 15]. Also, the altered lipid composition may affect the barrier function of the skin [3]. Other genes in which polymorphisms have been shown to associate with AD include genes involved in adaptive and innate immune responses, such as *IL4*, *IL4RA*, *SPINK5*, *CMA1*, *IL13*, *RANTES*, *CD14*, *DEFB1*, *GSTP1*, *IL18*, *NOD1*, and *TIM1* [3].

Allergens are known to engage and activate a variety of innate immunity receptors and drive strong Th2 responses [16]. Polymorphism in receptors TLR2 and TLR9 has been reported in AD patients, as well as attenuated TLR2 signalling [2, 17, 18], indicating that defective innate immunity mechanisms may play a role in the pathogenesis of AD.

AD patients are susceptible to skin infections, which may have consequences for the disease severity. Some of the AD patients display defects in antimicrobial peptide (AMP) expression [19, 20], most likely due to altered cytokine balance in the skin [2, 21]. Enhanced susceptibility for viral infection can also be partly due to an altered phenotype and/or lowered numbers of plasmacytoid DCs in AD lesions or decreased production of antiviral cytokines [22–24].

In addition to the aforementioned defects, many other factors, such as abnormally high expression of FcεRI on DCs or elevated numbers of skin-seeking CLA + T cells, have also been shown to have an effect on the pathomechanisms of AD [1, 25, 26].

Food-borne allergens are important triggers of AD responses, especially in children [27]. However, the role of food-borne allergens is very small in atopic hand eczema, with the exception of direct contact in food handling.

Airborne allergens can participate in the atopic inflammation through either their intrinsic proteolytic activity, which may impair the skin barrier or activate eosinophils and keratinocytes; activation of proteinase-activated receptor-2 (PAR-2), which is associated with barrier impairment and chronic itch; or IgE binding, which triggers the classical immediate-type response [28]. The role of airborne allergens is likely to be very small in atopic hand eczema.

Microbes can trigger inflammation in AD patients and exacerbate already ongoing inflammation. For example, skin-colonizing *Staphylococcus aureus* secrete toxins that can trigger inflammation through several mechanisms, such as inducing the production of toxin-specific IgE or inflammatory cytokines, activation of T cells, or inhibition of immunosuppressive Treg cells [29–34].

During times of stress, release of neurotransmitters and nerve growth factors in the blood and skin is increased, and this can enhance the inflammation induced by immune cells. In AD lesions, various changes in skin neurobiology are observed, strongly suggesting that the nervous system plays a significant role in the pathomechanisms of AD [35].

The genetic defects in AD patients interact with environmental triggers. For example, cat, but not dog, exposure during the first year of life predisposes only people with filaggrin deficiency to eczema [3]. Since genetic evolution is a slow process, the rapid increase in AD rates indicates that something in our environment has changed so that genetically prone people more often develop AD. There is strong evidence that reduced microbial exposure due to urbanization, improved hygiene, and efficient health-care measures may account for increased rates of allergic diseases. For example, the cord blood of neonates with mothers exposed to farm animals had a higher number of immunosuppressive Treg cells, and these children were clearly more protected from AD than children whose mothers were not exposed to farm animals during pregnancy [3, 36, 37].

12.3 Clinical Features

By definition, a patient with atopic hand eczema must have atopic eczema. For diagnosis of atopic eczema, the patient must have (1) itchy dermatitis (without itch the skin lesion is not atopic eczema) and (2) at least three out of five of the following: eczema in typical areas (flexural areas of legs and arms, upper body, neck, and head), eczema in typical areas earlier, dry skin, early onset of eczema (during first 12 months of life), and/or respiratory allergy and/or asthma [38].

Atopic eczema can be worsened intrinsically without apparent outside contributing factors. Such worsening is usually seen on all skin lesional sites in atopic eczema. The worsening can be enhanced by skin infections, especially *Staphylococcus aureus*, and contributing bacterial superantigens.

Atopic dry skin has a greater propensity for irritant dermatitis. This is especially common in hands, and atopic hand eczema is one of the most typical manifestations of atopic eczema in adulthood. Frequent washing and wet work are great risk factors for atopic hand eczema. Depending on the situation, the classification may be either atopic hand eczema, irritant hand dermatitis, or irritant atopic hand eczema or dermatitis. Irritant dermatitis can be diagnosed clinically by following the clinical outcome of change of work practices, homework, or other circumstances, in hand dermatitis.

Topical contact with protein allergens such as those in vegetables, due to cross-reaction from pollen allergy, may worsen and even cause atopic hand eczema. The contributing factors include IgE-mediated responses, cellular responses (protein contact dermatitis), irritation from proteolytic activities of some allergens, and wet conditions due to washing. Allergy to protein allergens can be diagnosed with prick tests.

Atopic hand eczema can be worsened also by allergic contact dermatitis (ACD). ACD develops in response to a hapten in sensitized individuals. ACD is not more common in atopic eczema patients, but it is not less common either. Th2 responses in atopic eczema seemingly do not protect against ACD. Also, atopic skin inflammation is very much driven by Th1 responses. ACD can be diagnosed with patch tests.

12.4 Treatment

The basic cause of atopic eczema, dry, sensitive skin, is a genetic phenomenon that cannot be healed. However, frequent use of emollients and avoidance of unnecessary wetting of the skin help in this regard [39].

Apart from the use of emollients, topical corticosteroids are the mainstay of treatment. Their use should be active in the beginning. The aim is to get the skin symptom-free. This usually takes 2–4 weeks. After that, a proactive treatment that consists of twice-a-week application for several months should be carried out, even though the skin is clinically normal. This prevents relapses and, according to studies, is not a major risk factor for thinning of the skin [40].

Topical calcineurin inhibitors, tacrolimus and pimecrolimus, are more useful in atopic hand eczema than in allergic and irritant hand dermatitis (though there may be an irritant component in certain cases of atopic hand eczema). Their use can be continuous, if needed [41]. The major obstacle for them has been their price, but as the patent has expired, the price will likely go down. There is a black box warning in the United States for these agents; therefore, topical corticosteroids should be tried first.

Light therapy with narrowband UVB can be useful, as can systemic treatments. However, for systemic treatments, the risk/benefit ratio should be considered. The systemic treatments include short-term corticosteroid administration [42], medium-term cyclosporine treatments [43], and, in some cases, longer-term azathioprine treatments [44].

Conclusion

Atopic hand eczema is a variant of hand eczema with its own etiologies and course. The chronicity of atopic eczema is a problem in treatment. However, careful treatment, especially with topical formulations, and avoidance of aggravating factors would benefit the patient greatly and usually enable a life without major obstacles from the disease.

References

1. Bieber T. Atopic dermatitis. Ann Dermatol. 2011;22: 125–37.
2. Novak N, Leung DY. Advances in atopic dermatitis. Curr Opin Immunol. 2011;23:778–83.
3. Boguniewicz M, Leung DY. Atopic dermatitis: a disease of altered skin barrier and immune dysregulation. Immunol Rev. 2011;242:233–46.
4. Barnes KC. An update on the genetics of atopic dermatitis: scratching the surface in 2009. J Allergy Clin Immunol. 2010;125:16–29. e1-11; quiz 30–1.
5. Palmer CN, Irvine AD, Terron-Kwiatkowski A, Zhao Y, Liao H, Lee SP, et al. Common loss-of-function variants of the epidermal barrier protein filaggrin are a major predisposing factor for atopic dermatitis. Nat Genet. 2006;38:441–6.
6. Spergel JM. From atopic dermatitis to asthma: the atopic march. Ann Allergy Asthma Immunol. 2010;105: 99–106. quiz 7–9, 17.
7. Kezic S, O'Regan GM, Yau N, Sandilands A, Chen H, Campbell LE, et al. Levels of filaggrin degradation products are influenced by both filaggrin genotype and atopic dermatitis severity. Allergy. 2011;66:934–40.
8. O'Regan GM, Kemperman PM, Sandilands A, Chen H, Campbell LE, Kroboth K, et al. Raman profiles of the stratum corneum define 3 filaggrin genotype-determined atopic dermatitis endophenotypes. J Allergy Clin Immunol. 2010;126:574–80.e1.
9. Henderson J, Northstone K, Lee SP, Liao H, Zhao Y, Pembrey M, et al. The burden of disease associated with filaggrin mutations: a population-based, longitudinal birth cohort study. J Allergy Clin Immunol. 2008;121:872–7.e9.
10. Marenholz I, Nickel R, Ruschendorf F, Schulz F, Esparza-Gordillo J, Kerscher T, et al. Filaggrin loss-of-function mutations predispose to phenotypes involved in the atopic march. J Allergy Clin Immunol. 2006;118:866–71.
11. De Benedetto A, Rafaels NM, McGirt LY, Ivanov AI, Georas SN, Cheadle C, et al. Tight junction defects in patients with atopic dermatitis. J Allergy Clin Immunol. 2011;127:773–86.e1-7.
12. Esparza-Gordillo J, Weidinger S, Folster-Holst R, Bauerfeind A, Ruschendorf F, Patone G, et al. A common variant on chromosome 11q13 is associated with atopic dermatitis. Nat Genet. 2009;41:596–601.
13. Henry J, Hsu CY, Haftek M, Nachat R, de Koning HD, Gardinal-Galera I, et al. Hornerin is a component of the epidermal cornified cell envelopes. FASEB J. 2011;25:1567–76.
14. Howell MD, Kim BE, Gao P, Grant AV, Boguniewicz M, Debenedetto A, et al. Cytokine modulation of atopic dermatitis filaggrin skin expression. J Allergy Clin Immunol. 2007;120:150–5.
15. Kim BE, Leung DY, Boguniewicz M, Howell MD. Loricrin and involucrin expression is down-regulated by Th2 cytokines through STAT-6. Clin Immunol. 2008;126:332–7.
16. Wills-Karp M. Allergen-specific pattern recognition receptor pathways. Curr Opin Immunol. 2010;22: 777–82.
17. Ahmad-Nejad P, Mrabet-Dahbi S, Breuer K, Klotz M, Werfel T, Herz U, et al. The toll-like receptor 2 R753Q polymorphism defines a subgroup of patients with atopic dermatitis having severe phenotype. J Allergy Clin Immunol. 2004;113:565–7.
18. Novak N, Yu CF, Bussmann C, Maintz L, Peng WM, Hart J, et al. Putative association of a TLR9 promoter polymorphism with atopic eczema. Allergy. 2007;62:766–72.
19. Nomura I, Goleva E, Howell MD, Hamid QA, Ong PY, Hall CF, et al. Cytokine milieu of atopic dermatitis, as compared to psoriasis, skin prevents induction of innate immune response genes. J Immunol. 2003;171:3262–9.
20. Ong PY, Ohtake T, Brandt C, Strickland I, Boguniewicz M, Ganz T, et al. Endogenous antimicrobial peptides and skin infections in atopic dermatitis. N Engl J Med. 2002;347:1151–60.
21. Howell MD, Boguniewicz M, Pastore S, Novak N, Bieber T, Girolomoni G, et al. Mechanism of HBD-3 deficiency in atopic dermatitis. Clin Immunol. 2006;121:332–8.
22. Lebre MC, van Capel TM, Bos JD, Knol EF, Kapsenberg ML, de Jong EC. Aberrant function of peripheral blood myeloid and plasmacytoid dendritic cells in atopic dermatitis patients. J Allergy Clin Immunol. 2008;122:969–76.e5.
23. Novak N, Allam JP, Hagemann T, Jenneck C, Laffer S, Valenta R, et al. Characterization of FcepsilonRI-bearing CD123 blood dendritic cell antigen-2 plasmacytoid dendritic cells in atopic dermatitis. J Allergy Clin Immunol. 2004;114:364–70.
24. Wollenberg A, Wagner M, Gunther S, Towarowski A, Tuma E, Moderer M, et al. Plasmacytoid dendritic cells: a new cutaneous dendritic cell subset with distinct role in inflammatory skin diseases. J Invest Dermatol. 2002;119:1096–102.
25. Boguniewicz M, Leung DY. Recent insights into atopic dermatitis and implications for management of infectious complications. J Allergy Clin Immunol. 2010;125:4–13. quiz 4–5.
26. Werfel T. The role of leukocytes, keratinocytes, and allergen-specific IgE in the development of atopic dermatitis. J Invest Dermatol. 2009;129:1878–91.
27. Hauk PJ. The role of food allergy in atopic dermatitis. Curr Allergy Asthma Rep. 2008;8:188–94.
28. Hostetler SG, Kaffenberger B, Hostetler T, Zirwas MJ. The role of airborne proteins in atopic dermatitis. J Clin Aesthet Dermatol. 2010;3:22–31.
29. Cardona ID, Goleva E, Ou LS, Leung DY. Staphylococcal enterotoxin B inhibits regulatory T cells by inducing glucocorticoid-induced TNF receptor-related protein ligand on monocytes. J Allergy Clin Immunol. 2006;117:688–95.

30. Laouini D, Kawamoto S, Yalcindag A, Bryce P, Mizoguchi E, Oettgen H, et al. Epicutaneous sensitization with superantigen induces allergic skin inflammation. J Allergy Clin Immunol. 2003;112:981–7.
31. Leung DY, Harbeck R, Bina P, Reiser RF, Yang E, Norris DA, et al. Presence of IgE antibodies to staphylococcal exotoxins on the skin of patients with atopic dermatitis. Evidence for a new group of allergens. J Clin Invest. 1993;92:1374–80.
32. Lin YT, Wang CT, Chao PS, Lee JH, Wang LC, Yu HH, et al. Skin-homing CD4+ Foxp3+ T cells exert Th2-like function after staphylococcal superantigen stimulation in atopic dermatitis patients. Clin Exp Allergy. 2011;41:516–25.
33. Miethke T, Wahl C, Heeg K, Echtenacher B, Krammer PH, Wagner H. T cell-mediated lethal shock triggered in mice by the superantigen staphylococcal enterotoxin B: critical role of tumor necrosis factor. J Exp Med. 1992;175:91–8.
34. Hong SC, Waterbury G, Janeway Jr CA. Different superantigens interact with distinct sites in the Vbeta domain of a single T cell receptor. J Exp Med. 1996; 183:1437–46.
35. Misery L. Atopic dermatitis and the nervous system. Clin Rev Allergy Immunol. 2011;41(3):259–66.
36. Schaub B, Liu J, Hoppler S, Schleich I, Huehn J, Olek S, et al. Maternal farm exposure modulates neonatal immune mechanisms through regulatory T cells. J Allergy Clin Immunol. 2009;123:774–82.e5.
37. Wills-Karp M, Santeliz J, Karp CL. The germless theory of allergic disease: revisiting the hygiene hypothesis. Nat Rev Immunol. 2001;1:69–75.
38. Williams HC, Burney PG, Hay RJ, Archer CB, Shipley MJ, Hunter JJ, et al. The U.K. working party's diagnostic criteria for atopic dermatitis. I. Derivation of a minimum set of discriminators for atopic dermatitis. Br J Dermatol. 1994;131:406–16.
39. Lodén M, Andersson AC, Lindberg M. Improvement in skin barrier function in patients with atopic dermatitis after treatment with a moisturizing cream (Canoderm). Br J Dermatol. 1999;140(2):264–7.
40. Van Der Meer JB, Glazenburg EJ, Mulder PG, Eggink HF, Coenraads PJ. The management of moderate to severe atopic dermatitis in adults with topical fluticasone propionate. The Netherlands Adult Atopic Dermatitis Study Group. Br J Dermatol. 1999;140(6):1114–21.
41. Reitamo S, Ortonne JP, Sand C, Cambazard F, Bieber T, Fölster-Holst R, et al. A multicentre, randomized, double-blind, controlled study of long-term treatment with 0.1% tacrolimus ointment in adults with moderate to severe atopic dermatitis. Br J Dermatol. 2005; 152(6):1282–9.
42. Hoare C, Li Wan Po A, Williams H. Systematic review of treatments for atopic eczema. Health Technol Assess. 2000;4(37):1–191.
43. Granlund H, Erkko P, Remitz A, Langeland T, Helsing P, Nuutinen M, et al. Comparison of cyclosporin and UVAB phototherapy for intermittent one-year treatment of atopic dermatitis. Acta Derm Venereol. 2001;81(1):22–7.
44. Meggitt SJ, Gray JC, Reynolds NJ. Azathioprine dosed by thiopurine methyltransferase activity for moderate-to-severe atopic eczema: a double-blind, randomised controlled trial. Lancet. 2006;367(9513):839–46.

Acute and Recurrent Vesicular Hand Eczema

13

Niels K. Veien

Contents

N.K. Veien, M.D., Ph.D.
Dermatology Clinic, Fyrkildevej 7,
Aalborg 9220, Denmark
e-mail: veien@dadlnet.dk

13.1 Definition

In this chapter, acute and recurrent vesicular hand eczema is defined as the infrequent or repeated eruption of vesicles on the palms, palmar aspects of the fingers, and/or sides of the fingers that cannot be explained by contact with external contactants.

13.2 Introduction

Acute and recurrent vesicular hand eczema is a morphological description of typically intensely pruritic hand eczema seen at the characteristic sites noted above. The eruption may also extend to the periungual area, and there may be simultaneous, similar eruptions on the soles.

The dermatitis is usually fairly symmetrical and on both hands. There is little or no inflammation unless frequent eruptions occur. In such cases, inflammation may gradually develop, in which case the dermatitis may mimic chronic hand eczema. Crops of tiny vesicles usually occur without external contact with allergens or irritants, and close inspection may be required in order to see the vesicles (Figs. 13.1, 13.2, and 13.3).

It is peculiar and characteristic that there are no lesions on adjacent forearm skin (Fig. 13.4).

Early descriptions included terms such as cheiropompholyx, dyshidrosis, dyshidrotic eczema, and pompholyx. The question of nomenclature has been dealt with in a thoughtful commentary by Storrs [1]. She concluded that the

A. Alikhan et al. (eds.), *Textbook of Hand Eczema*,
DOI 10.1007/978-3-642-39546-8_13, © Springer-Verlag Berlin Heidelberg 2014

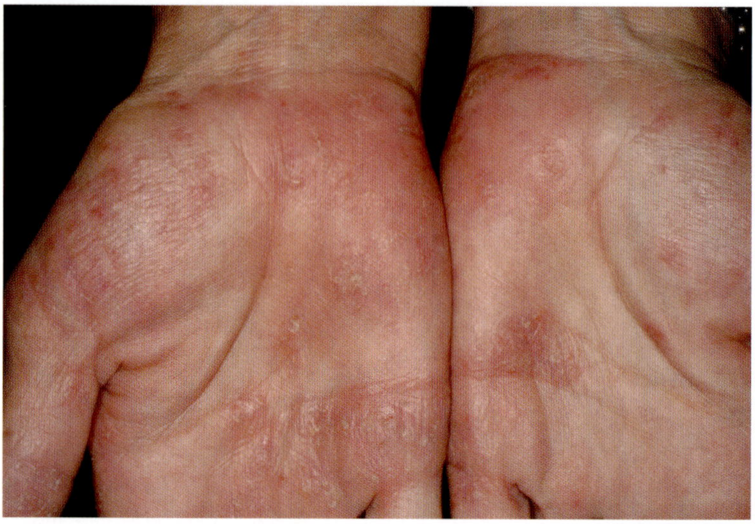

Fig. 13.1 Recurrent vesicular hand eczema with some inflammation

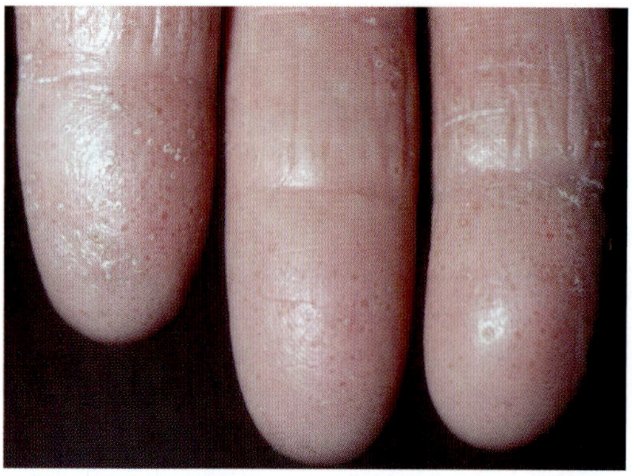

Fig. 13.2 Close-up photograph of a vesicular eruption

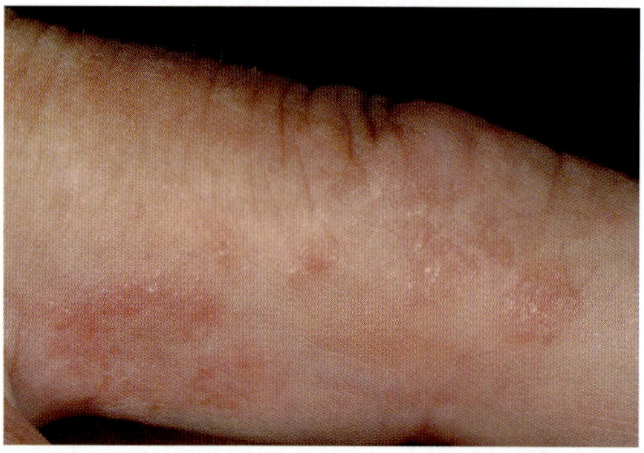

Fig. 13.3 Recurrent vesicular hand eczema on the side of a finger

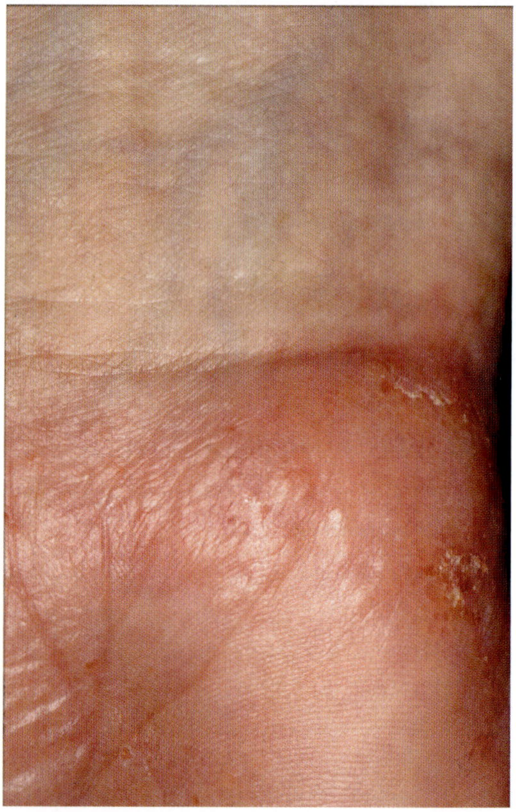

Fig. 13.4 Recurrent vesicular hand eczema. Note the crops of tiny vesicles and that the dermatitis is solely on palmar skin

term acute and vesicular hand dermatitis should be preferred over pompholyx and dyshidrosis and that we still do not know what causes this intriguing clinical manifestation. Throughout this chapter, the terminology used by the authors of the cited papers will be used.

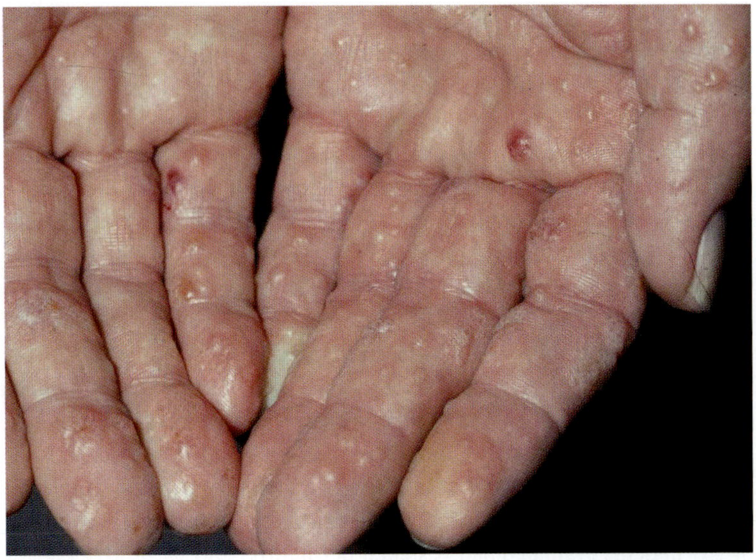

Fig. 13.5 Acute vesicular/bullous hand eczema as a rare, severe eruption

The term acute and recurrent vesicular hand eczema has been chosen, because there appear to be two clinical types of this dermatitis. One type is explosive, with eruptions of severe vesiculation or even bullous lesions (Fig. 13.5). This type is rare and best fits the initial descriptions of the dermatosis made in the late nineteenth century. Most of the cases described over the past 30 years are of a less severe type, with repeated eruptions of tiny, severely pruritic vesicles.

Although there have been many attempts to determine the etiology of acute and recurrent vesicular hand eczema, no general agreement has been reached. For many years, the eruptions were linked to nervousness or sweating in hot weather. It has been convincingly shown, however, that the vesicles are an expression of spongiosis as seen in acute eczema and that there is no connection with the acrosyringium [2]. Acute and recurrent vesicular hand eczema is, therefore, currently considered to be a variant of hand eczema that cannot be explained by external exposure to contact allergens or irritants on the involved skin.

Shelley [3] suggested the following possible causes of what he called dysidrosis (pompholyx): drug eruption, id reaction, mycotic infection, a psychosomatic cause, and/or an unknown cause.

After Christensen and Möller [4] showed that nickel-sensitive women often react with a vesicular eruption on palmar skin after oral challenge with nickel, a search was made for a connection between contact allergy and recurrent vesicular hand eczema. Numerous placebo-controlled oral challenge experiments, particularly among nickel-sensitive patients, have shown that it is possible in a dose-response fashion to reactivate vesicular hand eczema following an oral dose of nickel. Perhaps these investigations have uncovered a small part of what Shelley considered unknown etiology.

The topic has been reviewed several times, using the terms pompholyx-dyshidrotic eczema [5], dyshidrosis [6], pompholyx [7], acute and recurrent vesicular hand eczema (pompholyx) [8], and acute and recurrent vesicular hand eczema [9].

13.3 Epidemiology and Etiology

Few studies have dealt in detail with the morphology of hand eczema; therefore, it is difficult to estimate the epidemiology of acute and recurrent vesicular hand eczema. The question is further complicated by the lack of a common definition of this dermatitis.

In 1964–1965, Agrup [10] invited 141,444 persons in southern Sweden to have their hands and feet examined to determine whether they had a skin disease; 101,206 accepted the invitation. Of these, 1,551 had skin diseases on their hands, 827 had eczema, and 51 had acrovesiculatio recidivans.

Thelin and Agrup [11] described 83 patients with pompholyx seen in the same department of dermatology within a single year.

In a population-based study, 1,385 patients with hand eczema were examined by a dermatologist; 5 % had pompholyx [12].

Johansen et al. [13] carried out a prospective study of a consecutive group of 710 patients with hand eczema seen by dermatologists in the Danish Contact Dermatitis Group. The morphology of the eczema was determined based on photographs of six types of hand eczema. Thirty-three of 557 patients evaluated had vesicular dermatitis with infrequent eruptions, while 177 had vesicular dermatitis with repeated eruptions.

Diepgen et al. [14] suggested a clinical classification based upon both etiology and morphology and tested this classification on 416 hand eczema patients from ten European dermatology clinics. Thirty-seven of 396 patients (9 %) for whom a diagnosis was made had vesicular hand eczema. Another 30 had vesicular hand eczema in combination with specific etiological diagnoses.

Fourteen of 100 consecutive patients with hand eczema examined in a department of dermatology had pompholyx [15].

In a series of 364 consecutive patients, Meneghini and Angelini [16] failed to find evidence that microbial antigens caused pompholyx.

Lodi [17] studied 104 patients with pompholyx. No single definite cause was found.

A statistical relationship between vesicular eruptions on the hand and tinea pedis was found by Bryld et al. in a study of twins [18].

In a case-control study, multivariate analysis of 100 patients with pompholyx matched with 200 controls showed a statistically significant association between atopy and tinea pedis and vesicular hand eczema [19].

Guillet et al. [20] carried out a prospective study of 120 patients with pompholyx and found a significant number of patients with what they called allergic contact pompholyx. Many of the patch-test results that suggested this diagnosis were caused by shower gel or shampoo. It is difficult to test with such products, and no suitable controls were tested. A significant number of patients with contact dermatitis were included in the study, and many patients did not, therefore, fulfill the criteria for acute and recurrent hand eczema.

13.4 Atopy

It has been suggested that acute and recurrent vesicular hand eczema is a manifestation of atopic dermatitis. In fact, Schwanitz used the term *Das atopische palmoplantarekzem* in his study of 58 patients [21]. Lodi et al. found that 50 % of 104 patients with pompholyx had personal atopy or a family history of atopy, compared with 11.5 % in a control group ($p<0.001$). The number of patients or controls with atopic dermatitis was, however, not given [17].

In a prospective case-control study of 100 patients with pompholyx, personal atopy was statistically related to pompholyx [15].

Bryld et al. [18] found no statistical correlation between atopic dermatitis and vesicular eruptions on the hands among 283 twins with hand eczema.

13.5 Dermatophytid

The classical description of dermatophytid is a symmetrical, vesicular eruption on the palms, palmar skin of the fingers, and the sides of the fingers.

Kaaman and Torssander [22] described seven patients with vesicular id reactions on the hands documented by a positive trichophytin reaction. Most of the id reactions were caused by *Trichophyton (T.) mentagrophytes*.

Of 37 patients with vesicular id reactions on the hands, 28 had *T. mentagrophytes* on the feet, 9 had *T. rubrum* infection, and one had *Epidermophyton floccosum* infection [23].

A statistical correlation between vesicular eruptions on the hands and tinea pedis was seen in Bryld's twin study [18] and by Pitché et al. [19].

13.6 Drug Reactions

In a review of the literature, Gerstenblith et al. [24] identified 64 patients who had eczematous reactions following intravenous immunoglobulin therapy. Forty-eight of the patients had pompholyx either as the only manifestation or in combination with more widespread eczematous reactions.

Ekelund and Möller [25] challenged 12 patients with contact allergy to neomycin with oral neomycin and saw pompholyx in three patients following the challenge.

Menné and Weismann [26] noted a de novo vesicular eruption on the hands of a neomycin-sensitive patient after oral challenge with neomycin.

13.7 Systemic Contact Dermatitis

Systemic contact dermatitis is a flare of dermatitis in a contact-sensitized person after the hapten has been given orally, transcutaneously, rectally, intravenously, or following implantation. Examples of acute and recurrent vesicular hand eczema caused by systemic contact dermatitis are given above for the drug neomycin. Similar reactions have been seen following ingestion of pyrazinobutazone [27] and piroxicam [28].

Baeck et al. [29] studied 12 patients with contact allergy to inhaled corticosteroids in a tertiary referral center. Three of 12 patients had generalized cutaneous reactions following inhalation of corticosteroids.

It is curious that vesicular palmar eruptions are a common manifestation of systemic contact dermatitis caused by the metals nickel, cobalt, and chromium. This manifestation is not seen in patients with systemic contact dermatitis caused by topical steroids or gold [29, 30].

13.8 Allergic Contact Dermatitis

Food items may cause acute and recurrent hand eczema in contact-sensitized persons. An example of this is the recurrence of vesicular hand eczema after oral challenge with garlic in a garlic-sensitive patient [31].

The most common contact sensitization from plants is caused by Compositae plants. A flare of vesicular hand eczema was seen in one of four patients with contact sensitivity to lettuce after the ingestion of lettuce [32].

Three patients with contact allergy to spices had a flare of vesicular hand eczema following oral challenge with various spices [33].

Of 17 patients with contact sensitivity to balsam of Peru, four of four who had vesicular hand eczema experienced a flare of their dermatitis after oral challenge with balsam of Peru but not after placebo challenge [34].

Niinimäki [35] saw flares of vesicular hand eczema after oral challenge with balsam of Peru in 8 of 22 patients who had positive patch tests to balsam of Peru. The same author reported pompholyx reaction after oral challenge with various spices in three of seven patients (among 71 patients with positive patch tests to balsam of Peru) [36].

13.9 Metals

13.9.1 Implanted Metals

Implanted metals may have cutaneous side effects. Vesicular hand eczema is, however, not a common manifestation. The mechanism of cutaneous side effects of implanted metals is not clear. Cases of cutaneous delayed-type sensitization followed by elicitation of systemic contact dermatitis to the implanted metals have been reported. This mechanism does not, however, explain all the cases of cutaneous side effects caused by implanted metals [37].

Dental metals include wires used in orthodontic treatment, dental plates, and amalgam or gold in fillings or other types of dental restorations.

A boy developed palmar and plantar dermatitis after orthodontic treatment with wires containing nickel and chromium. He had positive patch tests to nickel and cobalt. The dermatitis faded after discontinuation of orthodontic treatment [38].

Of three girls with vesicular hand eczema undergoing orthodontic treatment with steel dental bands, one had a positive patch test to potassium dichromate. She experienced a flare of vesicular hand eczema after placebo-controlled oral challenge with 2.5 mg chromium given as potassium dichromate. The other two girls had negative patch tests, but the vesicular hand eczema of one of the two was reactivated after placebo-controlled oral challenge with 2.5 mg nickel; the other girl reacted to 2.5 mg chromium given as potassium dichromate. The dermatitis of two of the three girls faded after discontinuation of orthodontic treatment [39].

Infusion needles may release nickel. Two patients developed vesicular hand eczema after the use of such needles [40].

An ankle fracture repaired with a steel plate caused vesicular hand eczema. The patient in question had positive patch tests to nickel and chromate. The dermatitis improved after removal of the plate, which contained both nickel and chromium [41].

13.9.2 Ingested Metals

After Christensen and Möller in 1975 [4] demonstrated that vesicular hand eczema in nickel allergic patients might flare after placebo-controlled oral challenge with nickel, similar challenge studies have been performed in several centers.

Bedello et al. [42] challenged 49 nickel-sensitive patients with 2.24 mg nickel in a controlled study. Thirty-one patients reacted to the challenge. Fifteen of the patients who reacted to nickel had vesicular hand eczema.

Oral challenge with 1 or 3 mg nickel in a placebo-controlled study showed a dose-dependent flare of nickel patch-test sites. One patient also developed de novo vesicular hand eczema following challenge with 3 mg nickel [43].

Veien et al. [44] conducted a placebo-controlled study of 144 patients with positive patch tests to nickel and/or cobalt and a dermatitis thought to be consistent morphologically with systemic contact dermatitis. Of 97 patients sensitive only to nickel, 31 reacted to challenge with nickel, 8 reacted to nickel and cobalt, and 8 reacted to cobalt. Fifty-three of the 144 patients had vesicular hand eczema. Six of the 13 patients with positive patch tests to cobalt alone had vesicular hand eczema. Three of the six reacted to oral challenge with cobalt with a flare of dermatitis.

In another study [45], it was shown that four of six patients with vesicular hand eczema and positive patch tests only to cobalt experienced flares of dermatitis after placebo-controlled oral challenge with 1 mg cobalt given as cobalt chloride.

Disulfiram chelates nickel. Initiation of disulfiram treatment increases the concentration of nickel in serum. In the early phase of treatment, eruptions of vesicular hand eczema have been seen [46]. Similar eruptions of vesicular hand eczema have been seen following initiation of disulfiram treatment for chronic alcoholism in a cobalt-sensitive patient [47].

In another study, Yokozeki et al. [48] found that 20 % of 25 patients with pompholyx had positive patch tests to dichromate, while 16 % reacted to cobalt and 28 % to nickel. Four of six of the 25 patients reacted to oral challenge with either 2.5 mg nickel or 2.5 mg chromium.

In a placebo-controlled challenge experiment carried out for 31 patients with contact sensitivity to potassium dichromate, 11 of the patients who had vesicular hand eczema reacted to chromate, compared with 2 of 11 who did not have vesicular hand eczema. Close-up photographs taken prior to and 2 days after the challenge were compared in a blind fashion [49].

Eight of 12 patients with vesicular hand eczema reacted to oral challenge with 2.5 mg chromium in a double-blind, placebo-controlled study of 30 patients with contact sensitivity to potassium dichromate [50].

13.10 Other Causes

It has been suggested that acute and recurrent vesicular hand eczema could be induced by various food items.

Flood and Perry [51] described 30 patients with recurrent vesicular hand eczema. The dermatitis of these patients improved after they followed a strict diet, eliminating tuna, tomato, pineapple, American cheese, milk, egg, wheat, lamb, chocolate, and chicken.

The dermatitis of 21 patients who drank more than 10 cups of coffee a day improved after coffee consumption was reduced. Nine of the patients had recurrent, vesicular hand eczema. Five of the patients had no reaction to an oral challenge with caffeine [52].

Five patients developed pompholyx-like eruptions on the sides of the fingers after exposure to sunlight. The reactions were reproduced by UVA provocation on previously affected skin. No such reactions were seen in 10 control patients with idiopathic pompholyx [53].

Thirty-three patients with dyshidrotic eczema were trained to either increase or decrease skin conductance. Patients were randomized to receive either (a) training to decrease skin conductance or (b) training to increase skin conductance. Both groups received a Radio Shack kit NO. 28–182. This kit produces a tone that decreases in frequency as a relative function of decreased skin conductance. For group B, the same kit was wired to produce a decrease in tone as a relative function of increased skin conductance. Decreased skin conductance was followed by improvement of the dermatitis [54].

Biofeedback training led to an improvement of the dermatitis of five patients with dyshidrosis who had responded poorly to other treatments [55].

Fourteen of 23 individuals in a Chinese family had pompholyx. A gene located on chromosome 18q22.1–18q22.3 appeared to be the cause. The inheritance was autosomal dominant with 99.9 % penetrance [56].

13.11 Differential Diagnoses

The lesions of palmoplantar pustulosis may, in the early stages of the disease, appear as vesicles. In a matter of days, the content of the lesions becomes white or yellow as an expression of leukocyte content. Although severe eruptions may be painful, there is usually no pruritus.

Bullous pemphigoid has been known to mimic acute vesicular hand eczema. The diagnosis is based on histology and direct as well as indirect immunofluorescence consistent with findings in bullous pemphigoid [57, 58].

Dyshidrosis lamellosa sicca or recurrent palmar peeling is a very superficial scaling that may mimic a vesicular eruption. There is, however, no fluid in the initial lesions, and the individual lesions evolve into annular scaling. Repeated eruptions may lead to thinning of the stratum corneum and soreness of the skin (Figs. 13.6 and 13.7).

13.12 Severity

A score system for vesicular hand eczema known as dyshidrotic eczema area and severity index (DASI) was found to be useful in two clinical trials [59]. This scoring system is based on the scoring of four features: number of vesicles, erythema, desquamation, and itching. Each feature is scored arbitrarily as 0 = absent, 1 = mild, 2 = moderate, or 3 = severe. For vesicles, the total number is counted and divided by the affected area in cm^2.

13.13 Management

The most important aspect of the management of acute and recurrent vesicular hand eczema is the determination of the cause of the eruptions.

The history should include information about external and possible systemic exposures.

Vesicular eruptions have been described as occurring less than 1 h after exposure to proteins in persons with protein contact dermatitis.

Oral challenge with nickel has caused vesicular palmar eruptions after 1–3 days in nickel-sensitive patients. A history of exposures up to 3 days before the eruption of vesicular hand eczema is, therefore, an essential element in the diagnosis of this condition.

The history should include information regarding dermatophytosis of the feet, particularly that caused by *T. mentagrophytes* [23].

Patients with recurrent vesicular hand eczema should be patch tested with a standard tray, including the metals nickel, cobalt, and chromium, as well as balsam of Peru and perfume ingredients. When protein contact dermatitis is suspected, prick testing and prick-prick testing should be carried out with suspected food items.

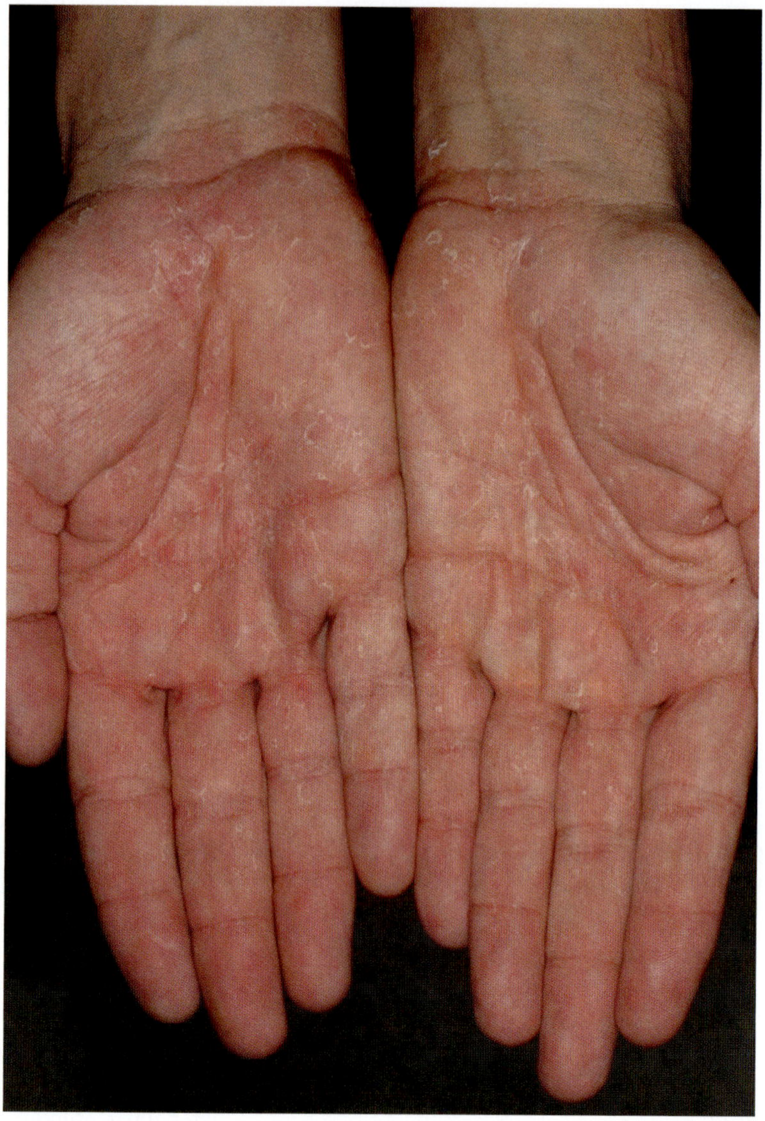

Fig. 13.6 Dyshidrosis lamellosa sicca or recurrent palmar peeling

Placebo-controlled oral challenge with haptens can be carried out in selected patients. It is particularly important to do controlled oral challenge if dietary restrictions are contemplated. Dietary restrictions may be difficult to adhere to and will have considerable impact on the daily life of the patient.

Diet trials in patients with hand eczema should last from 1 to 3 months. If improvement is not apparent, the diet trial should be discontinued. If improvement is seen, the diet should be moderated to make life easier for the patient.

Pharmacological treatment of acute and recurrent hand eczema is discussed further in Chaps. 27, 28, 29, 30, 31, 32, 33, 34, 35, 36, 37, 38, 39, 40, 41, and 42 of this book.

Topical and systemic treatment options for pompholyx were reviewed by Wollina [7]. He concluded that topical steroids are the cornerstone of treatment and that systemic corticosteroids should be used in severe cases. He scored treatment options according to level of evidence. The level of evidence of the value of various treatments of pompholyx is presented in Table 13.1 [7].

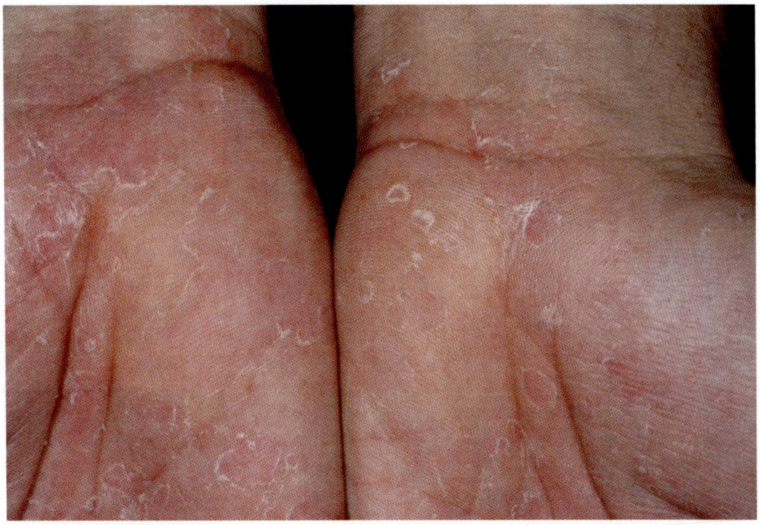

Fig. 13.7 Close-up photograph of the patient shown in Fig. 13.6

Table 13.1 Evidence-based medicine in pompholyx[a]

Treatments	Evidence level[b]
Botulinum toxin A	3[c]
Immunosuppressants (azathioprine, methotrexate, cyclosporine [ciclosporin], mycophenolate mofetil, corticosteroids, etc.)	4a[c]
Retinoids (alitretinoin)	2
PUVA	2
Radiotherapy	4a
Selective UVB phototherapy	3
Tap water iontophoresis	3[c]
Topical corticosteroids	2
Topical calcineurin inhibitors	2
Topical bexarotene plus mid-potency corticosteroid	2
UVA-1	2

PUVA psoralen plus UVA
[a]Reprinted with permission from Wollina [7]
[b]Levels of evidence-based medicine in clinical studies. Level 1: evidence is available for meta-analysis from several randomized controlled studies; level 2: evidence is available from at least one randomized controlled trial; level 4: evidence is available from good methodologic studies without randomization; level 4a: evidence is available from clinical case reports; level 4: this represents a consensus of respected experts or expert committees
[c]Mostly with topical corticosteroids

Conclusion

It is suggested that the term acute and recurrent vesicular hand eczema should be reserved for infrequent or recurrent pruritic vesicular eruptions solely on the palmar skin (palms, palmar aspects of the fingers, sides of the fingers, and/or periungual skin). The eruptions occur with no prior skin contact with contact allergens, irritants, or proteins. There is little or no inflammation following solitary eruptions, while repeated eruptions may be followed by inflammatory changes such as erythema, infiltration, and scaling. This makes it difficult to distinguish recurrent vesicular hand eczema from other types of hand eczema.

Acute and recurrent vesicular hand eczema is a nonspecific reaction pattern that may be associated with atopic dermatitis, drug eruptions, systemic contact dermatitis, id reactions, and probably other, as yet unidentified, sources.

Severe acute eruptions are rare. Therefore, most cases can be encompassed by the term recurrent vesicular hand eczema.

The terms dyshidrosis and dyshidrotic hand eczema are best abandoned, as there is no evidence of any relationship to the acrosyringium. The vesicles associated with acute and recurrent hand eczema are the result of spongiosis, as seen in acute dermatitis.

Pompholyx refers in the strictest sense to a rarely seen, severe eruption of vesicles or small bullae on palmar and possibly also on plantar skin. For many years, the term pompholyx has been used to describe recurrent vesicular hand eczema. As there is no clear definition of pompholyx, the term is not very useful.

References

1. Storrs F. Acute and recurrent vesicular hand dermatitis not pompholyx or dyshidrosis. Arch Dermatol. 2007;143(12):1578–80.
2. Kutzner H, Wurzel RM, Wolff HH. Are acrosyringia involved in the pathogenesis of "dyshidrosis"? Am J Dermatopathol. 1986;8(2):109–16.
3. Shelley WB. Dysidrosis (pompholyx). Arch Dermatol Syph. 1953;68:314–8.
4. Christensen OB, Möller H. External and internal exposure to the allergen in the hand eczema of nickel allergy. Contact Dermatitis. 1975;1(3):136–41.
5. Menné T, Hjorth N. Pompholyx – dyshidrotic eczema. Semin Dermatol. 1983;2(1):75–80.
6. Lofgren SM, Warshaw EM. Dyshidrosis: epidemiology, clinical characteristics and therapy. Dermatitis. 2006;17(4):165–81.
7. Wollina U. Pompholyx. A review of clinical features, differential diagnosis, and management. Am J Clin Dermatol. 2010;11(5):306–14.
8. Veien NK, Menné T. Acute and recurrent vesicular hand dermatitis (pompholyx). In: Menné T, Maibach H, editors. Hand eczema. 2nd ed. Boca Raton: CRC Press; 2000.
9. Veien NK. Acute and recurrent vesicular hand dermatitis. Dermatol Clin. 2009;27(3):337–53.
10. Agrup G. Hand eczema and other hand dermatoses in South Sweden [thesis]. Acta Derm Venereol. 1969;49 Suppl 61:1–91.
11. Thelin I, Agrup G. Pompholyx – a one year series. Acta Derm Venereol. 1985;65:214–7.
12. Meding B. Epidemiology of hand eczema in an industrial city [dissertation]. Acta Derm Venereol. 1990; Suppl 153:1–43.
13. Johansen JD, Hald M, Andersen BL, Laurberg G, Danielsen A, Avnstorp C, et al. Classification of hand eczema: clinical and aetiological types. Based on the guideline of the Danish Contact Dermatitis Group. Contact Dermatitis. 2011;65(1):13–21.
14. Diepgen TL, Andersen KE, Brandao FM, Bruze M, Bruynzeel DP, Frosch P, et al., on behalf of the European Environmental and Contact Dermatitis Research Group. Hand eczema classification: a cross-sectional, multicentre study of the aetiology and morphology of hand eczema. Br J Dermatol. 2008;160:353–58.
15. Handa S, Kaur I, Gupta T, Jindal R. Hand eczema. Correlation of morphologic patterns, atopy, contact sensitization and disease severity. Indian J Dermatol Venereol Lepro. 2012;78(2):153–8.
16. Meneghini CL, Angelini G. Contact and microbial allergy in pompholyx. Contact Dermatitis. 1979;5(1): 46–50.
17. Lodi A, Betti R, Charelli G, Urbani CE, Crosti C. Epidemiological clinical and allergological observations on pompholyx. Contact Dermatitis. 1992;26(1): 17–21.
18. Bryld LE, Agner T, Menné T. Relation between vesicular eruptions on the hands and tinea pedis, atopic dermatitis and nickel allergy. Acta Derm Venereol. 2003;83:186–8.
19. Pitché P, Boukari M, Tchangai-Walla K. Factors associated with palmoplantar or plantar pompholyx: a case-control study [in French]. Ann Dermatol Venereol. 2006;133(2):139–43.
20. Guillet MH, Wierzbicka E, Guillet S, Dagregorio G, Guillet G. A 3-year causative study of pompholyx in 120 patients. Arch Dermatol. 2007;143(12):1504–8.
21. Schwanitz HJ. Das atopische Palmoplantarekzem. Berlin: Springer; 1986.
22. Kaaman T, Torssander J. Dermatophytid – a misdiagnosed entity? Acta Derm Venerol. 1983;63(5):404–8.
23. Veien NK, Hattel T, Laurberg G. Plantar *Trichophyton rubrum* infections may cause dermatophytids on the hands. Acta Derm Venereol. 1994;74:403–4.
24. Gerstenblith MR, Antony AK, Junkins-Hopkins JM, Abuav R. Pompholyx and eczematous reactions associated with intravenous immunoglobulin therapy. J Am Acad Dermatol. 2011;66(2):312–6.
25. Ekelund A-G, Möller H. Oral provocation in eczematous contact allergy to neomycin and hydroxyquinolines. Acta Derma Venerol. 1969;49:422–6.
26. Menné T, Weismann K. Hämatogenes Kontaktekzem nach oraler Gabe von Neomyzin. Hautarzt. 1984; 35(6):319–20.
27. Dorado Bris JM, Aragues Montañes M, Sols Candela M, Garcia DA. Contact sensitivity to pyrazinobutazone (Carudol®) with positive oral provocation test. Contact Dermatitis. 1992;26(5):355–6.
28. Piqué E, Pérez JA, Benjumeda A. Oral piroxicam-induced dyshidrosiform dermatitis. Contact Dermatitis. 2004;50(6):382–3.
29. Baeck M, Pilette C, Drieghe J, Goossens A. Allergic contact dermatitis to inhalation steroids. Eur J Dermatol. 2010;20(1):102–8.
30. Möller H. Contact allergy to gold as a model for clinical-experimental research. Contact Dermatitis. 2010;62(4):193–200.
31. Burden AD, Wilkinson SM, Beck MH, Chalmers RJ. Garlic induced systemic contact dermatitis. Contact Dermatitis. 1994;30(5):299–300.
32. Oliwiecki S, Beck MH, Hausen BM. Compositae dermatitis aggravated by eating lettuce. Contact Dermatitis. 1991;24(4):318–9.
33. Dooms-Goosens A, Fubelloy R, Degreef H. Contact and systemic contact-type dermatitis to spices. Dermatol Clin. 1990;8(1):89–93.
34. Veien NK, Hattel T, Justesen O, Nørholm A. Oral challenge with balsam of Peru. Contact Dermatitis. 1985;12(2):104–7.
35. Niinimäki A. Delayed-type allergy to spices. Contact Dermatitis. 1984;11(1):34–40.

36. Niinimäki A. Double-blind placebo-controlled peroral challenges in patients with delayed-type allergy to balsam of Peru. Contact Dermatitis. 1995;33(2): 78–83.
37. Schalock PC, Menné T, Johansen JD, Taylor JS, Maibach HI, Lidén C, et al. Hypersensitivity reactions to metallic implants – diagnostic algorithm and suggested patch test series for clinical use. Contact Dermatitis. 2012;66(1):4–19.
38. Kerosuo H, Kanerva L. Systemic contact dermatitis caused by nickel in a stainless steel orthodontic appliance. Contact Dermatitis. 1997;36(2):112–3.
39. Veien NK, Borchorst E, Hattel T, Laurberg G. Stomatitis of systemically-induced contact dermatitis from metal wire on orthodontic materials. Contact Dermatitis. 1994;30(4):210–3.
40. Smeenk G, Teunissen PC. Allergische reacties op nickel uit infusie-toedieningssystemen [in Dutch]. Ned Tijdscht Geneeskd. 1977;121:4–9.
41. Kanerva L, Förström L. Allergic nickel and chromate hand dermatitis induced by orthopaedic metal implant. Contact Dermatitis. 2001;44(2):103–4.
42. Bedello PG, Goitre M, Cane D, Roncarolo G. Nichel: aptene ubiquitario. [in Italian]. G Ital Dermatol Venereol. 1985;120(4):293–6.
43. Hindsén M, Bruze M, Christensen OB. Flare-up reactions after oral challenge with nickel in relation to challenge dose and intensity and time of previous patch test reactions. J Am Acad Dermatol. 2001;44: 616–23.
44. Veien NK, Hattel T, Justesen O, Nørholm A. Oral challenge with nickel and cobalt in patients with positive patch tests to nickel and/or cobalt. Acta Derm Venereol. 1987;67:321–6.
45. Veien NK, Hattel T, Laurberg G. Placebo-controlled oral challenge with cobalt in patients with positive patch tests to cobalt. Contact Dermatitis. 1995;33(1): 54–5.
46. Lein LR, Fowler Jr JF. Nickel dermatitis recall during disulfiram therapy for alcohol abuse. J Am Acad Dermatol. 1992;26(4):645–6.
47. Menné T. Flare-up of cobalt dermatitis from Antabuse® treatment. Contact Dermatitis. 1985;12(1): 53.
48. Yokozeki H, Katayama I, Nishioka K, Kinoshita M, Nishiyama S. The role of metal allergy and local hyperhidrosis in the pathogenesis of pompholyx. J Dermatol. 1992;19(12):964–7.
49. Kaaber K, Veien NK. The significance of chromate ingestion in patients allergic to chromate. Acta Derm Venereol. 1977;57(4):321–3.
50. Veien NK, Hattel T, Laurberg G. Chromate-allergic patients challenged orally with potassium dichromate. Contact Dermatitis. 1994;31(3):137–9.
51. Flood JM, Perry DJ. Role of food allergy in eczematoid dermatitis. Arch Dermatol Syphilol. 1947;55: 493–506.
52. Veien NK, Hattel T, Justesen O. Dermatoses in coffee drinkers. Cutis. 1987;40:421–2.
53. Man I, Ibbotson SH, Ferguson J. Photoinduced pompholyx: a report of 5 cases. J Am Acad Dermatol. 2004;50(1):55–60.
54. Miller RM, Coger RW. Skin conductance conditioning with dyshidrotic eczema patients. Br J Dermatol. 1979;101:435–40.
55. Koldys KW, Meyer RP. Biofeedback training in the therapy of dyshidrosis. Cutis. 1979;24:219–21.
56. Chen J-J, Liang Y-H, Zhou F-S, Yang S, Wang J, Wang PG, et al. The gene for a rare autosomal dominant form of pompholyx maps to chromosome 18q22.1–18q22.3. J Invest Dermatol. 2006;126(2):300–4.
57. Patrizi A, Rizzoli L, Benassi L, Nerit I. Another case of dyshidrosiform pemphigoid. Eur Acad Dermatol Venereol. 2003;17:348–72.
58. Lupi F, Masini C, Ruffelli M, Puddu P, Cianchini G. Dyshidrosiform palmoplantar pemphigoid in a young man: response to dapsone. Acta Derm Venereol. 2010;90(1):80–1.
59. Vocks E, Plötz SG, Ring J. The dyshidrotic eczema area and severity index – a score developed for the assessment of dyshidrotic eczema. Dermatology. 1999;198(3):265–9.

Hyperkeratotic Eczema (Psoriasis) of the Palms

14

Steven R. Feldman and Arash Taheri

Contents

S.R. Feldman, M.D., Ph.D. • A. Taheri, M.D. (✉)
Dermatology, Wake Forest School of Medicine,
Medical Center Boulevard, Winston-Salem,
NC 27157-1071, USA
e-mail: sfeldman@wakehealth.edu;
ataheri@wakehealth.edu

14.1 Introduction

Hyperkeratotic eczema of the palms (also called hyperkeratotic hand eczema) is a relatively frustrating recalcitrant form of hand dermatitis. Although the nomenclature and the clinical and pathological presentations of the variants of hand eczema often overlap and render the diagnostic classification imprecise, this condition presents as chronic, scaly, slightly erythematous, hyperkeratotic, fissure-prone plaques on the palms. Typically, plaques are discrete, with relatively sharp margins (Fig. 14.1). They have a multifocal and symmetrical distribution. Sometimes the plaques coalesce together to cover most of the palmar surface. They typically occur on the central palms. The border of the palms and the volar surfaces of the fingers may also be involved. The eruption tends to spare dorsal hand and fingertips [1, 2]. Plantar involvement is present in some cases. Finding an eczematous eruption in other body areas is not common [1, 3].

The eruption may be asymptomatic; however, in nearly half of the patients, it is itchy [3]. When fissures are present, it may be painful. The symptoms may be severe and devastating in some patients. This chronic, incurable disease can cause significant functional, psychological, and social problems and severely impair a patient's quality of life [4].

Hyperkeratotic eczema of the palms may be clinically very similar to palmar psoriasis. We discuss the differentiation between these two entities later in this chapter.

A. Alikhan et al. (eds.), *Textbook of Hand Eczema*,
DOI 10.1007/978-3-642-39546-8_14, © Springer-Verlag Berlin Heidelberg 2014

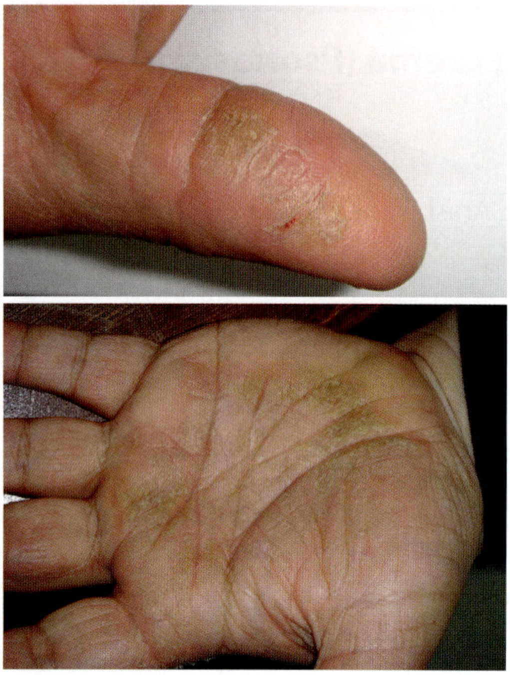

Fig. 14.1 Hyperkeratotic psoriasiform dermatitis of the palms in a middle-aged man

14.2 Epidemiology

Hyperkeratotic eczema of the palms constitutes 2–13 % of hand eczema [1, 5]. Its prevalence varies in different populations. Compared to other types of hand eczema, the hyperkeratotic type typically affects older age groups. It is most prevalent in people 40–60 years of age. This entity is more common in men than women [1, 3, 5, 6].

Hyperkeratotic eczema of the palms is usually considered a very chronic and recalcitrant eruption. Most of the patients encountered have a history of more than 3 years [3]. A review of 32 patients with hyperkeratotic hand eczema reexamined 10 years after initial presentation showed that in 29 patients the eruption had remained more or less unchanged [2]. The chronic, devastating course of the disease may lead to disability in manual workers.

14.3 Etiology

Hyperkeratotic eczema of the palms is considered an endogenous dermatitis. The etiology is unknown. As yet, genetics do not appear to play a major role in hyperkeratotic hand dermatitis. The patients usually have no relevant irritant exposure or contact sensitization [1, 7]. Patch tests are usually negative, and the incidence of atopy is not greater than in the general population. The prevalence of psoriasis in close relatives does not differ from what can be found in the general population [1, 2].

Although some authors consider hyperkeratotic hand dermatitis as an entity independent of mechanical irritation, some use the term "frictional hand dermatitis" to describe a subset of hyperkeratotic hand dermatitis that is precipitated by repeated mechanical trauma and friction to the hands [2, 8]. Frictional hand dermatitis is usually seen in manual workers and is more prominent on the dominant hand, where the mechanical stress is more severe. Once removed from the repeated mechanical trauma, the eruption improves after a few days to months, depending on the severity of the dermatitis. At least in some cases, what we call frictional hand dermatitis may actually be a form of chronic irritant contact dermatitis or maybe palmar psoriasis with Koebner phenomenon.

Some seasonal variability in severity of symptoms has been reported. In one study, 30 % of the patients with hyperkeratotic hand dermatitis experienced some degree of exacerbation in summers and 70 % in winters [3].

Most authors consider hyperkeratotic hand dermatitis and localized palmar psoriasis as two separate entities. However, differentiation between these two entities may be arbitrary. Clinical findings may be very similar. Some authors claim that psoriatic lesions have a thicker layer of silvery scale and are more inflammatory. However, we do not have any gold standard diagnostic measure to test this claim. Histopathological findings are usually nonspecific. In one study, only 10 % of the biopsies gave definitive diagnoses [9]. There is debate as to whether hyperkeratotic eczema of the palms is a truly eczematous condition or whether it represents manifestations of psoriasis.

14.4 Histopathology

The characteristic histologic features of hyperkeratotic hand eczema include spongiosis and psoriasiform hyperplasia of the epidermis, although the elongation of the rete ridges is usually not as regular as in typical cases of psoriasis. Overlying compact orthokeratosis with small foci of parakeratosis is typical. The dilated blood vessels in the upper dermis are surrounded by a moderately dense mononuclear cell infiltrate. Lymphocyte exocytosis may be prominent in the epidermis, but there are usually no neutrophils [10]. Histopathological findings cannot differentiate hyperkeratotic eczema of the palms from other types of chronic hand dermatitis.

Many features of eczematous palmar dermatitis overlap with those of plaque-type palmar psoriasis. Both dermatoses of this skin area share similar histologic features [9]. Some histologic features that have been suggested to be helpful in differentiating psoriasis from eczematous dermatitis include the absence of granular layer, regular epidermal hyperplasia, thinned suprapapillary plate, tortuous capillaries in the papillary dermis, and lack of spongiosis. However, both psoriasis and chronic eczematous conditions of the hands may show these features.

In 2007, Aydin et al. [11] conducted a study comparing histologic findings of palmoplantar psoriasis with those of palmoplantar eczema. The patients with eczema were not limited to hyperkeratotic type. Diagnostic criteria for distinguishing these two were not described, except for the presence of psoriatic lesions in other body areas in patients with psoriasis. Interestingly, in this study, spongiosis and vesiculation were more common in patients clinically classified as having palmoplantar psoriasis than in patients with dermatitis (Table 14.1). The authors concluded that histologic features of palmoplantar psoriasis and eczema overlap with each other.

Table 14.1 Distribution of histologic findings according to clinical diagnosis in Aydin et al. study [11]

	Palmoplantar psoriasis (%)	Palmoplantar eczema (%)
Spongiotic vesicles	76	60
Confluent parakeratosis	29	44
Multiple foci of parakeratosis	70	44
Neutrophils at the summits of parakeratosis	6	4
Loss of granular layer	41	36
Psoriasiform epidermal hyperplasia	88	80
Irregular epidermal hyperplasia	12	20
Thinned suprapapillary plate	59	40
Edema of the papillary dermis	29	12
Tortuous capillaries in the papillary dermis	53	44

14.5 Differential Diagnosis

Hyperkeratotic eczema of the palms is very similar clinically and histologically to localized palmar psoriasis. Evidence of psoriasis on other body areas, including the nails, can be used to help establish the diagnosis of psoriasis. At times, it can be difficult to determine whether psoriasiform hand dermatitis represents a chronic hyperkeratotic dermatitis or localized psoriasis. We tend to use the term "hyperkeratotic psoriasiform dermatitis of the palms" to describe these patients.

Other types of hand dermatitis such as contact dermatitis or atopic dermatitis may be hyperkeratotic in chronic stages. Distribution of lesions and sharp margins of plaques in hyperkeratotic eczema of the palms can help us to differentiate it from other types of hand eczema.

Acrokeratosis paraneoplastica (Bazex syndrome) may be difficult to distinguish from hyperkeratotic eczema of the palms and palmoplantar psoriasis clinically and histologically [12]. Distribution of lesions is usually a clue to the diagnosis. The lesions appear around the tips of the fingers and nail folds, dorsal hand and foot, the nose, and the conchae of the ears. Histologically, there is mild acanthosis and hyperkeratosis with scattered parakeratotic foci.

The term "keratoderma climactericum" is used to describe a condition that is sometimes similar to hyperkeratotic hand eczema clinically and pathologically, occurring on the soles in females over the age of 45 years. Pressure areas such as the heel and the forefoot are involved first. In severe cases, a thick yellowish hyperkeratotic layer may be seen with erythema and scaling at the margins [13]. Keratoderma climactericum is generally a clinical diagnosis, based on the age and sex of the patient and on typical clinical findings, including initial involvement of the feet. The relationship to endocrine function and hormonal levels remains uncertain [14]. There are reports of female patients in whom keratoderma climactericum arose following bilateral oophorectomy and was completely reversed by estrogen replacement [15].

A wide range of dermatoses may on occasion give palmar or plantar hyperkeratosis and erythema. Palmoplantar keratoderma is seen in a variety of genetic disorders and syndromes. Reiter's syndrome (keratoderma blennorrhagica), cutaneous T-cell lymphoma, palmoplantar pustulosis, lichen planus, pityriasis rubra pilaris, lupus erythematosus, Darier's disease, syphilis, and tinea manuum should be considered in differential diagnosis of hyperkeratotic hand dermatitis.

14.6 Treatment

Although hyperkeratotic hand dermatitis is not considered a form of contact dermatitis, traditionally, we recommend avoidance of irritants and aggressive use of emollients. Moisturizers and emollients, at least, help to reduce the symptoms significantly. Patch testing and searching for an allergen may be a wise approach when diagnosis is in question.

As for other types of chronic hand dermatitis, topical corticosteroids are usually first-line treatment for hyperkeratotic hand dermatitis and also for palmoplantar psoriasis. High-potency corticosteroids under occlusion are more effective. The optimal choice of vehicle is generally the one the individual patient likes and will most likely use. Long-term use is limited by local side effects, such as skin atrophy. Once initial control of the condition is achieved, perhaps after 2–3 weeks of daily use, patients should be transitioned to intermittent use to reduce the risk of skin atrophy. Considering the chronic course of hyperkeratotic eczema of the palms and problems with ruling out psoriasis, systemic corticosteroids are rarely used, though they may be prescribed intermittently when needed to control severe flares.

Topical vitamin D3 derivatives have been used with some success in treatment of hyperkeratotic hand eczema. In one study, the lesions almost disappeared after 2–8 weeks of treatment in four out of five patients and extremely improved with a 7-week treatment in one patient [16]. The authors of this book chapter have not seen this level of response in their personal experience.

Other topical treatments such as tar, calcineurin inhibitors (tacrolimus and pimecrolimus), and retinoids (bexarotene and tazarotene) have been used successfully in treating chronic hand eczema and psoriasis [17–20]. In one study, 39 % of patients with chronic severe hand dermatitis using bexarotene gel achieved 90 % or more clearance of hand lesions, and 79 % of patients achieved 50 % or more clinical improvement. Adverse events included stinging or burning (15 %), flare of dermatitis (16 %), and irritation (29 %) [21].

In another study comparing topical tazarotene cream with clobetasol propionate cream for palmoplantar psoriasis, the tazarotene group showed an 83 % mean severity score reduction compared to baseline at 12 weeks. Complete clearance was noted in 53 % of the patients. The clobetasol propionate group demonstrated an 89 % mean score reduction, with complete clearance in 61 % of the patients. Differences between the two groups were statistically insignificant. Side effects observed were initial irritation (41 %) in the tazarotene group and hypopigmentation (54 %) in the steroid-treated patients [22].

Using tazarotene in combination with a topical corticosteroid like clobetasol may be a better choice than either drug alone. This combination has the theoretical advantages of the topical steroid reducing the irritation of the vitamin A analog and the vitamin A analog potentially reducing the risk of atrophy associated with the topical corticosteroid.

Although topical treatments are first line in management of hyperkeratotic hand eczema, the response may not be satisfactory in some patients. In one study, 19 out of 32 patients considered they were somewhat improved by topical treatment including potent corticosteroids, bland ointments, and tar or Grenz rays, but the improvement was transient. Thirteen considered they were not improved at all by various topical treatments [2]. In a retrospective study on palmoplantar psoriasis, 17 of 62 patients showed marked improvement to topical agents, while the remaining patients required systemic agents or phototherapy [23]. The reason for unsatisfactory results of topical treatment of a palmar eruption may be poor penetration of the topical agent, but poor adherence to treatment should also be considered.

Systemic retinoids are effective in treatment of hyperkeratotic hand eczema. In one study, 59 % of the patients with hyperkeratotic hand eczema achieved a Physician Global Assessment rating of "clear" or "almost clear" hands with oral alitretinoin [24, 25]. In a multicenter trial of 1,032 patients with severe chronic hand dermatitis refractory to topical corticosteroids (most of whom had hyperkeratotic hand eczema), success, defined as clear or almost clear hands, was achieved in up to 48 % of patients treated with alitretinoin 30 mg/day, compared with 17 % for placebo; 75 % of patients experienced some reduction in disease signs and symptoms. Treatment was well tolerated, with dose-dependent adverse effects comprising headache, mucocutaneous events, hyperlipidemia, and decreased free thyroxine and thyroid-stimulating hormone. The median time to relapse, defined as recurrence of 75 % of initial signs and symptoms, was 5.5–6.2 months in the absence of anti-eczema medication [26].

Acitretin is considered an effective treatment for hyperkeratotic hand eczema and palmoplantar psoriasis. Acitretin is especially useful for thinning out thick hyperkeratotic areas and making the lesions more susceptible to other treatments such as topical agents and phototherapy. A 51 % reduction of all symptoms was observed among patients with hyperkeratotic hand eczema receiving 30 mg acitretin daily in one study [27]. A controlled study of comparative efficacy of oral acitretin, 25–50 mg/day, and topical betamethasone/salicylic acid ointment for chronic hyperkeratotic palmoplantar dermatitis showed that acitretin was significantly better than ointment after 30 days, and improvement persisted 5 months after suspension of treatment. Lesions improved more rapidly with acitretin, with minimal side effects. Patients were more satisfied with acitretin [28].

Phototherapy has been reported to work well for patients with hyperkeratotic hand eczema. Narrowband UVB (NB-UVB) may not be able to penetrate the thick stratum corneum of palm as well as UVA; therefore, photochemotherapy using UVA may, at least theoretically, be more effective than NB-UVB in this area. Evidence from clinical trials is mixed. The efficacies of oral PUVA and broadband UVB treatment in chronic eczematous dermatitis of the hands were compared in a randomized controlled study including 35 patients. One hand was exposed to light, and the other served as an untreated control. The dermatitis cleared on the treated hand in all PUVA patients, but in 9 out of 14 there was a relapse within 3 months. In the UVB group, clearing of the skin lesions was not achieved, but compared with the untreated hands, a statistically significant improvement was found at 12 weeks of treatment [29]. In a study of patients with palmoplantar psoriasis using NB-UVB irradiation on one side and paint-PUVA on the other side, there was a statistically significant improvement with both treatments. The difference in clinical response between the two treatment modalities was statistically significant, with the percentage reduction in severity index scores with the paint-PUVA treated side being 85 % compared with 61 % for the NB-UVB treated side [30]. In another study of 13 patients with chronic hand dermatitis treated with topical PUVA to one hand and broadband UVB to the other, however, no differences in clinical improvement between the two treatment modalities were found [31]. Furthermore, in a study of 15 patients with chronic hand eczema who received NB-UVB on one hand and paint-PUVA on the other hand, there was a similar 75 % reduction in total clinical scores in each treated side [32].

In a report of local bath PUVA for hyperkeratotic hand eczema, 43 % of patients cleared and 43 % improved substantially (reduction of extent by more than 50 %) [33]. In another study of 30 patients with palmoplantar eczema or psoriasis treated with 8 weeks of bath PUVA, 63 % showed a complete remission, and 23 % showed considerable improvement. Of note, palmoplantar psoriasis responded better than hyperkeratotic dermatitis to treatment [34]. In another study using bath PUVA treatment for palmoplantar dermatoses, the best results were found in patients with hyperkeratotic palmoplantar eczema, followed by patients with palmoplantar psoriasis. Among patients with hyperkeratotic palmoplantar eczema, 77 % had a good outcome (i.e., reduction of clinical symptoms by more than 50 %), as did 63 % of patients with palmoplantar psoriasis. After a mean follow-up interval of 4.3 years, the best long-term results were reported by patients with hyperkeratotic eczema. Of these who experienced an initial 50 % decrease or more in symptom intensity, 50 % remained asymptomatic, even years after treatment, while 33 % had significant improvement of the disease. In patients with palmoplantar psoriasis, 18 % reported long-term clearance, and 41 % had a good long-term clinical outcome [35].

Systemic administration of psoralen requires eye protection and may be associated with nausea. The limited area of involvement of hyperkeratotic eczema of the palms makes localized psoralen treatment a good option. Topical PUVA has theoretical advantages over systemic PUVA in terms of minimizing side effects. In one study on palmoplantar psoriasis, both bath PUVA and oral PUVA achieved a significant reduction of the mean initial severity index. Oral PUVA had a better effect at weeks 1–3; however, at the end of the fourth week, there was no significant difference between oral PUVA and bath PUVA [36].

In our experience, bath PUVA treatment can be associated with burns at the wrist; care should be taken to assure that the area exposed to psoralen and UV is consistent from treatment to treatment. The use of a cotton wristband placed at the identical location during each UV exposure may be useful.

A 308-nm monochromatic excimer light has shown promising results in treatment of palmoplantar psoriasis. In one study using a 308-nm excimer light, 54 patients affected by palmoplantar psoriasis were treated every 7–14 days. A mean number of 10 sessions was performed. After 4 months of treatment, a complete remission in 31 patients, a partial remission in 13 patients, and a moderate improvement in 10 patients were observed [37]. In another report, patients with palmoplantar psoriasis had a 52 % improvement in the mean severity index score after a total of 25 treatments (1/week) with only 7 % of patient achieving clearance [38].

Another study compared the efficacy of cream PUVA therapy with monochromatic excimer light therapy. Ten patients with psoriasis of the palms and soles were randomly assigned to receive cream PUVA on one side and 308-nm UVB on the contralateral side for 5 weeks. At the end of the treatment period, the test groups showed similar psoriasis area and severity index (PASI) score reduction (308-nm UVB, 64 %; cream PUVA, 65 %) [39].

Grenz rays are mainly absorbed in the epidermis and superficial portion of dermis [40]. They may be effective for treatment for hand dermatitis [41, 42]. However, a right–left hand comparison study found that Grenz was no more effective than placebo in the treatment of chronic hand eczema [43]. Another study of 25 patients with chronic hand dermatitis showed that conventional X-rays (300 rad) were superior to Grenz rays [44]. There are other reports of effectiveness of radiotherapy in hand eczema [45]. However, long-term side effects of radiotherapy may preclude its use as a first- or second-line treatment of palmoplantar dermatoses.

A right–left hand comparison study compared topical PUVA and conventional superficial radiotherapy for chronic hand dermatitis. Hands treated with superficial radiotherapy demonstrated rapid initial clearing; however, both groups showed similar improvement at 12 weeks' follow-up [46].

Methotrexate, cyclosporine, and mycophenolate mofetil, three systemic immunosuppressive agents, are effective in hand dermatitis [47–49]. Systemic immunosuppressants may be used in severe devastating cases of hyperkeratotic eczema of the palms unresponsive to topical drugs and phototherapy. Infliximab, alefacept, ustekinumab, and efalizumab have shown promising results in plaque-type palmoplantar psoriasis [50, 51]. In a randomized controlled trial, patients with palmoplantar psoriasis receiving infliximab showed 50 % reduction in the mean surface area of palmar and plantar lesions compared to an increase of 15 % in patients randomized to placebo. The difference was statistically significant [52]. In another report, an improvement in score from baseline of 50 % or more was observed in 51 % of patients with palmoplantar psoriasis treated with efalizumab [53].

Conclusion

Hyperkeratotic eczema of the palms is a chronic, frustrating disease. Clinical and histopathological findings and treatment modalities are very similar to palmoplantar psoriasis. The effects of the disease on the quality of life of the patient usually determine how far one should go in the treatment of hyperkeratotic psoriasiform hand eczema. As a step-by-step approach to the treatment of hyperkeratotic eczema of the palms and palmoplantar psoriasis, we recommend to proceed through the following stages:

1. Topical treatments, usually in combination or maybe one by one.
2. Systemic retinoids, phototherapy, or both together would be appropriate second-line treatments. They can be used in combination with topical treatments. Generally, the use of systemic retinoids should be avoided in women of child-bearing potential.
3. In severe, recalcitrant cases, addition of methotrexate, cyclosporine, mycophenolate mofetil, or biologic therapies should be considered.

A well-organized treatment protocol in conjunction with good patient adherence can significantly improve the rash appearance and quality of life in many patients. The patients should know that treatment may need to be continued for a long time. There are also some patients who may need to change their lifestyle or their work in order to adjust to their devastating situation.

References

1. Diepgen TL, Andersen KE, Brandao FM, Bruze M, Bruynzeel DP, Frosch P, et al. Hand eczema classification: a cross-sectional, multicentre study of the aetiology and morphology of hand eczema. Br J Dermatol. 2009;160(2):353–8.
2. Hersle K, Mobacken H. Hyperkeratotic dermatitis of the palms. Br J Dermatol. 1982;107(2):195–201.
3. Chopra A, Maninder, Gill SS. Hyperkeratosis of palms and soles: clinical study. Indian J Dermatol Venereol Leprol. 1997;63(2):85–8.
4. Pettey AA, Balkrishnan R, Rapp SR, Fleischer AB, Feldman SR. Patients with palmoplantar psoriasis have more physical disability and discomfort than patients with other forms of psoriasis: implications for clinical practice. J Am Acad Dermatol. 2003;49(2):271–5.
5. Veien NK, Hattel T, Laurberg G. Hand eczema: causes, course, and prognosis I. Contact Dermatitis. 2008;58(6):330–4.
6. Menné T, Johansen JD, Sommerlund M, Veien NK, Danish Contact Dermatitis Group. Hand eczema guidelines based on the Danish guidelines for the diagnosis and treatment of hand eczema. Contact Dermatitis. 2011;65(1):3–12.
7. Agner T, Andersen KE, Brandao FM, Bruynzeel DP, Bruze M, Frosch P, et al. Contact sensitisation in hand eczema patients-relation to subdiagnosis, severity and quality of life: a multi-centre study. Contact Dermatitis. 2009;61(5):291–6.
8. Wilkinson DS. Dermatitis from repeated trauma to the skin. Am J Ind Med. 1985;8(4–5):307–17.
9. Posada C, García-Doval I, de la Torre C, Cruces MJ. Value of palmar and plantar biopsies of hyperkeratotic and vesicular pustular lesions: a cross-sectional study. Actas Dermosifiliogr. 2010;101(1):103–5.
10. Weedon D. Skin pathology. 2nd ed. New York: Churchill Livingstone; 2002.

11. Aydin O, Engin B, Oğuz O, Ilvan S, Demirkesen C. Non-pustular palmoplantar psoriasis: is histologic differentiation from eczematous dermatitis possible? J Cutan Pathol. 2008;35(2):169–73.
12. Akhyani M, Mansoori P, Taheri A, Asadi KZ. Acrokeratosis paraneoplastica (Bazex syndrome) associated with breast cancer. Clin Exp Dermatol. 2004;29(4):429–30.
13. Enta T. Dermacase. Keratoderma climactericum. Can Fam Physician. 1996;42:629–31.
14. Bishop PM, Barber HW. Keratoderma climactericum (Haxthausen) treated with Oestrone. Proc R Soc Med. 1937;30(6):738–40.
15. Wachtel TJ. Plantar and palmar hyperkeratosis in young castrated women. Int J Dermatol. 1981;20(4): 270–1.
16. Egawa K. Topical vitamin D3 derivatives in treating hyperkeratotic palmoplantar eczema: a report of five patients. J Dermatol. 2005;32(5):381–6.
17. Schliemann S, Kelterer D, Bauer A, John SM, Skudlik C, Schindera I, et al. Tacrolimus ointment in the treatment of occupationally induced chronic hand dermatitis. Contact Dermatitis. 2008;58(5):299–306.
18. Menter A, Korman NJ, Elmets CA, Feldman SR, Gelfand JM, Gordon KB, et al. Guidelines of care for the management of psoriasis and psoriatic arthritis. Section 3. Guidelines of care for the management and treatment of psoriasis with topical therapies. J Am Acad Dermatol. 2009;60(4):643–59.
19. Jacobi A, Braeutigam M, Mahler V, Schultz E, Hertl M. Pimecrolimus 1% cream in the treatment of facial psoriasis: a 16-week open-label study. Dermatology. 2008;216(2):133–6.
20. Kumar B, Kumar R, Kaur I. Coal tar therapy in palmoplantar psoriasis: old wine in an old bottle? Int J Dermatol. 1997;36(4):309–12.
21. Hanifin JM, Stevens V, Sheth P, Breneman D. Novel treatment of chronic severe hand dermatitis with bexarotene gel. Br J Dermatol. 2004;150(3):545–53.
22. Mehta BH, Amladi ST. Evaluation of topical 0.1% tazarotene cream in the treatment of palmoplantar psoriasis: an observer-blinded randomized controlled study. Indian J Dermatol. 2011;56(1):40–3.
23. Adişen E, Tekin O, Gülekon A, Gürer MA. A retrospective analysis of treatment responses of palmoplantar psoriasis in 114 patients. J Eur Acad Dermatol Venereol. 2009;23(7):814–9.
24. Diepgen TL, Pfarr E, Zimmermann T. Efficacy and tolerability of alitretinoin for chronic hand eczema under daily practice conditions: Results of the TOCCATA open study comprising 680 patients. Acta Derm Venereol. 2012;92(3):251–5.
25. Schmitt-Hoffmann AH, Roos B, Sauer J, Spickermann J, Stoeckel K, Edwards D, et al. Pharmacokinetics, efficacy and safety of alitretinoin in moderate or severe chronic hand eczema. Clin Exp Dermatol. 2011;36 Suppl 2:29–34.
26. Ruzicka T, Lynde CW, Jemec GB, Diepgen T, Berth-Jones J, Coenraads PJ, et al. Efficacy and safety of oral alitretinoin (9-cis retinoic acid) in patients with severe chronic hand eczema refractory to topical corticosteroids: results of a randomized, double-blind, placebo-controlled, multicentre trial. Br J Dermatol. 2008;158(4):808–17.
27. Thestrup-Pedersen K, Andersen KE, Menné T, Veien NK. Treatment of hyperkeratotic dermatitis of the palms (eczema keratoticum) with oral acitretin. A single-blind placebo-controlled study. Acta Derm Venereol. 2001;81(5):353–5.
28. Capella GL, Fracchiolla C, Frigerio E, Altomare G. A controlled study of comparative efficacy of oral retinoids and topical betamethasone/salicylic acid for chronic hyperkeratotic palmoplantar dermatitis. J Dermatolog Treat. 2004;15(2):88–93.
29. Rosén K, Mobacken H, Swanbeck G. Chronic eczematous dermatitis of the hands: a comparison of PUVA and UVB treatment. Acta Derm Venereol. 1987;67(1):48–54.
30. Sezer E, Erbil AH, Kurumlu Z, Taştan HB, Etikan I. Comparison of the efficacy of local narrowband ultraviolet B (NB-UVB) phototherapy versus psoralen plus ultraviolet A (PUVA) paint for palmoplantar psoriasis. J Dermatol. 2007;34(7):435–40.
31. Simons JR, Bohnen IJ, van der Valk PG. A left-right comparison of UVB phototherapy and topical photochemotherapy in bilateral chronic hand dermatitis after 6 weeks' treatment. Clin Exp Dermatol. 1997; 22(1):7–10.
32. Sezer E, Etikan I. Local narrowband UVB phototherapy vs. local PUVA in the treatment of chronic hand eczema. Photodermatol Photoimmunol Photomed. 2007;23(1):10–4.
33. Schempp CM, Müller H, Czech W, Schöpf E, Simon JC. Treatment of chronic palmoplantar eczema with local bath-PUVA therapy. J Am Acad Dermatol. 1997; 36(5 Pt 1):733–7.
34. Behrens S, von Kobyletzki G, Gruss C, Reuther T, Altmeyer P, Kerscher M. PUVA-bath photochemotherapy (PUVA-soak therapy) of recalcitrant dermatoses of the palms and soles. Photodermatol Photoimmunol Photomed. 1999;15(2):47–51.
35. Bretterklieber A, Legat FJ, Wolf P, Hofer A. Retrospective long-term follow-up in patients with chronic palmoplantar dermatoses after good response to bath PUVA therapy. J Dtsch Dermatol Ges. 2012; 10(11):814–8.
36. Hofer A, Fink-Puches R, Kerl H, Quehenberger F, Wolf P. Paired comparison of bathwater versus oral delivery of 8-methoxypsoralen in psoralen plus ultraviolet: a therapy for chronic palmoplantar psoriasis. Photodermatol Photoimmunol Photomed. 2006;22(1): 1–5.
37. Nisticò SP, Saraceno R, Stefanescu S, Chimenti S. A 308-nm monochromatic excimer light in the treatment of palmoplantar psoriasis. J Eur Acad Dermatol Venereol. 2006;20(5):523–6.
38. Han L, Somani AK, Huang Q, Fang X, Jin Y, Xiang LH, et al. Evaluation of 308-nm monochromatic excimer light in the treatment of psoriasis vulgaris and palmoplantar psoriasis. Photodermatol Photoimmunol Photomed. 2008;24(5):231–6.

39. Neumann NJ, Mahnke N, Korpusik D, Stege H, Ruzicka T. Treatment of palmoplantar psoriasis with monochromatic excimer light (308-nm) versus cream PUVA. Acta Derm Venereol. 2006;86(1):22–4.
40. Edwards Jr EK, Edwards Sr EK. Grenz ray therapy. Int J Dermatol. 1990;29(1):17–8.
41. Lindelof B, Wrangsjo K, Liden S. A double-blind study of Grenz ray therapy in chronic eczema of the hands. Br J Dermatol. 1987;117(1):77–80.
42. Walling HW, Swick BL, Storrs FJ, Boddicker ME. Frictional hyperkeratotic hand dermatitis responding to Grenz ray therapy. Contact Dermatitis. 2008;58(1):49–51.
43. Cartwright PH, Rowell NR. Comparison of Grenz rays versus placebo in the treatment of chronic hand eczema. Br J Dermatol. 1987;117(1):73–6.
44. Fairris GM, Jones DH, Mack DP, Rowell NR. Constitutional superficial X-ray versus Grenz ray therapy in the treatment of constitutional eczema of the hands. Br J Dermatol. 1985;112(3):339–41.
45. Sumila M, Notter M, Itin P, Bodis S, Gruber G. Long-term results of radiotherapy in patients with chronic palmo-plantar eczema or psoriasis. Strahlenther Onkol. 2008;184(4):218–23.
46. Sheehan-Dare RA, Goodfield MJ, Rowell NR. Topical psoralen photochemotherapy (PUVA) and superficial radiotherapy in the treatment of chronic hand eczema. Br J Dermatol. 1989;121(1):65–9.
47. Egan CA, Rallis TM, Meadows KP, Krueger GG. Low-dose oral methotrexate treatment for recalcitrant palmoplantar pompholyx. J Am Acad Dermatol. 1999;40(4):612–4.
48. Granlund H, Erkko P, Reitamo S. Comparison of the influence of cyclosporine and topical betamethasone-17, 21-dipropionate treatment on quality of life in chronic hand eczema. Acta Derm Venereol. 1997;77(1):54–8.
49. Pickenacker A, Luger T, Schwarz T. Dyshidrotic eczema treated with mycophenolate mofetil. Arch Dermatol. 1998;134:378–9.
50. Lior S, Grigory K, Pnina S, Joseph S, Felix P. Therapeutic hotline. Alefacept in the treatment of hyperkeratotic palmoplantar psoriasis. Dermatol Ther. 2010;23(5):556–60.
51. Bulai Livideanu C, Lahfa M, Mazereeuw-Hautier J, Paul C. Efficacy of ustekinumab in palmoplantar psoriasis. Dermatology. 2010;221(4):321–3.
52. Bissonnette R, Poulin Y, Guenther L, Lynde CW, Bolduc C, Nigen S. Treatment of palmoplantar psoriasis with infliximab: a randomized, double-blind placebo-controlled study. J Eur Acad Dermatol Venereol. 2011;25(12):1402–8.
53. Katsambas A, Peris K, Vena G, Freidmann P, Wozel G, Daudén E, et al. Assessing the impact of efalizumab on nail, scalp and palmoplantar psoriasis and on quality of life: results from a multicentre, open-label, phase IIIb/IV trial. Arch Drug Info. 2009;2(4):66–70.

Hand Eczema in Hairdressers

15

Valeska Katinka Buder, Christoph Skudlik,
and Swen Malte John

Contents

V.K. Buder, M.D.
Institute for Health Service Research in Dermatology and Nursing Clinical Research-Health Care Research-Health Economics, University Medical Center Hamburg-Eppendorf, Martinistr.52, Hamburg 20246, Germany
e-mail: v.duder@uke.de

C. Skudlik, M.D. • S.M. John, M.D. (✉)
Department of Dermatology, Environmental Medicine and Health Theory, University of Osnabrueck, Sedanstr. 115, Osnabrueck 49090, Germany
e-mail: sjohn@uos.de; christoph.skudlik@uos.de

15.1 Introduction

In Germany, 25,056 new cases of occupationally related skin diseases were reported in 2011, and the number has risen by 25 % since a dermatological awareness campaign started in 2009. In 2009, there were 19,021 cases, while in 2010 there were 23,596. The number of eczema cases related to the hairdressing trade has also increased steadily over the past few years; in 2009, there were 1,045 reported cases, which increased to 1,251 by 2011. This is relative to the total of 236,606 full-time employees in the hairdresser trade in Germany in 2009 and 232,411 in 2011, respectively (Hartmann, K, 2013, Institution for Statutory Accident Insurance and Prevention in the Health and Welfare Services, Hamburg, Germany, Personal communication). Furthermore, it is safe to assume that there are a high number of unreported cases of occupational-related hand eczemas in Germany and other European countries.

15.2 Epidemiology

In Denmark, a register-based study published in 2011 of trained hairdressers (*n*=7,840) used a self-administered postal questionnaire, including

A. Alikhan et al. (eds.), *Textbook of Hand Eczema*,
DOI 10.1007/978-3-642-39546-8_15,

questions on hand eczema, to monitor occupational diseases. Of the 67.9 % (*n*=5,324) who responded, 2,186 have had hand eczema; 71.3 % of these were apprentices at the time of onset [1]. The majority (61.9 %) have had hand eczema several times, and 21.3 % have it (almost) all of the time, yet only 20.7 % had reported their hand eczema as being occupational to the National Board of Industrial Injuries (Denmark). Another 26.6 % did not report the occurrence of hand eczema because the "doctor did not tell me to," while 40.4 % "thought it would eventually get better." Overall, hand eczema can be considered a considerably under-reported occupational disease. The perception of hand eczema among hairdressers and the lack of reporting from doctors were defined as the main reasons for this [1]. This is rather remarkable because hand eczemas in hairdressers have been well documented for many decades and are a commonly reported risk of the occupation [2].

In the German FaSt study [3], which examined patch-tested workers in risky professions (*n*=1,842), the group of hairdressers showed the highest representation of occupational dermatoses (*n*=209, 11.3 %), which in most instances was hand eczema. Uter et al. followed 2,351 hairdressing apprentices in a prospective cohort study in Germany. Signs for irritant contact dermatitis were seen in 844 hairdressers (35.9 %) as early as within the first 6 weeks of training [4]. Schaad et al. evaluated the reasons why students in the Netherlands would drop out of hairdressing apprenticeship in the 1990s. Among the 872 dropouts of hairdressing schools, 486 (56 %) responded, and of these 190 (39 %) reported that skin disease was the reason for quitting [5]. Overall, hairdressers have a history of being highly vulnerable to skin alterations [4].

15.3 Causes of Hand Eczema in Hairdressers

Besides exposure to various irritants typical to the trade (e.g., repeated or continual wet work in combination with detergents and other irritating agents like H_2O_2), a high exposure to allergens increases an already high sensitization risk [6, 7]. Hairdressers have an intense exposure to water while washing the clients' hair or using occlusive gloves for several hours at a time. Furthermore, in addition to cutting hair, most of the hairdressers also do a high amount of coloring, styling, or permanent waving. In other words, hairdressers come into contact with chemical products while treating their clients' hairs and often do so without the added protection of gloves. Also, frequently the gloves used are unsuitable (e.g., polyethylene) or reused [8].

In the aforementioned Danish study, the reported daily wet work was quite high; 86.6 % had wet hands for more than 2 h and 54 % for more than 4 h. Glove use was fairly frequent for full head hair-coloring and bleaching procedures (93–97.7 %) but less frequent for high-/low-lighting procedures (49.7–60.5 %) and permanent waving (28.3 %). Gloves were rarely worn during hair washing (10 %), although this was frequently performed immediately after hair-coloring procedures (48.9 %). Recent publications underline the excessive amount of occupational skin exposure among hairdressers. The extent of wet work and chemical treatments is high. Glove use is inconsistent, especially for certain hair-coloring procedures and wet-work tasks.

These latest results can be used as an evidence for the appearance of the two main types of eczematous skin alterations common among hairdressers – irritant contact dermatitis and allergic contact dermatitis of the hands. Accordingly, in a recent study from North America, the rates for allergic and irritant contact dermatitis in a mixed hairdresser and cosmetologist cohort (*n*=432) were 72.7 % and 37.0 %, respectively [9].

15.4 Irritant Contact Dermatitis in Hairdressers

Irritant hand eczema is typically associated with the high amount of repeated or continual wet work a hairdresser is exposed to. German technical regulations on hazardous substances (TRGS 401) define wet work as more than 2 h of skin exposure to a humid environment or wearing impermeable gloves [10].

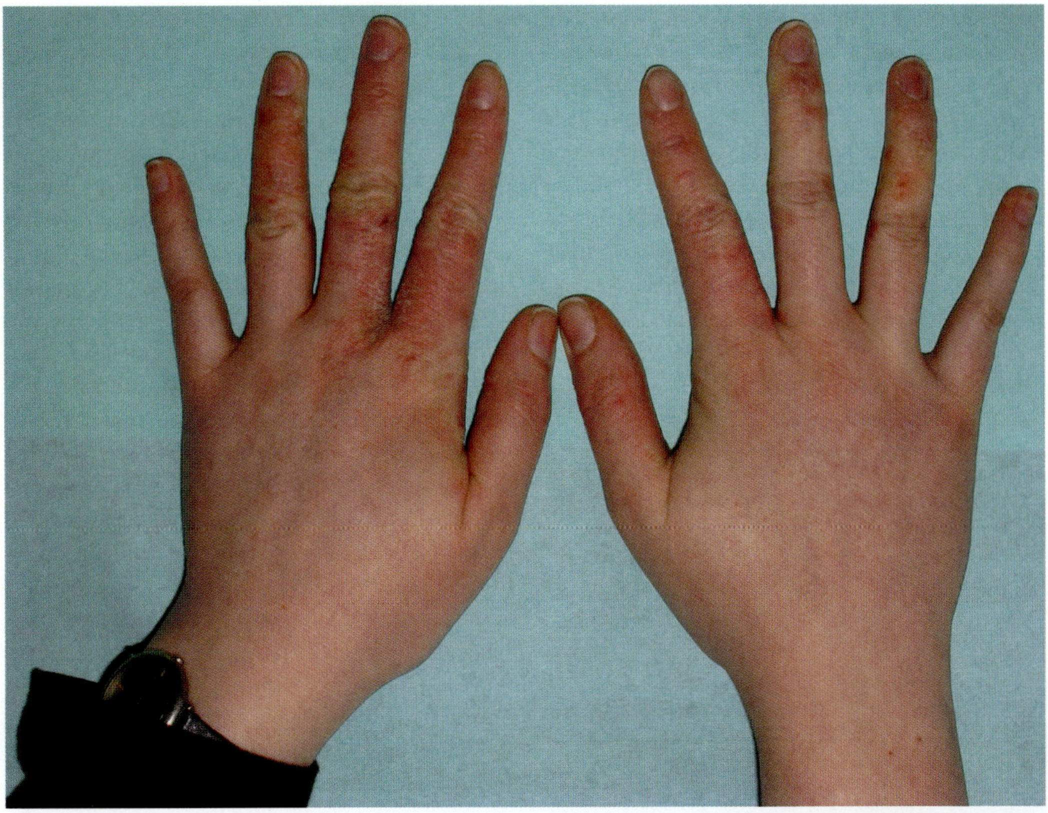

Fig. 15.1 Typical eczematous skin alterations in hand eczema in hairdressers affecting the second and third fingers of the serving hand

In a recent publication containing the initial results from the multicentre study "Rehabilitation of Occupational Skin Diseases – Optimization and Quality Assurance of Inpatient Management (ROQ)" concerning interdisciplinary integrated (inpatient/outpatient) rehabilitation measures for patients with severe occupational skin diseases (n=1,788), wet work was a frequent occupational hazard in all occupational groups [11]. Two hours or more wet work was most often reported by the hairdressers (96.7 %), followed by the "cleaning" group (91.4 %), the "food-handlers" group (87.4 %), and the "health care" group (82.1 %). Most hairdressers described a minimum of 3-4 h of wet work per day, although cases of 5-7 h of wet work were not uncommon. Also, in the recent North American study, shampoo, hair products, and non-skin cleansers were most commonly identified as irritant sources. It has to be kept in mind that water was not specifically coded in this study [9].

Most hairdressers prefer to cut their clients' hair while it is wet. Often the clients' hair is still wet from washing or from rinsing the dye from freshly colored hair. In this case, a right-handed person would use his/her right hand to cut the hair with a scissor while using the left hand as the "serving hand" [12]. Between the second and third fingers of the serving hand, a hairdresser presents a strand of hair to be cut.

As the second and third fingers of the serving hand are most exposed to the wet or freshly colored hair, these two particular fingers tend to develop the initial typical eczematous skin alterations (Fig. 15.1). Schwanitz and Uter [12] examined a prospective cohort study of 2,275 hairdressing apprentices in a median of 6 weeks after the start of their training in the years 1992, 1993, and 1994. Skin changes were noted in 821 (36 %). Most often the interdigital web space was affected (81 %, n=664) (Fig. 15.2). Furthermore, interdigital dermatitis is a concern and a potential precursor of severe hand dermatitis in hairdressers and is an important "sentinel" for secondary prevention. The interdigital dermatitis may consecutively spread to the back of the hands, fingers, and wrists. It was reported that at the beginning of an apprenticeship, weekends or holidays would provide enough time to let the skin recover. The longer the exposure lasts, the more barrier function impairment will occur and enable allergens and/or irritants an easier access to the deeper parts of the skin [12]. Sensitization will also be promoted by a proinflammatory milieu created by irritant skin damage.

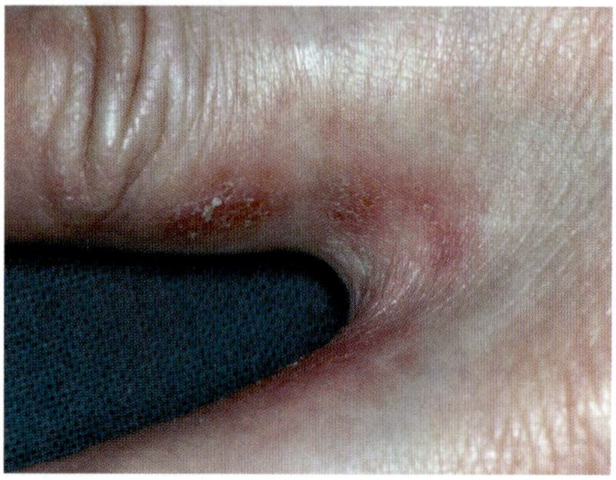

Fig. 15.2 Interdigital dermatitis caused by wet work in hairdressing

15.5 Allergic Contact Dermatitis in Hairdressers

Alongside irritant contact dermatitis, hairdressers often develop type IV allergic contact dermatitis due to their frequent use of hair colors, detergents, and permanent wave solutions. Often the allergic contact dermatitis is the direct result of previous irritant damage due to the high amount of wet work [12, 13].

In contrast to irritant contact dermatitis, allergic contact dermatitis frequently affects every part of the hands and includes the underarm and wrists or, if the hairdresser is applying color to his/her own hair, even regions of their own neck and face. The region on the body where the skin appears altered may even suggest which allergen is causing the reaction.

For example, fingertip dermatitis is often related to a type IV glyceryl monothioglycolate (GMTG) allergy. It has been observed that hairdressers check the quality of curls by using the dominant hand's fingers without any protection. In addition to irritant dermatitis, allergic contact dermatitis related to hair coloring may affect the second and third fingers of the hand (Fig. 15.3). These fingers would usually grip the hair and present them to the scissors during cutting after the coloring process [13].

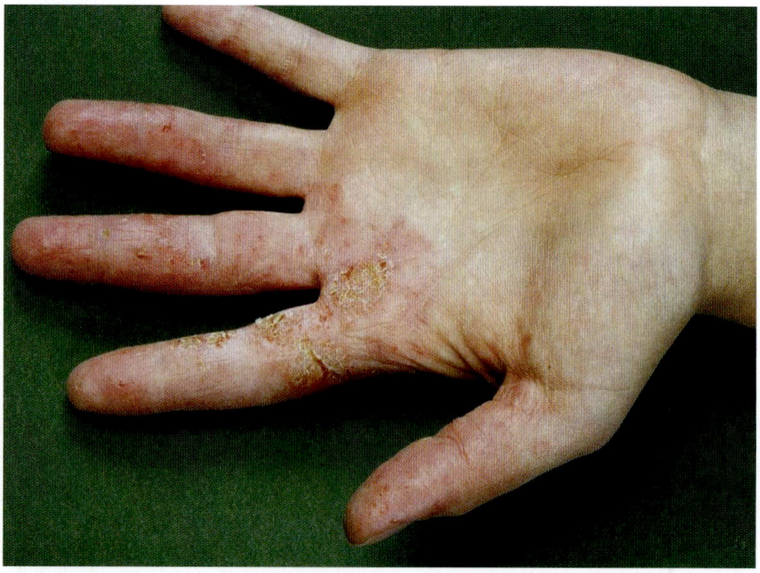

Fig. 15.3 Severe combined irritant and allergic hand eczema in hairdressers

Because of the frequent use of professional hair cosmetic products and due to their components, allergic contact dermatitis has developed in hairdressers and sometimes in their clients [6]. Alongside reducing agents, hair dyes, bleaching agents or preservatives, and fragrances used in hair products and even protective gloves (e.g., rubber accelerators) can cause allergic contact dermatitis in hairdressers. Therefore, a wide range of potential sensitizers in a patch test is needed to discover the underlying cause. Recommendations are given by the German Contact Dermatitis Research Group (DKG) for testing hairdressers using the test series "Standard," "Hairdresser," "Rubber," and "Preservative Agents in Externa" [14, 15].

15.6 Most Common Allergens in Hairdressers

Uter et al. [6] collected data on female patients (*n*=1260). Four hundred eighty of these women were still working or had been working for several years as hairdressers. The remaining 780 women had never worked as hairdressers but had contact dermatitis primarily due to their contact with hair cosmetics. In hairdressers, the most frequent allergens were ammonium persulfate (21.7 % positive), p-toluenediamine (19.6 % positive), p-phenylenediamine (PPD) (18.1 % positive), and GMTG (though it has decreased over time since it has not been used for (acid) permanent waves since 1995 (in 2005/2006, only 7.5 % positive). Biocides such as (chloro) methylisothiazolinone and methyldibromoglutaronitrile were also named as common allergens [6]. In the aforementioned recent study from North America, the most frequent currently relevant and occupationally related allergens were GMTG and PPD but also nickel sulfate, 2-hydroxyethyl-methacrylate, and quaternium-15. The differences between these studies (particularly relating to the last three allergens) could be explained by the mixed study cohort, which also contained cosmetologists [9].

15.6.1 Blonding Agents

Ammonium persulfate is used for hair-bleaching procedures. It may induce type IV and type I allergies. Cross-reactions are described with potassium persulfate and sodium persulfate.

15.6.2 Hair Dyes

Until the nineteenth century, the most common hair dye was henna [16]. It has since been replaced with PPD, which is still the main ingredient used in permanent hair color products (oxidative hair dyes). A study of the German Contact Dermatitis Research Group (DKG) [17] showed that a 1 % test concentration carried a risk of active sensitization through patch testing. Subsequently, PPD was removed from the standard series in Germany at the beginning of 2005 but is once again part of the hairdresser series at a 1 % test concentration. Additional allergies to other hair-dye ingredients, such as 2,5-diaminotoluene sulfate, 2-nitro-4-phenylenediamine, 5-aminophenol, 4-aminophenol, 4-aminodiphenylamine, and resorcinol, were also described.

15.6.3 Reducing Agents

GMTG is used as a reducing agent in acid perm solutions. Due to the hair fashion of the 1980s, it was used very often and showed a high sensitization potential. Since hair styles and fashion undergo a lot of changes and perm waves are no longer common, GMTG sensitization is less commonly reported than it was 20-30 years ago. For example, in Germany GMTG sensitization in hairdressers from 2005 to 2006 was 7.5 % [6]. In 1991, however, a survey by the German Institution for Statutory Accident Insurance and Prevention in the Health and Welfare Services (BGW – *Berufsgenossenschaft für Gesundheitsdienst und Wohlfahrtspflege*) reported that more than 50 % of examined hairdressers had been patch tested positive against GMTG. Furthermore, the overall sensitization rate for the hairdressing series within this survey was 34 %. Since 1995, the main producers and importers of hair products declared that they would voluntarily refrain from using GMTG. Shortly afterwards, it was legally banned in Germany and replaced by the much less immunogenic ammonium thioglycolate. Residual cases are considered probable "old sensitizations" [18–22]. This can be demonstrated by surveying the age groups of patch-tested hairdressers. Nowadays, in Germany, positive patch test reactions to GMTG cannot be found in the age group less than 20 years of age [23], an impressive example of successful primary prevention. It is remarkable that GMTG is not banned in most countries, even though a less harmful replacement is available (i.e., ammonium thioglycolate).

15.6.4 Surfactants, Preservatives, and Fragrances

Other potential allergens that might be important in hairdressers are the group of surfactants, preservatives, and fragrances. Cocamidopropyl betaine is an amphoteric tenside that can induce type IV allergies. It has a high irritant potential that sometimes may make it difficult to distinguish between irritant skin reactions and type IV allergies. Positive reactions to preservatives such as (chloro) methylisothiazolinone and parabens can also be found in hairdressers. In a study by Uter [6], 4.1 % of the hairdressers suffered from a type IV (chloro) methylisothiazolinone allergy, while the control group of clients showed only 1.8 % [6].

A wide variety of fragrances are used in professional hair cosmetics. The patch test with the standard series includes the fragrance mixes I and II in DKG series, although it may be difficult to determine whether an allergy to preservatives or a fragrance is developed during professional or private exposure.

15.6.5 Gloves

The friction and occlusive effect by gloves may not relieve but instead reinforce an irritant contact dermatitis. Additionally, the gloves used by hairdressers may contain mercaptobenzothiazole, thiuram, and carbamate compounds and can induce type IV allergies [20].

15.6.6 Type I Allergies in Hairdressers

Ammonium persulfate does not only elicit type IV allergic contact eczema but can also cause immediate reactions of the skin, mucous membranes, and the bronchial system. In rare cases, severe respiratory reactions and even anaphylactic shock have been reported [24]. While undertaking a patch test, a control of the patient's skin should be made 20 min after applying the test substance [25, 26]. Also, a prick and rub test with ammonium persulfate should be made if the patient describes dyspnea or skin prickling shortly after direct or indirect skin contact with bleaching solution.

15.7 Prevention of Hand Eczema

Wulfhorst et al. [27] estimated the annual economic costs for occupational dermatoses in general exceed €1.5 billion per year in Germany [27]. In the United States, the estimate was at least €10 billion per year, while the estimate in England was well over €230 million [27]. These figures include direct (e.g., treatment and worker's compensation) as well as indirect costs due to absenteeism (sick leave) and lack of productivity. The indirect costs constitute up to 90 % of the occupational contact dermatitis economic burden [27].

Career change and sick leave for a number of weeks a year are still the most common "cures" for hand eczema in hairdressers. In Germany, effective prevention strategies have been developed in the context of a hierarchical prevention concept (primary-secondary-tertiary prevention) (Fig. 15.4). The concept was scientifically evaluated and implemented throughout the country over several years [28], and a special ordinance for the hairdresser trade was issued (Technical Rule 530). Its purpose was to regulate the application of suitable personal protective equipment and make it possible to take allergens such as

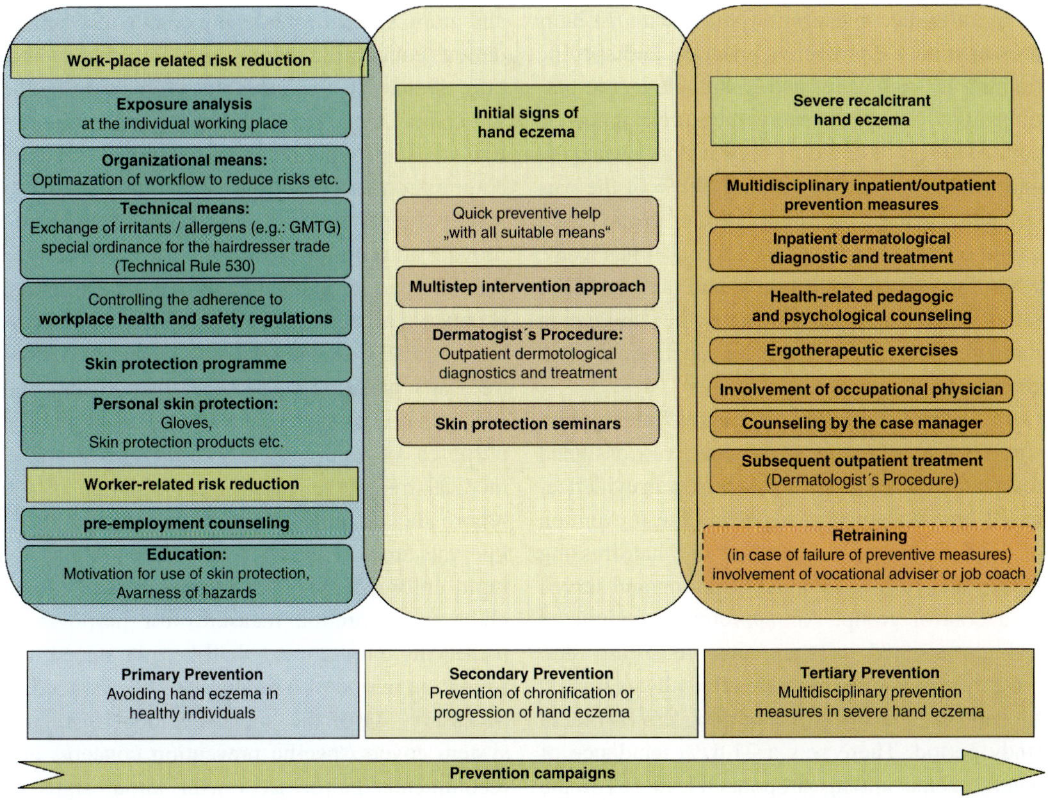

Fig. 15.4 Prevention concept (primary-secondary-tertiary prevention) in the hairdresser trade (Reprinted with permission from Skudlik C, John SM. Prevention and rehabilitation. In: Elsner P, John SM, Maibach I, Rustemeyer T, eds. Kanerva's occupational dermatology. 2nd ed. Heidelberg, Berlin: Springer; 2012: 1177–84)

GMTG largely off the market and to establish skin-health educational seminars and specific inpatient rehabilitation programs [28, 29].

15.8 Primary Prevention

Skin protection for hairdressers should start with primary prevention. Harmful exposure to chemicals such as GMTG or the use of rubber latex gloves should be eliminated or substituted. In addition, primary prevention should focus on worker-related strategies. Continuous health surveillance should be provided, and skin protection should be optimized by gloves [27, 29]. Furthermore, protective creams should be regularly applied to the skin of the hands. Individualized recommendations are given with regard to barrier creams for hairdressers, in the context of health educational training sessions, at our clinics. Individual risk factors were discussed, since the patient's motivation is important for the use and general application of barrier creams. The use of barrier creams before starting work and at the end of the breaks is recommended.

Several years ago, advertisements aimed at members of the hairdressing trade pitched the use of skin protective foam that was described as an "invisible glove." These attributes were misleading, since the foam is not protecting the skin from harm by irritants and type IV allergens. Also, the foam was based on stearic acid in the alkaline range that led to even more pronounced skin irritations (paradoxical effect [30]). Education and training, including updating vocational schools' curricula, should be provided to raise awareness of the first signs of hand eczema and effective preventive methods.

In an earlier intervention study with 73 hairdresser trainees, protective products and specific training lessons were made available to the participants. The effects were measured against a control group. It could be shown that toward the end of the first year of training, 90 % of the participants within the intervention group used cream on their hands more than four times a day, while the control group only had a compliance rate of 60 %. It was also shown that the intervention measure led to a significant decline in skin changes [31].

In a recent controlled prospective intervention study, 301 hairdressing apprentices were assigned to an intervention group and received an evidence-based training program regarding the prevention of hand eczema. Two hundred one hairdressing apprentices received standard training and served as a control group. All apprentices completed self-administered questionnaires regarding skin protection measures and were clinically examined for hand eczema three times during the 18-month study period. There was a 21.4 % incidence of hand eczema among dropouts (15.0 % in the intervention group and 25.5 % in the control group; p=0.3). Of note, more apprentices from the intervention group used gloves during wet-work procedures. In summary, it could be shown that primary prevention is able to increase the use of gloves and reduce the incidence of hand eczema in hairdressing apprentices [32].

15.9 Secondary Prevention

The target group of secondary prevention is hairdressers with initial signs of occupational contact dermatitis. Secondary prevention aims at early disease detection, thereby increasing opportunities for interventions to prevent hand eczema chronification or the progression of symptoms.

In Germany, even if there is only a slight suspicion that a dermatosis may be work related, a dermatologist's report (Hautarztbericht) may be filed with the respective employers' liability insurance institution [33]. This report requires the consent of the person concerned. It is based on a detailed examination, including patch tests and atopy screening. It also includes recommendations concerning therapy, personal skin protection, after-work skin care, and even changing the workplace. Once the insurer has been notified, it will – if an occupational cause is likely – usually commission the reporting dermatologist to follow up the patient with regular consultations and provide all required treatments for a consecutive 6-month period. In an attempt to handle potential occupational dermatoses as quickly and unbureaucratically as possible, this so-called dermatologist's procedure was recently updated, and the dermatologist's fees have been raised. For the purposes of optimal early intervention, rapid medical treatment following completion of the report and documentation of progress at close intervals are now required, as a rule. In doing so, rapid enforcement of an insured person's legal claim to prevention measures for purposes of preserving employment shall be guaranteed; the follow-up period of 6 months can be extended, if necessary. Also, the social accident insurance system covers specific prevention concepts and recommends hairdressers with initial signs of occupational hand eczema to take part in special work-related skin protection seminars free of charge [28, 33].

The skin protection plans and operating instructions issued in Germany by the BGW follow these scientifically based preventive measures and promote the consistent use of glove protection (e.g., gloves made of vinyl or nitrile; see also www.bgw-online.de).

In the hairdressing trade, an almost tenfold reduction in occupational skin diseases was observed due to a systematic preventive program [34, 35].

Several intervention studies in the hairdressing trade have produced fair-quality evidence that prevention is effective [27]. Wulfhorst et al. [36] followed 215 hairdressers from 1994 to 1997 who suffered from occupational contact dermatitis. They attended a 6-month combined dermatological and educational program that included counseling as well as an intervention in the respective hairdressers' shops. The intervention group (IG, n=215) and the control group (CG, n=85, received solely dermatological treatment) were sent follow-up questionnaires 9 months and 5 years after their participation. A subset of the IG was followed up again 10 years after participation. The follow-up survey after 9 months showed that 71.8 % ($n=117$) of the IG could remain at work, while only 60.0 % of the CG did. In the IG group, 12.8 % stopped working after 5 years due to occupational contact dermatitis versus 27.3 % of the CG; this difference was significant [36]. Besides the criteria of "remaining" or "not remaining" at work, the results showed that the interdisciplinary intervention program led to an increased and sustained knowledge about occupational contact dermatitis and resulted in improved preventive measures by the individual at the work place.

15.10 Tertiary Prevention

The intensified comprehensive measures of tertiary prevention are indicated when, due to severe recalcitrant occupational contact dermatitis, a hairdresser's occupation is threatened [11, 28]. Therefore, the Osnabrueck model, which was implemented in a multicenter study of the German Statutory Accident Insurance (DGUV), comprises a rehabilitation program for hairdressers and other occupation groups [11, 37].

Occupational hand eczema is a high-cost factor for the statutory employers' liability insurance bodies in Germany. Several studies clearly show that hairdressers show the highest representation of occupational dermatoses. Nevertheless, due to systematic multistep prevention procedures, a significant number of hairdressers can carry on in their profession. Most important is the implementation of early prevention strategies [11, 27].

Conclusion

- Hand eczema is a chronic disease with a high socioeconomic burden and has a negative impact on quality of life.
- Hand eczema in hairdressers is an often reported occupational drawback.
- Two main types of eczematous skin alterations are common in hairdressers: irritant contact dermatitis and allergic contact dermatitis of the hands.
- Patch testing with several hairdressing-related allergens is necessary after observing signs of hand eczema in hairdressers.
- Several intervention studies have shown preventive strategies are effective for hairdressers.
- Skin protection for hairdressers should start with primary prevention.

References

1. Lysdal SH, Søsted H, Johansen JD. Do hairdressers in Denmark have their hand eczema reported as an occupational disease? Results from a register-based questionnaire study. Contact Dermatitis. 2011;66(2):72–8.
2. Borelli S, Moormann J, Duengemann H, Manok M. Results of a 4-year serial test on apprentices of the hairdresser profession. Berufsdermatosen. 1965;13(4):216–38.
3. Geier J, Uter W, Lessmann H, Schnuch A. FaSt-Frühzeitige Erkennung allergener Stoffe bei beruflicher und nicht beruflicher Exposition. Göttingen: Abschlussbericht Informationsverbund Dermatologischer Kliniken (IVDK); 2002.
4. Uter W, Pfahlberg A, Gefeller O, Schwanitz HJ. Prevalence and incidence of hand dermatitis in hairdressing apprentices: results of the POSH study. Prevention of occupational skin disease in hairdressers. Int Arch Occup Environ Health. 1998;71(7):92–487.
5. Schaad J, de Jonge JFM. Te vroeg uit de kappersopleiding. Leiden: TNO; 1992.
6. Uter W, Lessmann H, Geier J, Schnuch A. Contact allergy to hairdressing allergens in female hairdressers and clients- current data from IVDK, 2003–2006. J Dtsch Dermatol Ges. 2007;5:993–1001.
7. Van der Walle HB. Hairdressers. In: Kanerva L, Elsner P, Wahlberg JE, Maibach HI, editors. Handbook of occupational dermatology, vol. 1. Berlin: Springer; 2001. p. 960–8.
8. Lysdal SH, Søsted H, Flyvholm MA, Johansen JD. A quantification of occupational skin exposures and the use of protective gloves among hairdressers in Denmark. Contact Dermatitis. 2012;66:323–34.
9. Warshaw EM, Wang MZ, Mathias CG, Maibach HI, Belsito DV, Zug KA, et al. Occupational contact dermatitis in hairdressers/cosmetologists: retrospective analysis of North American contact dermatitis group data, 1994 to 2010. Dermatitis. 2012;23(6):258–68.
10. Wetzky U, Bock M, Wulfhorst B, John SM. Short- and long-term effects of single and repetitive glove occlusion on the epidermal barrier. Arch Dermatol Res. 2009;301:595–602.
11. Skudlik C, Weisshaar E, Scheidt R, Elsner P, Wulfhorst B, Schoenfeld M, et al. First results from the multicentre study rehabilitation of occupational skin diseases – optimisation and quality assurance of

inpatient management (ROQ). Contact Dermatitis. 2012;66(3):140–7.

12. Schwanitz HJ, Uter W. Interdigital dermatitis: sentinel skin damage in hairdressers. Br J Dermatol. 2000; 142:1011–2.
13. Stenveld H. Hairdressers. In: Rustemeyer T, Elsner P, John SM, Maibach HI, editors. Kanerva's occupational dermatology. Berlin: Springer; 2012. p. 1507–19.
14. Uter W, Brehler R, Eck E, Geier J, Koch P, Peters KP, et al. Berufsspezifische Epikutantestung bei Friseuren – Empfehlungen der Arbeitsgruppe "Berufs-Testreihen" der Deutschen Kontaktallergie-Gruppe. Dermatosen. 1999;47:26–9.
15. Geier J, Krautheim A, Lessmann H. Allergologische Diagnostik und aktuelle Allergene in der Berufsdermatologie. Hautarzt. 2009;60:708–17.
16. Handa S, Mahajan R, De D. Contact dermatitis to hair-dye: an update. Indian J Dermatol Venereol Leprol. 2012;78(5):583 90.
17. Hillen U, Jappe U, Frosch PJ, Becker D, Brasch J, Lilie M, German Contact Dermatitis Research Group, et al. Late reactions to the patch-test preparations para-phenylenediamine and epoxy resin: a prospective multicentre investigation of the German Contact Dermatitis Research Group. Br J Dermatol. 2006; 154(4):665–70.
18. Peters KP, Frosch PJ, Uter W, Schnuch A, Arnold R, Bahmer F. Type IV-Allergien auf Friseurberufsstoffe. Ergebnisse des Informationsverbundes Dermatologischer Kliniken (IVDK). Dermatosen. 1994;42:711–50.
19. Schnuch A, Geier J. Glycerylmonothioglykolat-Sensibilisierung bei Friseurkunden. Dermatosen. 1995;43:29.
20. Uter W. Epidemiologie und Prävention von Handekzemen in Feuchtberufen am Beispiel des Friseurhandwerks. Osnabrück: Universitätsverlag Rasch; 1999.
21. Uter W, Geier J, Schnuch A. For the IVDK study group. Downward trend of sensitization to glyceryl monothioglycolate in German hairdressers. Dermatology. 2000;200:3–132.
22. Uter W, Lessmann H, Geier J, Schnuch A. Contact allergy to ingredients of hair cosmetics in female hairdressers and clients – an 8-year analysis of IVDK data. Contact Dermatitis. 2003;49:236–40.
23. Uter W, Geier J, Lessmann H, Schnuch A. Is contact allergy to glyceryl monothioglycolate still a problem in Germany? Contact Dermatitis. 2006;55:54–6.
24. Babilas P, Landthaler M, Szeimies RM. Anaphylactic reaction following hair bleaching. Hautarzt. 2005;56: 1152–5.
25. Aalto-Korte K, Mäkinen-Kiljunen S. Specific immunoglobulin E in patients with immediate persulfate hypersensitivity. Contact Dermatitis. 2003;49:22–5.
26. Leino T, Tammilehto L, Hytönen M, Sala E, Paakkulainen H, Kanerva L. Occupational skin and respiratory diseases among hairdressers. Scand J Work Environ Health. 1998;24:398–406.
27. Wulfhorst B, Bock M, Skudlik C, Wigger-Alberti W, John SM. Prevention of hand eczema: gloves, barrier creams and workers' education 2011. In: Johansen JD, Frosch PJ, Lepoittevin J-P, editors. Contact dermatitis. Berlin: Springer; 2011. p. 985–1011.
28. Skudlik C, John SM. Prevention and rehabilitation. In: Elsner P, John SM, Maibach HI, Rustemeyer T, editors. Textbook of Kanerva's occupational skin diseases, vol. 2. Berlin: Springer; 2012. p. 1177–84.
29. Skudlik C, John SM. Skin protection for hairdressers. In: Schliemann S, Elsner P, editors. Skin protection, practical applications in the occupational setting, vol. 34. Basel: Karger; 2007. p. 133–7.
30. Frosch PJ, Schulze-Dirks A, Hoffmann M, Axthelm I. Efficacy of skin barrier creams (II). Ineffectiveness of a popular "skin protector" against various irritants in the repetitive irritation test in the guinea pig. Contact Dermatitis. 1993;29:74–7.
31. Riehl U. Interventionsstudie zur Prävention von Hauterkrankungen bei Auszubildenden des Friseurhandwerks. In: Schwanitz HJ, editor. Studien zur Prävention in Allergologie, Berufs- und Umweltdermatologie (ABU). Band III. Osnabrück: Universitätsverlag Rasch; 2000.
32. Bregnhøj A, Menné T, Johansen JD, Søsted H. Prevention of hand eczema among Danish hairdressing apprentices: an intervention study. Occup Environ Med. 2012;69(5):6–310.
33. John SM, Skudlik C, Römer W, Blome O, Brandenburg S, Diepgen TL, et al. Recommendation: dermatologist's procedure. Recommendations for quality assurance of the German Society of Dermatology (DDG) and the task force on occupational and environmental dermatology (ABD). J Dtsch Dermatol Ges. 2007;5(12): 1146–8.
34. Dickel H, Kuss O, Schmidt A, Diepgen TL. Impact of preventive strategies on trend of occupational skin disease in hairdressers: population based register study. Br J Dermatol. 2002;324:1422–3.
35. Nienhaus A, Rojahn K, Skudlik C, Wulfhorst B, Dulon M, Brandenburg S. Secondary individual prevention and rehabilitation in female hairdressers suffering from skin diseases. Gesundheitswesen. 2004;66: 759–64.
36. Wulfhorst B, Bock M, Gediga G, Skudlik C, Allmers H, John SM. Sustainability of an interdisciplinary secondary prevention program for hair dressers. Int Arch Occup Environ Health. 2010;83:165–71.
37. Weisshaar E, Skudlik C, Scheidt R, Matterne U, Wulfhorst B, Schönfeld M, et al. Multicentre study "rehabilitation of occupational skin diseases - optimization and quality assurance of inpatient management (ROQ)" – results from 12-month follow-up. Contact Dermatitis. 2013;68(3):169–74.

Hand Eczema from Metalworking Fluids

16

Johannes Geier

Contents

J. Geier, M.D.
Information Network of Departments of Dermatology (IVDK), University of Goettingen, von-Siebold-Str. 3, Goettingen 37075, Germany
e-mail: jgeier@gwdg.de

16.1 Introduction

In metal processing, metalworking fluids (MWF) are used for lubricating and cooling workpieces and tools and for flushing away metal chips. Two groups of MWF have to be differentiated. Water-based MWF (wb MWF) are prepared on site at the metalworking company by aqueous dilution of a concentrate delivered by the lubricant producer. Neat oils are non-water-miscible oily preparations used as purchased from the manufacturer. MWF have a complex composition, which is commonly based on mineral oils or (semi-)synthetic hydrocarbon compounds. Emulsifiers, buffers, stabilizers, antifog additives, foam inhibitors, corrosion inhibitors, biocides, and other admixtures are usually added, according to the respective needs [1–4]. During the working process, biocides other than those contained in the original wb MWF may be added. MWF may be contaminated by slideway oils or hydraulic oils leaking from the processing machines [3–5].

Occupational contact dermatitis (OCD) frequently occurs in metalworkers exposed to MWF [6–16]. In cross-sectional studies from the Netherlands and Sweden, prevalence of OCD, mainly hand dermatitis, among metalworkers exposed to MWF was 26 % and 14 %, respectively [8, 9, 12]. In the Swiss Prospective Metal Worker Eczema Study (PROMETES), the 2.5-year incidence of hand dermatitis was 23 % [7]. The 3 year incidence of hand eczema was 15 %

A. Alikhan et al. (eds.), *Textbook of Hand Eczema*,
DOI 10.1007/978-3-642-39546-8_16, © Springer-Verlag Berlin Heidelberg 2014

among metalworker apprentices in the German prospective cohort study in the car industry (PACO-study) [10]. In a retrospective survey from Finland, 20 % of the metalworkers reported hand or forearm dermatitis during the past 12 months [15]. Current skin symptoms were reported by 10 % of metalworkers and were associated with frequent use of oil-based metalworking fluids and organic solvent/degreasing agents in two large European prospective cohort studies [16].

Irritant contact dermatitis (ICD) is more frequently reported than allergic contact dermatitis (ACD) in most studies on OCD in metalworkers. However, ICD promotes and often precedes sensitization [17]; therefore, the prevalence of ACD depends on the average duration of exposure and skin disease. Additionally, other factors, such as atopy, also have to be considered [3, 11, 13, 14], and very often OCD is a combination of irritant, allergic, and possibly endogenous factors, as pointed out by Grattan et al. [11].

OCD due to MWF mostly presents as vesicular or rhagadiform eczema of the web spaces, the lateral aspects of the fingers, and the backs of the hands. In the course of the disease, the dermatitis tends to spread to the palms and the wrists up to the forearms. Bacterial superinfections are possible [2, 6, 13, 14]. MWF dermatitis may have an unsatisfactory prognosis. Pryce et al. performed a follow-up study on 121 metalworkers and found that skin symptoms in more than 70 % of the patients were still present after 2 years, partly in spite of job discontinuation [13]. Shah et al. had similar findings [18]. However, the outcome depends very much on the individuals concerned, particularly on the patients' understanding of the cause of the disease and on their willingness to change their behavior in the workplace [13, 18]. A recent study on 1,355 metalworkers in Germany showed that the acceptance of skin-protective measures, in particular of barrier creams, was very low, which certainly contributed to recalcitrant dermatitis [19].

16.2 Irritant Contact Dermatitis Caused by Metalworking Fluids

Skin irritation by wb MWF is mainly caused by wet work, alkaline pH (usually 8.5–9.6), emulsifiers, and biocides [4, 13, 14]. Prevention is hampered by the fact that wearing protective gloves is prohibited at most MWF workplaces because of the risk of injury from rotating tools. Mostly, there is no continuous, but repetitive, exposure to wb MWF (e.g., when changing the workpiece). Splashes of wb MWF are usually not removed when other operations, such as control measurements, are performed. On the skin, the wb MWF dries up within a few minutes, resulting in an increased concentration and enhanced irritancy [20]. Additionally, mechanical factors, such as pressure and friction, and exposure to metal dust play a role in the damage of the epidermal barrier in metalworkers [7]. In contrast, lipopolysaccharides (endotoxins) from bacteria in the MWF apparently do not have any irritant effect on the skin [21].

16.3 Contact Allergens in Metalworking Fluids

In several studies on OCD in metalworkers, the most frequently observed MWF allergens were formaldehyde and other biocides, particularly formaldehyde releasers. Additionally, sensitization to colophonium/abietic acid, p-phenylenediamine (PPD), p-aminoazobenzene (PAAB), dichromate, and cobalt have been described, but the clinical relevance of these findings could not always be confirmed [6, 9, 11, 12, 22–27]. In case reports, a variety of other allergens in MWF have been described, such as diglycolamine [28]; ethylenediamine [29]; MEA [30, 31]; alkanolamineborates [32]; a condensate of boric acid, MEA, and fatty acids [33]; fatty acid polydiethanolamide [34]; oleyl alcohol [30]; tertiary-butylhydroquinone [35]; imazalil [36]; iodopropynyl butylcarbamate [37]; sodium

Table 16.1 MWF allergens to be patch-tested in metalworkers with suspected MWF dermatitis[a]

MWF series of the German Contact Dermatitis Research Group				
No.	Substance	Occurrence in MWF	Function in MWF	Patch test concentration
1	7-Ethylbicyclooxazolidine (Bioban CS 1246)	wb MWF	Biocide, formaldehyde releaser	1 % pet.
2	Benzylhemiformal	wb MWF	Biocide, formaldehyde releaser	1 % pet.
3	4,4-Dimethyl-1,3-oxazolidine/3,4,4-trimethyl-1,3-oxazolidine (Bioban CS 1135)	wb MWF	Biocide, formaldehyde releaser	1 % pet.
4	Octylisothiazolinone	wb MWF	Biocide	0.025 % pet.
5	N,N'-Methylene-bis-5-methyl-oxazolidine	wb MWF	Biocide, formaldehyde releaser	1 % pet.
6	Iodopropynyl butylcarbamate (IPBC)	wb MWF	Biocide	0.2 % pet.
7	Sodium-2-pyridinethiol-1-oxide (sodium omadine)	wb MWF	Biocide	0.1 % aq.
8	1,2-Benzisothiazolin-3-one, sodium salt	wb MWF	Biocide	0.1 % pet.
9	4-(2-Nitrobutyl) morpholine/4,4'-(2-ethyl-2-nitro-trimethylene) dimorpholine (Bioban P 1487)[b]	wb MWF	Biocide, formaldehyde releaser	1 % pet.
10	Methylisothiazolinone	wb MWF	Biocide	0.05 % aq.
11	Morpholinyl mercaptobenzothiazole (MOR)[b]	wb MWF	Rust preventive	0.5 % pet.
12	1,3,5-Tris(2-hydroxyethyl)-hexahydrotriazine (Grotan BK)	wb MWF	Biocide, formaldehyde releaser	1 % pet.
13	Monoethanolamine (MEA)	wb MWF	Rust preventive	2 % pet.
14	Abietic acid	wb MWF	Emulsifier/surfactant	10 % pet.
15	Diethanolamine (DEA)[b]	wb MWF	Rust preventive	2 % pet.
16	p-tert-Butylphenol	neat oils	Antioxidant	1 % pet.
17	2-Phenoxyethanol	wb MWF	Biocide	1 % pet.
18	Diglycolamine (2-(2-aminoethoxy)ethanol)	wb MWF	Emulsifier	1 % pet.
19	Triethanolamine (TEA)	wb MWF	Rust preventive	2.5 % pet.
20	Glyoxal trimer (dihydrate)	wb MWF	Biocide; possibly formed during usage	1 % pet.
21	Benzotriazole	wb MWF and neat oils	Rust preventive	1 % pet.
Baseline series				
No.	Substance	Occurrence in MWF	Function in MWF	Patch test concentration
22	Formaldehyde[c]	wb MWF	Top up biocide	1 % aq.
23	(Chloro-)methylisothiazolinone (MCI/MI)	wb MWF	Top up biocide	0.01 % aq.
24	Lanolin alcohol	wb MWF	Anti-wear additive	30 % pet.
25	Zinc diethyldithiocarbamate (ZDEC)[d]	neat oils	Anti-wear additive	1 % pet.
26	Cetearyl alcohol	wb MWF	Stabilizer/anti-wear additive	20 % pet.
27	Colophonium[e]	wb MWF	Emulsifier/surfactant	20 % pet.
28	Mercaptobenzothiazole	wb MWF	Rust preventive	2 % pet.

wb MWF water-based metalworking fluid, *pet.* petrolatum
[a]Modified from [3, 5, 23]
[b]Used until about 1995. No current usage in MWF
[c]Released from formaldehyde releasers
[d]Tested as a marker for sodium diethyldithiocarbamate
[e]Allergic reaction indicates contact allergy to oxidation products of resin acids

pyrithione [38, 39]; ethylhexylzinc dithiophosphate [34, 40]; oak moss resin [31]; glyoxal [41]; 2,5-dimercapto-1,3,4-thiadiazole [42]; and phenyl-alpha-naphthylamine [42]. Based on literature reports, information from the lubricant and metalworking industry, and patch test results of the Information Network of Departments of Dermatology (IVDK), patch testing with the allergens listed in Table 16.1 can be recommended [5, 27]. The most important allergens are described in detail in the following sections.

16.3.1 Monoethanolamine, Diethanolamine, and Triethanolamine

In wb MWF, MEA, diethanolamine (DEA), and triethanolamine (TEA) serve as rust-preventive agents with emulsifying properties, while diglycolamine is an emulsifier [43]. In two German studies, MEA ranked first among the MWF allergens [23, 27]. It has been suspected that many positive reactions to the test preparation MEA 2 % pet. are false-positive reactions. However, it could be shown that these reactions truly indicate contact allergy [44]. Due to a potential formation of carcinogenic N-nitrosamines, the use of DEA in wb MWF has declined since the mid-1990s, leading to a far lower frequency of sensitizations to DEA compared to MEA [23, 27]. TEA, which is also a frequent component of creams and cosmetics, was found to be a rare MWF allergen, although it is widely being used in MWF.

16.3.2 Colophonium/Abietic Acid

Oxidation products of abietic acid and other resin acids are the main sensitizers in colophonium [45]. MWF do not contain colophonium but distilled tall oil (DTO). According to industry information, about 30 % of the DTO are resin acids; of these, about one-third are abietic acid. On exposure to air, which occurs during normal use of wb MWF, the resin acids oxidize rather quickly [46–48]. The formation of alkanolamine salts from resin acids in wb MWF probably has no influence on the oxidation because different parts of the resin acid molecules are involved in salt formation and the oxidation process, respectively [47]. Although the concentration of resin acids in the wb MWF may be rather low, usually the wb MWF dries up on the contaminated skin, and the concentration rises within minutes [20]. If the irritant damage to the epidermal barrier of the exposed skin is also taken into account, occupational exposure to wb MWF carries a high risk of sensitization. This is illustrated by epidemiological data. In a German study, metalworkers with OCD and exposure to wb MWF had an eightfold increased risk of sensitization to colophonium when compared to metalworkers with OCD who were *not* exposed to wb MWF [23].

16.3.3 Fragrances

In the same study, metalworkers exposed to wb MWF with OCD had an increased risk of sensitization to fragrance mix and Balsam of Peru, when compared to metalworkers with OCD who were *not* exposed to wb MWF [23]. Until about 1990, fragrances or odor masks, even Balsam of Peru, were mentioned as common components of wb MWF [9, 14, 49]. Nowadays, however, no fragrances are added to the MWF concentrate, according to information from the lubricant-producing industry. However, it cannot be excluded that so-called odor masks are added by the metalworking companies during the usage of the wb MWF. Corresponding products are being offered on the market. Of course, this does not imply that *every* fragrance allergy in metalworkers is acquired by contact with wb MWF. In every individual case, a complete history has to be taken, particularly with respect to other allergen sources (aftershave, deodorant, etc.). Sometimes, however, this investigation will reveal occupational causation of fragrance allergy induced or at least elicited by wb MWF [31].

16.3.4 Cobalt, Nickel, and Chromium

Some studies on cobalt, nickel, and dichromate in MWF have been published [50–55]. In most of these, it was not clear whether the content of metal particles (introduced by abrasion of tools or workpieces) or the concentration of metal ions was determined. Thus, data on the valence state of the metal ions and the "bioavailability" are lacking. Hence, it cannot be excluded that, in some cases, hardly soluble metal oxides or metal sulfides were measured, which are not as important from the allergologic point of view. The results of these studies can be summarized as follows: cobalt, nickel, and chromium are not present in fresh, unused MWF. In used MWF, the cobalt concentration was usually below 3 ppm, if no cobalt-containing hard metals were processed. Only if hard metals containing cobalt were processed, cobalt concentrations up to 300 ppm – in single cases, even more – were found. The elicitation threshold in patients allergic to cobalt is regarded to range from 100 to 1,000 ppm cobalt ions [56, 57]. In pre-damaged skin, reactions could even be elicited with 10 ppm cobalt [58]. Hence, if cobalt is present in MWF as dissolved ions, those concentrations found in hard metal processing could be sufficient to elicit an allergic reaction, possibly even to induce sensitization. In the aforementioned studies, concentrations of nickel and chromium in used MWF usually were below 1 ppm. However, in a few exceptional cases, concentrations were found that might suffice to elicit an allergic reaction in highly sensitized individuals, if the metals are present in a suitable, ionized form. In a multifactorial analysis of data from the IVDK of more than 80,000 patients, Uter et al. could not find an increased risk of sensitization to cobalt, nickel, or dichromate in metalworkers [59], indicating that occupational relevance of contact allergy to the metal ions mentioned is an exceptional phenomenon. Hence, in every case of contact allergy to these metals in metalworkers exposed to MWF, it is mandatory to elucidate the source of exposure and to establish the clinical relevance of the positive test reaction. Occupational exposure other than MWF (e.g., workpieces, tools, handles) or private exposure (e.g., jeans button, costume jewelry, piercing) has to be considered.

16.3.5 Formaldehyde and Formaldehyde Releasers

Formerly, it was common to use formaldehyde solution for additional preservation of wb MWF during usage. Nowadays, formaldehyde releasers primarily are used for preservation of wb MWF and in system cleansers [5, 60]. The amount of formaldehyde released depends on various factors, such as pH, temperature, microbial contamination, and so on [61]. Peak formaldehyde concentrations may arise from additional preservation during the usage. An increased frequency of sensitization to formaldehyde among metalworkers with OCD exposed to wb MWF has been described in several studies [9, 11, 23, 59]. Allergic reactions to formaldehyde releasers may be caused by the whole molecule or by the formaldehyde released. However, there is only a limited correlation between the ability to release formaldehyde and concomitant patch test reactions to formaldehyde and the releaser [61]. Studies on this subject are hampered by the fact that patch test reactions to this type of biocides are often weak and poorly reproducible [22, 61].

16.3.6 Methylchloroisothiazolinone/Methylisothiazolinone

Methylchloroisothiazolinone/methylisothiazolinone (MCI/MI) is not used as a preservative in the MWF concentrate, but it may be added to the wb MWF at the workplace as additional biocide [5]. This poses a risk for the metalworkers: a single skin contact with concentrated MCI/MI may cause sensitization [62]. In the 1980s, MCI/MI was widely used as preservative in body-care products at relatively high concentrations, which led to an "epidemic" of MCI/MI sensitization. As a consequence, its use concentration was strictly limited and its usage was reduced, leading to declining sensitization rates [63]. Nowadays, MCI/MI is being used in skin-care products at very low concentrations that probably will not induce new sensitizations [64, 65]. Hence, the individual exposure to MCI/MI has to be established in every metalworker sensitized to MCI/

MI with special regard to additional preservation of the wb MWF during its use. Although MCI has a much higher allergenic potency than MI, isolated sensitizations to MI have been observed [66, 67]. Recently, increasing rates of sensitization to MCI/MI as well as to MI were observed, probably due to the increased usage of MI, leading to primary sensitization to MI with cross-reactivity to MCI [68]. Benzisothiazolinone (BIT) and octylisothiazolinone (OIT), which are also currently used for preservation of wb MWF, do not cross-react with MCI/MI [69].

16.4 Patch Testing with MWF from the Patient's Workplace

As patch testing with MWF patch test series does not cover all potentially allergenic MWF components, MWF from the patient's workplace and their components should be tested in every case concerned [6, 9, 11, 12]. However, test concentrations and vehicles recommended for patch testing with MWF vary a lot [2, 6, 9, 11, 12, 70–72].

An interdisciplinary working party on allergy diagnostics in the metal industry published recommendations on how to patch test MWF from the patient's workplace in 2002 (in German language only) [4]. The essential points of these recommendations are the following: both fresh and used MWF should be patch-tested. In the case of wb MWF, a sample of the fresh, undiluted MWF concentrate should be obtained. The sample of the used MWF must be taken from the inflows of the machines (and not from the so-called sumps) to avoid contamination with metal chips, which might cause irritant patch test reactions. Samples of used wb MWF must be stored in a refrigerator and tested within less than 5 days; otherwise microbial contamination will change or even destroy the emulsion. Fresh concentrate of the wb MWF should be tested 5 % aq. Used wb MWF can be patch-tested as is, provided the concentration at the workplace is ≤8 %. In the case of higher workplace concentrations, further dilution to an end concentration of 4–8 % is recommended. The pH must be checked before patch testing. Usually, wb MWF are alkaline (pH 8.6–9.5), but experience shows that this is tolerated. Neat oils should be tested 50 % in olive oil. Used wb MWF samples must be accompanied by information about concentration and pH at the time of sampling, date of the last change of the MWF, system cleaner used, date of last preservation, name of bactericide and fungicide used, name of other additives and date of addition, material processed in the machine, and possible influx of hydraulic oils, slideway oils, or other oils by leakage. For neat oils, only data on the last change of the MWF, additives, material processed in the machine, and possible influx of other oils needs to be documented. The interdisciplinary working party emphasizes that false-negative test reactions to MWF may occur even under the recommended conditions [4]. Allergenic components in the MWF may be diluted too much and thus may elicit no reaction on patch testing in the intact skin of the upper back, although they may cause ACD on the pre-damaged skin of the hands under workplace conditions. Hence, patch testing with the single components of the MWF should be performed not only in case of a positive patch test reaction to the MWF from the workplace but also in clinically suspected cases, in which no test reaction to the individual MWF could be seen.

16.5 Preventive Measures

In addition to the general rules for the prevention of skin damage from wet work, some particular measures when working with wb MWF should be considered. If the skin is wetted with MWF only intermittently, the MWF should not dry up on the skin but should be removed, in order to avoid a rise in concentration by vaporization of water. Cleaning cloths used for tools or workpieces should easily be distinguishable from those for wiping off the hands. Skin contact with MWF should be minimized by automation, encapsulation of machines, and so forth. For degreasing workpieces, suitable devices such as hooks and sieves should be used for immersing, thus reducing the alternating skin irritation by MWF and solvents.

Pollution of the MWF by dirt, food, and so on has to be avoided. Workplaces have to be kept clean. Concentration and pH of the MWF have to be controlled weekly in order to recognize and eliminate any increase of concentration or pH in time. Bacterial contamination itself does not affect skin irritancy of the MWF. However, there is an indirect effect because in case of a high microbial colonization, additional preservation is necessary for technical reasons. Every addition of preservatives has to be documented exactly (e.g. date, amount, product used). Most suitably, additional preservation is performed after the last shift on Friday, so the biocide is almost completely dispersed at the beginning of work on Monday morning. In companies without a weekend break, as few metalworkers as possible should be exposed to the maximum biocide concentration, and all workers must be informed about the higher preservative content. System cleansers should not be used during operation hours, because they contain high concentrations of biocides. The same precautions as with additional preservation have to be taken.

Conclusion

Metalworking fluids (MWF) are a frequent cause of occupational hand eczema in metalworkers. Working with water-based MWF involves wet work, thus irritating the skin. Additionally, the alkaline pH, emulsifiers, and biocides increase irritancy. Together with mechanical cofactors, this leads to chronic irritant hand dermatitis in metalworkers. However, MWF also contain sensitizers causing ACD. The most important are monoethanolamine, colophonium/abietic acid, formaldehyde and formaldehyde releasers, and other biocides such as isothiazolinones. Because allergens not fully covered by the commercially available patch test series may be in the individual MWF, patch testing with MWF brought in by the patient is important. Good working hygiene, workers' education, and, in particular, avoidance of letting water-based MWF dry up on the skin are essential preventive measures. Unfortunately, metalworkers' adherence to skin protection is not very high, and gloves are not allowed in many workplaces because of the danger of severe injury by rotating tools.

References

1. Anonymus. Kühlschmierstoffe. In: Greim H, editor. Gesundheitsschädliche Arbeitsstoffe. Toxikologisch-arbeitsmedizinische Begründungen von MAK-Werten. 31. Weinheim: Lieferung VCH; 2000.
2. Foulds IS. Cutting fluids. In: Kanerva L, Elsner P, Wahlberg JE, Maibach HI, editors. Handbook of occupational dermatology. Berlin: Springer; 2000. p. 691–700. Chapter 86.
3. Geier J, Lessmann H, Schmidt A, Englitz H-G, Schnuch A. Kontaktekzeme durch Kühlschmierstoffe in der Metallindustrie. Akt Dermatol. 2003;29:185–94.
4. Tiedemann K-H, Zoellner G, Adam M, Becker D, Boveleth W, Eck E, et al. Empfehlungen für die Epikutantestung bei Verdacht auf Kontaktallergie durch Kühlschmierstoffe. 2. Hinweise zur Arbeitsstofftestung. Dermatol Beruf Umwelt. 2002;50:180–9.
5. Geier J, Lessmann H, Schumacher T, Eckert C, Becker D, Boveleth W, et al. Vorschlag für die Epikutantestung bei Verdacht auf Kontaktallergie durch Kühlschmierstoffe. 1. Kommerziell erhältliche Testsubstanzen. Dermatol Beruf Umwelt. 2000;48:232–6.
6. Alomar A, Conde-Salazar L, Romaguera C. Occupational dermatoses from cutting oils. Contact Dermatitis. 1985;12:129–38.
7. Berndt U, Hinnen U, Iliev D, Elsener P. Hand eczema in metalworker trainees – an analysis of risk factors. Contact Dermatitis. 2000;43:327–32.
8. de Boer EM, van Ketel WG, Bruynzeel DP. Dermatoses in metal workers. (I). Irritant contact dermatitis. Contact Dermatitis. 1989;20:212–8.
9. de Boer EM, van Ketel WG, Bruynzeel DP. Dermatoses in metal workers. (II). Allergic contact dermatitis. Contact Dermatitis. 1989;20:280–6.
10. Funke U, Fartasch M, Diepgen TL. Incidence of work-related hand eczema during apprenticeship: first results of a prospective cohort study in the car industry. Contact Dermatitis. 2001;44:166–72.
11. Grattan CEH, English JSC, Foulds IS, Rycroft RJG. Cutting fluid dermatitis. Contact Dermatitis. 1989;20:372–6.
12. Gruvberger B, Isaksson M, Frick M, Pontén A, Bruze M. Occupational dermatoses in a metalworking plant. Contact Dermatitis. 2003;48:80–6.
13. Pryce DW, Irvine D, English JSC, Rycroft RJG. Soluble oil dermatitis: a follow-up study. Contact Dermatitis. 1989;21:28–35.
14. Pryce DW, White I, English JSC, Rycroft RJG. Soluble oil dermatitis: a review. J Soc Occup Med. 1989;39:93–8.
15. Suuronen K, Jolanki R, Luukkonen R, Alanko K, Susitaival P. Self-reported skin symptoms in metal workers. Contact Dermatitis. 2007;57:259–64.

16. Mirabelli MC, Zock J-P, Bircher AJ, Jarvis D, Keidel D, Kromhout H, et al. Metalworking exposures and persistent skin symptoms in the ECRHS II and SAPALDIA 2 cohorts. Contact Dermatitis. 2009;60:256–63.
17. Hornstein OP. Ekzemkrankheiten. Therapiewoche. 1984;34:400–9.
18. Shah M, Lewis FM, Gawkrodger DJ. Prognosis of occupational hand dermatitis in metalworkers. Contact Dermatitis. 1996;34:27–30.
19. Kütting B, Weistenhöfer W, Baumeister T, Uter W, Drexler H. Current acceptance and implementation of preventive strategies for occupational hand eczema in 1355 metalworkers in Germany. Br J Dermatol. 2009;161:390–6.
20. Krbek F, Schäfer T. Untersuchungen an Tropfen und Rückständen von wassermischbaren Kühlschmierstoffen. Arbeitsmed Sozialmed Präventivmed. 1991;26:411–6.
21. Becker D. Hautirritationen durch Endotoxine in Kühlschmierstoffen. Ergebnisbericht zu einem Projekt der Süddeutschen Metall-Berufsgenossenschaft und der Universitäts-Hautklinik Mainz, 2004.
22. Brinkmeier T, Geier J, Lepoittevin J-P, Frosch PJ. Patch test reactions to Biobans in metal workers are often weak and not reproducible. Contact Dermatitis. 2002;47:27–31.
23. Geier J, Lessmann H, Schnuch A, Uter W. Contact sensitizations in metalworkers with occupational dermatitis exposed to water-based metalworking fluids. Results of the research project "FaSt.". Int Arch Occup Environ Health. 2004;77:543–51.
24. Nethercott JR, Rothman N, Holness DL, O'Toole T. Health problems in metal workers exposed to a coolant oil containing Kathon 886 MW. Am J Contact Derm. 1990;1:94–9.
25. Uter W, Schaller S, Bahmer FA, Brasch J, et al. Contact allergy in metal workers – a one-year analysis based on data collected by the "Information Network of Dermatological Clinics" (IVDK) in Germany. Derm Beruf Umwelt. 1993;41:220–7.
26. Uter W, Geier J, Ippen H. Nachrichten aus dem IVDK: Aktuelle Sensibilisierungshäufigkeiten bei der DKG-Testreihe "Metallverarbeitung". Derm Beruf Umwelt. 1996;44:34–6.
27. Geier J, Lessmann H, Dickel H, Frosch PJ, Koch P, Becker D, et al. Patch test results with the metalworking fluid series of the German contact dermatitis research group (DKG). Contact Dermatitis. 2004;51:118–30.
28. Geier J, Lessmann H, Graefe A, Fuchs T. Contact allergy to diglycolamine in a water-based metalworking fluid. Contact Dermatitis. 2002;46:121.
29. Crow KD, Peachey RDG, Adams JE. Coolant oil dermatitis due to ethylenediamine. Contact Dermatitis. 1978;4:359–61.
30. Koch P. Occupational allergic contact dermatitis from oleyl alcohol and monoethanolamine in a metalworking fluid. Contact Dermatitis. 1995;33:273.
31. Owen CM, August PJ, Beck MH. Contact allergy to oak moss resin in a soluble oil. Contact Dermatitis. 2000;43:112.
32. Bruze M, Hradil E, Eriksohn I-L, Gruvberger B, Widström L. Occupational allergic contact dermatitis from alkanolamineborates in metalworking fluids. Contact Dermatitis. 1995;32:24–7.
33. Jensen CD, Andersen KE. Allergic contact dermatitis from a condensate of boric acid, monoethanolamine and fatty acids in a metalworking fluid. Contact Dermatitis. 2003;49:45–6.
34. Kanerva L, Tupasela O, Jolanki R. Occupational allergic contact dermatitis from ethylhexylzinc dithiophosphate and fatty acid polydiethanolamide in cutting fluids. Contact Dermatitis. 2001;44:193–4.
35. Meding B. Occupational contact dermatitis from tertiary-butylhydroquinone (TBHQ) in a cutting fluid. Contact Dermatitis. 1996;34:224.
36. Piebenga WP, van der Walle HB. Allergic contact dermatitis from 1–[2-(2,4-dichlorophenyl)-2–(2-propenyloxy) ethyl]-1H-imidazole in a water-based metalworking fluid. Contact Dermatitis. 2003;48:285–6.
37. Majoie IML, van Ginkel CJW. The biocide iodopropynyl butylcarbamate (IPBC) as an allergen in cutting oils. Contact Dermatitis. 2000;43:238–40.
38. Isaksson M. Delayed diagnosis of occupational contact dermatitis from sodium pyrithione in a metalworking fluid. Contact Dermatitis. 2002;47:248–9.
39. Le Coz C-J. Allergic contact dermatitis from sodium pyrithione in metalworking fluid. Contact Dermatitis. 2001;45:58–9.
40. Isaksson M, Frick M, Gruvberger B, Pontén A, Bruze M. Occupational allergic contact dermatitis from the extreme pressure (EP) additive, zinc, bis ((O, O'-di-2-ethylhexyl)dithiophosphate) in neat oils. Contact Dermatitis. 2002;46:248–9.
41. Aalto-Korte K, Mäkelä EA, Huttunen M, Suuronen K, Jolanki R. Occupational contact allergy to glyoxal. Contact Dermatitis. 2005;52:276–81.
42. Aalto-Korte K, Suuronen K, Kuuliala O, Jolanki R. Contact allergy to 2,5-dimercapto-1,3,4-thiadiazole and phenyl-*alpha*-naphthylamine, allergens in industrial greases and lubricant oils – contact allergy to water-insoluble greases is uncommon but needs to be considered in some workers. Contact Dermatitis. 2008;58:93–6.
43. Lessmann H, Uter W, Schnuch A, Geier J. Skin sensitizing properties of the ethanolamines mono-, di-, and triethanolamine. Data analysis of a multicentre surveillance network (IVDK) and review of the literature. Contact Dermatitis. 2009;60:243–55.
44. Geier J, Lessmann H, Schnuch A, Uter W. Diagnostic quality of the patch test preparation monoethanolamine 2% pet. Contact Dermatitis. 2005;52:171–3.
45. Hausen BM, Brinkmann J, Dohn W. Lexikon der Kontaktallergene, 6. Ergänzungs-Lieferung, Kolophonium, K 4. Landsberg: Ecomed. 1998. p. 1–15.
46. Hausen BM, Krohn K, Budianto E. Contact allergy due to colophonium. (VII). Sensitizing studies with oxidation products of abietic and related acids. Contact Dermatitis. 1990;23:352–8.
47. Hausen BM, Börries M, Budianto E, Krohn K. Contact allergy due to colophonium. (IX). Sensitization studies with further products isolated after oxidative degradation of resin acids and colophonium. Contact Dermatitis. 1993;29:234–40.

48. Karlberg A-T. Air oxidation increases the allergenic potential of tall-oil rosin. Colophonium contact allergens also identified in tal-oil rosin. Am J Contact Dermat. 1991;2:43–9.
49. Ippen H. Allergische Hautschäden bei der Metallbearbeitung. Derm Beruf Umwelt. 1979;27:71–4.
50. Einarsson Ö, Kylin B, Lindstedt G, Wahlberg JE. Chromium, cobalt and nickel in used cutting fluids. Contact Dermatitis. 1975;1:182–3.
51. Einarsson Ö, Eriksson E, Lindstedt G, Wahlberg JE. Dissolution of cobalt from hard metal alloys by cutting fluids. Contact Dermatitis. 1979;5:129–32.
52. Lehmann E, Fröhlich N. Kühlschmierstoffe – Zusätzliche Belastungen durch Metallionen? Amtliche Mitteilungen der Bundesanstalt für Arbeitsschutz, January. 1993. p. 1–7.
53. Minkwitz R, Fröhlich N, Lehmann E. Untersuchungen von Schadstoffbelastungen an Arbeitsplätzen bei der Herstellung und Verarbeitung von Metallen – Beryllium, Cobalt und deren Legierungen, Fb. 367. Dortmund: Schriftenreihe der Bundesanstalt für Arbeitsschutz; 1983.
54. Pfeiffer W, Breuer D, Blome H, Deninger C, et al. BIA-report 7/96 Kühlschmierstoffe. Sankt Augustin: Hauptverband der gewerblichen Berufsgenossenschaften (HVBG); 1996.
55. Wahlberg JE, Lindstedt G, Einarsson Ö. Chromium, cobalt and nickel in Swedish cement, detergents, mould and cutting oils. Berufsdermatosen. 1977;25:220–8.
56. Rystedt I. Evaluation and relevance of isolated test reactions to cobalt. Contact Dermatitis. 1979;5:233–8.
57. Wahlberg JE. Thresholds of sensitivity in metal contact allergy. 1. Isolated and simultaneous allergy to chromium, cobalt, mercury and-or nickel. Berufsdermatosen. 1973;21:22–33.
58. Allenby CF, Basketter DA. Minimum eliciting patch test concentrations of cobalt. Contact Dermatitis. 1989;20:185–90.
59. Uter W, Gefeller O, Geier J, Lessmann H, Pfahlberg A, Schnuch A. Untersuchungen zur Abhängigkeit der Sensibilisierung gegen wichtige Allergene von arbeitsbedingten sowie individuellen Faktoren. Bremerhaven: Schriftenreihe der Bundesanstalt für Arbeitsschutz und Arbeitsmedizin, Forschung, Fb 949, Wissenschaftsverlag NW; 2002.
60. Thamm H. Formaldehyd und Formaldehydabspalter in Kühlschmierstoffen: Aktueller Stand. Allergologie. 1997;20:232–8.
61. Geier J, Lessmann H, Schnuch A, Fuchs T. Kontaktallergien durch formaldehydabspaltende biozide. Eine analyse der daten des IVDK aus den Jahren 1992 bis 1995. Allergologie. 1997;20: 215–24.
62. Kanerva L, Tarvainen K, Pinola A, Leino T, Granlund H, Estlander T, et al. A single accidental exposure may result in a chemical burn, primary sensitization and allergic contact dermatitis. Contact Dermatitis. 1994;31:229–35.
63. Mowad CM. Methylchloroisothiazolinone revisited. Am J Contact Dermat. 2000;11:114–8.
64. Fewings J, Menné T. An update of the risk assessment for methylchloroisothiazolinone/methylisothiazolinone (MCI/MI) with focus on rinse-off products. Contact Dermatitis. 1999;41:1–11.
65. Robinson MK, Gerberick GF, Ryan CA, McNamee P, White IR, Basketter DA. The importance of exposure estimation in the assessment of skin sensitization risk. Contact Dermatitis. 2000;42:251–9.
66. Thyssen JP, Sederberg-Olsen N, Thomsen JF, Menné T. Contact dermatitis from methylisothiazolinone in a paint factory. Contact Dermatitis. 2006;54: 322–4.
67. Gruvberger B, Isaksson M, Dubnika I, Hindsén M, Pontén A, Svedman C, et al. Patch testing with isothiazolinones. Contact Dermatitis. 2006;55(1):13.
68. Geier J, Lessmann H, Schnuch A, Uter W. Recent increase in allergic reactions to methylchloroisothiazolinone/methylisothiazolinone: is methylisothiazolinone the culprit? Contact Dermatitis. 2012;67:334–41.
69. Geier J, Schnuch A. No cross sensitization between MCI/MI, benzisothiazolinone, and octylisothiazolinone. Contact Dermatitis. 1996;34:148–9.
70. Frosch PJ, Pilz B, Peiler D, Dreier B, Rabenhorst S. Die Epikutantestung mit patienteneigenen Produkten. In: Plewig G, Przybilla B, editors. Fortschritte der praktischen dermatologie und venerologie 15. Berlin: Springer; 1997. p. 166–81.
71. Jolanki R, Estlander T, Alanko K, Kanerva L. Patch testing with a patient's own materials handled at work. In: Kanerva L, Elsner P, Wahlberg JE, Maibach HI, editors. Handbook of occupational dermatology. Berlin: Springer; 2000. p. 375–83. Chapter 47.
72. Geier J, Uter W, Lessmann H, Frosch PJ. Patch testing with metalworking fluids from the patient's workplace. Contact Dermatitis. 2004;51:172–9.

Hand Eczema from Acrylate Compounds in Dentistry

17

Anthony T.J. Goon and Marléne A.I. Isaksson

Contents

A.T.J. Goon, MBBS, MRCP, FRCP, Ph.D. (✉)
National Skin Centre, 1 Mandalay Road, Singapore 308205, Singapore
e-mail: anthonygoon@nsc.gov.sg

M.A.I. Isaksson, M.D., Ph.D.
Department of Occupational and Environmental Dermatology, Lund University, Skåne University Hospital, Jan Waldenströms Gata 18 Ingang 73, Plan 5, Malmö SE 20502, Sweden
e-mail: marlene.isaksson@skane.se

17.1 Introduction

Hand eczema is not uncommon among dental professionals, whether they are dentists, dental technicians, or dental nurses. In addition to endogenous hand eczema and irritant contact dermatitis, allergic contact dermatitis is also a common diagnosis in these professionals. Implicated allergens include sensitizers present in the baseline or standard patch test series (e.g., metals, fragrance, rubber, colophony). Furthermore, among the most common allergens causing contact allergy in this group of patients are the (meth) acrylate monomers, which are not in the baseline series of most patch test centers.

17.2 Acrylates

The term “acrylates” needs further clarification. It may refer to esters of acrylic acid exclusively, or it may include esters of both acrylic acid and

A. Alikhan et al. (eds.), *Textbook of Hand Eczema*,
DOI 10.1007/978-3-642-39546-8_17, © Springer-Verlag Berlin Heidelberg 2014

methacrylic acid as well as some of their other derivatives. In this chapter, the term "acrylate" will be used for esters of acrylic acid only and "acrylate/methacrylate" or "(meth)acrylate" for esters of acrylic and/or methacrylic acid.

Acrylate and methacrylate plastics can be either thermoplastics or thermoset plastics, depending on the type of monomer that has been used. Polymers made from monomers that only have one functional group (acrylate or methacrylate group) will form thermoplastic polymers after hardening (polymerization). Polymers made from monomers with two or more functional groups will form thermoset polymers. Polymers made from mixtures of monomers of which one has one functional group and the other two or more functional groups can form polymers with varying degrees of thermoplastic/thermoset characteristics, depending on the proportions of these monomers.

Contact allergy to (meth)acrylates among dental professionals has been well studied, [1-8] and there are numerous epidemiologic studies available in the medical literature. These cases would usually manifest clinically with hand eczema.

17.3 Chemistry of Acrylates

The acrylates are characterized by the vinyl unsaturated radical, CH_2=CH–. This vinyl radical is present in the large family of monomers used for the production of vinyl plastics, which also include polystyrenes and polyvinyls.

The basic chemical structures of acrylic and methacrylic acid are shown in Fig. 17.1.

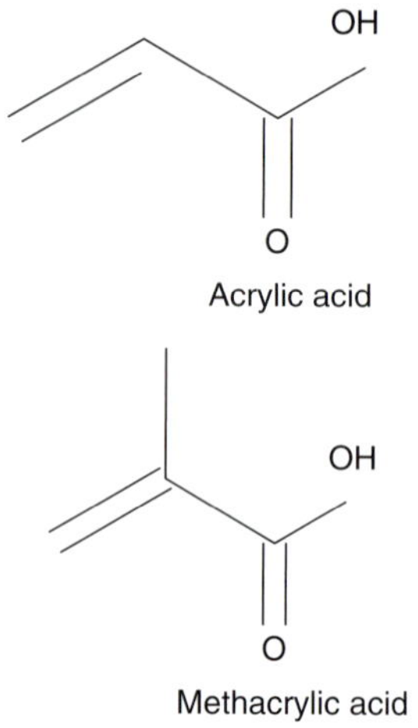

Fig. 17.1 Basic chemical structures of acrylic and methacrylic acid

(Meth)acrylates, in general, are α (alpha), β (beta)-unsaturated carbonyl compounds attached to an adjacent carbonyl group. The oxygen atom of the carbonyl group is more electronegative than the carbon atom and thus draws electron density away from the carbon atom to increase the >C=O bond's polarity. Therefore, the carbon atom becomes electrophilic and thus more reactive with nucleophiles, while the electronegative oxygen atom can react with an electrophile. When this double bond is activated, the group reacts readily with electrophiles, nucleophiles, and free radicals.

Methacrylates have an extra methyl group bound to the α (alpha) carbon of the –C=C– double bond. This extra methyl group donates electrons to the double bond, thus stabilizing it. Furthermore, the methyl group acts as steric hindrance. These factors render methacrylates less reactive than their corresponding acrylates, and this is reflected in their lower sensitizing capacity.

Acrylic and methacrylic polymers are obtained by polymerization of monomeric derivatives of acrylic acids. This group includes acrylic and methacrylic acids, their esters, amides, salts, halides, and nitriles, with the esters being the most important. These esters polymerize under the influence of heat, light, oxygen, and oxygen-yielding substances such as sodium peroxide, hydrogen peroxide, and benzoyl peroxide. The basic structures of these polymers are chains of varying lengths or network structures formed by linking together the original monomeric molecules.

Monomers of acrylic and methacrylic resins may have one or more functional groups. Monofunctional monomers contain only one functional acrylate or methacrylate group on each monomer molecule. Multifunctional monomers have two or more functional groups per monomer molecule and are called di-, tri-, and tetra-acrylates or methacrylates. Increasing the number of functional groups will increase the viscosity of the resin as well as increase the number of cross-links in the finished product, which may be desirable for certain applications, such as in adhesives and dental composite resins.

During the polymerization process, several other chemicals are required besides the monomers themselves. Initiators (e.g., benzoyl peroxide) are required to release free radicals in order to start the process. These initiators enter into the chemical reaction and become part of the final chemical compound and, hence, are not catalysts. Self-curing resins require heat activation by activators (e.g., tertiary amines) to break the initiator into free radicals at ambient temperature. The activator forms a complex with the initiator, reducing the thermal energy (and thus the temperature) needed to split benzoyl peroxide into two free radicals. Newer visible light-cured dental resin systems utilize camphoroquinone and an organic amine to generate free radicals when irradiated by blue-violet light.

In order to improve storage stability and working time for dental resins, inhibitors (e.g., methyl ether of hydroquinone) are added to prevent spontaneous polymerization during storage and slow down the process of polymerization to allow adequate time for mixing and placement of the resin.

Two or more chemically different monomers may be combined to yield specific desired physical properties. These combined polymers are termed copolymers. An acrylate/methacrylate monomer may be copolymerized with other acrylate/methacrylate monomers and/or non-acrylate monomers.

17.4 Historical Aspects

In 1843, Redtenbacher first obtained acrylic acid from the air oxidation of acrolein [9]. Acrolein (systematic name: propenal) is the simplest unsaturated aldehyde. Its chemical formula is CH_2=CH–CHO.

This was followed by the first synthesis of methacrylic acid in 1865. Polymerization of acrylics was subsequently observed by Dr. Otto Röhm in Darmstadt, Germany, in 1901, and polymethyl acrylate manufacture by Röhm and Haas of Philadelphia began in 1927 [9]. The mid-1930s saw the first production of polymethylmethacrylate and its marketing as Perspex, Lucite, and Plexiglas. Further developments and the introduction of more derivatives of acrylic compounds were made after extensive research by Imperial Chemical Industries (I.C.I.) Ltd. of London, E.I. DuPont de Nemours & Co., Inc., and Röhm and Haas Co. in the United States [10].

Acrylics were first used in dentistry in 1935, and by 1937 their use had become more widespread. By the 1940s, acrylates/methacrylates had been extensively used for removable dental prostheses, individual impression trays, orthodontic devices, occlusal splints, fixed crowns, and bridges [11]. Hypersensitivity to methyl methacrylate (MMA) was first reported by Stevenson [12] and Moody [13] in 1941. They described allergic, eczematous, contact dermatitis of the hands and faces of dentists caused by the acrylic resin monomer. Stoy [14] cited several dental laboratory technicians with local dermatitis caused by this monomer. In 1954, Fisher reported on two dentists and two dental technicians with hand eczema and allergic contact dermatitis from MMA. In those patients MMA was patch tested at 100 %! [15]

17.5 Which Types of Acrylates Are Used in the Dental Profession?

For the last 20 years, acrylics (acrylates and methacrylates) have replaced amalgam in dental restorations. Methacrylates, in particular, have been identified as major occupational contact sensitizers. Three groups of acrylics are important in dentistry:

1. Monofunctional methacrylates, such as MMA and 2-hydroxyethyl methacrylate (2-HEMA), the latter being common in bonding products. Both are semi-volatile
2. Multifunctional methacrylates, such as ethylene glycol dimethacrylate (EGDMA),

triethylene glycol dimethacrylate (TREGDMA), and triethyleneglycol diacrylate (TREGDA)
3. Acrylated and methacrylated prepolymers, such as 2,2-bis[4–(2–hydroxy-3-methacryloxypropoxy)phenyl]-propane (bis-GMA) (Bowen resin) and urethane dimethacrylate (UEDMA), the former in dentin bonding products and both present in dental filling materials [16]

Dental prostheses, dentin bonding agents, and dental composite resins all contain various acrylics. They are a common cause of occupational allergic contact dermatitis in dental personnel. The frequency of contact allergy to methacrylates is lower in dental patients than in dental personnel, because patients are exposed to uncured acrylics for shorter durations.

17.5.1 Dental Prostheses

Plastics or polymers are often used in dentures or prostheses, fixed bridges and crowns, facades, orthodontic devices, models, trays, and occlusal splints. Dental technicians previously handled methacrylates with bare hands [17] but nowadays use protective gloves whenever possible but less often than dentists and dental nurses. The MMA and polymethyl methacrylate (PMMA) system is the most important system for removable prostheses or dentures. Polymethyl methacrylate denture base has dominated the market for over 50 years [18]. The basement sheets are made from liquid MMA, which is mixed with PMMA powder, resulting in a mass that is molded manually or mechanically. The powder may contain copolymers of other acrylates, such as polyisobutyl acrylate or polystyrene [19]. In the powder, there may also be organic peroxide initiators, x-ray contrast substances, pigments, cadmium and ferric salts, iron oxides, titanium dioxide to control translucency, and dyed synthetic fibers for esthetics [17]. Potential allergens are dyes, nylon fibers, pigments, and zinc or titanium oxides.

The liquid may contain other monomers such as n-butyl methacrylate, isobutyl methacrylate, or lauryl methacrylate. Other components may include a hydroquinone inhibitor, dimethacrylates or cross-linking agents such as EGDMA, an organic amine accelerator if cold-curing or self-curing, and UV absorbers [17, 19]. After the molding process, the polymerization starts by means of heat, chemicals, UV radiation, or visible light. In the heat-polymerization process, the monomer solution may contain cross-linking bifunctional (meth)acrylates such as 1,4-butanediol dimethacrylate, 1,4-butanediol diacrylate, ethylene glycol methacrylate, or EGDMA [17]. Cross-linking helps the dilution of high-viscosity monomers and makes the three-dimensional structure more rigid [17]. The monomer solution, which is polymerized chemically, may contain N,N-dimethyl-p-toluidine as an accelerator. Another amine accelerator is 4-tolyldiethanolamine [17]. Hypoallergenic denture base materials exist, and significantly lower residual MMA monomer content was found when comparing these denture base materials to PMMA [18]. Other alternatives for prosthetic materials are polymers such as polyvinyl chloride, polyvinyl acetate, polystyrene and polystyrene copolymers, phenol formaldehyde resins, polyamides, and polyurethanes. Polycarbonates can also have this function.

Dental technicians nowadays use more complex light-cured acrylics, which are similar to dental composite resins (DCR) in composition. Hence, they are exposed to methacrylates with a higher sensitizing potential than MMA and thus have a higher risk of contracting occupational contact dermatitis [20].

An orthodontist developed pulpitis because of exposure to MMA liquid when remodelling children's dental devices with cold-curing acrylics without protective gloves. She was allergic to MMA, which was her only exposure, but reacted also to butyl acrylate, ethyl acrylate, and 2-hydroxypropyl methacrylate, possibly due to cross-reactivity with MMA [17]. Animal studies showed that animals sensitized to methacrylates may show cross-reactivity to acrylates but not vice versa [21]. A dental technician with hand eczema was allergic to MMA when patch tested and also to MMA liquid 1 % pet. and PMMA powder 100 %, which is very uncommon, as this is polymerized material and should not contain more than minute amounts of monomer [17].

Crowns and bridges or facades are made from PMMA powder and MMA liquid or paste. The liquid contains monomers of MMA, tetrahydrofurfuryl methacrylate (the cross-linkers), the dimethacrylate monomers EGDMA, TREGDMA, and 1,4-butanediol dimethacrylate; and the prepolymer, urethane dimethacrylate. The inhibitor, hydroquinone, stabilizes the monomers, and the activator N,N-dimethyl-p-toluidine acts as an initiator. The powder is usually PMMA with inorganic fillers.

The light- and heat-polymerizing dental materials can contain dimethacrylates, diacrylates, trimethacrylic monomers, and oligomers containing several urethane and dimethacrylate groups in the molecule.

17.5.2 Dentin Bonding Agents

Dentin bonding agents are plastics without fillers; they are also called resins. The first dentin bonding agent was N-phenyl glycine glycidyl methacrylate, Bowen's resin. Bonding systems formerly contained a primer and an adhesive, but nowadays it is usually a one-step procedure. After etching the surface to be treated with 37 % phosphoric acid, the dentin is covered by the bonding agent (adhesive), which is pressed out into the cavity with pressurized air. Polymerization is then accomplished by blue visible light, and subsequently the DCR is applied to the cavity of the tooth in layers and cured either with chemicals or with the same visible light as above. 2-HEMA is most often present in bonding systems because it is water soluble and does not damage the pulp. Bis-GMA, TREGDMA, and UEDMA can also be present. Because bis-GMA may be used in dentin bonding agents, DGEBA resin may also be present as an impurity in these resins.

In Malmö, we had seen a dentist with pulpitis who had been allergic to his bonding resin containing 2-HEMA (Fig. 17.2). He had also been using a dual-function spatula without wearing protective gloves. A brush in one end of the spatula had been dipped into uncured resin before he placed it into the cavity of the tooth. He then turned the spatula around and used the other end to level out the DCR placed into the tooth just after he had used pressurized air to inject the DCR from a pistol-like device. Thus, his skin was directly exposed to the bonding resin, and when the eczema appeared on his dorsal hand, he immediately suspected that this had been due to the bonding agent (Fig. 17.3).

From Finland, it was reported that a female dentist repeatedly developed pharyngitis at work. A chamber provocation test indicated that her symptoms were caused by acrylics. Prick tests with acrylics were negative while patch tests were strongly positive, without the patient having any skin lesions [22]. Also from Finland came a report of a dental laboratory worker developing symptoms of conjunctivitis. He was exposed to chemical-curable and light-curable methacrylates and was sensitized to multiple methacrylates, including MMA, 2-HEMA, EGDMA, and TREGDMA. Conjunctivitis may thus be caused by type IV allergy to methacrylates [23]. Acrylate compounds are reported to also cause occupational laryngitis [24].

17.5.3 Dental Composite Resins

Dental composite resins based on bisphenol A and glycidyl (meth)acrylates have been used since 1962 [25]. Bis-GMA is the most commonly used. This resin can also be manufactured by an addition reaction between diglycidyl ether of bisphenol A (DGEBA) resin and methacrylic acid. Therefore, bis-GMA can be classified as a dimethacrylated epoxy, even though it does not contain a reactive epoxy group [16]. DCR may, as a result, contain DGEBA resin as an impurity. Hence, a person sensitized to DGEBA resin may react to bis-GMA or vice versa, especially if that person has a strong hypersensitivity to DGEBA resin and/or bis-GMA (i.e., reacts to low concentrations of the allergen when it is patch tested in a serial dilution) [26].

One of our patients in Malmö, previously sensitized to DGEBA resin, had severe stomatitis adjacent to a newly made DCR restoration (containing bis-GMA) in the mouth as well as eczema

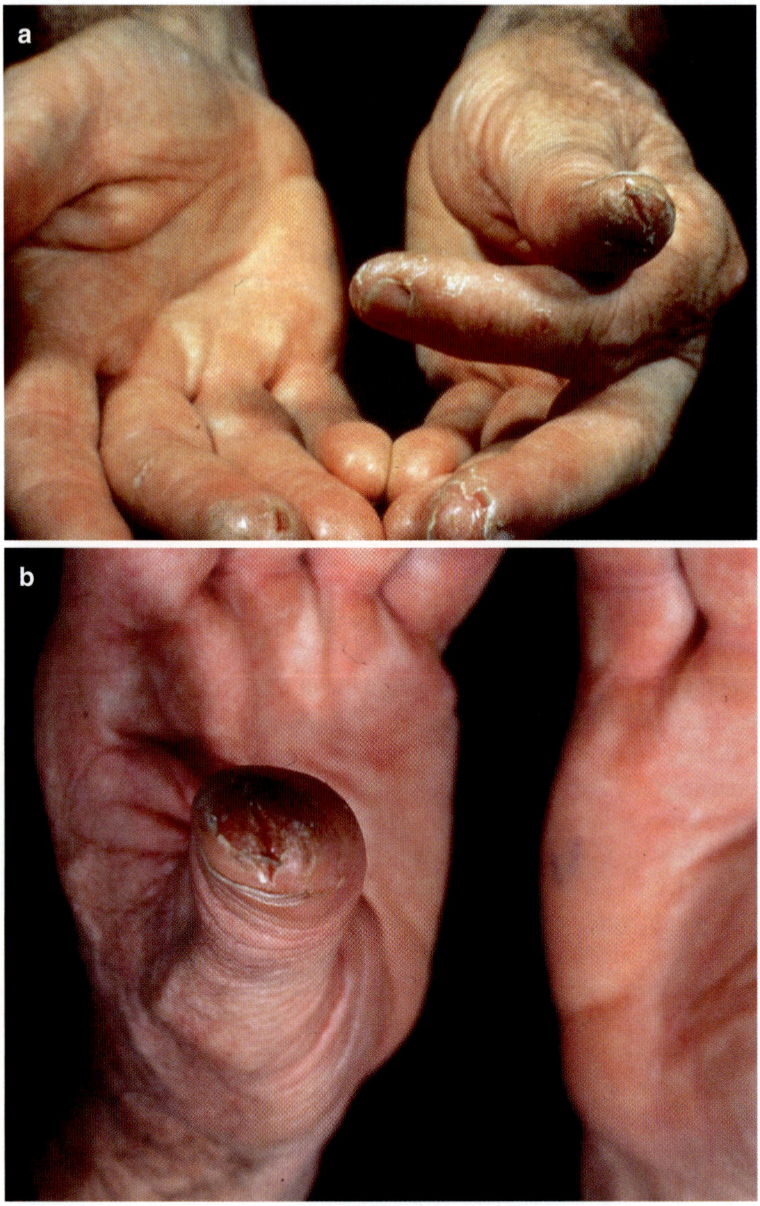

Fig. 17.2 (**a**) and (**b**) A dentist with allergic contact dermatitis (pulpitis) from 2-hydroxyethyl methacrylate (2-HEMA) in a bonding product

on the cheek just overlying the DCR filling. Some authors have discussed cross-reactivity between DGEBA resin and epoxy acrylates, but a lack of cross-reactivity between these two compounds has also been reported [27].

(Meth)acrylated urethanes are also used in DCR but to a lesser extent. The aliphatic urethane methacrylates such as UEDMA are the most common, but aromatic urethanes are also used. Contact allergy to methacrylated urethanes and bis-GMA is rare. Both have a high molecular weight and a relatively high viscosity. To dilute these monomers, other methacrylates or dimethacrylates of lower viscosity are added (e.g., MMA, TREGDMA, and EGDMA) [28].

In the 1980s in Finland, four dental nurses were sensitized to bis-GMA and epoxy diacrylate, resulting in occupational allergic contact dermatitis [29]. Since then, a few new cases from dental practice have been reported [30, 31].

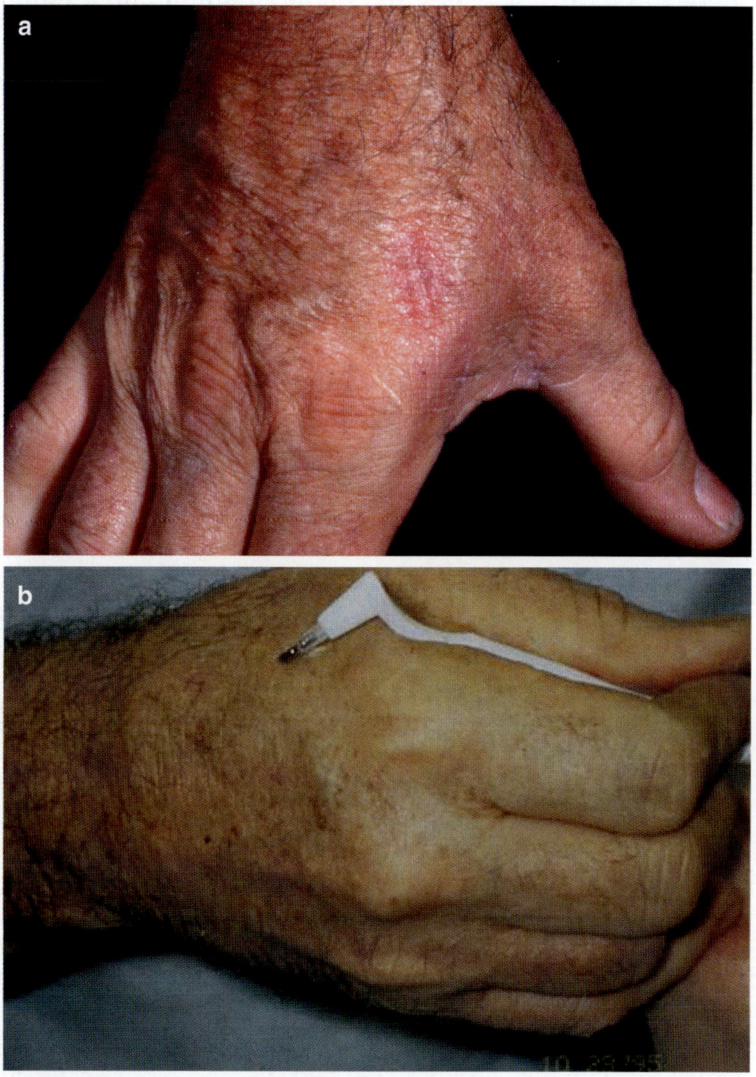

Fig. 17.3 (**a**) and (**b**) Allergic contact dermatitis on the dorsal hand of the same dentist as in Fig. 17.2 due to contamination of the unprotected skin by a brush previously dipped in uncured bonding resin

17.5.4 Additional Substances that may be Present in Dental Acrylics

17.5.4.1 Additives in Dental Acrylics: Activators, Initiators, Stabilizers, and Inhibitors

At room temperature, cold-cured or self-cured acrylics need an activator or accelerator for the polymerization reaction. The activator most used is the tertiary aromatic amine N,N-dimethyl-p-toluidine. There has been one report of a dentist with occupational allergic contact dermatitis from 4-tolyl diethanolamine [32], a rare sensitizer.

Benzoyl peroxide is an initiator and catalyst for acrylic and polyester resins. Few cases of contact allergy have been reported in the dental profession. Two cases of patients with allergic contact dermatitis in the manufacture of dental prostheses have been published [33], as well as a case of a dentist who was allergic to benzoyl peroxide and mercury [34]. False-positive reactions may be seen when patch testing with benzoyl peroxide, as it also is an irritant.

Another initiator is camphoroquinone, used in visible-light-cured dental acrylic composite materials and primers. So far, no dental contact allergy has been reported, but a case of patch test sensitization has been reported [35].

The inhibitors hydroquinone and methyl hydroquinone are used to prevent unintended spontaneous polymerization. *p*-Methoxyphenol and butylated cresols are also inhibitors. 2,6-di-(tert-Butyl)-4-methylphenol (BHT) is another inhibitor that is a rare sensitizer [36].

17.5.4.2 UV Absorbers

To improve color stability of a plastic and to prevent it from yellowish discoloration and darkening with age, UV stabilizers are added [28]. These may be benzophenones, such as 2,2-dihydroxy-4-methoxybenzophenone (UV9, Eusolex 4360), 2-hydroxy-4-methoxybenzophenone, and 2,4-dihydroxybenzophenone; or 2(2-hydroxy-5-methylphenyl)benzotriazole (Tinuvin P), phenyl salicylate, methyl salicylate, resorcinol monobenzoate, or stilbene [37]. 2,2-Dihydroxy-4-methoxybenzophenone (Eusolex 4360) may be present in DCR. Allergic contact dermatitis and photocontact dermatitis from sunscreens have been reported, but there have been no reports on occupational allergic contact dermatitis in dental personnel.

17.5.4.3 Plasticizers

Plasticizers are added to plastics to improve the flexibility and pliability. Dibutyl phthalate may be added to the solution in prosthetic and rebasing materials [17]. There are no reports of contact allergy in dental practice.

17.5.4.4 Bisphenol A and DGEBA Resin

Bisphenol A is used in the production of epoxy resins and polycarbonates but is also used as an additive in the manufacture of PVC plastics. It is a rare sensitizer in dental care. A dental assistant with hand eczema was allergic to bisphenol A, which was found in the DCR she handled by means of chemical analysis. She became free of symptoms after avoiding exposure to DCR [38].

17.5.5 Ethyl Cyanoacrylate Glue

Cyanoacrylates are widely used as instant contact adhesives for metal, glass, rubber, and plastics. Dental technicians use this type of glue regularly [39]. Cyanoacrylates polymerize almost instantaneously in air at room temperature and bond immediately and strongly to surface keratin. Due to this, many authors have considered allergic reactions virtually impossible. However, there have been a few cases published, although not from the dental field.

17.5.6 Ionomers and Compomers

An example of a resin-modified glass ionomer cement is triple-cured hybrid-glass ionomer, which was introduced in the 1990s. This ionomer contains the same sensitizing methacrylates as DCR and bonding agents. Conventional glass ionomer cements are mixed with acrylate monomers, which should be water soluble and hence would contain 2-HEMA and initiators. The mixture thus contains 2-HEMA and, often, modified polyacrylic acid linked to methacrylate units. They are polymerized by light, when 2-HEMA and the methacrylate units link together. This gives better strength and better esthetic properties. If mixed manually, there is a risk of occupational sensitization, which is why a no-touch technique should be applied.

A Finnish dental nurse suffered from pulpitis from the acrylic tri-cure glass ionomer that she worked with. The light-cured hybrid-glass ionomer system was composed of a powder, a primer, and a liquid. The latter two contained 2-HEMA, to which she reacted during patch testing. She also reacted to the hybrid-glass ionomer primer and liquid, tested at 1 % pet. [40]. Compomers are composite plastics where the acrylate monomer is modified with carboxylic acid groups and the filler is glass – much the same as in ionomers. Compomers are used as filling material and cement. When used, it should be preceded by a bonding plastic.

17.6 Epidemiology of Hand Eczema and Contact Allergy Among Dental Workers: Dentists, Nurses, and Technicians

The prevalence of skin problems is high compared to other groups of professionals. In the case of occupational contact dermatitis, dental professionals present with hand eczema [41]. The frequency of occupational contact dermatitis in dental personnel was considered to be about 40 % some 20 years ago [42], and according to the Finnish Register of Occupational Diseases (FROD), the occurrence of occupational diseases among dental personnel increased threefold in the 1990s due to the increased usage of acrylics [43, 44]. Figures from the FROD from the 1990s showed that more than two-thirds of reported contact dermatitis cases in dentists and dental nurses were allergic in origin, the most common sensitizers being methacrylates, disinfectants and antimicrobials, rubber chemicals, and mercury. Most of these diseases were hand dermatitis [43, 44]. Dental personnel are also exposed to other contact allergens, the most important being fragrances, formaldehyde, and metals.

The frequency of occupational contact allergy was estimated to be 1 % in dental occupations overall [45]. A 10-year retrospective study on patch test results from Swedish dental personnel and dental patients tested with dental series containing acrylics showed 2.3 % of dental patients and 5.8 % of dental personnel had reacted to methacrylates. The most common allergen for both groups was 2-HEMA, followed by EGDMA and triethylene glycol dimethacrylate (TREGDMA) [7].

Methacrylate and acrylate allergy (36 acrylic monomers) in dental personnel was summarized from 12 years of patch testing at the Finnish Institute of Occupational Health (FIOH). 2-HEMA was the most important allergen in dentists and dental nurses, whereas MMA and EGDMA dominated among dental technicians [46].

In one Swedish study, the 1-year prevalence of hand eczema was 14 % in 527 dental personnel. Of 72, 41 were patch tested and 4 were allergic to acrylics [47]. In a survey of 700 Swedish dentists, dental nurses, and dental technicians, a frequency of 8 % occupational skin allergy was reported, and 3 % overall had a dermatitis due to allergy to acrylics [31, 48]. Among 174 Swedish dental personnel referred for screening for occupational skin disease, hand eczema was diagnosed in 63 %. Of these, 67 % were classified as irritant contact dermatitis and 33 % as allergic. Twenty-two percent (24/109) tested to the dental series had positive reactions to methacrylates, the majority reacting to several preparations. Reactions to 2-HEMA, EGDMA, and MMA occurred most frequently. Two-thirds of those with acrylate allergy gave a history of having had hand eczema at some time. Almost two-thirds of the dental personnel with occupational hand eczema who were hypersensitive to an acrylic were also positive to one of the allergens in the baseline, mainly nickel [31].

A questionnaire study given to Danish dentists revealed a 1-year prevalence of skin reactions related to occupation of 21.4 %. The main causes reported were hand washing and soaps, latex gloves, and (di)methacrylate-containing materials, occurring at point prevalences of 7.1 %, 1.3 %, and 1.7 %, respectively. Specifically, dentists were seriously affected (4 % methacrylate allergy) [49], while dental technicians had lower figures (2 % methacrylate allergy) [49].

In a Swedish survey of dentists, the 1-year prevalence of self-reported hand eczema was 15 %. The hand eczema diagnosis was confirmed in 94 % of the dentists examined, yielding a minimum 1-year prevalence of 11.6 %. Five percent of the dentists with hand eczema during the previous 12 months had positive reactions to acrylics, and all these were to 2-HEMA, with six also reacting to EGDMA. The prevalence of contact allergy to acrylics was below 1 % in the population of responding dentists, and these cases did not have any serious medical, social, or occupational consequences [3].

Out of 923 Finnish female dental nurses, 799 answered a questionnaire. Of the 328 (almost one-third) who reported work-related dermatitis on their hands, forearms, or face, 245 participated in an interview. One hundred seven were chosen for further examination, and both patch tests and prick tests were performed in 86. The prevalence of occupational skin disease was 6.5 % in the surveyed dental nurse population. Allergic contact dermatitis was the most common diagnosis (3.6 %), with methacrylates (1.3 %) and rubber chemicals (1.3 %) being the most common causes [50].

In a questionnaire study in the early 1990s comprising 1,132 German dental technicians, 29 % reported skin lesions attributed to work and 36 % suspected plastic materials as the primary cause. Among the 55 dental technicians who were examined and patch tested, 64 % had allergic contact dermatitis and 24 % had irritant contact dermatitis. Seventy-four percent of the allergens were found in plastic materials. Contact allergy to MMA, 2-HEMA, and EGDMA was seen in 16 %, 33 %, and 27 %, respectively [1].

A retrospective cohort study among former dental technician students in Sweden showed the risk of hand eczema to be more than doubled compared to controls and that the job involved frequent and unprotected exposure to acrylates and wet work [51].

To summarize, dental personnel are exposed to a variety of contact allergens, the most important being acrylics, rubber additives, fragrances, formaldehyde, and metals.

17.7 Clinical Presentation of Irritant Contact Dermatitis of the Hands in Dental Personnel

Dental personnel are exposed to a variety of irritants such as contact with plastics and (meth) acrylates [1]. In dental technicians, physical irritation when polishing plastic materials was one of the major causes of irritant contact dermatitis in several surveys [1, 52]. In Denmark a study on dental technicians showed acrylates to be the major culprit; of 69 technicians with hand eczema, 64 used MMA and cyanoacrylate glues on a regular basis, often daily [37]. Therefore, working in dental practice poses a risk of contracting irritant contact dermatitis [1]. The dorsum of fingers, especially on the dominant hand, the finger webs, and the lateral aspects of fingers are the most common sites of irritant contact dermatitis in dental personnel. Eighty percent of the dermatitis was present on the dorsum of fingers and around 70 % on the lateral aspects of fingers in a study investigating dental technicians. Symptoms and signs range from pain and stinging to scaling, erythema, dry skin with fissures, vesicles, and hyperkeratosis.

17.8 Clinical Presentation of Allergic Contact Dermatitis of the Hands

17.8.1 In Dental Personnel

In occupational acrylic contact allergy, the fingertips were most often affected (93 % of cases) [1]. Pulpitis is a common clinical presentation, usually affecting the first three fingers. Also in over 80 % of cases, the lateral aspects of the fingers were affected, while the dorsal aspects of the fingers and the backs of the hands were affected in 68 % and 46 %, respectively [1]. Signs and symptoms range from very dry skin, scaling, fissures, rhagades, vesicles, bullae, hyperkeratosis, and erythema to itching, smarting, pain, stinging, burning, tingling, slight numbness of the fingertips, and reduced sensitivity. Mild paresthesia may persist for weeks or months after the dermatitis has subsided. Paresthesia may also develop without any contact allergy. Paresthesia is caused by a local effect of acrylics on the peripheral nerves without systemic neural effects [53]. Nail folds may become swollen and red [54].

17.8.2 In a Dental Patient

In Malmö, one of our patients suffered from a systemic contact dermatitis with vesicular hand eczema for many weeks after she had a DCR restoration made containing bis-GMA. She was occupationally sensitized to DGEBA resin several years before this occasion.

17.9 Contact Urticaria of the Hands in Dental Personnel

Immediate reactions may be allergic or nonallergic. Allergic reactions are IgE-mediated reactions, usually caused by proteins. However, certain low-molecular-weight chemicals may also elicit similar immediate hypersensitivity reactions caused by both allergic and unknown mechanisms. Contact urticaria due to acrylates is not usually seen, but edema of the hands [55] has been described as an atypical form of contact allergic reaction to acrylic dental prostheses.

17.10 Other Considerations

When diagnosing and managing patients with hand eczema from dental acrylates, it is essential to consider other causal and/or contributory factors in the pathogenesis of the patient's clinical presentation. Atopic predisposition, endogenous hand eczema, domestic factors, hobbies, supplementary jobs, and other causes of irritation would have to be taken into account. Other differential diagnoses to keep in mind include other hand dermatoses, such as psoriasis and id reactions.

As mentioned before, cases of fingertip paresthesia [53, 56] caused by acrylate/methacrylate contact allergy, have also been reported, and this may occur even without allergic contact dermatitis [57].

17.11 Indications for Patch Testing for Acrylate/Methacrylate Contact Allergy and Screening for Contact Allergy to Acrylics

In dental professionals, those with evident or suspected occupational contact dermatitis or worsening of an endogenous dermatitis in dental work should at least be patch tested with the baseline series and a dental series as well as the patient's own samples whenever possible to confirm contact allergies or to rule them out. In more complex cases, the diagnosis and conclusion after patch testing may have to be made in collaboration with the patient's dentist.

Furthermore, many centers have separate dental series for dental personnel and dental patients. MMA was previously a standard allergen for screening for (meth)acrylate allergy. However, it is a weak sensitizer and not a very good screening substance for such allergies. The newer (meth) acrylates are much more potent sensitizers than MMA.

It is the current common practice to test methacrylates at a concentration of 2 % pet. and acrylates at 0.1 % pet. These doses have been found to be less likely to cause active sensitization.

Another consideration is the material of the patch test chambers used. Aluminum oxide, which may be present in metal chambers, may cause rapid polymerization of the monomers. If the vehicle is petrolatum, a metal chamber (e.g., the Finn chamber) works fine, but if the acrylic is diluted in acetone or some other solvent, a plastic chamber should be used so as to not risk polymerization of the acrylic monomers, leading to a false-negative patch test reaction [58].

Because acrylate/methacrylate patch test preparations are not included in the baseline series of most centers, most dermatologists would have to rely on and remember to apply supplementary series containing these allergens in order to pick up patients with these contact allergies. Commercial series vary in the number of allergens available. In the most recent catalogues, Chemotechnique Diagnostics (Vellinge, Sweden) has various supplementary series containing up to 24 acrylate/methacrylate allergens, while Trolab Hermal (Hamburg, Germany) has 6 allergens.

Patch test centers around the world may have similar series, some of which may have in excess of 30 allergens. Shorter acrylate/methacrylate screening series for patients with exposure to dental and other applications have been used with some success in some centers [7, 59-62]. In

Malmö, we have seen that 2-HEMA would have picked up all our dental personnel looking at figures 10 years back [7]. A study in Malmö and Singapore has screened for contact allergy to acrylics in the baseline series during more than 2 years of testing. The tested acrylics were 2-HEMA, MMA, EGDMA, TREGDA, and 2-hydroxypropyl acrylate (2-HPA). The prevalence of acrylate allergy was 1.4 % in Malmö and 1.0 % in Singapore. The positive reactions in the baseline series in Malmö, in order of frequency, were 2-HEMA, TREGDA, 2-HPA, EGDMA, and MMA. In Singapore, the substances (in order of frequency) were TREGDA, EGDMA, and 2-HEMA [62]. When comparing these figures with older figures from Singapore, we saw that only two allergens were common in both centers (unpublished data) and that over time, the frequencies for the various allergens change [61]. However, such shortened series are center specific and there is no single short series that can be applied to all centers. These series would also vary with time as the pattern of acrylate/methacrylate use changes.

It is essential to perform two patch test readings (on days 3 or 4 and day 7), as late reactions may occur with many allergens seen in the dental setting. Acrylates/methacrylates [63], gold, [64], and mercury [65, 66] are some of the dental allergens that tend to show late positive readings. Concerning mercury, 30 % of contact allergy would have been missed without a reading on day 7 [66]. In one study [7], positive reactions to 2-HEMA would have been missed in 25 % of patients if the day 2 reading had been omitted. In many studies looking at contact allergy frequency, day 7 readings have not been performed consistently.

When available, testing to the patient's own samples is recommended. Dilution to a level of 0.1 % pet. for acrylates and 2.0 % for methacrylates is essential in order to prevent active sensitization, as acrylate allergens are strong sensitizers and should never be tested undiluted. Hence, information on the concentration of the allergen in the sample would be ideal; unfortunately, this is only rarely available in clinical practice. Therefore, if it is only known that a product contains acrylates but the percentage is unknown, one has to assume that it contains 100 % acrylate monomers and subsequently dilute the product to 0.1 % pet.

17.12 Patch Test Sensitization

Active sensitization is iatrogenic sensitization to a chemical induced by application of a patch test. Some acrylics have been incriminated in active sensitization. Ethyl acrylate, 2-hydroxypropyl acrylate, and 2-hydroxyethyl acrylate sensitized patients in Finland, resulting in their patch test concentrations being lowered, while some other substances even had to be removed from the test series [67]. Acrylics are strong allergens and should never be applied undiluted to the skin, because a single such exposure can induce sensitization [68]. Therefore, patch testing patients with undiluted acrylic products may be hazardous and requires knowledge on the sensitizing potential of the tested substance. A dental patient had been actively sensitized to acrylics by her dentist, who performed a "use test" on intact skin with undiluted glass ionomer containing sensitizing acrylics (e.g., 2-HEMA). According to some authors, dentists should be warned against performing use tests with dental acrylics [68].

Conclusion

Acrylates/methacrylates are still frequently reported as causes of occupational skin disease in the dental profession. Because of their desirable properties in these applications, no suitable substitutes are available to replace them entirely. Hence, we will likely continue to see occupational allergic contact dermatitis affecting the finger pulps, sides of fingers, palms, and dorsal hands in these professionals in the years to come. Direct skin contact while working with monomers or accidental skin contamination will easily lead to sensitization, more so for the acrylates than the methacrylates. Patch testing is still unwieldy, with most centers using large supplementary series to confirm or rule out contact allergy to these substances. Abbreviated series published so far are center specific, and we may not extrapolate these to be equally applicable to other patch test populations. Dilution of patch test preparations to a level of 0.1 % pet. for acrylates and 2.0 % for methacrylates is essential in order to prevent active sensitization. When testing to a product with unknown concentration of these substances, one has to assume that it contains 100 % acrylate monomers and subsequently dilute the product to 0.1 % pet.

References

1. Rustemeyer T, Frosch PJ. Occupational skin diseases in dental laboratory technicians. (I). Clinical picture and causative factors. Contact Dermatitis. 1996;34:125–33.
2. Kiec-Swierczynska MK. Occupational allergic contact dermatitis due to acrylates in Lodz. Contact Dermatitis. 1996;34:419–22.
3. Wallenhammar LM, Ortengren U, Andreasson H, Barregard L, Bjorkner B, Karlsson S, et al. Contact allergy and hand eczema in Swedish dentists. Contact Dermatitis. 2000;43:192–9.
4. Geukens S, Goossens A. Occupational contact allergy to (meth)acrylates. Contact Dermatitis. 2001;44:153–9.
5. Wrangsjo K, Swartling C, Meding B. Occupational dermatitis in dental personnel: contact dermatitis with special reference to (meth)acrylates in 174 patients. Contact Dermatitis. 2001;45:158–63.
6. Lindberg M, Silverdahl M. The use of protective gloves and the prevalence of hand eczema, skin complaints and allergy to natural rubber latex among dental personnel in the county of Uppsala, Sweden. Contact Dermatitis. 2000;43:4–8.
7. Goon AT, Isaksson M, Zimerson E, Goh CL, Bruze M. Contact allergy to acrylate/methacrylate in the dental series in southern Sweden: simultaneous positive patch test reaction patterns and possible screening allergens. Contact Dermatitis. 2006;55:219–26.
8. Aalto-Korte K, Alanko K, Kuuliala O, Jolanki R. Methacrylate and acrylate allergy in dental personnel. Contact Dermatitis. 2007;57:324–30.
9. Fink JK. Acrylic resins. In: Ebnesajjad S, editor. Reactive polymers fundamentals and applications: a concise guide to industrial polymers. Norwich: William Andrew Inc./Plastics Design Library; 2005. p. 349–72.
10. Schwartz JB. The acrylics. In: The acrylic plastics in dentistry. Brooklyn: Dental Items of Interest Publishing Company; 1950. p. 107–134.
11. Kanerva L, Estlander T, Jolanki R, Tarvainen K. Occupational allergic contact dermatitis caused by exposure to acrylates during work with dental prostheses. Contact Dermatitis. 1993;28:268–75.
12. Stevenson WJ. Methyl-methacrylate dermatitis. Contact Point. 1941;18:171.
13. Moody WL. Severe reaction from acrylic liquid. Dent Digest. 1941;47:305.
14. Stoy PJ. Denture sore mouth with particular reference to acrylics. J Irish Dent A. 1952;7:13.
15. Fisher AA. Allergic sensitization of skin and oral mucosa to acrylic denture materials. J Am Med Assoc. 1954;156:238–42.
16. Kanerva L, Estlander T, Jolanki R. Occupational skin allergy in the dental profession. Dermatol Clin. 1994;12:517–32.
17. Kanerva L, Estlander T, Jolanki R, Tarvainen K. Occupational allergic contact dermatitis caused by exposure to acrylates during work with dental prostheses. Contact Dermatitis. 1993;28:268–75.
18. Pfeiffer P, Rosenbauer E-U. Residual methyl methacrylate monomers, water sorption, and water solubility of hypoallergenic denture base materials. J Prosthet Dent. 2004;92:72–8.
19. Finnish Advisory Board of Chemicals. Acrylate compounds: uses and evaluation of health effects. Helsinki: Government Printing Centre; 1992.
20. Kanerva L, Estlander T, Jolanki R, Tarvainen K. Dermatitis from acrylates in dental personne. In: Menné T, Maibach HI, editors. Hand eczema. Boca Raton: CRC Press; 1994.
21. Van der Walle HB. Sensitizing potential of acrylic monomers in guinea pig. Thesis, Katholieke Universiteit te Nijmegen, Krips Repro Meppel. 1982. p. 1–112.
22. Kanerva L, Estlander T, Jolanki R, Pekkarinen E. Occupational pharyngitis associated with allergic patch test reactions from acrylics. Allergy. 1992;47:571–3.
23. Estlander T, Kanerva L, Kari O, Jolanki R, Mölsä K. Occupational conjunctivitis associated with type IV allergy to methacrylates. Allergy. 1996;51:56–9.
24. Sala E, Hytönen M, Tupasela O, Estlander T. Occupational laryngitis with immediate allergic or immediate type specific chemical hypersensitivity. Clin Otolaryngol Allied Sci. 1996;21:42–8.
25. Bowen RL. Dental filling material comprising vinyl silane treated fused silica and a binder consisting of the reaction product of bisphenol A and glycidyl acrylate. 1962. US Patent 3,066,112.
26. Isaksson M, Zimerson E, Svedman C. Occupational airborne allergic contact dermatitis from methacrylates in a dental nurse. Contact Dermatitis. 2007;57:371–5.
27. Nethercott JR. Allergic contact dermatitis due to an epoxy acrylate. Br J Dermatol. 1981;104:697–703.
28. Axéll T, Björkner B, Fregert S, Niklasson B. Standard patch test series for screening of contact allergy to dental materials. Contact Dermatitis. 1983;9:82.
29. Kanerva L, Estlander T, Jolanki R. Allergic contact dermatitis from dental composite resins due to aromatic epoxy acrylates and aliphatic acrylates. Contact Dermatitis. 1989;20:201–11.
30. Geukens S, Goossens A. Occupational contact allergy to (meth)acrylates. Contact Dermatitis. 2001;44:153–9.

31. Wrangsjö K, Swartling C, Meding B. Occupational dermatitis in dental personnel: contact dermatitis with special reference to (meth)acrylates in 174 patients. Contact Dermatitis. 2001;45:158–63.
32. Kanerva L, Jolanki R, Estlander T. Dentist's occupational allergic contact dermatitis caused by coconut diethanolamide, N-ethyl-4-toluene sulphonamide and 4-tolyldiethanolamine. Acta Derm Venereol (Stockh). 1993;73:126–9.
33. Calnan CD, Stevenson CJ. Studies in contact dermatitis XV. Dental materials. Trans St John's Hosp Dermatol Soc. 1963;49:9–26.
34. Kanerva L, Tarvainen K, Estlander T, Jolanki R. Occupational allergic contact dermatitis caused by mercury and benzoyl peroxide. Eur J Dermatol. 1994;4:359–61.
35. Malanin K. Active sensitization to camphoroquinone and double active sensitization to acrylics with long-lasting patch test reactions. Contact Dermatitis. 1993;29:284–5.
36. Estlander T, Rajaniemi R, Jolanki R. Hand dermatitis in dental technicians. Contact Dermatitis. 1984;10: 201–5.
37. Björkner B, Niklasson B. Contact allergy to the UV absorber Tinuvin P in a dental restorative material. Am J Contact Dermatitis. 1997;8:6–7.
38. Jolanki R, Kanerva L, Estlander T. Occupational allergic contact dermatitis caused by epoxy diacrylate in ultraviolet-light-cured paint, and bisphenol a in dental composite resin. Contact Dermatitis. 1995;33:94–9.
39. Mürer AJL, Poulsen OM, Roed-Petersen J. Tüchsen. Skin problems among Danish dental technicians. A cross-sectional study. Contact Dermatitis. 1995;33: 42–7.
40. Kanerva L, Estlander T, Jolanki R. Occupational allergic contact dermatitis caused by acrylic tri-cure glass ionomer. Contact Dermatitis. 1997;37:49–50.
41. Gawkrodger DJ. Investigation of reactions to dental materials. Br J Dermatol. 2005;153:479–85.
42. Rustemeyer T, Frosch PJ. Occupational contact dermatitis in dental personnel. In: Kanerva L, Elsner P, Wahlberg JE, Maibach HI, editors. Handbook of occupational dermatology. Berlin/Heidelberg: Springer; 2000.
43. Kanerva L, Lahtinen A, Toikkanen J, Forss H, Estlander T, Susitaival P, et al. Increase in occupational skin diseases of dental personnel. Contact Dermatitis. 1999;40:104–8.
44. Kanerva L, Alanko K, Estlander T, Jolanki R, Lahtinen A, Savela A. Statistics on occupational dermatitis from (meth)acrylates in dental personnel. Contact Dermatitis. 2000;42:175–6.
45. Uveges RE, Grimwood RE, Slawsky LD, Marks Jr JG. Epidemiology of hand dermatitis in dental personnel. Mil Med. 1995;160:335–8.
46. Aalto-Korte K, Alanko K, Kuuliala O, Jolanki R. Methacrylate and acrylate allergy in dental personnel. Contact Dermatitis. 2007;57:324–30.
47. Lindberg M, Silverdahl M. The use of protective gloves and the prevalence of hand eczema, skin complaints and allergy to natural rubber latex among dental personnel in the county of Uppsala, Sweden. Contact Dermatitis. 2000;43:4–8.
48. Ohlson C-G, Svensson L, Mossberg B, Hök M. Prevalence of contact dermatitis among dental personnel in a Swedish rural county. Swed Dent J. 2001;25:13–20.
49. Munksgaard EC, Hansen EK, Engen T, Holm U. Self reported occupational dermatological reactions among Danish dentists. Eur J Oral Sci. 1996;104: 396–402.
50. Alanko K, Susitaival P, Jolanki R, Kanerva L. Occupational skin diseases among dental nurses. Contact Dermatitis. 2004;50:77–82.
51. Meding B, Hosseiny S, Wrangsjö K, Andersson E, Hagberg S, Torén K, et al. Hand eczema, skin exposure and glove use in dental technicians. Contact Dermatitis. 2004;50:203.
52. Estlander T, Rajaniemi R, Jolanki R. Hand dermatitis in dental technicians. Contact Dermatitis. 1984;10: 201–5.
53. Kanerva L, Mikola H, Henriks-Eckerman ML, Jolanki R, Estlander T. Fingertip paresthesia and occupational allergic contact dermatitis caused by acrylics in a dental nurse. Contact Dermatitis. 1998;38:114–6.
54. Kanerva L, Henriks-Eckerman ML, Estlander T, Jolanki R. Dentist's occupational allergic paronychia and contact dermatitis caused by acrylics. Eur J Dermatol. 1997;7:177–80.
55. Bauer A, Wollina U. Denture-induced local and systemic reactions to acrylate. Allergy. 1998;53: 722–3.
56. Fisher AA, Baran RL. Adverse reaction to acrylate sculptured nails with particular reference to prolonged paresthesia. Am J Contact Dermatitis. 1991;2: 38–42.
57. Baran RL, Schibli H. Permanent paresthesia to sculptured nails: a distressing problem. Dermatol Clin. 1990;8:139–41.
58. Bruze M, Björkner B, Lepoittevin JP. Occupational allergic contact dermatitis from ethyl cyanoacrylate. Contact Dermatitis. 1995;32:156–9.
59. Constandt L, Hecke EV, Naeyaert J-M, Gossens A. Screening for contact allergy to artificial nails. Contact Dermatitis. 2005;52:73–7.
60. Koppula SV, Fellman JH, Storrs FJ. Screening allergens for acrylate dermatitis associated with artificial nails. Am J Contact Dermatitis. 1995;6:18–85.
61. Goon AT, Bruze M, Zimerson E, Goh CL, Isaksson M. Contact allergy to acrylates/methacrylates in the acrylate and nail acrylics series in southern Sweden: simultaneous positive patch test reaction patterns and possible screening allergens. Contact Dermatitis. 2007;57:21–7.
62. Goon AT, Bruze M, Zimerson E, Goh CL, Soo-Quee Koh D, Isaksson M. Screening for acrylate/methacrylate allergy in the baseline series: our experience in

Sweden and Singapore. Contact Dermatitis. 2008;59:307–13.
63. Isaksson M, Lindberg M, Sundberg K, Hallander A, Bruze M. The development and course of patch-test reactions to 2-hydroxyethyl methacrylate and ethyleneglycol dimethacrylate. Contact Dermatitis. 2005;53:292–7.
64. Bruze M, Hedman H, Björkner B, Möller H. The development and course of test reactions to gold sodium thiosulfate. Contact Dermatitis. 1995;33: 386–91.
65. Gawkrodger DJ. Investigation of reactions to dental materials. Br J Dermatol. 2005;153:479–85.
66. Jalili S, Bruze M, Isaksson M. Contact allergy to mercury in amalgam. Malmö: Elective study Faculty of Medicine, Lund University; 2008.
67. Kanerva L, Estlander T, Jolanki R. Sensitization to patch test acrylates. Contact Dermatitis. 1988;18: 10–5.
68. Kanerva L, Lauerma AI. Iatrogenic acrylate allergy complicating amalgam allergy. Contact Dermatitis. 1988;38:58–9.

Hand Eczema in the Hospital and Medical Industry

18

Ana M. Giménez-Arnau

Contents

A.M. Giménez-Arnau, M.D., Ph.D.
Department of Dermatology, Hospital del Mar, Universitat Autònoma i Pompeu Fabra, Barcelona, Passeig Maritim 25-29, Barcelona 08003, Spain
e-mail: 22505aga@comb.cat

18.1 Introduction

Health-care personnel are quite susceptible to contact dermatitis. An average annual incidence of occupational skin diseases of 7.3 per 10,000 workers has been described [1]. Contact dermatitis of the hands is by far the most frequent condition suffered by people involved directly in health-care tasks. The situation described by Stingeni et al. in 1995 constantly recurs in most countries of the world [2]. Contact dermatitis of the hands and forearms was reported at that time in 21.2 % of 1,301 hospital employees; it occurs significantly more frequently in women, subjects less than 31 years of age, workers in internist or surgical departments, cleaners, and nurses. Irritant contact dermatitis was originally present in the majority of those cases (94.9 %), induced mainly by disinfectants and gloves. Atopy was already suggested as a relevant factor to favor hand dermatitis. Consequently, the need to develop and implement effective primary and secondary preventive measures has become a challenge for occupational dermatology.

This chapter will review hand eczema as a condition suffered by health-care workers. Usually hand eczema is due to exogenous inducers that cause dermatitis, but endogenous factors can also be involved. Epidemiologic, clinical appearance, diagnostic, etiologic, and preventive knowledge regarding hand eczema in health-care personnel is updated.

A. Alikhan et al. (eds.), *Textbook of Hand Eczema*,
DOI 10.1007/978-3-642-39546-8_18, © Springer-Verlag Berlin Heidelberg 2014

18.2 Epidemiology

The 1-year prevalence of hand eczema reported in the general population was 9.7 % and 11.8 % in Sweden [3, 4], with a point prevalence of 5.4 % [4]. Health-care workers show a far higher point prevalence of hand eczema (17–30 %) [5, 6]. A population-based register study of occupational skin diseases developed in Northern Bavaria showed an annual hand eczema incidence rate of 7.3 cases per 10,000 health-care workers [7]. Hand eczema was screened using a self-administered questionnaire based on the Nordic Occupational Skin Questionnaire (NOSQ-2002) in an unselected hospital population [8]. From a total of 1,909 employees, 23 % reported hand eczema within the past 12 months. Assistant nurses (32 %), nurses (30 %), and nursing aides (27 %) showed the highest frequencies, which occurred mainly in medical and surgical departments [8].

Nurses are the category of health workers that suffer the highest prevalence of hand eczema. This is supported by different studies. An incidence of 6.5 cases/1,000 person-month in nurses compared with 1 case/1,000 person-month in office employees was estimated in a retrospective study [9]. As hand eczema is a worldwide condition, its prevalence in nurses was checked in different countries. The prevalence reported were as follows: United States (25.9–55.6 %) [10–12], the Netherlands (between 29.4 % and 32.0 %) [6], Japan (35–53.3 %) [13, 14], Italy (21.2 %) [2], Poland (46 %) [15], China (17.7 %) [16], Hong Kong (22.1 %) [17], Taiwan (22 %) [18], Australia (43.2–59.3 %) [19], and Turkey (47.5 %) [20]. Hand eczema tends to be more frequent in nurses involved in intensive care units (65 %) [12] or surgical units (48 %) [13]. Hand eczema in nurses is an occupational-related dermatitis. Any type of eczema (atopic, contact, or dyshidrotic) can be developed alone or in combination with others, but irritant and allergic contact dermatitis are the most frequent [21].

18.3 Risk Factors

Atopy, dry skin, wet work, contact irritants, stress, or certain genetic markers were studied as potential risk factors to develop hand eczema.

A history of allergic diseases and especially of atopic eczema is the main risk factor for hand eczema [13]. The increased risk varied from 3.76- to 5.3-fold [16, 22] compared with nonatopic subjects. TNF-α (alpha) polymorphism at −308 (AA/GA than GG) coupled with the atopic history favors the severity of irritation and impairs the recovery from exposure response to treatment in chronic irritant hand dermatitis and normal skin [23]. Dry skin is defined as rough skin with fine desquamation. It can be conditioned by endogenous (filaggrin mutations, cutaneous lipid impairment, or atopy), exogenous (wet work or irritant contact) factors, or both. Wet-work activities as repeated washing of hands with soap can induce irritant contact dermatitis [24].

The development of a standardized consensus-based methodology for the assessment of wet-work-induced hand dermatitis is still a global challenge. The exposure to toxic and irritant skin agents with the inappropriate use of occlusive gloves is very common. According to Jungbauer et al. [25] nursing home, followed by regular, intensive care, and dialysis nurses, showed a decreased frequency of wet-work activities assessed by direct observation. Wet work in intensive care units accounted for 24 % of the overall morning shift duration. This was 16 % in dialysis wards and 9 % in regular wards. The mean duration of occlusion by gloves was not very long – 3.1 min on regular wards and 6.7 min in intensive care units. These observations demonstrate how the characteristics of the wet work are not the same in different hospital departments; therefore, a reduction in wet-work exposure, decreased frequency of hand washing, and use of gloves for patient washing were measures recommended by the authors [25]. Recently, a wet-work sampler with the objective of assessing the duration and frequency of wet work was developed at the University of Aberdeen with poor success because there was not a good correlation between the sampler results and the observer assessment [26]. The instrument measures the difference of temperature generated by evaporative cooling between two sensors: one sensor on the skin and a second one placed 2 mm above the skin. The optimal temperature difference to discern wet and dry skin differed considerably between individual nurses, with a median sensitivity of 78 % and 62 % and a median specificity of 79 % and 68 % for indicating wet skin and glove use, respectively [26].

Health-care workers are usually exposed to activities that lead to an impaired barrier function. These activities include continuous exposure to moisture, contact with irritants (water by itself and/or aggressive surface disinfectants), and occlusive gloves. Clinical irritation becomes apparent, often in the interdigital spaces. Aggravating factors also include certain climatic conditions. When mild irritation is present and the regenerating mechanism of the skin fails because of continuous irritant exposure or endogenous factors such as atopic diathesis, the epidermal barrier gets more and more disrupted, and hand eczema becomes chronic and severe [27].

Hand eczema can be classified based on its etiology and morphology as allergic, irritant, atopic, vesicular, or hyperkeratotic. Sometimes its trigger factor is unknown. The identification of new contributing factors responsible of chronic eczema continues to be a subject of research. One thousand seven hundred forty-four hospital workers were asked to answer a questionnaire in order to assess whether occupational stress factors and psychological problems through occupational stress factors were associated with skin disorders. High job demands, low social support, high strain, and high iso-strain were all associated with a higher prevalence of reported hand dermatitis. Although depression and anxiety were also associated with a higher risk of hand dermatitis, they do not appear to be the mechanisms behind this association [28].

The involvement of these risk factors in the development of hand eczema in health-care workers, especially in nurses, has been confirmed in many studies all over the world [13–20].

18.4 Clinical Types and Diagnosis

Eczema and dermatitis are used many times as synonyms. Clinically, eczema is a polymorphic eruption that can present as macules/patches, papules/plaques, and vesicles. Among the secondary findings are oozing, crusting, scaling, lichenification, and fissuring. Pruritus is common in all types of eczema/dermatitis. Pathological changes in the epidermis include intercellular edema, spongiosis, acanthosis, and parakeratosis. In the upper dermis a perivascular infiltrate of lymphocytes tends to migrate into the epidermis. Although irritant and allergic contact hand dermatitis are different in etiology and clinical expression, sometimes the signs and symptoms do not allow one to distinguish between the two. It is not rare for patients to suffer both irritant and allergic contact eczema at the same time. The initial episode of irritant contact dermatitis can precipitate an allergic contact dermatitis from agents previously tolerated.

Irritant contact dermatitis is caused by chemicals, with or without contributing physical factors such as friction or mechanical abrasion. The skin lesions are present only at sites where there has been contact with irritants. Patients with irritant contact dermatitis may complain of burning, mild itching, or pain. Mild cases are typically characterized as red and scaly patches in the interdigital webs and on the knuckles of the dorsal hand. Moderate to severe cases show more affected areas, and the entire hand can be affected. As severity increases, the lesions are increasingly dry, hyperkeratotic, scaly, fissured, and erythematous (Fig. 18.1). In contrast to irritant contact dermatitis, the allergic type tends to spread beyond the contact area and presents as an extremely itchy, erythematous reaction with

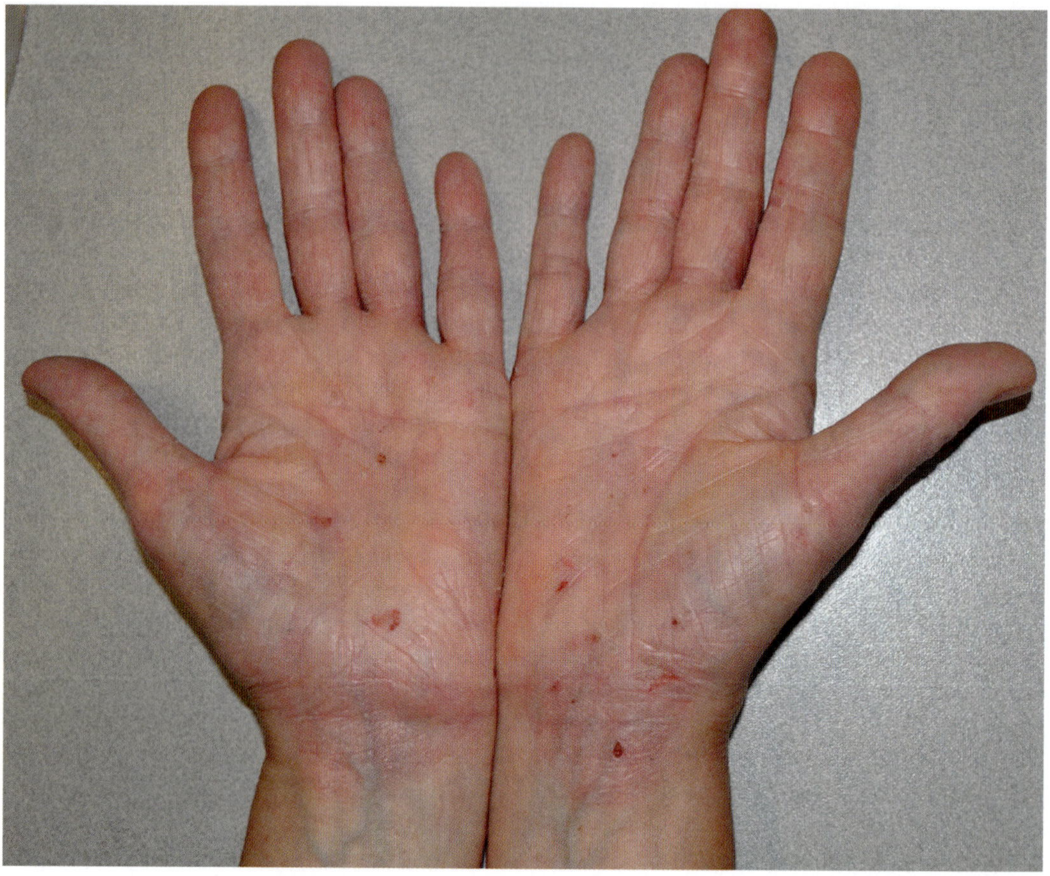

Fig. 18.1 Occupational chronic hand contact eczema affecting palms of the hands. Dry skin and fissured, itchy lesions with a negative patch test suggest an irritant origin

vesicles and sometimes confluent bullae. Patients often complain of severe itching with lesions that appear on every part of the hand that have even indirect contact with the eliciting allergen. The allergic reaction may spread to adjacent parts of the skin or even generalize to the wrist or arms (Fig. 18.2). Clinically, irritant contact dermatitis and allergic contact dermatitis can sometimes be differentiated by history and location, although usually complementary diagnostic tools are required.

Diagnosis involves a complete medical history which should include occupation, possible repeated exposures at work and home (including estimated frequency of hand washing and cleansing agent used), time course of the disease, individual work habits, skin care habits, use of protective gloves, and previous diagnoses and treatments (including self-treatment). Irritant contact dermatitis is diagnosed mainly by supporting history and clinical findings. No specific diagnostic test is available. A patch test with sodium lauryl sulfate has been postulated as a useful method to assess individual skin susceptibility to irritancy, although irritant contact dermatitis pathogenesis is based on the combination of individual predisposition with external irritation. Diagnostic patch testing is recommended for all patients with hand eczema of more than 3 months and/or relapse, to identify the role of contact allergens in the environment [29]. Patch testing is the only test that can confirm the diagnosis of allergic contact eczema, and it can also identify the causative contact allergen [30]. Several diseases, such as atopic hand dermatitis, *tinea manuum*, aquagenic syringeal acrokeratoderma (Fig. 18.3), and hand psoriasis may occasionally mimic contact dermatitis of the hands. Some diagnostic procedures may be needed. These include diagnostic

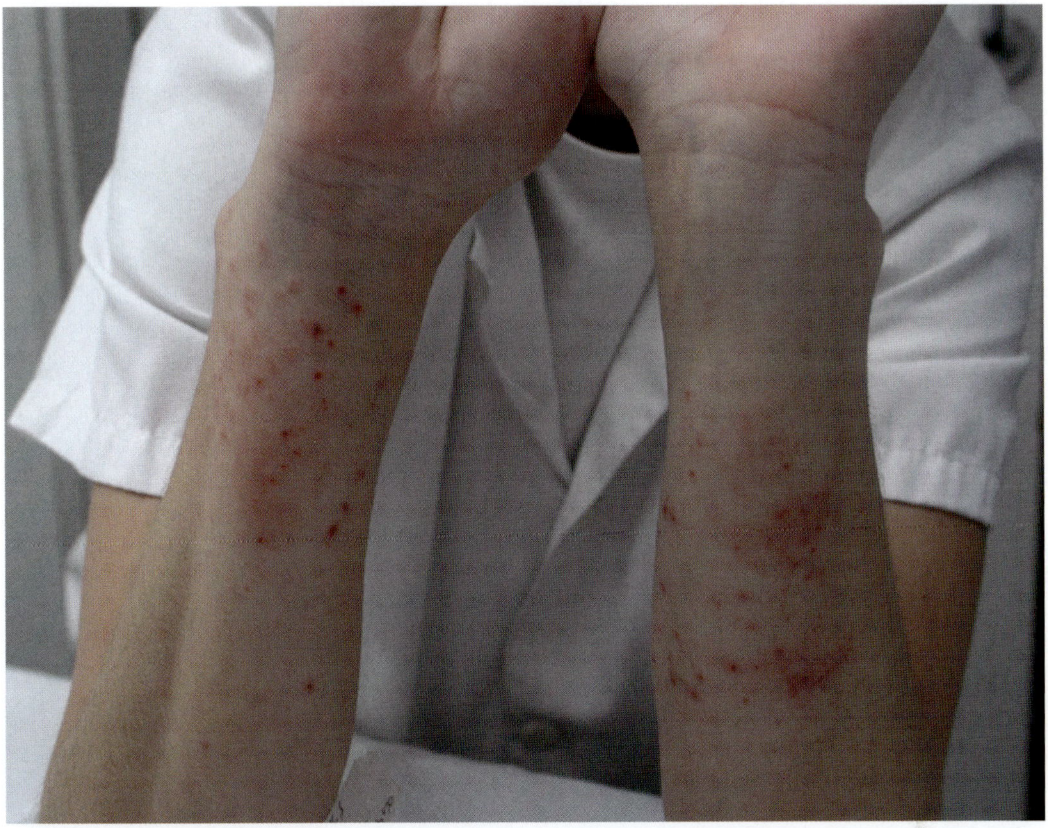

Fig. 18.2 Occupational contact allergic eczema to glutaraldehyde suffered by a nurse working at the gastroenterology sterilization department. Itchy erythema with papules and vesicles involving the wrists and forearms

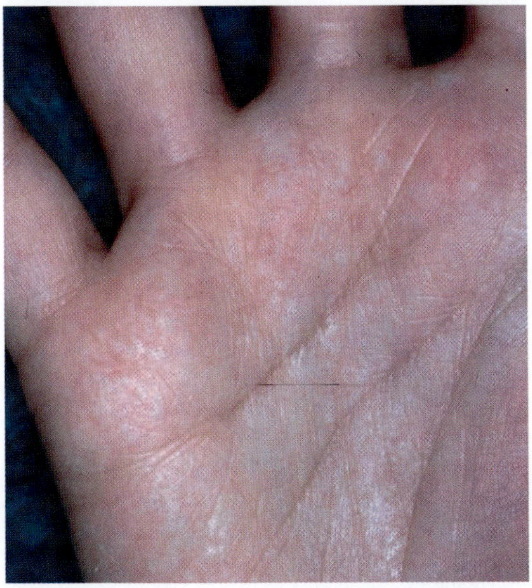

Fig. 18.3 Aquagenic syringeal acrokeratoderma. Painful transient, small, confluent papules with dilated puncta appearing on the palms after exposure to water (corresponding to dilated eccrine ostia)

patch tests, skin prick tests, microbial tests, and skin biopsies.

Allergic hand eczema can be induced by low molecular weight chemicals but also by proteins. Exposure to natural rubber latex can be responsible for immediate hypersensitivity reactions (contact urticaria and protein contact dermatitis) in health-care workers. Published latex sensitization prevalence rates range from 2.9 % to 22 % among health-care workers [31]. In a study of 532 workers, sensitization was more frequent ($p<0.05$) among atopic (81.3 %) than nonatopic (59.5 %) workers [31]. Work-related hand eczema was more common in the latex glove users (23.4 %) than in nonusers (4.9 %), as was hand urticaria (9.9 % and 2.1 %, respectively) [31]. Latex sensitization can be assessed by measuring specific immunoglobulin E and by prick testing.

In order to standardize occupational hand eczema, a “7-step consultation plan” was proposed by Soost et al. [32]. The protocol involved physicians, occupational therapists, and occupational consultants considering dermatological, educational, and occupational aspects. Hand contact eczema in health-care workers must be managed via multidisciplinary health resources.

18.5 Etiology

The most frequent cause of hand dermatitis in the general population seems to be irritant contact dermatitis, followed by atopic dermatitis and allergic contact dermatitis. The most common type of contact dermatitis in health workers is irritant contact dermatitis. The frequent use of disinfectant solutions, detergents, and soaps for hand washing can induce stratum corneum lipid disturbances and, consequently, a skin barrier defect [33]. Transepidermal water loss (TEWL) is increased by brush washing compared to simple hand washing [34]. Cumulative irritant contact dermatitis readily favors sensitization to a broad number of commonly employed substances. A variety of different contact allergens is responsible for hand eczema (Table 18.1) [35–38].

Table 18.1 Etiology of hand eczema in health-care workers: list of substances involved in the development of contact hand eczema [35–39]

Nurses, clinical assistants, and cleaners
Ampholytics, surfactants, and soaps
9-lauryl-3,6,9-triazanonanoic acid
7-dilauryl-1,4,7-triazaheptane
Bis (aminopropyl)-laurylamine
Chloramine-T (sodium *p*-toluenesulphonchloramine)
Dimethyl didecyl ammonium chloride
Dinitrochlorobenzene, nitrogen mustards
Didecyldimethylammonium chloride qualenium 12
Dodecyldiaminoethylglycine hydrochloride
Methyldibromo glutaronitrile
N,N-bis (3-aminopropyl) dodecylamine
Squaric acid diethylester
Undecylenamide diethanolamide
Diisocyanates
Drugs
Antibiotics
Cephalosporins
Meropenem
Penicillins
Streptomycin
Boldo (diuretic herbal medicine)
Cascara (anthraquinone stimulant laxative)
Chlorpromazine
Cyanamide
Diacetylmorphine
Dipyridamole
Ethylenediamine
Meclofenoxate
Meglumine diatrizoate
Mesna
Methylprednisolone
Neoplastic drugs
Ammonium hexachloroplatinate
Ammonium tetrachloroplatinate
Cisplatin
Methotrexate
Mitomycin
Nitrogen mustards
Nitrosoureas
Papain
Propacetamol
Ranitidine
Tylosin
Vitamin B_6
Gloves
Natural rubber latex
PVC gloves, benzoisothiazolinone
Thiuram
Mercaptobenzothiazole
Glutaraldehyde
Thiomersal
Surgeons
Antiseptic Components
Benzalkonium chloride
Benzydamine hydrochloride
Chlorhexidine
Dibromosalicylanilide
Dichlorophene G 4
Dowicides
Fentichlor
Hexachlorophene G 11
Imidazolidinyl urea (preservative)
p-cresol
Sodium hypochlorite
Sodium hyposulfite
Colophony
Gloves
Thiuram
Mercaptobenzothiazole
Polymethyl methacrylate

Table 18.1 (continued)

Laboratory personnel
2-Aminophenyl disulfide
3-4-Dicarbethoxyhexane-2,5-dione
Alcohols: amyl, butyl, ethyl, methyl, and isopropyl
Bisphenolic epoxy resins
Dicyclohexyl carbodiimide
Diisopropyl carbodiimide
Dimethylaminopropylethyl carbodiimide
Drugs
Azathioprine
Cephalosporins
Codeine
Cytosine arabinoside
N-acetyl-cysteine
Simvastatin
Vitamin A
Vitamin K_3
Ethyl-2-bromo-*p*-methoxyphenylacetate
Ethyl chloro oximido acetate
Isothiazolinone
Limonene (dipentene – hydroperoxides in autoxidized *d*-limonene)
Propylene oxide
Pyridine in Karl Fischer reagent
Sodium bisulfite
Other therapies
Benzydamine hydrochloride, in topical nonsteroidal anti-inflammatory agent
Lavender fragrance, in topical nonsteroidal anti-inflammatory agents
Isothiazolinone, in radiographic developing solutions
Metaproterenol unit
Benzoyl peroxide in a hardener substance (orthopedic technician)

18.6 Prevention

Primary and secondary preventive measures to avoid hand eczema, both irritant and allergic, are strongly recommended [29]. Skin care programs have shown a significant positive effect in the prevention of hand eczema in workers involved in health-care tasks [39–45]. Effective hand care includes the proper use of gloves, good hand hygiene measures, and correct use of emollients and moisturizers.

The management of hand hygiene in health-care settings is reviewed in extensive guidelines

Table 18.2 Preparations used for hand hygiene

Plain (non-antimicrobial) soap
Alcohols
Chlorhexidine
Chloroxylenol
Hexachlorophene
Iodine and iodophors
Quaternary ammonium compounds
Triclosan
Hypochlorite
Silver-containing polymers to ethanol carrier

[46, 47]. Some of the more common principles of hand hygiene are listed in Table 18.2. Hand decontamination is crucial to control nosocomial infections. The products used for hand decontamination should have good antimicrobial effectiveness and be accepted by hospital staff. Low-irritation disinfectants were developed and their antimicrobial properties were demonstrated. Alcohol-based hand solutions were studied thoroughly and are recommended as replacements for traditional soaps for hand washing in the health-care system [48]. Alcohol-based hand solutions have faster antimicrobial activity, a broad spectrum of antimicrobial activity, and better skin tolerance, all factors that support their inclusion in hand hygiene protocols. In Europe these products are classified as drugs and therefore subject to drug laws [49]. Alcohol-based hand solutions induce less epidermal barrier disruption than lauryl sulfate [50]. Skin patch test with 1-propanol, 2-propanol, and ethanol (all 60–90 % w/w) showed normal TEWL but did have a slight decrease of corneometry values, indicating loss of skin hydration [51]. Although these solutions are better tolerated than standard detergents, the addition of an emollient improves their acceptance. Sometimes nurses complain about burning sensation when using alcohol-based solutions and wrongly attribute the symptom to an allergic reaction [52]. A study of 2,750 health-care workers assessing the safety of an alcohol-based solution (70 % isopropyl alcohol) reported that only 0.47 % developed irritant contact dermatitis [53]. Additionally, a 60 % n-propanol solution was demonstrated safe in a patch test study performed on healthy and

Table 18.3 Recommendations for hand washing and use of alcohol-based solutions

1. The product should only be applied to dry and clean skin
2. The product should be rubbed until the skin is dry (approximately 30 s)
3. Hands should not be washed immediately after the hand disinfection
4. Between applications of hand rubs, hands should be washed only when they are visibly soiled
5. A mild nonalkaline soap should be used
6. Water for a hand wash should be cold
7. The duration of the hand wash should remove visible contamination and be as short as possible
8. Residual soap should be rinsed off completely
9. Brushes should not be used
10. Skin care lotions and creams should be used between hand hygiene procedures
11. Hands should be dry before gloves are put on

pre-irritated skin [27]. Table 18.3 presents a summary of how to use alcohol-based solutions [27]. An interventional study implementing hand hygiene measures in 521 trainees from 14 nursing schools in Central Germany helped the health workers led to an increase in use of alcohol-based solutions and a reduction of hand washing. These measures helped to improve skin conditions [54].

As in other occupations in which wet work is an important trigger factor for hand eczema, the correct use of adequate protective gloves is required. The correct use of gloves is not the objective of this chapter; it is reviewed in depth in other chapters of this book. Commonly, protective measures against hand eczema are applied simultaneously. A study conducted with healthy volunteers showed less skin irritation by glove occlusion when the time of using gloves was reduced, the use of soaps was decreased, and the use of alcohol-based lotions increased [55].

In order to obtain alternative measures to improve hand skin care, new useful tools were described. A water-based hand disinfectant (Desisoft, Oy Soft Protector, Finland) based on polyhexamethylene guanidine demonstrated a statistically significant decrease in colonization of the fingertips before and after disinfection ($p<0.001$) [56]. Users of the water-based hand disinfectant reported dry skin more often than did control subjects, but visual inspection and the results of the moisture measurement showed no difference between both groups [56]. Aloe vera-coated gloves prevented also skin irritation and improved the compliance with hand hygiene requirements in a pilot study [57].

18.7 Treatment

The treatment of hand eczema in health-care workers does not differ from that of eczema in other at-risk professions. According to the guidelines from the European Society of Contact Dermatitis, acute hand eczema should be treated promptly, the causative exogenous factors should be identified, and the use of moisturizers /emollients shows a grade of recommendation A with a level of evidence 2 [29].

Although different moisturizers and emollients are available, there is not enough evidence to recommend one or the other. Few prospective and comparative studies were conducted assessing the efficacy of emollients and/or barrier creams. A barrier skin cream including glycerin, isopropyl myristate, triethanolamine, stearic acid, dimethicone, 2-bromonitropropane, 1.3 diol acrylates C-10/C-, and alcyl acrylate cream (Hand Sense, North American Safety Products Inc, Orange, CA, USA) was compared to a fragrance-free, oil-containing hand lotion (control group) (Lubriderm, Warner Lambert Consumer Health Care, Morris Plains, NJ, USA) in health-care workers with severe hand irritation [58]. Subjects in both groups experienced a significant improvement in scaling, cracking, and pain. Subjects using the oil-containing lotion showed greater improvement than the experimental group [58]. Sixty-nine percent of subjects who used the control lotion showed complete resolution of full-thickness integumentary breaks and pain, compared to 52 % of subjects who used the barrier cream ($p=0.26$) [58].

Irritant hand dermatitis (subclinical or incipient) can be managed by minimizing wet work and hydrating with high lipid content products and alcohol-based solutions [59, 60]. Acute and chronic hand eczema (irritant or allergic) may require topical (corticosteroids or topical calcineurin inhibitors), physical (phototherapy), or systemic (alitretinoin, systemic corticosteroids, cyclosporine, azathioprine, methotrexate, or acitretin) treatment. Potent topical corticosteroids are the first choice for treatment, and the use of other drugs does not differ from hand eczema developed in the general population or in other occupations [29].

18.8 Further Research and Conclusions

Contact dermatitis of the hands is likely the most frequent condition suffered by health-care workers. Among health workers, nurses suffer the highest prevalence of hand eczema. Occupational hand eczema is a worldwide condition. Atopy, wet work, and a previous history of hand eczema are risk factors for hand eczema. Irritant contact dermatitis of the hands and allergic contact dermatitis of the hands can be suffered simultaneously, although an initial episode of irritant contact dermatitis can precipitate an allergic contact dermatitis to agents previously tolerated. Patch testing is the only way to confirm the diagnosis of allergic contact eczema. Educational activities related to skin care have demonstrated a significant effect in preventing hand eczema in health-care workers. These training courses include hand hygiene, glove use, and recommendations on emollient/moisturizer use. Acute hand eczema should be treated promptly, the causative exogenous factors should be identified, and the use of moisturizers/emollients is recommended. Potent topical corticosteroids are the first choice for treatment.

Studies are ongoing to investigate the effects of hand eczema classification and individual counseling on health-care workers with hand eczema [61] and to assess the effectiveness of implementing prevention strategies against hand eczema in health-care workers [62]. It would be useful to develop prospective studies to assess the long-term effectiveness of multifactorial skin care educational training, to compare periodic questionnaires with questionnaires plus cutaneous examination-based health surveillance programs, or to assess the prevalence of infection in health-care workers with or without dermatitis [63]. Hand eczema is a worldwide problem, which requires a global approach.

References

1. Mahler V, Bruckner T, Schmidt A, Diepgen TL. Occupational contact dermatitis in health care workers. (ESCD Meeting. Copenhagen). Contact Dermatitis. 2004;50:158–9.
2. Stingeni L, Lapomarda V, Lisi P. Occupational hand dermatitis in hospital environment. Contact Dermatitis. 1995;33:172–6.
3. Meding B, Jarvholm B. Hand eczema in Swedish adults-changes in prevalence between 1983 and 1996. J Invest Dermatol. 2002;118:719–23.
4. Meding B, Swanbeck G. Epidemiology of different types of hand eczema in an industrial city. Acta Derm Venereol. 1990;153(Suppl):1–43.
5. Kavli G, Angell E, Moseng D. Hospital employees and skin problems. Contact Dermatitis. 1987;17:156–8.
6. Smit HA, Burdorf A, Coenraads PJ. Prevalence of hand dermatitis in different occupations. Int J Epidemiol. 1993;22:288–93.
7. Dickel H, Huss O, Schmidt A, Kretz J, Diepgen T. Importance of irritant contact dermatitis in occupational skin disease. Am J Clin Dermatol. 2002;3:283–9.
8. Flyholm M-A, Bach B, Rose M, Jepsen KF. Self-reported hand eczema in a hospital population. Contact Dermatitis. 2007;57:110–5.
9. Smit HA, Coenraads PJ. A retrospective cohort study on the incidence of hand dermatitis in nurses. Int Arch Occup Environ Health. 1993;64:541–4.
10. Larson E, Friedman C, Cohran J, Treston-Aurand J, Green S. Prevalence and correlates of skin damage on the hands of nurses. Heart Lung. 1997;26:404–12.
11. Forrester BG, Roth VS. Hand dermatitis in intensive care units. J Occup Environ Med. 1998;40:881–5.
12. Lampel HP, Patel N, Boyse K, O'Brien SH, Zirwas MJ. Prevalence of Hand Dermatitis in patients nurses at a United States Hospital. Dermatitis. 2007;18:140–2.
13. Smith DR, Ohmura K, Yamagata Z. Prevalence and correlates of hand dermatitis among nurses in a Japanese teaching hospital. J Epidemiol. 2003;13:157–61.
14. Smith DR, Adachi Y, Mihashi M, Kawano S, Ishitake T. Hand dermatitis risk factors among clinical nurses in Japan. Clin Nurs Res. 2006;15:197–208.
15. Szepietwski J, Salomon J. Hand dermatitis: a problem commonly affecting nurses. SaRloocmznoink iJ Akademii Medycznej w Białymstoku. 2005;50 Suppl 1:46–8.
16. Smith DR, Wei N, Zhao L, Wang R-S. Hand dermatitis among nurses in a newly developing region of Mainland China. Int J Nurs Stud. 2005;42:13–9.

17. Luk N-MT, Lee H-CS, Luk C-KD, Cheung Y-YA, Chang M-C, Chao V-K, et al. Hand eczema among Hong Kong nurses: a self-report questionnaire survey conducted in a regional hospital. Contact Dermatitis. 2011;65:329–35.
18. Lan C-CE, Feng W-W, Lu Y-W, Wu C-S, Hung S-T, Hsu H-Y, et al. Hand eczema among University Hospital Nursing staff: identification of high-risk sector and impact on quality of life. Contact Dermatitis. 2008;59:301–6.
19. Smith DR, Smyth W, Leggat PA, Wang R-S. Prevalence of hand dermatitis among hospital nurses working in a tropical environment. Aust J Adv Nurs. 2005;22:28–32.
20. Özyazicioglu N, Sürenler S, Tanriverdi G. Hand dermatitis among pediatric nurses. J Clin Nurs. 2010;19: 1597–603.
21. Strauss RM, Gawkrodger DJ. Occupational Contact dermatitis in nurses with hand Desisoft; Soft Protector eczema. Contact Dermatitis. 2001;44:293–6.
22. Lan C-CE, Tu H-P, Lee C-H, Wu C-S, Ko Y-C, Yu H-S, et al. Hand dermatitis among university hospital nursing staff with and without atopic eczema: assessment of risk factors. Contact Dermatitis. 2010;64:73–9.
23. Davis JA, Visscher MO, Wickett RR, Hoath SB. Influence of tumor necrosis factor-α polymorphism-308 and atopy on irritant contact dermatitis in healthcare workers. Contact Dermatitis. 2010;63:320–33.
24. Sacleux P, Bozec A, Veyres P, Negrin N, Vandenbos F, Bondiau PY, et al. Etude des facteurs de risque de sécheresse et dírritation des mains du personnel dans neuf établisssements de soins. Med Mal Infect. 2011;41:126–34.
25. Jungbauer FHW, Steenstra FR, Groothoff JW, Coenraads PJ. Characteristics of wet work in nurses. Int Arch Occup Environ Health. 2005;78:248–51.
26. Visser MJ, Behroozy A, Verberk MM, Semple S, Kezic S. Quantification of wet-work exposure in nurses using a newly developed wet-work exposure monitor. Ann Occup Hyg. 2011;55:810–6.
27. Kampf G, Löffler H. Dermatological aspects of a successful introduction and continuation of alcohol-based hands rubs for hygienic hand disinfection. J Hosp Infect. 2003;55:1–7.
28. Magnavita N, Elovainio M, Heponiemi T, Magnavita AM, Bergamaschi A. Are skin disorders related to work strain in hospital workers? A cross-sectional study. BMC Public Health. 2011;11:600.
29. Diepgen T, Andersen KE, Chosidow O, Coenraads PJ, Elsner P, English J, et al. Guidelines for diagnosis, treatment and prevention of hand eczema. Contact Dermatitis. 2013. www.escd.org.
30. Yang Y, Zirwas M. Hand dermatitis in primary care: A nurse practitioner's role in management. J Am Acad Nurs Pract. 2009;21:671–6.
31. Page E, Esswein E, Petersen M, Lewis D, Bledsoe T. Natural rubber latex: glove use, sensitization, and airborne and latent dust concentrations at a Denver Hospital. J Occup Environ Med. 2000;42:613–20.
32. Soost S, Graupner I, Morch-Röder A, Pohrt U, Worm M. A 7-step consultation plan for health care workers and hairdressers. JDDG. 2007;5:756–60.
33. Kikuchi-Numagami K, Saishu T, Fukaya M, Kanazawa E, Tagami H. Irritancy of scrubbing up for surgery with or without a brush. Acta Derm Venereol. 1999;79:230–2.
34. Hachem JP, De Paepe K, Sterckx G, Kaufman L, Rogiers V, Roseeuw D. Evaluation of biophysical and clinical parameters of skin barrier function among hospital workers. Contact Dermatitis. 2002;46:220–3.
35. Giménez-Arnau A. Occupational contact dermatitis: health personnel. In: Duus Johanssen J, Frosch PJ, Lepoittevin J-P, editors. Contact dermatitis. 5th ed. Berlin/Heidelberg: Springer; 2011. p. 841–51.
36. Suneja T, Belsito DV. Occupational dermatoses in health care workers evaluated for suspected allergic contact dermatitis. Contact Dermatitis. 2008;58:285–90.
37. Aalto-Korte K, Ackermann L, Henriks-Eckerman ML, Väljmaa J, Reinikka-Railo H, Leppänen E, et al. 1,2-Benzisothiazolin-3-one in disposable polyvinyl chloride gloves for medical use. Contact Dermatitis. 2007;57:365–70.
38. Sasseville D, Thériault M. Occupational contact urticaria caused by polyvinylchloride gloves. Contact Dermatitis. 2011;66:46–52.
39. Held E, Wolff C, Gyntelberg F, Agner T. Prevention of work-related skin problems in student auxiliary nurses: an intervention study. Contact Dermatitis. 2001;44:297–303.
40. Held E, Mygind K, Wolff C, Gyntelberg F, Agner T. Prevention of work related skin problems: an intervention study in wet work employees. Occup Environ Med. 2002;59:556–61.
41. Weisshaard E, Radulescu M, Bock M, Albrecht U, Zimmermann E, Diepgen TL. Skin protection and skin disease prevention courses for secondary prevention in health care workers: first results after two year of implementation. JDDG. 2005;3:33–8.
42. Loeffler H, Brucker T, Diepgen T, Effendi I. Primary prevention in health care employees: a prospective intervention study with a 3-year training period. Contact Dermatitis. 2006;54:202–9.
43. Weisshaard E, Radulescu M, Soder S, Apfelbacher CJ, Bock M, Grundmann JU, et al. Secondary individual prevention of occupational skin diseases in health care workers, cleaners and kitchen employees: aims, experiences and descriptive results. Int Arch Occup Environ Health. 2007;80:477–84.
44. Appelbacher CJ, Soder S, Diepgen TL, Weisshaar E. The impact of measures for secondary individual prevention of work-related skin diseases in health care workers: 1–year follow-up study. Contact Dermatitis. 2009;60:144–9.
45. Dulon M, Pohrt U, Skudlik C, Nienhaus A. Prevention of occupational skin disease: a workplace intervention study in geriatric nurses. Br J Dermatol. 2009;161: 337–44.

46. Boyce JM, Pittet D. Guideline for hand hygiene in health–care settings. Recommendations of the Healthcare Infection Control Practices Advisory Committee and the HICPAC/SHEA/APIC/IDSA Hand Hygiene Task Force. MMWR Recomm Rep. 2002;51:1–44.
47. Kampf G, Kramer A. Epidemiologic background of hygiene and evaluation of the most important agents for scrubs and rubs. Clin Microbiol Rev. 2004;17: 863–93.
48. Winnefeld M, Richard MA, Drancourt M, Grob JJ. Skin tolerance and effectiveness of two hand decontamination procedures in everyday hospital use. Br J Dermatol. 2000;143:546–50.
49. Kampf G, Löffler H. Prevention of irritant contact dermatitis among health care workers by using evidence-based hand hygiene practices: a review. Ind Health. 2007;45:645–52.
50. Löffler H, Effendy I, Happle R. The sodium lauryl sulfate test. A noninvasive functional evaluation of skin hypersensitivity. Hautarzt. 1996;47(11):832–8.
51. Löffler H, Kampf G, Schmermund D, Maibach HI. How irritant is alcohol? Br J Dermatol. 2007;157(1): 74–81.
52. Stutz N, Becker D, Jappe U, John SM, Ladwig A, Spornraft-Ragaller P, et al. Nurses'perceptions of the benefits and adverse effects of hand disinfection: alcohol-based rubs vs. hygienic handwashing: a multicenter questionnaire study with additional patch testing by the German Contact Dermatitis Research Group. Br J Dermatol. 2009;160:565–72.
53. Graham M, Nixon R, Burrell LJ, Bolger C, Johnson PDR, Grayson ML. Low rates of cutaneous adverse reactions to alcohol-based hand hygiene solution during prolonged use in a large teaching hospital. Antimicrob Agents Chemother. 2005;49:4404–5.
54. Löffler H, Bruckner T, Diepgen T, Effendy I. Primary prevention in health care employees: a prospective intervention study with a 3-year training period. Contact Dermatitis. 2006;54(4):202–9.
55. Jungbauer FHW, van der Harst JJ, Groothoff JW, Coenraads PJ. Skin protection in nursing work: promoting the use of gloves and hand alcohol. Contact Dermatitis. 2004;51:135–40.
56. Agthe N, Terho K, Kurvinen T, Routamaa M, Peltonen R, Litinen K, Kanerva M. Microbial efficacy and tolerability of a new, non-alcohol-based hand disinfectant. Infect Control Hosp Epidemiol. 2009;30:685–90.
57. Korniewicz DM, El Masri M. Effect of Aloe-vera Impregnated gloves on hand hygiene attitudes of health care workers. Medsurg Nurs. 2007;16:247–52.
58. McCormick RD, Buchman TL, Maki DG. Double-blind, randomized trial of scheduled use of a novel barrier cream and an oil-containing lotion for protecting the hands of health care workers. AJIC Am J Infect Control. 2000;28:302–10.
59. Batalla A, Garcia-Doval I, de la Torre C. Products for hand hygiene and antisepsis: use by health professionals and relationship with hand eczema. Actas DemoSifiliogr. 2012;103:192–7.
60. Visscher M, Davis J, Wickett R. Effect of topical treatments on irritant hand dermatitis in health care workers. Am Infect Control. 2009;37:842–50.
61. Ibler KS, Agner T, Hansen JL, Gluud C. The hand eczema trial (HET): design of a randomized clinical trial of the effect of classification and individual counseling versus no intervention among health-care workers with hand eczema. BMC Dermatol. 2010;10:8.
62. Van der Meer EWC, Al Boot C, Jungbauer FHW, van der Klink JJL, Rustenmeyer T, Coenraads PJ, et al. Hands 4U: a multifaceted strategy to implement guideline-based recommendations to prevent hand eczema in health care workers: design of randomized controlled trial and (cost) effectiveness evaluation. BMC Public Health. 2011;11:669.
63. Smedley J, Williams S, Peel P, Pedersen K, on behalf of the Dermatitis Guideline Development Group. Management of occupational dermatitis in healthcare workers: a systematic review. Occup Environ Med 2012;69:276–9

19 Hand Eczema from Rubber Gloves

Curtis P. Hamann, Kim M. Sullivan, and Peggy Wright

Contents

C.P. Hamann, M.D. (✉) • K.M. Sullivan • P. Wright
SmartPractice, 3400 E. McDowell Rd,
Phoenix, AZ 85008, USA
e-mail: hamann@smarthealth.com;
sullivan@smarthealth.com;
mwright1438@comcast.net

19.1 Introduction

The predominant causes of glove-related eczema are contact with chemicals that penetrate the glove barrier, environmental conditions, and/or the processing chemicals that remain in the gloves in sufficient quantities to sensitize or elicit a reaction in sensitized individuals [1]. Manufacturers' efforts to reduce total natural rubber latex (NRL) proteins in gloves due to concerns about type I latex allergies have not necessarily reduced the amount of residual processing chemicals. The primary sensitizers are sulfur-containing chemicals, such as thiurams, dithiocarbamates, and mercaptobenzothiazole derivatives used to accelerate the vulcanization process for both natural and synthetic rubber gloves. These chemicals are found alone or in varying combinations and can cause irritant and allergic contact dermatitis [2, 3]. Furthermore, chemicals used in conjunction with glove use and/or on the skin prior to donning gloves, such as lotions or powders, impact the skin barrier and/or the physical properties of the gloves. The repetitive use of an occlusive polymer layer on the hand may also contribute to irritant or allergic contact dermatitis. Individuals suffering from glove-related dermatitis often randomly switch brands or select a synthetic rubber or plastic glove over an NRL product in an attempt to resolve their hand eczema. Switching gloves with no understanding of the causative allergen(s) is unlikely to permanently resolve the problem and may exacerbate the situation.

A. Alikhan et al. (eds.), *Textbook of Hand Eczema*,
DOI 10.1007/978-3-642-39546-8_19, © Springer-Verlag Berlin Heidelberg 2014

19.2 Hand Eczema in Glove Users

Dermatitis from rubber gloves poses a significant burden in occupational medicine and reportedly is on the rise. The distribution of the skin's reaction and the correlation between the use of gloves and deterioration from dermatitis make it easy to link gloves to the disease. It is often more difficult to determine the specific causative allergen(s) and make informative glove recommendations without patch testing.

The chronic course of glove-related dermatitis typically involves long treatment (frequently inadequate), use of sick leave, risk of job loss, increased exposure to pathogens, and a negative impact on the quality of life [4]. The disease spectrum related to glove use includes irritant contact dermatitis (ICD), allergic contact dermatitis (ACD), and allergic contact urticaria (ACU). Chemical, mechanical, thermal, and climatic effects may cause or exacerbate chronic ICD and ACD associated with glove use. Risk factors are varied and may occur independently or in combination (Table 19.1).

19.2.1 Glove-Related ICD

The occlusive nature of a glove may induce alterations in transepidermal water loss (TEWL),

Table 19.1 Risk factors for occupational, glove-related contact dermatitis

Risk factor	Contributors to hand dermatitis
Wet work[a]	Spend 1/4 of the daily shift (2 h) with hands in a wet environment, increasing susceptibility to dermatitis
	Spend a corresponding amount of time wearing moisture-proof protective gloves that create an occlusive environment. Occlusion is known to enhance absorption of drugs through the skin and may increase penetration of chemicals and antigens, resulting in ACD or ICD [5]
	Frequently clean hands, with exposure to detergents possibly aggravating the irritant skin response
Chemical exposure	Use soaps and/or disinfectants in combination with glove use, which can heighten susceptibility to dermatitis
	Use cleaning products that are strongly related to the worsening of hand eczema [6]
	Wear gloves as recommended to avoid getting hands wet or dirty, resulting in frequent or prolonged use, increasing vulnerability to dermatitis because of occlusion
	Use alcohol-based disinfectants as recommended instead of water/soap when hands are not visibly dirty [7]
	Have contact with a variety of chemicals, such as glutaraldehyde, acrylates, and solvents that have the potential to contribute to the dermatitis. Both glutaraldehyde and formaldehyde break through both rubber and vinyl surgical and examination gloves in a few minutes to hours, depending on the glove's thickness and formulation [8]
Duration of glove wear	Wear gloves for prolonged periods, possibly facilitating skin irritation of the hands. This practice may be related to occlusion, friction, and maceration from the glove [9]. See wet work above
	Frequently wash hands, with exposure to detergents and surgical scrubs before glove use, possibly further aggravating the irritant skin response
	Wear gloves for short periods, resulting in glove occlusion that significantly impacts skin irritation [10]
	Wear gloves for long periods, resulting in a negative impact on the water-barrier function of normal skin [10]
Glove powder	Use glove powder, which contributes to irritation (friction, alkaline pH) and affects skin roughness, one measure of skin irritation [11]
Moisturizers/ barrier creams	Use these products, which may impact water-barrier function and hydration level of the skin [9]. Studies on barrier creams remain contradictory and inconclusive based on the effect that creams have on the integrity of the polymer itself, the ability of the cream to enhance or protect the hand from transport of allergens. Sensitizers in products used for hand washing and disinfection as well as in creams and emollients also frequently cause hand eczema in glove users [12]

[a]Flyvholm and Lindberg [7]

affecting skin-barrier function and causing ICD [10, 13]. Additionally, scientists know that occlusion enhances absorption of drugs through the skin, and gloves may contribute to the occurrence of ICD and ACD due to increased penetration of chemicals [5, 14]. The clinical spectrum of ICD is highly variable, but is typically characterized by redness, dryness, roughness, scaling, and infiltration [11].

Studies on glove-related causes of ICD, however, are contradictory, which may reflect the methods of testing or the gloves used. Some researchers have examined the effects of glove occlusion on the barrier function of normal skin and have found a correlation between the pattern of glove wear and ICD [10, 13]. Others have reported that short- and long-term glove occlusion, whether during single or repetitive use, are not risk factors for the development of hand dermatitis [15–17]. One of those studies, however, determined that both occlusion and water exposure were capable of inducing higher susceptibility to irritation from sodium lauryl sulfate (SLS), and although occlusion did not induce measurable alterations in skin physiology, water exposure did cause a significant increase in TEWL [17].

19.2.2 Glove-Related ACD

ACD related to glove use typically presents with localization of the eczema on the dorsal side of the fingers and hands and on the flexor or extensor surfaces of the forearms, not extending beyond the glove's contact with the skin. Although a time lag of several hours to several days from exposure to symptoms is usual, rubber-glove contact with delicate skin, such as the periorbital areas, may induce itching and edema a few hours after exposure, causing misinterpretation as a type I reaction [18].

The frequency of type I hypersensitivity to NRL has diminished since the 1990s due to increased awareness of the allergenic potential of NRL proteins, reduction in the amount of total protein and antigenic protein levels in NRL products, and the increased replacement with *latex-free* gloves [19, 20]. *Low-protein* gloves, however, are not necessarily low in allergens or in chemical content [21, 22].

Prior to the 1990s, researchers did not consider NRL to be a type IV sensitizer. Cases of type IV hypersensitivity to NRL – without ACU and a negative skin-prick test for the NRL protein – have been reported [23–25]. It is important to note, however, that NRL patch test preparations may contain rubber processing chemicals not known to the supplier. Because NRL is highly perishable, producers add preservatives to it immediately after tapping the trees. These preservatives (typically ammonia or formaldehyde) are used to de-ammoniate the NRL. Secondary preservatives, such as zinc oxide, may also be used before transporting the latex to the manufacturer [26, 27]. Medical practitioners should cautiously interpret patch test results when using nonstandardized NRL allergens, patch testing with ammoniated latex samples from glove manufacturers, or making their own eluates from glove samples.

19.2.3 Occupational Sectors

The most frequent diagnosis for occupational hand eczema is ICD, primarily associated with wet work and glove-wearing occupations, including health care, hairdressing, cleaning service, and food processing [11, 28]. ACD induced by rubber additives is also common and responsible for 40–70 % of the cases of occupational dermatitis [29]. Some glove users present with concomitant reactions, such as ACD to rubber chemicals and ACU from NRL [30].

19.2.3.1 Health-Care Workers

Researchers estimate that the prevalence of occupational skin disorders among health-care workers (HCWs) ranges from 7.9 % to 30.7 %, with nurses having the highest prevalence [2, 12, 31]. Hand involvement, female gender, and a history of atopy appear to be traits that are significantly more common among HCWs with dermatitis than non-HCWs [12, 32].

For HCWs, wet work, with 20–40 hand washes per day, is a contributing factor, as is duration of glove wear [33]. Thiurams are the most frequently reported rubber allergen, and approximately 8.87–13.0 % of HCW are patch test positive to thiurams [2, 12].

On a daily basis, HCWs often come into contact with a variety of chemical irritants and allergens, such as disinfectants, acrylates, and antibiotics, while wearing examination gloves rather than the appropriate, chemically resistant utility gloves. The resulting permeation of these chemicals through the gloves can contribute to dermatitis [8]. Dental personnel (56 %) have experienced higher rates of glutaraldehyde ACD compared to other HCWs (5 %), most likely as a result of exposure levels and inappropriate glove selection [32–34].

19.2.3.2 Cleaners

Hand dermatitis is a major problem for cleaners, reportedly affecting as many as 81.6 % in this vocation [35]. The primary risks, in addition to individual susceptibility and female gender, are wet work, frequent contact with detergents and cleaning chemicals, and the need to use occlusive gloves for up to one-third of the work day [36, 37]. The most common allergens in this occupational sector are rubber-glove accelerators – thiurams, zinc diethyldithiocarbamate, mercaptobenzothiazole – and disinfectants [36]. Reportedly, cleaners have a 3.1-fold elevated risk for acquiring a thiuram allergy [36, 38].

Although gloves contribute to dermatitis for this sector, they also are essential in preventing it. In 2006, Mygind et al. studied hand eczema among gut cleaners in a Danish swine slaughterhouse and found that the group using a high-fat moisturizer, cotton inner gloves, and outer protective gloves had the lowest risk of eczema [39].

19.2.3.3 Hairdressers

Occupational contact dermatitis is common among hairdressers, who are routinely exposed to water, irritants, and sensitizers, and their use of gloves is often inadequate [40, 41]. In 2003, Nettis et al. evaluated hairdressers for type I and type IV glove-related sensitization and found that 98.4 % of participants displayed skin symptoms and 34.4 % showed respiratory and/or conjunctival symptoms associated with the use of NRL gloves [42]. The most frequent positive patch test results involved paraphenylenediamine; although a rubber additive, this chemical appeared not to be related to glove use but rather to permanent hair dye. The most common sensitizing accelerators were thiuram mix (8.2 %), tetramethylthiuram monosulfide (8.2 %), and carba mix (8.2 %). Although all hairdressers are at risk for developing hand eczema, apprentice hairdressers are most commonly affected [40]. Hairdressers' awareness of hazards and selection of appropriate gloves are essential to minimizing the risk of hand eczema.

19.2.3.4 Food Service Workers

Food service workers are at risk from both ICD and ACD due to continuous exposure to liquids, food ingredients, soaps, detergents, and disinfectants. The main allergens in this group are food related or linked to the use of protective gloves, with this group generally having a 1.8-fold increased risk of being sensitized to thiurams, with cooks having the highest (2.5-fold) relative risk [43].

19.3 Accelerators in Gloves

Manufacturers use several hundred additives to facilitate rubber-glove processing. These chemicals include accelerators, antioxidants, antimicrobials, emulsifiers, and biocides (Table 19.2). Accelerators include thiurams, dithiocarbamates, thiazoles, and thioureas, all of which may induce ACD in humans. Geier et al. concluded that the responsible accelerators in rubber gloves have not changed substantially in the past 17 years [2, 44]. For North America, the European Union, and Australia, some studies show that 5–10 % of the population is allergic to rubber additives, primarily due to increased glove use [57]. Other studies have found higher percentages in particular populations: 31.7 % of patch test patients with suspected rubber allergy [31] and 19.60 % of patients with hand eczema [6].

Table 19.2 Sensitizing chemicals used in production of NRL or synthetic rubber gloves[a]

Type of sensitizer	
Accelerators	Chemical
Thiurams	Dipentamethylenethiuram disulfide (DPTD) Tetrabutylthiuram disulfide (TBTD) Dipentamethylenethiuram tetrasulfide (PTT) Tetraethylthiuram disulfide (TETD) Tetramethylthiuram monosulfide (TMTM) Tetramethylthiuram disulfide (TMTD) Tetramethyl/tetraethyl thiuram disulfide (MET) Tetrabenzyl thiuram disulfide (TBzTD)
Dithiocarbamates	Zinc dibenzyldithiocarbamate (ZBED) Zinc dibutyldithiocarbamate (ZDBC) Zinc diethyldithiocarbamate (ZDEC) Zinc dimethyldithiocarbamate (ZDMC) Zinc dipentamethylene dithiocarbamate (ZPC) Zinc diisobutyl dithiocarbamate (ZDiBC) Piperidine pentamethylene dithiocarbamate Copper dimethyl dithiocarbamate (CUDD)
Guanidines	Diphenylguanidine (DPG) Diortho tolyguanidine (DOTG)
Benzothiazoles/benzothiazolesulfenamides	Dibenzothiazyl disulfide (MBTS) N-cyclohexyl-2-benzothiazolesulfenamide (CBS) Mercaptobenzothiazole (MBT) Morpholino mercaptobenzothiazole (MMBT) Zinc mercaptobenzothiazole (ZMBT) Mercaptobenzimidazole (MBI) Morpholinyl mercaptobenzothiazyl (MOR) N-oxydiethylene-2-benzothiazole sulfenamide (OBTS) N-cyclohexyl benzothiazole-2-sulfenamide (CZ-CBS) N,N-dicyclohexyl-2-benzothiazole sulfenamide (DCBS) 2,2′-dithio dibenzothiazole (DM-MBTS) 4-morpholinyl-2-benzothiazole disulfide (MBD) N-oxydiethylene-2-benzothiazole sulfenamide (NOBS) N-t-butyl-2-benzothiazolesulfenamide (NS-TBBS) N-tert-butyl-2-benzothiazole sulfenamide (TBBS) Benzothiazyl-2-dicyclohexyl sulfenamide (DCBS)
Thioureas	Dibutylthiourea (DBTU) Diethylthiourea (DETU) Diphenylthiourea (DPTU) Ethylenethiourea (ETU) Dimethylthiourea (DMTU) Thiourea (TU)
Preservatives/antimicrobials	Sorbic acid Epichlorhydrin Cetylpyridinechloride Formaldehyde and formaldehyde releasers

(continued)

Table 19.2 (continued)

Type of sensitizer Accelerators	Chemical
Antioxidants	4,4′-thio*bis* (6-*tert*-butyl-*meta*-cresol) (Lowinox 44S36) Butylated hydroxyanisole (BHA) 4,4′-Dihydroxydiphenyl ether (DHDE) N-isopropyl-N'-phenyl-paraphenylenediamine (IPPD) N-cyclohexyl-N'-phenyl paraphenylenediamine (CTP)
Other antigens	Acryloyl morpholine (ACMO) Aniline Diaminodiphenylmethane (DDM) Dibutylamine (DBA) Diethylamine (DEA) Dihydroxybiphenyl (BPL) Dimethylamine (DMA) Dimethylbutylphenyl-p-phenylenediamine (DMBPPD) Diphenyl-p-phenylenediamine (DPPD) Dithiodimorpholine (DTDM) n-Dodecylmercaptan (NDDM) Ethylenediamine dihydrochloride Hexamethylenetetramine Hydrochinonmonobenzylether Iodopropynyl butylcarbamate Isopropylphenylenediamine or black rubber mix (IPPD) Methenamine N-ethylanine (EAN) Phenyl-beta-naphthylamine (PBN) Piperidine (PP) Tert-butylcatechol Trimethyldihydroquinoline

[a]Created with data from [2, 31, 44–56]

In 2002, De Jong et al. ranked the allergenic potency of 15 different accelerators commonly used in production of NRL medical gloves by lymph node assay and identified 14 chemicals as sensitizers. The researchers concluded that the chemicals of choice for glove production were tetrabutylthiuram disulfide (TBTD) among the thiuram compounds, zinc dibutyldithiocarbamate (ZDBC) among the carbamates, and zinc 2-mercaptobenzothiazole (ZMBT) among the benzothiazoles, with the total amount of residual chemicals and the chemical's potency being important for allergy induction. Guanidines and thioureas, also known sensitizers, were not tested [58] (Fig. 19.1).

The variations observed in sensitization frequencies to rubber allergens over time and geographically involve (1) the number of people using a particular glove at a particular time, (2) the length of particular manufacturers' leach time for gloves, and (3) changes in the use of particular chemicals or use of new chemicals and the resulting new reactions between chemicals that occur (see Table 19.2).

19.3.1 Thiurams/Thiuram Mix

Thiuram derivatives are used in the production of NRL, nitrile, and chloroprene rubber gloves and, historically, have accounted for 70–80 % of the cases of glove-related contact reactions [45, 57, 59, 60]. Although most commonly identified as the primary cause of rubber ACD, thiurams are less frequently identified in the contents

Fig. 19.1 Allergenic potency of accelerators, listed from greatest to least (Adapted from [58])

1. Zinc diethyldithiocarbamate (ZDEC)	Dithiocarbamate	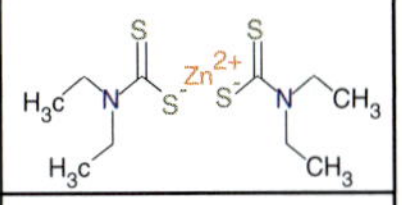
2. Tetramethylthiuram disulfide (TMTD)*	Thiuram	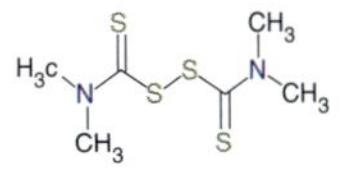
3. Tetraethylthiuram disulfide (TETD)*	Thiuram	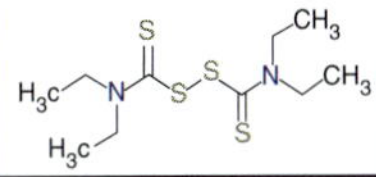
4. Zinc dipentamethylene dithiocarbamate (ZPC)	Dithiocarbamate	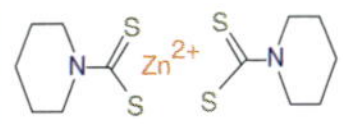
5. Zinc dimethyldithiocarbamate (ZDMC)	Dithiocarbamate	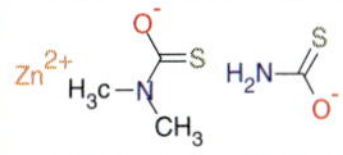
6. Dibenzothiazyl disulfide (MBTS)	Benzothiazole	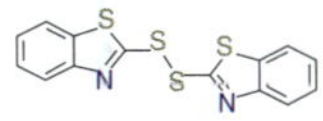
7. Dipentamethylenethiuram disulfide (DPTD)*	Thiuram	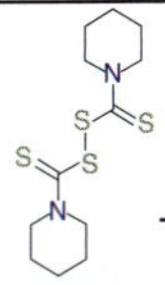
8. Tetramethylthiuram monosulfide (TMTM)*	Thiuram	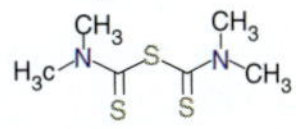
9. Mercaptobenzothiazole (MBT)	Benzothiazole	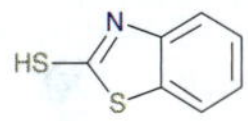
10. Mercaptobenzimidazole (MBI)	Benzothiazole	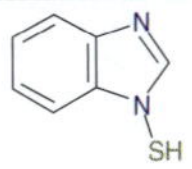
11. Dipentamethylenethiuram tetrasulfide (DPTT)	Thiuram	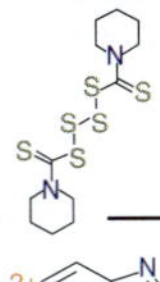
12. Zinc mercaptobenzothiazole (ZMBT)	Benzothiazole	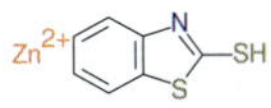
13. Tetrabutylthiuram disulfide (TBTD)**	Thiuram	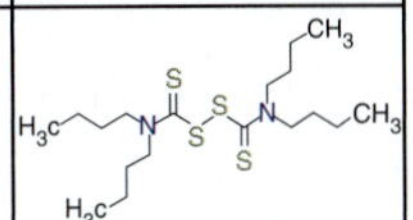
14. Diethylamine (DEA)	Amine	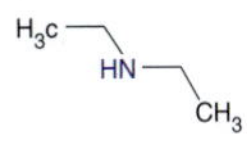
15. Zinx dibutyldithio carbamate (ZDBC)	Carbamate	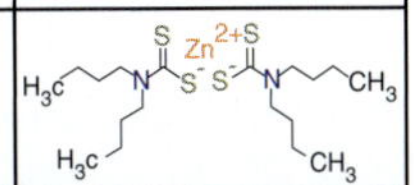
*In Thiuram Mix		
**Additional in some Thiuram Mixes		

of either surgical or examination gloves [3, 22, 46, 61, 62]. In an effort to reduce thiuram sensitization, manufacturers now often substitute carbamates, thiuram tetrasulfides, or butylated thiuram derivatives for thiurams in glove production [46, 63, 64]. Thiuram-free gloves are available and recommended for high-risk groups such as HCWs and food processors. Although glove use is the primary contact source, airborne thiuram contact dermatitis has been reported in a thiuram-sensitive HCW [65]:

- Since the 1990s, some studies have shown a significant decline in the frequency of positive reactions to the thiuram mix among HCWs, theoretically due to reduced residual accelerator content [38, 61]. However, other studies have reported no such decline [2, 12, 31]. Bhargava et al. reported no change in thiuram positivity in HCW from 1980 to 2006, but did show a significant decline among housewives [47]. Geier et al. also reported that thiurams are still commonly used in both natural and synthetic rubber examination gloves due to their relatively low cost and remain a primary sensitizer [2] (Table 19.3).

Worldwide, standard patch-testing trays use the thiuram mix containing tetramethylthiuram disulfide (TMTD), tetraethylthiuram disulfide (TETD),

Table 19.3 Review of patch-testing results with thiurams

Who (n)	Allergen	Patch test preparation	Prevalence (%)	Reference
IVDK – patients with occupational contact dermatitis and suspected glove allergy, $n=1{,}976$	Thiurams	At least 1positive to any thiuram	15.1	Geier (2003) 1995–2001 [44]
IVDK – patients with occupational contact dermatitis and suspected glove allergy, $n=3{,}306$	Thiurams	At least 1positive to any thiuram	13.0	Geier (2012) 2002–2010 [2]
IVDK-HCW with occupational contact dermatitis and suspected glove allergy, $n=1{,}019$	Thiurams	At least 1positive to any thiuram	15.0	Geier (2012) 2002–2010 [2]
Female cleaners in dermatology departments in Germany, Switzerland, and Austria, $n=803$	Thiurams	At least 1positive to any thiuram	11.6	Liskowsky (2011) [36]
Thiuram mix				
Patients with hand eczema in Brazil, $n=250$	Thiuram mix	TMTD, TMTM, TETD, DPTM (025 % each) 1 % pet	7.2	Duarte (2003) 1993–1995 [6]
Patients tested by the NACDG, $n=3{,}435$	Thiuram mix	TMTD, TMTM, TETD, DPTD (0.25 % each) 1 % pet	6.9	Zug (2009) 1996–1998 [66]
Patients tested by the NACDG, $n=5{,}830$	Thiuram mix	TMTD, TMTM, TETD, DPTD (0.25 % each) 1 % pet	4.7	Zug (2009) 1998–2000 [66]
IVDK – patients with occupational contact dermatitis and suspected glove allergy, $n=1{,}916$	Thiuram mix	TMTD, TMTM, TETD, DPTD (0.25 % each) 1 % pet	12.9	Geier (2003) 1995–2001 [44]
Non-HCW patch tested by the NACDG, $n=13{,}568$	Thiuram mix	TMTD, TMTM, TETD, DPTD (0.25 % each) 1 % pet	0.9	Warshaw (2008) 1998–2004 [12]
Patients tested by the NACDG, $n=4{,}907$	Thiuram mix	TMTD, TMTM, TETD, DPTD (0.25 % each) 1 % pet	4.5	Zug (2009) 2001–2002 [66]

Table 19.3 (continued)

Who (n)	Allergen	Patch test preparation	Prevalence (%)	Reference
Patients tested by the NACDG, n=5,141	Thiuram mix	TMTD, TMTM, TETD, DPTD (0.25 % each) 1 % pet	4.6	Zug (2009) 2003–2004 [66]
Patients tested by the NACDG, *n*=4,443	Thiuram mix	TMTD, TMTM, TETD, DPTD (0.25 % each) 1 % pet	3.9	Zug (2009) 2005–2006 [66]
Non-HCW with ACD in Kansas, USA, *n*=685	Thiuram mix	TMTD, TMTM, TETD, DPTD (0.25 % each) 1 % pet	6.9	Suneja (2008) 1994–2006 [32]
IVDK – patients with occupational contact dermatitis and suspected glove allergy, *n*=3,070	Thiuram mix	TMTD, TMTM, TETD, DPTD (0.25 % each) 1 % pet	11.1	Geier (2012) 2002–2010 [2]
ESSCA patch test patients (11 EU countries), *n*=25,181	Thiuram Mix	TMTD, TMTM, TETD, DPTD (0.25 % each) 1 % pet	Range: 0.6–2.7 %	Uter (2012) 2007–2008 [67]
Patients with suspected ACD from rubber by Mayo Group, *n*=739	Thiuram Mix	TMTD, TMTM, TETD, DPTD (0.25 % each) 1 % pet	7.6	Bendewald (2010) 2000–2007 [31]
HCW patch tested by the NACDG, *n*=1,252	Thiuram mix	TMTD, TMTM, TETD, DPTD (0.25 % each) 1 % pet	8.87	Warshaw (2008) 1998–2004 [12]
HCW with ACD in Kansas, USA, *n*=53	Thiuram mix	TMTD, TMTM, TETD, DPTD (0.25 % each) 1 % pet	24.5	Suneja (2008) 1994–2006 [32]
IVDK-HCW with occupational contact dermatitis and suspected glove allergy, *n*=936	Thiuram mix	TMTD, TMTM, TETD, DPTD (0.25 % each) 1 % pet	13.0	Geier (2012) 2002–2010 [2]
Tetraethylthiuram (TETD)				
IVDK – patients with occupational contact dermatitis and suspected glove allergy, *n*=1,412	TETD	0.25 % pet	10.3	Geier (2003) 1995–2001 [44]
IVDK – patients with occupational contact dermatitis and suspected glove allergy, *n*=2,474	TETD	0.25 % pet	9.3	Geier (2012) 2002–2010 [2]
Patients with suspected ACD from rubber by Mayo Group, *n*=772	TETD	1 % pet	4.5	Bendewald (2010) 2000–2007 [31]
IVDK-HCW with occupational contact dermatitis and suspected glove allergy, *n*=832	TETD	0.25 % pet	10.7	Geier (2012) 2002–2010 [2]
Tetramethylthiuram monosulfide (TMTM)				
IVDK – patients with occupational contact dermatitis and suspected glove allergy, *n*=1,423	TMTM	0.25 % pet	8.1	Geier (2003) 1995–2001 [44]

(continued)

Table 19.3 (continued)

Who (n)	Allergen	Patch test preparation	Prevalence (%)	Reference
Patients with suspected ACD from rubber by Mayo Group, $n=771$	TMTM	1 % pet	5.4	Bendewald (2010) 2000–2007 [31]
IVDK – patients with occupational contact dermatitis and suspected glove allergy, $n=2{,}478$	TMTM	0.25 % pet	7.5	Geier (2012) 2002–2010 [2]
IVDK-HCW with occupational contact dermatitis and suspected glove allergy, $n=834$	TMTM	0.25 % pet	7.2	Geier (2012) 2002–2010 [2]
Tetramethylthiuram disulfide (TMTD)				
IVDK – patients with occupational contact dermatitis and suspected glove allergy, $n=1{,}420$	TMTD	0.25 % pet	7.1	Geier (2003) 1995–2001 [44]
Patients with suspected ACD from rubber by Mayo Group, $n=772$	TMTD	1 % pet	3.1	Bendewald (2010) 2000–2007 [31]
IVDK – patients with occupational contact dermatitis and suspected glove allergy, $n=2{,}479$	TMTD	0.25 % pet	5.2	Geier (2012) 2002–2010 [2]
IVDK-HCW with occupational contact dermatitis and suspected glove allergy, $n=834$	TMTD	0.25 % pet	5.2	Geier (2012) 2002–2010 [2]
Dipentamethylenethiuram disulfide (DPTD)				
IVDK – patients with occupational contact dermatitis and suspected glove allergy, $n=1{,}916$	DPTD	0.25 % pet	5.1	Geier (2003) 1995–2001 [44]
Patients with suspected ACD from rubber by Mayo Group, $n=772$	DPTD	1 % pet	2.7	Bendewald (2010) 2000–2007 [31]
IVDK – patients with occupational contact dermatitis and suspected glove allergy, $n=2{,}479$	DPTD	0.25 % pet	3.6	Geier (2012) 2002–2010 [2]
IVDK-HCW with occupational contact dermatitis and suspected glove allergy, $n=836$	DPTD	0.25 % pet	4.8	Geier (2012) 2002–2010 [2]
Occupation: cleaners				
Occupation: health-care worker (HCW)				

tetramethylthiuram monosulfide (TMTM), and dipentamethylenethiuram disulfide (DPTD), each at 0.25 %, as a marker for contact allergies from rubber accelerators. An alternative thiuram mix is available that adds TBTD as a fifth component. The thiuram mix does not detect all cases of thiuram allergy, and it is advisable to use both the standard series and the rubber series for a suspected rubber-glove allergy [2].

19.3.2 Dithiocarbamates/Carba Mix

Dithiocarbamates (carbamates) are accelerators used in NRL, nitrile, and chloroprene gloves and are sensitizing agents [2, 48, 62, 63]. Zinc diethyldithiocarbamate (ZDEC) and ZDBC are the most common accelerators found in gloves [22, 44, 63]. In 2012, Geier et al. reported that dithiocarbamates elicit positive reactions in 3.5 % of those with glove-related allergy, with ZDEC continuing to be the most prominent dithiocarbamate allergen in both examination and surgical gloves. Chipinda et al. found that the critical functional group in ZDEC's allergenicity is the thiol and that haptenation occurs primarily through chelation of metalloproteins and formation of mixed disulfides [48]. Prevalence rates range from 0.87 % in the general population to 7.4 % among those with suspected rubber allergy to

15.1 % among HCWs depending on the studies reported [12, 31, 68] (Table 19.4).

Researchers have confirmed cross-reactivity between dithiocarbamates and thiurams [2, 69]. Almost all patients who react to ZDEC will also react to TETD [2]. Oxidation of dithiocarbamates may form thiurams on and in the skin, and sensitization to dithiocarbamates is almost always combined with thiuram sensitization, yet only a portion of persons sensitive to thiurams also react to dithiocarbamates [2, 46]. A strong correlation exists between the degree of reactivity to thiurams and the likelihood of reacting to ZDEC [46].

Table 19.4 Review of patch-testing results with dithiocarbamates

Who (n)	Allergen	Patch test preparation	Prevalence (%)	Reference
Dithiocarbamates				
IVDK – patients with occupational contact dermatitis and suspected glove allergy, $n = 1987$	Dithiocarbamates	At least 1 to any dithiocarbamate	3.4	Geier (2003) 1995–2001 [44]
IVDK – patients with occupational contact dermatitis and suspected glove allergy, $n = 3,319$	Dithiocarbamates	At least 1 to any dithiocarbamate	3.5	Geier (2012) 2002–2010 [2]
IVDK-HCW with occupational contact dermatitis and suspected glove allergy, $n = 1,022$	Dithiocarbamates	At least 1 to any dithiocarbamate	3.2	Geier (2012) 2002–2010 [2]
Carba mix				
Patients with hand eczema in Brazil, $n = 252$	Carba mix	DPG 3 % pet	5.2	Duarte (2003) 1993–1995 [6]
Non-HCW with ACD in Kansas, USA, $n = 685$	Carba mix	DPG, ZDEC, ZDBC 3 % pet	5.4	Suneja (2008) 1994–2006 [32]
Non HCW patch tested by the NACDG, $n = 13,568$	Carba mix	DPG, ZDEC, ZDBC 3 % pet	0.87	Warshaw (2008) 1998–2004 [12]
Patients tested by the NACDG, $n = 3,437$	Carba mix	DPG, ZDEC, ZDBC 3 % pet	7.3	Zug (2009) 1996–1998 [66]
Patients tested by the NACDG, $n = 5,829$	Carba mix	DPG, ZDEC, ZDBC 3 % pet	4.8	Zug (2009) 1998–2000 [66]
Patients tested by the NACDG, $n = 4,907$	Carba mix	DPG,ZDEC,ZDBC (1 % each) 3 % pet	4.9	Zug (2009) 2001–2002 [66]
Patients tested by the NACDG, $n = 5,142$	Carba mix	DPG, ZDEC, ZDBC 3 % pet	4.0	Zug (2009) 2003–2004 [66]
Patients tested by the NACDG, $n = 4,443$	Carba mix	DPG, ZDEC, ZDBC (1 % each) 3 % pet	3.9	Zug (2009) 2005–2006 [66]
Patients with suspected ACD from rubber by Mayo Group, $n = 739$	Carba mix	DPG, ZDEC, ZDBC (1 % each) 3 % pet	7.4	Bendewald (2010) 2000–2007 [31]
HCW with ACD in Kansas, USA, $n = 53$	Carba mix	DPG, ZDEC, ZDBC (1 % each) 3 % pet	15.1	Suneja (2008) 1994–2006 [32]
HCW patch tested by the NACDG, $n = 1,252$	Carba mix	DPG, ZDEC, ZDBC (1 % each) 3 % pet	5.43	Warshaw (2008) 1998–2004 [12]
Zinc diethyldithiocarbamate (ZDEC)				
IVDK – patients with occupational contact dermatitis and suspected glove allergy, $n = 1,987$	ZDEC	1 % pet	3.3	Geier (2003) 1995–2001 [44]

(continued)

Table 19.4 (continued)

Who (n)	Allergen	Patch test preparation	Prevalence (%)	Reference
IVDK – patients with occupational contact dermatitis and suspected glove allergy, n=3,119	ZDEC	1 % pet	3.6	Geier (2012) 2002–2010 [2]
IVDK-HCW with occupational contact dermatitis and suspected glove allergy, n=952	ZDEC	1 % pet	3.4	Geier (2012) 2002–2010 [2]
Patients with suspected ACD from rubber by Mayo Group, n=762	ZDEC	1 % pet	1.2	Bendewald (2010) 2000–2007 [31]
Zinc dibutyldithiocarbamate (ZDBC)				
IVDK – patients with occupational contact dermatitis and suspected glove allergy, n=1,377	ZDBC	1 % pet	0.4	Geier (2003) 1995–2001 [44]
Patients with suspected ACD from rubber by Mayo Group, n=760	ZDBC	1 % pet	0.5	Bendewald (2010) 2000–2007 [31]
IVDK-HCW with occupational contact dermatitis and suspected glove allergy, n=841	ZDBC	1 % pet	0.1	Geier (2012) 2002–2010 [2]
IVDK – patients with occupational contact dermatitis and suspected glove allergy, n=2,495	ZDBC	1 % pet	0.2	Geier (2012) 2002–2010 [2]
Zinc dibenzyldithiocarbamate (ZBED)				
IVDK – patients with occupational contact dermatitis and suspected glove allergy, n=2,303	ZBED	1 % pet	0.2	Geier (2012) 2002–2010 [2]
IVDK-HCW with occupational contact dermatitis and suspected glove allergy, n=739	ZBED	1 % pet	0.3	Geier (2012) 2002–2010 {11992)
Patients with suspected ACD from rubber by Mayo Group, n=97	ZBED	1 % pet	1.0	Bendewald (2010) 2000–2007 [31]
Zinc dimethyldithiocarbamate (ZDMC)				
Patients with suspected ACD from rubber by Mayo Group, n=772	ZDMC	1 % pet	1.6	Bendewald (2010) 2000–2007 [31]

Patients may acquire this co-sensitization to thiurams and dithiocarbamates by co-exposure to both groups of chemicals through wearing different brands of gloves [2]. Due to glove use in the presence of strong oxidizing chemicals such as disinfectants, iodine, hydrogen peroxide, and bleach, other oxidation products may also occur and are potential sensitizers [48].

Great variability exists in the amount of allergen found in gloves. Even different lots of the same brand of glove may contain significant differences in residual chemical content [70]. Nitrile gloves contain considerable amounts of allergen and reportedly can contain the highest amount of dithiocarbamates [70]. Medical practitioners should exercise caution when recommending a synthetic rubber glove over an NRL glove to patients allergic to rubber chemicals without understanding the residual chemical content of the recommended glove [70].

19.3.3 1,3-Diphenylguanidine

Although 1,3-diphenylguanidine (DPG) is used in the production of NRL, nitrile, and chloroprene rubber gloves, it has been identified as "playing a minor role in rubber glove contact allergies" [44]. It is reported to be a problem allergen with a low reaction index, making irritant and allergic reactions somewhat difficult to differentiate when patch testing [44, 45]. In 2012, Geier et al. found

Table 19.5 Review of patch-testing results with guanidines

Who (n)	Allergen	Patch test preparation	Prevalence (%)	Reference
1,3-Diphenylguanidine (DPG)				
IVDK – patients with occupational contact dermatitis and suspected glove allergy, $n = 1{,}455$	DPG	1 % pet	1.9	Geier (2003) 1995–2001 [44]
IVDK – patients with occupational contact dermatitis and suspected glove allergy, $n = 2{,}578$	DPG	1 % pet	3.0	Geier (2012) 2002–2010 [2]
IVDK-HCW with occupational contact dermatitis and suspected glove allergy, $n = 841$	DPG	1 % pet	2.1	Geier (2012) 2002–2010 [2]
Patients with suspected ACD from rubber by Mayo Group, $n = 759$	DPG	1 % pet	7.5	Bendewald (2010) 2000–2007 [31]

that 3.0 % of all occupational dermatitis patients were sensitive to DPG but again reiterated the low diagnostic quality of common test preparations of DPG (1 % pet) (Table 19.5).

In 2010, the Mayo Clinic Group found that DPG, one of the three components of carba mix, was the third most common source of allergic reactions, with 7.5 % of their 759 patients with suspected rubber allergy testing positive [31]. This is almost twice the rate of other comparative studies. Because carba mix (which contains DPG) has a low sensitivity for detecting diphenylguanidine allergy, testing with both the carba mix and DPG is recommended [31]. To avoid the possibility of false-positive readings, it is also recommended that sodium lauryl sulfate (SLS) be used as an irritant control [2].

19.3.4 Mercaptobenzothiazole/Mercapto Mix

Mercapto compounds are accelerators and/or antioxidants used in the manufacture of NRL, nitrile, and polychloroprene surgical, examination, and utility gloves [63, 71]. The prevalence of positive reactions to either mercaptobenzothiazole (MBT) or the mercapto mix components has declined over the past 35 years and is now a relatively uncommon allergen [72, 73]. Consequently, the North American Contact Dermatitis Group (NACDG) dropped mercapto mix from its standard tray in 2013 (Table 19.6).

Despite the fact that allergy to mercapto compounds has diminished, it continues to be used in the production of many products, including rubber gloves and shoes, and everyday exposure continues. Internationally, the prevalence of allergy to mercapto compounds varies by country and regional exposure; however, the global, pooled, weighted average of allergy to MBT and its derivatives among patch test patients is at least 1.7 %, but could be as high as 3.0 % [2, 73].

Concomitant reactivity exists between MBT and mercapto mix, and researchers recommend testing with both in cases of suspected glove dermatitis [2]. Because testing with MBT alone would miss about 20–25 % of relevant patch test reactions and testing with mercapto mix alone would miss about 22–33 % of reactions, some research groups have added mercaptobenzothiazole to the mercapto mix (each of the four components, dibenzothiazyl disulfide [MBTS], N-cyclohexyl-2-benzothiazolesulfenamide [CBS], MBT, morpholino mercaptobenzothiazole [MMBT] at 0.5 % each) and recommend testing with both MBT and the mercapto mix as part of the standard series [2, 75]. It is also recommended with suspected MBT allergy to test with the expanded rubber series, including the three single components, because 14 % of contact allergy to any MBTs are missed if only testing with MBT and mercapto mix [2, 76].

Degradation of the mercapto mix has been reported to occur within weeks at room temperature, with the remaining component being

Table 19.6 Review of patch-testing results with mercaptobenzothiazole and derivatives

Who (n)	Allergen	Patch test preparation	Prevalence (%)	Reference
Mercaptobenzothiazole and derivatives				
IVDK – patients with occupational contact dermatitis and suspected glove allergy, $n = 1{,}984$	Mercaptobenzothiazole and derivatives	At least 1 to any mercapto derivative	2.9	Geier (2003) 1995–2001 [44]
IVDK – patients with occupational contact dermatitis and suspected glove allergy, $n = 3{,}323$	Mercaptobenzothiazole and derivatives	At least 1 to any mercapto derivative	3.0	Geier (2012) 2002–2010 [2]
IVDK-HCW with occupational contact dermatitis and suspected glove allergy, $n = 1{,}021$	Mercaptobenzothiazole and derivatives	At least 1 to any mercapto derivative	2.3	Geier (2012) 2002–2010 [2]
Mercapto mix				
Patients with hand eczema in Brazil, $n = 250$	Mercapto mix	NA	2.8	Duarte (2003) 1993–1995 [6]
IVDK – patients with occupational contact dermatitis and suspected glove allergy, $n = 106$	Mercapto mix	2 % pet	0.0	Geier (2003) 1995–2001 [44]
IVDK – patients with occupational contact dermatitis and suspected glove allergy, $n = 1{,}815$	Mercapto mix	1 % pet	2.2	Geier (2003) 1995–2001 [44]
HCW patch tested by the NACDG, $n = 1{,}254$	Mercapto mix	CBS, MBTS, MMBT- (0.333 each) 1 % pet	0.4	Warshaw (2008) 1998–2004 [12]
Non HCW patch tested by the NACDG, $n = 13{,}573$	Mercapto mix	CBS, MBTS, MMBT- (0.333 each) 1 % pet	0.26	Warshaw (2008) 1998–2004 [12]
Patients tested by the NACDG, $n = 5{,}834$	Mercapto mix	CBS, MBTS, MMBT – (0.333 each) 1 % pet	1.3	Zug (2009) 1998–2000 [66]
Patients tested by the NACDG, $n = 4{,}908$	Mercapto mix	CBS, MBTS, MMBT – (0.333 each) 1 % pet	0.7	Zug (2009) 2001–2002 [66]
Patients tested by the NACDG, $n = 5{,}143$	Mercapto mix	CBS, MBTS, MMBT – (0.333 each) 1 % pet	0.9	Zug (2009) 2003–2004 [66]
Patients tested by the NACDG, $n = 4{,}444$	Mercapto mix	CBS, MBTS, MMBT – (0.333 each) 1 % pet	0.8	Zug (2009) 2005–2006 [66]
Patients with suspected ACD from rubber by Mayo Group, $n = 738$	Mercapto mix	CBS, MBTS, MMBT – (0.333 each) 1 % pet	1.2	Bendewald (2010) 2000–2007 [31]
Rubber allergen sensitive patients in Brazil, $n = 222$	Mercapto mix	NA	21.17	Scherrer (2008) 1999–2007 [74]
ESSC – patch test patient (11 EU countries), $n = 9{,}882$	Mercapto mix (with MBT)	1 % pet	Range 0.0–1.1 %	Uter (2012) 2007–2008 [67]
ESSCA – patch test patient (11 EU countries), $n = 12{,}746$	Mercapto mix (without MBT)	2 % pet	Range 0.3–1.0 %	Uter (2012) 2007–2008 [67]
IVDK – patients with occupational contact dermatitis and suspected glove allergy, $n = 3{,}070$	Mercapto mix	MBTS, CBS, MBT, MMBT 1 % pet	2.1	Geier (2012) 2002–2010 [2]
IVDK-HCW with occupational contact dermatitis and suspected glove allergy, $n = 932$	Mercapto mix	MBTS, CBS, MBT, MMBT 1 % pet	1.4	Geier (2012) 2002–2010 [2]

Table 19.6 (continued)

Who (n)	Allergen	Patch test preparation	Prevalence (%)	Reference
Mercaptobenzothiazole (MBT)				
Patients with hand eczema in Brazil, $n=251$	MBT	1 % pet	2.8	Duarte (2003) 1993–1995 [6]
IVDK – patients with occupational contact dermatitis and suspected glove allergy, $n=106$	MBT	2 % pet	2.0	Geier (2003) 1995–2001 [44]
IVDK – patients with occupational contact dermatitis and suspected glove allergy, $n=1{,}815$	MBT	1 % pet	2.2	Geier (2003) 1995–2001 [44]
Non HCW patch tested by the NACDG, $n=13{,}572$	MBT	1 % pet	0.38	Warshaw (2008) 1998–2004 [12]
HCW patch tested by the NACDG, $n=1{,}254$	MBT	1 % pet	0.72	Warshaw (2008) 1998–2004 [12]
Patients tested by the NACDG, $n=5{,}834$	MBT	1 % pet	2.0	Zug (2009) 1998–2000 [66]
Patients tested by the NACDG, $n=4{,}907$	MBT	1 % pet	0.9	Zug (2009) 2001–2002 [66]
Patients tested by the NACDG, $n=5{,}143$	MBT	1 % pet	0.9	Zug (2009) 2003–2004 [66]
Patients tested by the NACDG, $n=4{,}442$	MBT	1 % pet	0.9	Zug (2009) 2005–2006 [66]
Patients with suspected ACD from rubber by Mayo Group, $n=753$	MBT	1 % pet	2	Bendewald (2010) 2000–2007 [31]
Patients with suspected ACD from rubber by Mayo Group, $n=376$	MBT	2 % pet	2.7	Bendewald (2010) 2000–2007 [31]
ESSCA – patch test patients (11 EU countries), $n=25{,}181$	MBT	2 % pet	Range 0.2–1.4 %	Uter (2012) 2007–2008 [67]
IVDK – patients with occupational contact dermatitis and suspected glove allergy, $n=3{,}112$	MBT	2 % pet	2.3	Geier (2012) 2002–2010 [2]
IVDK-HCW with occupational contact dermatitis and suspected glove allergy, $n=948$	MBT	2 % pet	1.6	Geier (2012) 2002–2010 [2]
N-cyclohexyl-2-benzothiazyl sulfenamide (CBS)				
IVDK – patients with occupational contact dermatitis and suspected glove allergy, $n=1{,}439$	CBS	1 % pet	1.8	Geier (2003) 1995–2001 [44]
IVDK – patients with occupational contact dermatitis and suspected glove allergy, $n=2{,}480$	CBS	1 % pet	1.6	Geier (2012) 2002–2010 [2]
IVDK-HCW with occupational contact dermatitis and suspected glove allergy, $n=833$	CBS	1 % pet	1.1	Geier (2012) 2002–2010 [2]
Dibenzothiazyl disulfide (MBTS)				
IVDK – patients with occupational contact dermatitis and suspected glove allergy, $n=1{,}439$	MBTS	1 % pet	1	Geier (2003) 1995–2001 [44]
Patients with suspected ACD from rubber by Mayo Group, $n=771$	MBTS	1 % pet	1.2	Bendewald (2010) 2000–2007 [31]

(continued)

Table 19.6 (continued)

Who (n)	Allergen	Patch test preparation	Prevalence (%)	Reference
IVDK – patients with occupational contact dermatitis and suspected glove allergy, $n=2{,}481$	MBTS	1 % pet	1.0	Geier (2012) 2002–2010 [2]
IVDK-HCW with occupational contact dermatitis and suspected glove allergy, $n=834$	MBTS	1 % pet	0.6	Geier (2012) 2002–2010 [2]
Morpholinyl mercaptobenzothiazole (MMBT)				
Patients with suspected ACD from rubber by Mayo Group, $n=770$	MMBT	1 % pet	2.2	Bendewald (2010) 2000–2007 [31]
IVDK – patients with occupational contact dermatitis and suspected glove allergy, $n=2{,}556$	MMBT	1 % pet	2.2	Geier (2012) 2002–2010 [2]
IVDK-HCW with occupational contact dermatitis and suspected glove allergy, $n=833$	MMBT	1 % pet	1.2	Geier (2012) 2002–2010 [2]

NA information not available

MBTS; this indicates that the nature of the mix may vary depending on duration and conditions of storage [77].

Mercapto compounds do not typically cross-react outside of their own group, and although some animal studies have shown cross-sensitization with morpholine, researchers have reported no such cross-sensitization in humans. Cronin has described co-sensitization of TMTD and MBT: 12.1 % of patients in the study reacted to both, but only 7.3 % reacted to MBT alone and 80.6 % to thiuram alone [73, 78]. Mercapto mix appears to have the highest likelihood of occurrence with other allergens, having a high multiple-sensitivity index with a strong association with N-isopropyl-N'-phenyl-p-phenylenediamine, thiuram mix, ZDEC, and p-tert-butylphenol formaldehyde [79].

19.3.5 Thioureas

The use of thioureas as antidegradants and accelerators in rubber-glove production, particularly for polychloroprene (Neoprene), is not as common as use of thiurams, dithiocarbamates, or MBT [49, 80–82]. Thioureas are infrequent allergens, with only 0.1–0.4 % positive reactions in those with suspected glove allergy [2], and the rate is not significantly higher for HCWs [12]. In the EU, prevalence of sensitivity to a variety of thiourea mixtures ranges from 0.1 % to 1.2 % [81] (Table 19.7). Thioureas are the responsible allergen in most cases of ACD from chloroprene [49].

The NACDG has reported that men are significantly more likely to be sensitized (with high clinical relevance) to mixed dialkyl thioureas (MDTU) than other standard-series allergens, with high clinical relevance [49]. In addition to shoes, gloves are one of the most common sources [49], particularly chloroprene sports gloves and medical examination and surgical gloves [81, 82].

The compounds documented to cause contact allergy include diethylthiourea (DETU), dibutylthiourea (DBTU), diphenylthiourea (DPTU), ethylenethiourea (ETU), dimethylthiourea (DMTU), and thiourea (TU) [2, 49, 83, 84].

Patch testing is typically done using mixed dialkyl thioureas (MDTU); however, the mix components are not always the same:

- Two-component MDTUs, which include diethylthiourea and dibutylthiourea [49]
- Three-component MDTUs, which include diethylthiourea, dibutylthiourea, and diphenylthiourea [81]
- Four-component MDTUs, which contain diethylthiourea, dibutylthiourea, diphenylthiourea, and ethylenethiourea [84]

Table 19.7 Review of patch-testing results with thioureas

Who (n)	Allergen	Patch test preparation	Prevalence (%)	Reference
IVDK – patients with occupational contact dermatitis and suspected glove allergy, $n = 1444$	Thioureas	At least 1 to any thiourea	0.4	Geier (2003) 1995–2001 [44]
IVDK– patients with occupational contact dermatitis and suspected glove allergy, $n = 2,487$	Thioureas	At least 1 to any thiourea	0.4	Geier (2012) 2002–2010 [2]
IVDK-HCW with occupational contact dermatitis and suspected glove allergy, $n = 837$	Thioureas	At least 1 to any thiourea	1.0	Geier (2012) 2002–2010 [2]
Mixed dialkyl thioureas (MDTU)				
HCW patch tested by the NACDG, $n = 1,250$	MDTU	1 % pet	0.32	Warshaw (2008) 1998–2004 [12]
Non HCW patch tested by the NACDG, $n = 13,542$	MDTU	DBTU and DETU 1 % pet	0.13	Warshaw (2008) 1998–2004 [12]
Patients tested by the NACDG, $n = 5,807$	MDTU	DBTU and DETU 1 % pet	1.1	Zug (2009) 1998–2000 [66]
Patients tested by the NACDG, $n = 4,897$	MDTU	DBTU and DETU 1 % pet	0.8	Zug (2009) 2001–2002 [66]
Patients tested by the NACDG, $n = 5,140$	MDTU	DBTU and DETU 1 % pet	1	Zug (2009) 2003–2004 [66]
Patients tested by the NACDG, $n = 4,430$	MDTU	DBTU and DETU 1 % pet	1.0	Zug (2009) 2005–2006 [66]
Patients with suspected ACD from rubber by Mayo Group, $n = 738$	MDTU	DBTU and DETU 1 % pet	1.5	Bendewald (2010) 2000–2007 [31]
Diphenylthiourea (DPTU)				
IVDK – patients with occupational contact dermatitis and suspected glove allergy, $n = 1,443$	DPTU	1 % pet	0.3	Geier (2003) 1995–2001 [44]
Patients with suspected ACD from rubber by Mayo Grou, $n = 771$	DPTU	1 % pet	0.4	Bendewald (2010) 2000–2007 [31]
IVDK – patients with occupational contact dermatitis and suspected glove allergy, $n = 2,479$	DPTU	1 % pet	0.3	Geier (2012) 2002–2010 [2]
IVDK-HCW with occupational contact dermatitis and suspected glove allergy, $n = 833$	DPTU	1 % pet	0.5	Geier (2012) 2002–2010 [2]
Dibutylthiourea (DBTU)				
IVDK – patients with occupational contact dermatitis and suspected glove allergy, $n = 1,436$	DBTU	1 % pet	0.1	Geier (2003) 1995–2001 [44]
Patients with suspected ACD from rubber by Mayo Group, $n = 770$	DBTU	1 % pet	0.9	Bendewald (2010) 2000–2007 [31]
IVDK – patients with occupational contact dermatitis and suspected glove allergy, $n = 2,473$	DBTU	1 % pet	0.2	Geier (2012) 2002–2010 [2]
IVDK-HCW with occupational contact dermatitis and suspected glove allergy, $n = 834$	DBTU	1 % pet	0.6	Geier (2012) 2002–2010 [2]

When reviewing prevalence rates among international groups, prevalence ranges from 0.03 % to 3.5 %, which may be reflective of this difference in the mixes used for patch testing [12, 31].

McCleskey and Swerlick have reported that using MDTU containing only DETU and DBTU in testing for ACD may underestimate the prevalence, missing up to 25 % of thiourea-induced rubber ACD; this suggests that additional thioureas be tested either in the mix or individually [85].

Warshaw et al. have reported 24.9 % of their MDTU-positive patients have co-sensitization to another rubber chemical [49], while Comfere et al. found that up to 50 % of their patients with patch test reactions to thiourea also reacted to other rubber chemicals, with carba mix and thiuram mix the most common co-reactors [84]. Liippo et al. also reported concurrent reactions to other rubber chemicals, including thiuram, DPG, carbamates, MBT, components of black rubber mix, and diaminodiphenylmethane in 24 % of their MDTU-positive patients [81].

19.3.6 Other Allergens in Gloves

19.3.6.1 Xanthates

Sasseville et al. reported in 2007 that 50 % of patients sensitized to carbamates, thiurams, or mercaptobenzothiazole exhibit cross-reactions with xanthates. Xanthates are irritants, and it has been recommended that patch test concentrations be lowered to 5 % or less [69]. Further, the researchers hypothesized that, if cross-reactivity works both ways, 50 % of those in the mining industry with xanthate allergy could be at risk for developing contact dermatitis when exposed to carbamates, thiurams, and MBT [69].

19.3.6.2 Dithiodimorpholine

Dithiodimorpholine (DTDM) is a vulcanizing agent reported to be the cause of ACD in two HCWs with nitrile glove–related dermatitis [64]. The Mayo Group found that 4,4-dithiodimorpholine produced the highest proportion of positive reactions [31].

19.3.6.3 Disproportionated Rosins

Researchers have identified chemical species consistent with the composition of disproportionated rosins (dehydroabietic acid [DHA], didehydroabietic acid, and other pimaric or isopimaric species) in dichloromethane extracts of four brands of chloroprene gloves. Despite this DHA exposure, researchers have not established a potential association with ACD from gloves [71]. Dermatologists might consider patch-testing glove-allergic patients with (oxidized) colophony or disproportionated rosin in addition to other allergenic accelerators in chloroprene gloves [71].

19.3.6.4 Glove Powder

Accelerator content may be lower in powder-free (PF) gloves, because of the methods used to produce them. The powder from the glove containing the highest recorded amount of accelerator, however, did not contain measurable accelerator in the powder fraction, suggesting that these hydrophobic accelerators do not selectively partition to the powder, as do the water-soluble latex-protein allergens [3].

19.3.6.5 Formaldehyde

Researchers have found emissions of formaldehyde from flock-lined PVC, nitrile, and NRL household gloves [14, 50]. The investigator reported that the inside of the glove generally emitted the most formaldehyde.

19.3.6.6 Antioxidants

Antioxidants used in NRL examination gloves include 4,4-thiobis (6-tert-butyl-meta-cresol) (Lowinox 44S36) and butylhydroxyanisole, and researchers have reported them to cause ACD [86]. One study has reported 2,2′-methylene-bis-(4-methyl-6-tert-butylphenol) as a source of sensitization from a nitrile glove [51].

19.3.6.7 Antimicrobials

Cetyl peridinium chloride is a quaternary ammonium compound used as an antimicrobial in some gloves. Several reports have implicated this chemical in glove allergies from NRL [87, 88].

19.3.7 ACD to PVC

The market for PVC gloves has expanded remarkably owing to concern over NRL protein allergy. Although not as common as ACD from rubber examination gloves, researchers have reported contact dermatitis to PVC in both examination and household gloves, as follows:

- Bisphenol A – antioxidant and inhibitor [52, 53]
- Irgalite orange – organic pigments [89]
- Formaldehyde [50]
- Adipic polyester – plasticizer [54]
- Poly(adipic acid-*co*-1,2-propylene glycol)-plasticizer [54, 55]
- Benzisothiazolinone (BIT) – slimicide and antimicrobial [90]

- Di-(*n*-octyl)tin-bis(2-ethylhexylmaleate) – stabilizer [55, 91]
- Tricresyl phosphate [92]
- Triphenyl phosphate [93]
- Methyldiclorobenzenesulfonate [92]
- Diisodecyl phthalate (DIDP) – plasticizer [94]

Ponten et al. tested three types of gloves (PVC, nitrile, and NRL) and showed delayed reactions were just as common for PVC industrial gloves as for rubber, at least for the reusable glove with flocked lining [50].

Conclusion

Both the chemicals in gloves and the chemicals to which particular professions expose individuals can cause hand dermatitis. Health-care workers, cleaners, hairdressers, and food service workers are particularly at risk because of frequent and/or prolonged exposure to water and/or chemical irritants and allergens. Use of gloves in itself has risks because some chemicals in gloves are known allergens. Since manufacture of protective gloves will always require use of chemicals, some individuals will always develop sensitivity to them. The primary sensitizers in gloves are sulfur-containing chemicals, such as thiurams, dithiocarbamates, and MBT derivatives. All individuals using protective gloves and their dermatologists need to be aware that random selection of a different type of glove will not necessarily resolve current or prevent future dermatitis. Successful treatment requires identification of the causative allergen(s) and selection of gloves that do not contain that allergen.

References

1. Wrangsjo K. IgE-mediated latex allergy and contact allergy to rubber in clinical occupational dermatology. Stockholm: National Institute of Occupational Health; 1993.
2. Geier J, Lessmann H, Mahler V, Pohrt U, Uter W. Occupational contact allergy caused by rubber gloves – nothing has changed. Contact Dermatitis. 2012;67(3):149–56.
3. Depree GJ, Bledsoe TA, Siegel PD. Survey of sulfur-containing rubber accelerator levels in latex and nitrile exam gloves. Contact Dermatitis. 2005;53(2):107–13.
4. Apfelbacher CJ, Soder S, Diepgen TL, Weisshaar E. The impact of measures for secondary individual prevention of work-related skin diseases in health care workers: 1-year follow-up study. Contact Dermatitis. 2009;60(3):144–9.
5. Zhai H, Maibach HI. Skin occlusion and irritant and allergic contact dermatitis: an overview. Contact Dermatitis. 2001;44(4):201–6.
6. Duarte I, Nakano JT, Lazzarini R. Hand eczema: evaluation of 250 patients. Dermatitis. 1998;9(4):216–23.
7. Flyvholm MA, Lindberg M. OEESC-2005 summing up on the theme irritants and wet work. Contact Dermatitis. 2006;55(6):317–21.
8. Makela EA, Vainiotalo S, Peltonen K. The permeability of surgical gloves to seven chemicals commonly used in hospitals. Ann Occup Hyg. 2003;47(4):313–23.
9. Held E, Jorgensen LL. The combined use of moisturizers and occlusive gloves: an experimental study. Dermatitis. 1999;10(3):146–52.
10. Ramsing DW, Agner T. Effect of glove occlusion on human skin (II): long-term experimental exposure. Contact Dermatitis. 1996;34:258–62.
11. Brehler R, Voss W, Muller S. Glove powder affects skin roughness, one parameter of skin irritation. Contact Dermatitis. 1998;39(5):227–30.
12. Warshaw EM, Schram SE, Maibach HI, Belsito DV, Marks JG, Fowler JF, et al. Occupation-related contact dermatitis in North American health care workers referred for patch testing: cross-sectional data, 1998 to 2004. Dermatitis. 2008;19(5):261–74.
13. Burke FJT, Wilson NHF, Cheung SW. Factors associated with skin irritation of the hands experienced by general dental practitioners. Contact Dermatitis. 1995;32:35–8.
14. Ponten A, Dubnika I. Delayed reactions to reusable protective gloves. Contact Dermatitis. 2009; 60(4):227–9.
15. Boyle DK, Forsyth A, Bagg J, Stroubou K, Griffiths CE, Burke FJ. An investigation of the effect of prolonged glove wearing on the hand skin health of dental healthcare workers. J Dent. 2002;30(5–6):233–41.
16. Wetzky U, Bock M, Wulfhorst B, John SM. Short- and long-term effects of single and repetitive glove occlusion on the epidermal barrier. Arch Dermatol Res. 2009;301:595–602.
17. Fartasch M, Taeger D, Broding HC, Schoneweis S, Gellert B, Pohrt U, et al. Evidence of increased skin irritation after wet work: impact of water exposure and occlusion. Contact Dermatitis. 2012;67(4):217–28.
18. Wrangsjo K, Meding B. Hospital workers. Clin Dermatol. 1997;15(4):573–8.
19. Filon FL, Radman G. Latex allergy: a follow up study of 1040 healthcare workers. Occup Environ Med. 2006;63(2):121–5.
20. Latza U, Haamann F, Baur X. Effectiveness of a nationwide interdisciplinary preventive programme for latex allergy. Int Arch Occup Environ Health. 2005;78(5):394–402.
21. Mahler V, Fischer S, Fuchs T, Ghannadan M, Valent P, Fartasch M, et al. Prevention of latex allergy by

selection of low-allergen gloves. Clin Exp Allergy. 2000;30(4):509–20.
22. Brehler R, Rutter A, Kutting B. Allergenicity of natural rubber latex gloves. Contact Dermatitis. 2002;46(2):65–71.
23. Lezaun A, Marcos C, Martin JA, Quirce S, Gomez M. Contact dermatitis from natural latex. Contact Dermatitis. 1992;27(5):334–5.
24. Wyss M, Elsner P, Wuthrich B, Burg G. Allergic contact dermatitis from natural latex without contact urticaria. Contact Dermatitis. 1993;28:154–6.
25. Wilkinson SM, Beck MH. Allergic contact dermatitis from latex rubber. Br J Dermatol. 1996;134(5):910–4.
26. Mellstrom GA, Boman AS. Gloves: types, materials, and manufacturing. In: Mellstrom GA, Wahlberg JE, Maibach HI, editors. Protective gloves for occupational use. Boca Raton: CRC Press; 1994. p. 21–35.
27. Truscott W. Manufacturing methods sought to eliminate or reduce sensitivity to natural rubber products. In: Food and Drug Administration Center for Devices and Radiological Health, editor. Program and Proceedings. International latex conference: sensitivity to latex in medical devices, Baltimore, 1992, p. 66.
28. Skoet R, Olsen J, Mathiesen B, Iversen L, Johansen JD, Agner T. A survey of occupational hand eczema in Denmark. Contact Dermatitis. 2004;51(4):159–66.
29. Boman A, Estlander T, Wahlberg JE. Protective gloves for occupational use. 2nd ed. Boca Raton: CRC Press; 2005.
30. Holness DL, Mace SR. Results of evaluating health care workers with prick and patch testing. Am J Contact Dermat. 2001;12(2):88–92.
31. Bendewald MJ, Farmer SA, Davis MDP. An 8-year retrospective review of patch testing with rubber allergens: the Mayo Clinic experience. Dermatitis. 2010;21(1):33–40.
32. Suneja T, Belsito DV. Occupational dermatoses in health care workers evaluated for suspected allergic contact dermatitis. Contact Dermatitis. 2008;58(5):285–90.
33. Andreasson H, Boman A, Johnsson S, Karlsson S, Barregard L. On permeability of methyl methacrylate, 2-hydroxyethyl methacrylate and triethyleneglycol dimethacrylate through protective gloves in dentistry. Eur J Oral Sci. 2003;111(6):529–35.
34. Ravis SM, Shaffer MP, Shaffer C, Dehkharghani S, Belsito D. Glutaraldehyde-induced and formaldehyde-induced allergic contact dermatitis among dental hygienists and dental assistants. J Am Dent Assoc. 2003;134:1072–8.
35. Mirabelli MC, Vizcaya D, Martí Margarit A, Antó JM, Arjona L, Barreiro E, et al. Occupational risk factors for hand dermatitis among professional cleaners in Spain. Contact Dermatitis. 2012;66(4):188–96.
36. Liskowsky J, Geier J, Bauer A. Contact allergy in the cleaning industry: analysis of contact allergy surveillance data of the Information Network of Departments of Dermatology. Contact Dermatitis. 2011;65(3):159–66.
37. Jungbauer FHW, van der Harst JJ, Schuttelaar ML, Groothoff JW, Coenraads PJ. Characteristics of wet work in the cleaning industry. Contact Dermatitis. 2004;51(3):131–4.
38. Uter W, Hegewald J, Pfahlberg A, Lessmann H, Schnuch A. Contact allergy to thiurams: multifactorial analysis of clinical surveillance data collected by the IVDK network. Int Arch Occup Environ Health. 2010;83:675–81.
39. Mygind K, Sell L, Flyvholm MA, Jepsen KF. High-fat petrolatum-based moisturizers and prevention of work-related skin problems in wet-work occupations. Contact Dermatitis. 2006;54(1):35–41.
40. Nixon R, Roberts H, Frowen K, Sim M. Knowledge of skin hazards and the use of gloves by Australian hairdressing students and practising hairdressers. Contact Dermatitis. 2006;54(2):112–6.
41. Lysdal SH, Johansen JD, Flyvholm MA, Sosted H. A quantification of occupational skin exposures and the use of protective gloves among hairdressers in Denmark. Contact Dermatitis. 2012;66(6):323–34.
42. Nettis E, Dambra P, Soccio AL, Ferrannini A, Tursi A. Latex hypersensitivity: relationship with positive prick test and patch test responses among hairdressers. Allergy. 2003;58(1):57–61.
43. Andrea B, Geier J, Elsner P. Type-IV allergy in the food processing industry: sensitization profiles in bakers, cooks and butchers. Contact Dermatitis. 2002;46(4):228–35.
44. Geier J, Lessmann H, Uter W, Schnuch A. Occupational rubber glove allergy: results of the Information Network of Departments of Dermatology (IVDK), 1995–2001. Contact Dermatitis. 2003;48(1):39–44.
45. Rose RF, Lyons P, Horne H, Wilkinson SM. A review of the materials and allergens in protective gloves. Contact Dermatitis. 2009;61(3):129–37.
46. Knudsen BB, Hametner C, Seycek O, Heese A, Koch HU, Peters KP. Allergologically relevant rubber accelerators in single-use medical gloves. Contact Dermatitis. 2000;43(1):9–15.
47. Bhargava K, White IR, White ML. Thiuram patch test positivity 1980–2006: incidence is now falling. Contact Dermatitis. 2009;60(4):222–3.
48. Chipinda I, Hettick JM, Simoyi RH, Siegel PD. Zinc diethyldithiocarbamate allergenicity: potential haptenation mechanisms. Contact Dermatitis. 2008;59(2):79–89.
49. Warshaw EM, Cook JW, Belsito DV, DeLeo VA, Fowler JF, Maibach HI, et al. Positive patch-test reactions to mixed dialkyl thioureas: cross-sectional data from the north American contact dermatitis group, 1994 to 2004. Dermatitis. 2008;19(4):190–201.
50. Ponten A. Formaldehyde in reusable protective gloves. Contact Dermatitis. 2006;54(5):268–71.
51. Horn HM, Aldridge RD. Contact urticaria due to nitrile gloves. Contact Dermatitis. 2003;49(3):163–4.
52. Aalto-Korte K, Alanko K, Henriks-Eckerman ML, Estlander T, Jolanki R. Allergic contact dermatitis from bisphenol A in PVC gloves. Contact Dermatitis. 2003;49(4):202–5.
53. Matthieu L, Godoi AFL, Lambert J, van Grieken R. Occupational allergic contact dermatitis from

bisphenol A in vinyl gloves. Contact Dermatitis. 2003;49(6):281–3.
54. Sowa J, Kobayashi H, Tsuruta D, Sugawara K, Ishii M. Allergic contact dermatitis due to adipic polyester in vinyl chloride gloves. Contact Dermatitis. 2005;53(4):243–4.
55. Ueno M, Adachi A, Horikawa T, Inoue N, Mori A, Sasaki K. Allergic contact dermatitis caused by poly(adipic acid-co-1,2-propylene glycol) and di-(n-octyl) tin-bis(2-ethylhexylmaleate) in vinyl chloride gloves. Contact Dermatitis. 2007;57(5):349–51.
56. Kligman AM. The spectrum of contact urticaria: wheals, erythema, pruritus. Dermatol Clin. 1990;8(1):57–60.
57. von Hintzenstern J, Heese A, Koch HU, Peters K-P, Hornstein OP. Frequency, spectrum and occupational relevance of type IV allergies to rubber chemicals. Contact Dermatitis. 1991;24:244–52.
58. De Jong WH, Van Och FM, Den Hartog Jager CF, Spiekstra SW, Slob W, Vandebriel RJ, et al. Ranking of allergenic potency of rubber chemicals in a modified local lymph node assay. Toxicol Sci. 2002;66(2):226–323.
59. Estlander T, Jolanki R, Kanerva L. Allergic contact dermatitis from rubber and plastic gloves. In: Mellstrom GA, Wahlberg JE, Maibach HI, editors. Protective gloves for occupational use. Boca Raton: CRC Press; 1994. p. 221–39.
60. Frosch PJ, Born M, Schutz R. Contact allergy to rubber, surgical and vinyl gloves [Kontaktallergien auf gummi-, operations und vinylhandschuhe]. Hautarzt. 1987;38(4):210–7.
61. Knudsen B, Lerbaek A, Johansen JD, Menne T. Reduction in the frequency of sensitization to thiurams. A result of legislation? Contact Dermatitis. 2006;54(3):170–1.
62. Kaniwa M, Isama K, Nakamura A, Kantoh H, Hosono K, Itoh M, et al. Identification of causative chemicals of allergic contact dermatitis using a combination of patch testing in patients and chemical analysis application to cases from rubber gloves. Contact Dermatitis. 1994;31(2):65–71.
63. Siegel PD, Fowler JFJ, Storrs FJ, Sasseville D, Pratt M, Bledsoe TA, et al. Allergen content of patient problem and nonproblem gloves: relationship to allergen specific patch test findings. Dermatitis. 2010;21(2):77–83.
64. Silvestri DL. Rubber glove dermatitis and allergy to dithiodimorpholine. Dermatitis. 2012;23(4):187–8.
65. Jensen P, Menne T, Thyssen JP. Allergic contact dermatitis in a nurse caused by airborne rubber additives. Contact Dermatitis. 2011;65(1):54–5.
66. Zug KA, Warshaw EM, Fowler JFJ, Maibach HI, Belsito DL, Pratt MD, et al. Patch test results of the North American Contact Dermatitis Group 2005–2006. Dermatitis. 2009;20(3):149–60.
67. Uter W, Aberer W, Armario-Hita JC, Fernandez-Vozmediano JM, Ayala F, Balato A, et al. Current patch test results with the European baseline series and extensions to it from the European Surveillance System on Contact Allergy Network, 2007–2008. Contact Dermatitis. 2012;67(1):9–19.
68. Utas S, Ferahbas A, Yildiz S. Patients with vulval pruritus: patch test results. Contact Dermatitis. 2008;58(5):296–8.
69. Sasseville D, Mowza AS, Moreau L. Cross-reactions between xanthates and rubber additives. Dermatitis. 2007;18(3):150–4.
70. Bergendorff O, Persson C, Hansson C. High-performance liquid chromatography analysis of rubber allergens in protective gloves used in health care. Contact Dermatitis. 2006;55(4):210–5.
71. Siegel PD, Law BF, Fowler JF, Fowler LM. Disproportionated rosin dehydroabietic acid in neoprene surgical gloves. Dermatitis. 2010;21(3):157–9.
72. Adams AK, Yiannias JA. Mercaptobenzothiazole and mercapto mix. Dermatitis. 2008;19(5):E39–41.
73. Adams AK, Warshaw EM. Allergic contact dermatitis from mercapto compounds. Dermatitis. 2006;17(2):56–70.
74. Scherrer MA, Fialho E. Rubber contact allergy: evaluation in patients patch tested from 1999 to 2007 in Brazil. 2008 Annual ACDS meeting abstracts: oral presentations dermatitis: May/June 2008;19(3):172.
75. Diepgen TL, Bruynzeel DP, Andersen KE, Brandao FM, Bruze M, Goncalo M, et al. Mercaptobenzothiazole or the mercapto-mix: which should be in the standard series? Contact Dermatitis. 2006;55(1):36–8.
76. Geier J, Uter W, Schnuch A, Brasch J. Diagnostic screening for contact allergy to mercaptobenzothiazole derivatives. Am J Contact Dermat. 2002;13(2):66–70.
77. Hansson C, Agrup G. Stability of mercaptobenzothiazole compounds. Contact Dermatitis. 1993;28(1):29–34.
78. Cronin E. Shoe dermatitis. Br J Dermatol. 1966;78:618–25.
79. Dickel H, Taylor JS, Bickers DR, Merk HF, Bruckner TM. Multiple patch-test reactions: a pilot evaluation of a combination approach to visualize patterns of multiple sensitivity in patch-test databases and a proposal for a multiple sensitivity index. Am J Contact Dermat. 2003;14(3):148–53.
80. Scheman A, Jacob S, Zirwas M, Warshaw E, Nedorost S, Katta R, et al. Contact allergy: alternatives for the 2007 North American Contact Dermatitis Group (NACDG) standard screening tray. Dis Mon. 2008;54(1–2):7–156.
81. Liippo J, Ackermann L, Hasan T, Laukkanen A, Rantanen T, Lammintausta K. Sensitization to thiourea derivatives among Finnish patients with suspected contact dermatitis. Contact Dermatitis. 2010;63(1):37–41.
82. Kohli N, Habbal S. Occupational allergic contact dermatitis due to thioureas. Dermatitis. 2010;21(1):E5–6.
83. Dooms-Goossens A, Chrispeels MT, de Veylder H, Roelandts R, Willems L, Degreef H. Contact and photocontact sensitivity problems associated with thiourea and its derivatives: a review of the literature and case reports. Br J Dermatol. 1987;116(4):573–9.

84. Comfere NI, Davis MDP, Fett DD. Patch test reactions to thioureas are frequently relevant. Dermatitis. 2005;16(3):121–3.
85. McCleskey PE, Swerlick RA. Clinical review: thioureas and allergic contact dermatitis. Cutis. 2001;68(6):387–96.
86. Rich P, Belozer ML, Norris P, Storrs FJ. Allergic contact dermatitis to two antioxidants in latex gloves: 4,4-thiobis (6-tert-butyl-meta-cresol) (Lowinox 44S36) and butylhydroxyanisole. J Am Acad Dermatol. 1991;24(1):37–43.
87. Castelain M, Castelain PY. Allergic contact dermatitis from cetyl pyridinium chloride in latex gloves. Contact Dermatitis. 1993;28(2):118.
88. Steinkjer B. Contact dermatitis from cetyl pyridinium chloride in latex surgical gloves. Contact Dermatitis. 1998;39(1):29–30.
89. Kanerva L, Jolanki R, Estlander T. Organic pigment as a cause of plastic glove dermatitis. Contact Dermatitis. 1985;13(1):41–3.
90. Aalto-Korte K, Ackermann L, Henriks-Eckerman ML, Valimaa J, Reinikka-Railo H, Leppanen E, et al. 1,2-Benzisothiazolin-3-one in disposable polyvinyl chloride gloves for medical use. Contact Dermatitis. 2007;57(6):365–70.
91. Ito A, Imura T, Sasaki K, Kakihara K, Mori A, Ito M. Allergic contact dermatitis due to mono(2-ethylhexyl) maleate in di-(n-octyl)tin-bis(2-ethylhexyl maleate) in polyvinyl chloride gloves. Contact Dermatitis. 2009;60(1):59–61.
92. Estlander T, Jolanki R, Kanerva L. Dermatitis and urticaria from rubber and plastic gloves. Contact Dermatitis. 1986;14(1):20–5.
93. Suuronen K, Pesonen M, Henriks-Eckerman ML, Aalto-Korte K. Triphenyl phosphite, a new allergen in polyvinylchloride gloves. Contact Dermatitis. 2012;68:42–9.
94. Lensen GJ, Jungbauer FHW, Coenraads PJ, Schuttelaar MLA. Contact allergy to di-isodecyl phthalate. Contact Dermatitis. 2012;66(4):230–1.

Hand Eczema in the Construction Industry

20

Johannes Geier

Contents

J. Geier, M.D.
Information Network of Departments of Dermatology (IVDK), University of Goettingen, von-Siebold-Str. 3, Goettingen 37075, Germany
e-mail: jgeier@gwdg.de

20.1 Introduction

Occupational hand eczema occurs frequently among bricklayers, construction workers, tile setters, and others working in the building trade. In this chapter, four items are presented: (1) specific exposure, including allergens and irritants; (2) particular clinical aspects; (3) frequent contact sensitizers and resulting patch test recommendations; and (4) preventive measures.

20.2 Specific Exposure

20.2.1 Cement and Concrete

From the viewpoint of occupational dermatology, cement is still one of the most important occupational contact materials in the construction industry. It is produced by burning ground raw materials (limestone, clay, etc.) at up to 1,500 °C to cement clinker, which consists mainly of calcium silicates, -aluminates, and -ferrites. The clinker is mixed with calcium sulfate, forming the proper cement. Cement contains chromate as a result of contamination of the raw materials or abrasion from steel surfaces during the production process. Cement also may contain traces of cobalt and nickel [1–6]. Cement is a constituent of concrete, mortar, plaster, and screed. Concrete is a mixture of cement, stones, additives, and water. Additives are liquefiers, setting retarders or accelerators, sealants, and so forth. Lignin sulfonates or sulfonates of melamine-, naphthalene-,

A. Alikhan et al. (eds.), *Textbook of Hand Eczema*,
DOI 10.1007/978-3-642-39546-8_20, © Springer-Verlag Berlin Heidelberg 2014

or phenol-formaldehyde condensates, and polyacrylates are used as liquefiers. Tributyl phosphate serves as an antifoaming agent. Sealants are often metal salts of stearic acid or oleic acid. Concrete additives may be preserved with formaldehyde releasers, isothiazolinones, or phenols [3, 7, 8].

Wet cement is alkaline (pH > 12), owing to its content of calcium oxide, which reacts to calcium hydroxide with water. In addition, cement is hygroscopic and abrasive. Therefore, cement may cause irritant contact dermatitis with skin exsiccation [9–12]. Being hygroscopic, cement dust on sweaty skin may form "wet" cement and act as an irritant. Hardened cement is generally recognized as safe with regard to irritant or allergic reactions [9, 10, 13].

The most important allergen in cement is hexavalent chromium (i.e., chromate; Cr VI). Water-soluble Cr VI penetrates the skin easily. In the skin, it is reduced to trivalent chromium and bound to protein complexes, which probably are the actual hapten [14–16]. Chromate contents of cement may vary a lot; up to 25 ppm have been found in the past [17]. According to Avnstorp, more than 2 ppm of Cr VI is necessary to induce allergic sensitization, while the elicitation threshold is about 1 ppm [1]. By adding ferrous sulfate to the cement, Cr VI is reduced to Cr III, which in the alkaline milieu of cement is present as hardly soluble chromium hydroxide/oxide. The concentration of water-soluble Cr VI is kept below 2 ppm this way. This has been practiced in Scandinavian countries for decades and has proved to successfully prevent allergic contact eczema to cement [11, 12, 18, 19].

Cobalt in cement occurs as hardly soluble cobalt oxide. In the presence of free amino acids, water-soluble cobalt complexes are formed, which can elicit positive patch test reactions in sensitized individuals [5]. In eczematous skin, the epidermal barrier is damaged, and there are more free amino acids than in healthy skin. Therefore, secondary contact allergy to cobalt is frequent among patients with allergic cement eczema, who are primarily sensitized to chromate [5].

In contrast, acquiring contact allergy to nickel by handling cement is very unlikely because nickel in cement is only present as non-water-soluble nickel oxide, which is not transformed to a water-soluble state [5, 6, 18].

20.2.2 Resins and Glues

Tile setters, floor layers, and others are not only exposed to cement-containing products but also to resins and glues such as epoxy resin systems, formaldehyde resins, and polyurethanes [9, 20]. Epoxy resin systems are used for floor and wall coatings, for concrete repair, and for filling cracks in stone and concrete. An epoxy resin system consists of the basic resin, reactive diluents to adjust viscosity, and hardeners. Additionally, filler materials, pigments, and other additives may be present. Contact allergens in these systems are not only the basic resins, mostly based on diglycidyl ether of bisphenol A or F, but also hardeners, such as m-xylidene diamine or isophorone diamine, and reactive diluents such as 1,6-hexanediol diglycidyl ether and other glycidyl ethers [17, 20–22]. Amine hardeners may also irritate the skin [10]. Phenol-formaldehyde resins and urea-formaldehyde resins are used as adhesives for wood and floor coatings [22, 23]. Adhesives may be preserved, for instance, with isothiazolinones [23–25]. For insulation in hollow spaces, and in fitting of windows and door cases, polyurethane foams are used; polyurethane adhesives are common in floor laying [23, 25]. Polyurethanes are reaction products of polyalcohols with di- or polyvalent isocyanates. The latter are skin and airway sensitizers [21, 22, 26].

20.2.3 Additional Exposure

Many tools, in particular those for tile setting, have rubber handles or are made of rubber. Contact with rubber allergens in the construction industry also occurs through gloves, hoses, gaskets, and so forth. [11, 12, 27].

Insulation material made from mineral wool (glass wool, rock wool) is being used widely. It usually contains at least 90 % artificial mineral fibers, up to 7 % artificial resins (phenol- or urea-formaldehyde resins), and about 1 % oils and other additives. The resins are cured in a hot air stream, which removes volatile components like phenol or formaldehyde from the product [28]. Mineral wool may cause a specific type of irritant dermatitis (see below).

Removing residual lime or shades of cement from tiles and cleaning stone, clinker, or concrete surfaces is often done using phosphorous acid, hydrochloric acid, sulfamido acid, solvents, or detergents, which may be irritating to the skin [8, 9].

Generally, employees working in the building trade used to have contact with solvents, gasoline, technical oils, greases, and the like. Solvents are misused as hand cleaning agents [23].

Pitch and tar, which can cause phototoxic reactions and folliculitis, were in use until the 1970s for insulation of roofs, basements, and floors [23]. Nowadays, bitumen is used for these purposes.

20.3 Clinical Aspects of Occupational Hand Eczema in the Building Trade

Skin irritated by cement is dry, sclerotic, and fissured. Nails often are tarnished and brittle. Chronic allergic contact dermatitis to cement often presents as dry, infiltrated, pachydermic, sometimes hyperkeratotic eczema with fissures and rhagades [9–12]. A mycological investigation should be performed because not infrequently secondary tinea manuum complicates the skin disease [29]. Cement also may cause acute damage to the skin; fortunately, however, cement burns are rare events and usually do not affect the hands [30]. These burns often start hours after contact with a dark erythema or a bluish livid discoloration of the skin. Within 24–48 h, blisters, ulcers, or necroses develop. In most cases, cement burns occur after intense contact with wet cement under pressure, for instance, when kneeling in wet cement or when wet cement contaminates the inside of shoes [9, 10]. Prolonged and intense contact with wet cement may also lead to toxic paronychia and subungual necrosis [9, 10, 21].

Dermatitis caused by artificial mineral fibers is itchy and presents with little papules, folliculitis, or petechiae; however, it rarely affects the hands, but rather the flexures or regions with intense contact with contaminated clothes [9, 10, 23].

20.4 Contact Sensitizers and Patch Test Recommendations

In Scandinavian countries, chromate-reduced cement with less than 2 ppm hexavalent chromium has been used since the 1980s. Since then, allergic cement eczema has declined significantly, and contact allergy to chromate is no longer a specific and urgent problem in the construction industry [18, 19]. In other European countries, however, it took much longer to convince cement producers, employers, and responsible authorities of the advantages of chromate-reduced cement. It was not before 2000 that a corresponding voluntary trade agreement was signed in Germany [27]. Since 2003, a European Union (EU) regulation makes the use of chromate-reduced cement containing less than 2 ppm Cr VI mandatory when direct skin contact cannot be excluded [31]. Since then, chromate sensitization has declined significantly in the building trade [32]. However, according to current (2009–2011) data from the Information Network of Departments of Dermatology (IVDK) in Germany, Switzerland, and Austria, contact allergy to chromate still occurs frequently, probably due to earlier sensitization [33].

IVDK data analyses from the 1990s showed that the following allergens were most important in bricklayers, construction workers, tile setters, and others in the building industry with occupational dermatitis: chromate; cobalt; rubber chemicals such as thiurams, mercaptobenzothiazole, and its derivatives; N-isopropyl-N'-phenyl-p-phenylenediamine (IPPD); and epoxy resin [34, 35]. A multifactorial data analysis based on data from 1992 to 2000 confirmed that even when potential confounders were taken into consideration, sensitization to chromate, cobalt, epoxy resin, thiurams, and IPPD was significantly increased among these patients [36, 37]. Furthermore, a strong association between chromate and cobalt sensitization could be noted [36, 37]. Similar findings were made in a register of occupational skin disease in Northern Bavaria, Germany [38]. Notably, there is no association between nickel allergy and cement eczema [18, 37]. The spectrum of rubber allergens and the association between sensitizations to chromate and cobalt have been confirmed in IVDK data from 2009 to 2011 [33].

Current IVDK data reveal that contact allergy to epoxy resin has been increasing during the last decade [33, 39]. In 2009 to 2011, sensitization to epoxy resin was almost as frequent as sensitization to chromate among bricklayers, construction workers, tile setters, and so on with occupational dermatitis [33]. About two-thirds of these patients were not only sensitized to the basic resin based on diglycidyl ether of bisphenol A or F (DGEBA or DGEBF), but also to reactive diluents and amine hardeners. Among the diluents, 1,6-hexanediol diglycidyl ether and 1,4-butanediol diglycidyl ether were the leading allergens, with a high proportion of concomitant reactions. However, sensitization to aromatic glycidyl ethers such as phenyl glycidyl ether (PGE), cresyl glycidyl ether, and p-tert-butylphenyl glycidyl ether was also found. Here, too, concomitant reactions among this group were frequent, probably due to immunological cross-reactivity [33]. Cross-reactions of epoxy resin based in DGEBA and PGE may occur, due to immunological cross-reactivity [40, 41]. Among the amine hardeners used in epoxy resin systems, m-xylidene diamine (MXDA) is the most frequent allergen, far more frequent than isophorone diamine (IPDA) [33, 42, 43].

4,4′-Diaminodiphenylmethane (syn. 4,4′-methylenedianiline or MDA) is a suspected carcinogen and, therefore, no longer in use in epoxy resin systems. However, contact sensitization to MDA is frequently found in construction workers with occupational dermatitis [33]. In these patients, positive patch test reactions to MDA probably indicate sensitization to diphenylmethan-4,4′-diisocyanate (MDI) [44]. The underlying mechanism is as follows. Like all diisocyanates, MDI is very reactive. On contact with water (or humidity, e.g., on the skin), the corresponding amine, namely, MDA, is formed. In addition, MDA may be formed from MDI in the skin [45]. Patch test preparations with isocyanates are rather unstable owing to their high reactivity. Hence, the diisocyanate content of these preparations is often far below the declared concentration, and patch testing with these components is rather uncertain [46]. Therefore, patch testing with MDA as a surrogate is recommended [44, 45]. Sensitization to MDI in the construction industry may be acquired by handling two-component polyurethane glues, foams, and so forth.

Among the preservatives, currently methylisothiazolinone (MI) is of outstanding allergological importance, not only in general, but also in construction workers with occupational dermatitis [33, 47]. The recent increase in sensitization to this biocide is probably due to its increased use in industrial and skin care products. A high proportion of patients sensitized to MI this way also react to methylchloroisothiazolinone/methylisothiazolinone (MCI/MI) [47].

Considering frequent and important allergens in this branch, the German Contact Dermatitis Research Group (Deutsche Kontaktallergie-Gruppe; DKG) recommends to patch test the baseline series, the rubber series, and the DKG series "construction industry" (Table 20.1) in bricklayers, tile setters, construction workers, and so on with suspected occupational contact allergy [48].

20.5 Preventive Measures

As mentioned above, the most important preventive measure to reduce allergic contact eczema to cement is lowering the content of water-soluble Cr VI to less than 2 ppm. According to studies from the 1990s, wearing gloves did not efficiently prevent allergic cement dermatitis [11, 12, 18]. This is no surprise, because in the construction industry gloves consisting primarily of leather and textile fabric are worn, which are easily soaked and penetrated and do not protect against any harmful substance. When working with cement or concrete, it is recommended that nitrile-coated cotton gloves be worn [49]. However, these gloves do not protect against allergens in

Table 20.1 Patch test series "construction industry" recommended by German Contact Dermatitis Research Group (DKG). To be tested in addition to the baseline series and the rubber series

No.	Allergen	Concentration
Components of epoxy resin systems		
1	Diethylenetriamine	1 % pet.
2	4,4′-Diaminodiphenyl methane	0.5 % pet.
3	Isophorone diamine	0.5 % pet.
4	Butyl glycidyl ether	0.25 % pet.
5	Cresyl glycidyl ether	0.25 % pet.
6	Phenyl glycidyl ether	0.25 % pet.
7	1,4-Butanediol diglycidyl ether	0.25 % pet.
8	1,6-Hexanediol diglycidyl ether	0.25 % pet.
9	Trimethylhexane-1,6-diamine	0.5 % pet.
10	p-tert-Butylphenyl glycidyl ether	0.25%pet.
11	m-Xylylene diamine	0.1 % pet.
12	Trimethylolpropane triglycidyl ether	0.25 % pet.
Components of other resins		
13	p-tert-Butylcatechol	0.25 % pet.
14	Phenol-formaldehyde resin (novolak)	5 % pet.
15	Hydroxyethylacrylate	0.1 % pet.
Biocides/preservatives		
16	1,2-Benzisothiazolin-3-one, sodium salt	0.1 % pet.
17	Methylisothiazolinone	0.05 % aqu.

epoxy resin systems. No general recommendation for this exposure can be given, because it depends on many factors (e.g., solvent contents) to determine which gloves are protective and resistant against the epoxy resin system in use. As a rule of thumb, nitrile gloves of more than 0.4 mm thickness are suitable for many solvent-free epoxy resin systems [50]. Because skin contact with epoxy resins may induce sensitization very quickly, workers' education right from the beginning is crucial. Avoiding skin contact, good working hygiene and comprehensive knowledge of the hazards are the best ways to prevent occupational allergic contact dermatitis from epoxy resin systems in the construction industry.

Conclusion

Occupational hand eczema occurs frequently in bricklayers, tile setters, construction workers, and others working in the building trade. Responsible irritants are cement, acidic cleaning agents, and detergents. The most frequent contact allergens are chromate, cobalt, epoxy resin system components, and thiurams. Usage of chromate-reduced cement has significantly decreased the frequency of allergic cement eczema due to chromate allergy in Scandinavian countries. However, in the rest of Europe, corresponding measures followed with a delay of about 20 years, and chromate is still a frequent occupational allergen there. Cobalt, which is also contained in cement, frequently leads to secondary sensitization in chromate-allergic individuals. Contact allergens of increasing importance are components of epoxy resin systems: basic resins, reactive diluents, and amine hardeners. Thiuram allergy is frequently acquired by wearing rubber gloves. Improvement in working hygiene and wearing adequate thiuram-free protective gloves are the most urgently needed approaches to prevent hand eczema in the construction industry.

References

1. Avnstorp C. Risk factors for cement eczema. Contact Dermatitis. 1991;25:81–8.
2. Avnstorp C. Cement eczema. In: Menné T, Maibach HI, editors. Exogenous dermatoses: environmental dermatitis. Boca Raton: CRC Press; 1991. p. 401–14.
3. Falbe J, Regitz M, editors. Römpp chemie lexikon. 9th ed. Stuttgart: Georg Thieme; 1989. p. 405–6. 3593–3594, 5115–5117.
4. Fregert S, Gruvberger B. Chemical properties of cement. Berufsdermatosen. 1972;20:238–48.
5. Fregert S, Gruvberger B. Solubility of cobalt in cement. Contact Dermatitis. 1978;4:14–8.
6. Schubert HJ, Lück H, Auermann E. Nickel dermatitis in construction workers. In: Frosch PJ, Dooms-Goossens A, Lachapelle JM, et al., editors. Current topics in contact dermatitis. Berlin: Springer; 1989. p. 191–4.
7. Industrieverband Bauchemie und Holzschutzmittel. e.V. Sachstandsbericht. Betonzusatzmittel und Umwelt, Frankfurt, 1993.
8. Reul H. Handbuch der bauchemie. Augsburg: Verlag für Chemische Industrie, H. Ziolkowski KG; 1991.
9. Adams RM. Occupational skin disease. 2nd ed. Philadelphia: W.B. Saunders; 1990. p. 16–7. 601–603, 606, 665, 672.
10. Fisher AA. Contact dermatitis. 3rd ed. Philadelphia: Lea & Febiger; 1986. p. 500. 566–569, 762–772.

11. Avnstrop C. Cement workers. In: Kanerva L, Elsner P, Wahlberg JE, Maibach HI, editors. Handbook of occupational dermatology. Berlin/Heidelberg: Springer; 2000. p. 875–7.
12. Avnstrop C. Construction workers. In: Kanerva L, Elsner P, Wahlberg JE, Maibach HI, editors. Handbook of occupational dermatology. Berlin/Heidelberg: Springer; 2000. p. 890–2.
13. Burrows D. Chromate dermatitis. In: Maibach HI, editor. Occupational and industrial dermatology. 2nd ed. Chicago: Year Book Medical Publishers; 1987. p. 403–5.
14. Mali JWH, van Kooten WJ, van Neer FCJ. Some aspects of the behaviour of chromium compounds in the skin. J Invest Dermatol. 1963;41:111–22.
15. Mali JWH, van Kooten WJ, van Neer FCJ, Spruit D. Quantitative aspects of chromium sensitization. Acta Derm Venereol (Stockh). 1964;44:44–8.
16. Siegenthaler U, Laine A, Polak L. Studies on contact sensitivity to chromium in the guinea pig. The role of valence in the formation of the antigenic determinant. J Invest Dermatol. 1983;80:44–7.
17. Rühl R, Kluger N. Handbuch der Bau-Chemikalien. Hrsg. von den Berufsgenossenschaften der Bauwirtschaft. Landberg am Lech: Ecomed Verlagsgesllschaft; 1995: Chapter I-1, p. 1; Chapter II-1.1 - II-1.3, p. 6; Chapter II-3.6, p. 5–9; Chapter II-1.6.613, p. 1–3; Chapter IV-3, p. 1–10; Chapter IV-3.10, p. 1–2; Chapter IV-3.11, p. 1–2; Chapter IV-6.13.1.1, p. 1–2.
18. Avnstorp C. Cement eczema – an epidemiological intervention study. Acta Derm Venereol (Stockh). 1992;179(Suppl):1–22.
19. Roto P, Sainio H, Reunala T, Laippala P. Addition of ferrous sulfate to cement and risk of chromium dermatitis among construction workers. Contact Dermatitis. 1996;34:43–50.
20. Geier J, Uter W, Lessmann H, Hillen U, Goergens U, Kersting K, et al. Kontaktallergien gegen Epoxidharze – ein unterdiagnostiziertes problem. Allergo J. 2003;12:323–8.
21. Zschunke E. Grundriß der Arbeitsdermatologie. Berlin: VEB Verlag Volk und Gesundheit; 1985. p. 44–51. 57–59, 68–87.
22. Björkner B, Frick-Engfeldt M, Pontén A, Zimerson E. Plastic materials. In: Johansen JD, Frosch PJ, Lepoittevin JP, editors. Contact dermatitis. 5th ed. Berlin/Heidelberg: Springer; 2011. p. 695–728.
23. Fregert S. Construction work. In: Maibach HI, editor. Occupational and industrial dermatology. 2nd ed. Chicago: Year Book Medical Publishers; 1987. p. 403–5.
24. Geier J, Kleinhans D, Peters K-P. Kontaktallergien durch industriell verwendete biozide. Dermatosen Beruf Umwelt. 1996;44:154–9. Erratum in: Dermatosen Beruf Umwelt 1996;44:256.
25. Hillen U, Lessmann H, Grabbe S, Geier J. Kontaktsensibilisierungen gegen bestandteile von klebstoffen unter berücksichtigung beruflicher kontaktsensibilisierungen. Dermatologie Beruf Umwelt. 2007;55:10–9.
26. Rothe A. Zur Frage arbeitsbedingter Hautschädigungen durch polyurethanchemikalien. Berufsdermatosen. 1976;24:7–24.
27. Geier J, Lessmann H. BK Nr. 5101 – Maurer. In: Szliska C, Brandenburg S, John SM, editors. Berufsdermatosen, 1. Austauschlieferung. München: Dustri-Verlag Deisenhofen; 2006. p. 217–31.
28. Anonymous. Umgang mit Mineralwolle-Dämmstoffen (Glaswolle, Steinwolle). Herausgegeben von: Fachvereinigung Mineralfaserindustrie e.V., Deutscher Abbruchverband e.V., Hauptverband der Deutschen Bauindustrie e.V., Industriegewerkschaft Bauen-Agrar-Umwelt, Industriegewerkschaft Bergbau, Chemie, Energie, Zentralverband des Deutschen Baugewerbes e.V., unter Mitarbeit von: Arbeitsgemeinschaft der Bau-Berufsgenossenschaften, Berufsgenossenschaft der keramischen und Glas-Industrie, Berufsgenossenschaftliches Institut für Arbeitssicherheit, Länderausschuss für Arbeitsschutz und Sicherheitstechnik. Stand: 05/2002. Verlag, Wiesbaden.
29. Reichenberger M. Katamnestische Untersuchungen bei Angehörigen des Baugewerbes. Berufsdermatosen. 1972;20:271–94.
30. Kleinhans D. Verätzung durch Zementmörtel (Gutachtenfall). Dermatosen Beruf Umwelt. 1984;32: 97–9.
31. European Commission. Directive 2003/53/EC of the European Parliament and of the Council of 18 June 2003 amending for the 26th time Council Directive 76/769/EEC relating to restrictions on the marketing and use of certain dangerous substances and preparations (nonylphenol, nonylphenol ethoxylate and cement). Off J Eur Union. 2003;178/24e178/28.
32. Stocks SJ, McNamee R, Turner S, Carder M, Agius RM. Has European Union legislation to reduce exposure to chromate in cement been effective in reducing the incidence of allergic contact dermatitis attributed to chromate in the UK? Occup Environ Med. 2012;69:150–2.
33. Geier J, Lessmann H, Skudlik C, Ballmer-Weber B, Weisshaar E, Uter W, Schnuch A. Berufsbedingte Kontaktallergie bei Maurern, Fliesenlegern und Angehörigen verwandter Berufe. Aktuelles Sensibilisierungsspektrum und Entwicklungen der letzten Jahre. Dermatologie Beruf Umwelt 2012;60: 136–50.
34. Geier J, Schnuch A. A comparison of contact allergies among construction and non-construction workers attending contact dermatitis clinics in Germany. Results of the IVDK from November 1989 until July 1993. Am J Contact Dermat. 1995;6:86–94.
35. Geier J, Schnuch A. Kontaktallergien im Bau-Hauptgewerbe. Eine Auswertung der Daten des Informationsverbunds Dermatologischer Kliniken (IVDK) 1994–1996. Dermatosen Beruf Umwelt. 1998;46:109–14.
36. Uter W, Rühl R, Pfahlberg A, Geier J, Schnuch A, Gefeller O. Kontaktallergien bei Bauarbeitern. Ergebnisse einer multifaktoriellen Analyse von

IVDK-Daten. Dermatologie Beruf Umwelt. 2003;51:D47–55.
37. Uter W, Rühl R, Pfahlberg A, Geier J, Schnuch A, Gefeller O. Contact allergy in construction workers: results of a multifactorial analysis. Ann Occup Hyg. 2004;48:21–7.
38. Bock M, Schmidt A, Bruckner T, Diepgen TL. Occupational skin disease in the construction industry. Br J Dermatol. 2003;149:1165–71.
39. Geier J, Krautheim A, Uter W, Lessmann H, Schnuch A. Occupational contact allergy in the building trade in Germany: influence of preventive measures and changing exposure. Int Arch Occup Environ Health. 2011;84:403–11.
40. Pontén A, Zimerson E, Bruze M. Sensitizing capacity and cross-reactivity of phenyl glycidyl ether. Contact Dermatitis. 2004;50:166.
41. Pontén A, Zimerson E, Bruze M. Can simultaneous contact allergies to phenyl glycidyl ether and epoxy resins of the bisphenol A/F-types be explained by contamination of the epoxy resins? Contact Dermatitis. 2008;59:273–9.
42. Geier J, Lessmann H, Hillen U, Jappe U, Dickel H, Koch P, Frosch PJ, Schnuch A, Uter W. An attempt to improve diagnostics of contact allergy due to epoxy resin systems. First results of the multicentre study EPOX 2002. Contact Dermatitis. 2004;51:263–72.
43. Geier J. Kontaktallergie gegen Epoxidharze aus der Perspektive des Informationsverbundes Dermatologischer Kliniken (IVDK) und der Deutschen Kontaktallergie-Gruppe (DKG). Gefahrstoffe-Reinhaltung Luft. 2010;70:7–9.
44. Aalto-Korte K, Suuronen K, Kuuliala O, Henriks-Eckerman M-L, Jolanki R. Occupational contact allergy to monomeric isocyanates. Contact Dermatitis. 2012;67:78–88.
45. Frick-Engfeldt M, Isaksson M, Zimerson E, Bruze M. How to optimize patch testing with diphenylmethane diisocyanate. Contact Dermatitis. 2007;57:138–51.
46. Frick M, Zimerson E, Karlsson D, Marand A, Skarping G, Isaksson M, Bruze M. Poor correlation between stated and found concentrations of diphenylmethane-4,4′-diisocyanate (4,4′-MDI) in petrolatum patch-test preparations. Contact Dermatitis. 2004;51:73–8.
47. Geier J, Lessmann H, Schnuch A, Uter W. Recent increase in allergic reactions to methylchloroisothiazolinone/methylisothiazolinone: is methylisothiazolinone the culprit? Contact Dermatitis. 2012;67:334–41.
48. Geier J. Änderungen der DKG-Testreihen, September 2010. Dermatologie Beruf Umwelt. 2010;58:141–4.
49. Struppek K, Ludwig S. Prävention des Chromat-Ekzems im Baugewerbe. Dermatosen Beruf Umwelt. 1999;47:13–5.
50. Ziegler C, Kersting K. Tätigkeiten mit Epoxidharzen. Handschuhempfehlungen und Sensibilisierungspotential. Sicherheitsingenieur. 2012;2:30–2.

Hand Eczema in Janitorial and Related Industries

21

Elke Weisshaar and Thomas L. Diepgen

Contents

E. Weisshaar, M.D., Ph.D. (✉) • T.L. Diepgen
Department of Clinical Social Medicine, Occupational and Environmental Medicine, Heidelberg University Hospital, Thibautstr. 3, Heidelberg 69115, Germany
e-mail: elke.weisshaar@med.uni-heidelberg.de

21.1 Description of Janitorial and Related Industries

A person working in the janitorial or a related industry may be called a janitor, janitress (female), caretaker, maintenance man/woman, facility manager, custodian cleaner, or concierge. People working in related industries are maids and cleaning personnel. In these jobs, cleaning duties are dominant. This comprises cleaning bathrooms, sinks, lunch rooms, kitchens, tables, hotel rooms, and so on. Basic cleaning tasks may differ strongly among enterprises.

In most countries, a job in the janitorial and related industry is not a recognized occupation requiring formal training. Some countries, like Germany, for example, offer certified training courses for janitors. Persons may have simply learned a trade. Working in the janitorial industry requires physical fitness, manual skills, and the ability to communicate.

A janitor can be a caretaker of buildings such as residential houses, hospitals, schools, swimming pools, or companies. This entails maintenance, repair work, service operation, and, in some cases, security duties. Janitors frequently carry out duties such as maintenance and repair of, for example, buildings, equipment, expendable materials, and supplies. The janitorial industry comprises tasks such as cleaning of floors, windows, cellars, vehicle halls, underground garages, and bathrooms; emptying trash; picking up litter; maintaining illumination of buildings and air conditioning; setting up rooms; dusting equipment and furniture; and other tasks. Janitors may also be responsible for

A. Alikhan et al. (eds.), *Textbook of Hand Eczema*,
DOI 10.1007/978-3-642-39546-8_21, © Springer-Verlag Berlin Heidelberg 2014

taking care of park and recreation areas, watering plants, winter services, cleaning of sidewalks, and moving activities.

All this explains the great variety of duties in this profession and the variable nature of the jobs. The exact task of a janitor depends on his/her contract and the individual workplace. Especially in larger workplaces/organizations, some duties may be outsourced. Janitorial work is often performed in the afternoon, evening, or overnight. In bigger organizations such as corporations and hospitals, they work the day shift. A janitor frequently works on his/her own. He/she may be employed or be a self-employed person with his/her own janitorial company.

21.2 Potential Hazardous Materials

The great diversity of tasks in the janitorial industry leads to contact with the following materials/procedures:

- Water and wet work
- Wearing gloves
- Tools (e.g., metal, plastic, rubber, nails, screws)
- Detergents
- Disinfectants
- Cleaning cloths
- Colors, cement, and adhesives
- Grit
- Lubricating grease
- Electronic bulbs
- Neon lamps
- Plants
- Vacuum cleaners and cleaning machines
- Mowing machines

21.3 Clinical Aspects of Chronic Hand Eczema in the Janitorial and Related Industries

Chronic hand eczema (CHE), also called chronic hand dermatitis, is an inflammation of the skin of the hands [1] that can affect janitors. It is common, with a point prevalence of 4 % among adults in the general population; the 1-year prevalence is around 10 % [2] (also see Chap. 7). There are no epidemiological studies on how frequently janitors and employees in related industries are affected by CHE. The Carpe registry is a CHE registry on long-term patient management containing 1,163 patients with CHE. Janitors are included in the occupation group "Distribution, Warehouse," accounting for 2.3 % of all documented occupations [3].

Classification of CHE is based on clinical and etiological factors (also see Chaps. 3 and 6). Also, in the janitorial industry, cases are classified according to cause when possible. CHE frequently presents as irritant contact dermatitis of the hands. This is caused by wet work, repeated exposure to irritants like detergents and lubricating grease, and an increased amount of manual activities. Irritant contact dermatitis, especially if untreated or not sufficiently treated, predisposes one to acquire additional contact allergy. This may lead to allergic contact dermatitis of the hands. It can be caused by a variety of substances, such as rubber additives (e.g., gloves), chromate (e.g., leather, cement), preservatives or fragrances (e.g., detergents, creams) [4], fluids (e.g., lubricating grease), and plastics. In daily clinical practice, CHE frequently presents as a mixture of irritant and allergic contact dermatitis of the hands (Figs. 21.1 and 21.2).

There are no specific studies in janitors concerning diagnosis and contact allergy. One study about cleaning and kitchen employees ($n=124$) showed 49.2 % to have atopic skin diathesis. In 8.9 %, CHE was severe. Nearly 50 % suffered from irritant contact dermatitis, and around 7 % had allergic contact dermatitis [5]. Twenty-seven percent had a mixture of irritant, atopic, and allergic contact dermatitis of the hands [5]. A 1-year follow-up study of 212 cleaning and kitchen employees revealed that 46.2 % of employees had irritant contact dermatitis and 35.4 % had a mixture of all [6]; 4.7 % had atopic hand dermatitis, and 3 % had allergic contact dermatitis of the hands [6].

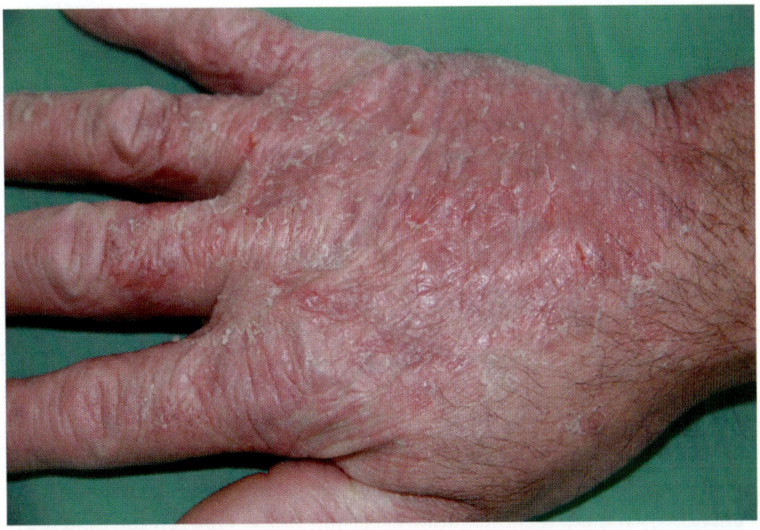

Fig. 21.1 Chronic irritant hand eczema in a 56-year-old janitor working in a chemical company

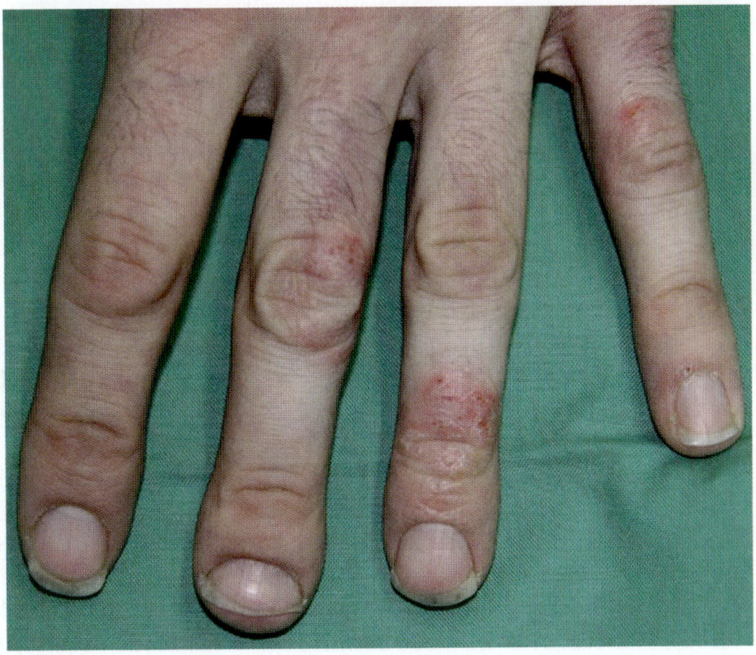

Fig. 21.2 Chronic irritant (vesicular) hand eczema with a nummular eczema pattern in a 43-year-old janitor working in a university hospital

21.4 Differential Diagnoses and Diagnostics

Differential diagnosis needs to consider the diversity of tasks and contact with hazardous materials. This is why taking a patient's history and elucidating a precise job description are of utmost importance. History of asthma, hay fever, and childhood eczema must also be considered. As the barrier function of atopic skin is comprised, patients are predisposed to irritant contact dermatitis. About one-third to one-half of patients with CHE may have atopy, and this is considered as the most important risk factor for CHE [1, 2, 7] (also see Chap. 8).

Diagnostics include obtaining the patient's history and a precise job description, thorough clinical investigation of the whole skin, and allergy testing. Patch testing in janitors and employees of related industries should include standard series, disinfectants, rubber materials, preservative agents, fragrances, adhesive and glues, colors, and cements. Patch test material can be acquired from commercial patch test material suppliers. Since commercially available test substances can never cover all potential contact allergens, patch testing of patients' own materials handled at work is an important measure in identifying contact allergens (also see Chaps. 24 and 25). In janitors, the testing of gloves, lubricating grease, tools, detergents, adhesives and glues, and skin care protection agents should be considered. Patch testing with patients' own materials must follow certain rules and consider safety regulations [8]. In our own studies, reviewing the charts of 212 cleaning and kitchen employees identified the following most common contact allergens: nickel (II) sulfate (29.7 %), cobalt (II) chloride (10.4 %), fragrance mix (9.9 %), thiuram mix (8.5 %), p-phenylenediamine (6.1 %), potassium dichromate (5.7 %), and wool wax alcohol (5.2 %) [6].

21.5 Treatment, Prevention, and Prognosis of CHE in Janitorial and Related Industries

Treatment includes the general and specific measures for treatment of CHE [9] (also see Chaps. 30, 31, 32, 33, 34, 35, 36, 37, 38, 39, and 40). For severe cases, an interdisciplinary integrated inpatient rehabilitation measure may be necessary [10, 11]. This comprises a 3-week intensive dermatological treatment including diagnostic procedures and patient education. A very recent prospective study of 1,788 individuals showed that this rehabilitation measure is associated with sustained improvements in terms of ability to work, quality of life, prognosis, and reductions in days of absence from work. Additionally, the use of topical corticosteroids could be significantly reduced [11].

Detecting an underlying contact allergy is necessary in case of contact dermatitis of the hands in janitors. If any contact allergens are identified, they must be substituted (e.g., change of gloves, lubricating grease, cream). As in any profession exposed to irritants, prevention is of great importance (also see Chaps. 26, 27, and 28). This includes varying protective gloves, using skin-protecting creams [12], and moisturizing the skin regularly. Especially in janitors, choosing the right galenics is of high importance. If a fatty lotion or ointment is recommended, people may not use it because it will stain their tools. Measures of secondary individual prevention include educational intervention and the so-called skin courses for secondary prevention or skin protection courses. Secondary individual prevention courses have been established for different professions, such as hairdressers, health care workers, cleaners, and kitchen employees [5, 6, 13, 14]. These skin protection courses have been shown to have a positive impact on the patients' skin disease, well-being, skin health, and quality of life [6, 14–16].

There are no studies focussing on prognosis of CHE in janitorial and related industries. It depends on substitution of contact allergens if identified and patients' motivation to implement and sustain skin protection measures as well as success of therapy. Our data showed that 81.5 % of cleaning and kitchen employees were able to change skin care habits [6]; 86.2 % employed protective measures; 71.5 % wore gloves [6]; and 26.9 % reduced the frequency of washing hands. One may assume that prognosis is better than in other professions because the janitorial and related industries consist of several variable and diverse tasks. One must assume that in the case of maids and cleaners, the proportion of wet work is significantly higher than in other employees of the janitorial industry.

Conclusion

Janitors and workers in related industries frequently fulfill a great variety of tasks, which may cause them to come in contact with different skin irritants, such as wet work, gloves, and variable materials (e.g., detergents, metal, plastic, rubber, fluids). Differential diagnoses need to consider the diversity of tasks, which is why taking a patient's history and obtaining a precise job description are of utmost importance in this profession. Irritant contact dermatitis appears to be the most frequent type of hand eczema in janitors, but contact allergy always needs to be ruled out. Patch testing should consider disinfectants, rubber materials, preservative agents, fragrances, adhesive and glues, colors, cements, and so on. Patch testing of patients' own materials handled at work may be necessary. Prognosis depends on sufficient therapy, substitution of contact allergens, if identified, and patients' motivation to implement and sustain skin protection measures.

References

1. Coenraads PJ. Hand eczema. N Engl J Med. 2012;367(19):1829–37.
2. Thyssen JP, Gimenez-Arnau E, Lepoittevin JP, Menne T, Boman A, Schnuch A. The critical review of methodologies and approaches to assess the inherent skin sensitization potential (skin allergies) of chemicals. Part III. Contact Dermatitis. 2012;66(1):53–70.
3. Apfelbacher CJ, Molin S, Weisshaar E, Bauer A, Elsner P, Mahler V, Weiss M, Ruzicka T, Diepgen TL. Characteristics and provision of care in patients with chronic hand eczema: updated data from the carpe registry. Acta Derm Venereol. 2013. doi: 10.2340/00015555-1632. [Epub ahead of print]
4. Tanko Z, Shab A, Diepgen TL, Weisshaar E. Polyvalent type IV sensitizations to multiple fragrances and a skin protection cream in a metal worker. J Dtsch Dermatol Ges. 2009;7(6):541–3.
5. Weisshaar E, Radulescu M, Soder S, Apfelbacher CJ, Bock M, Grundmann JU, et al. Secondary individual prevention of occupational skin diseases in health care workers, cleaners and kitchen employees: aims, experiences and descriptive results. Int Arch Occup Environ Health. 2007;80(6):477–84.
6. Soder S, Diepgen TL, Radulescu M, Apfelbacher CJ, Bruckner T, Weisshaar E. Occupational skin diseases in cleaning and kitchen employees: course and quality of life after measures of secondary individual prevention. J Dtsch Dermatol Ges. 2007;5(8):670–6.
7. Diepgen TL. Occupational skin diseases. J Dtsch Dermatol Ges. 2012;10(5):297–313. quiz 4–5. Epub 2012/03/30.
8. Krautheim A, Lessmann H, Geier J. Patch testing with patient's own materials handled at work. In: Rustemeyer T, Elsner P, John SM, Maibach HI, editors. Kanerva's occupational dermatology. Berlin: Springer; 2012. p. 919–33.
9. Diepgen TL, Elsner P, Schliemann S, Fartasch M, Kollner A, Skudlik C, et al. Guideline on the management of hand eczema ICD-10 Code: L20. L23. L24. L25. L30. J Dtsch Dermatol Ges. 2009;7(3):S1–16.
10. Skudlik C, Weisshaar E, Scheidt R, Elsner P, Wulfhorst B, Schonfeld M, et al. First results from the multicentre study rehabilitation of occupational skin diseases – optimization and quality assurance of inpatient management (ROQ). Contact Dermatitis. 2012;66(3):140–7.
11. Weisshaar E, Skudlik C, Scheidt R, Matterne U, Wulfhorst B, Schonfeld M, Elsner P, Diepgen TL, John SM; ROQ Study Group. Multicentre study 'rehabilitation of occupational skin diseases – optimization and quality assurance of inpatient management (ROQ)'-results from 12-month follow-up. Contact Dermatitis. 2013;68(3):169–74. doi: 10.1111/j.1600-0536.2012.02170.x. Epub 2012 Oct 10.
12. Kutting B, Baumeister T, Weistenhofer W, Pfahlberg A, Uter W, Drexler H. Effectiveness of skin protection measures in prevention of occupational hand eczema: results of a prospective randomized controlled trial over a follow-up period of 1 year. Br J Dermatol. 2010;162(2):362–70.
13. Weisshaar E, Radulescu M, Bock M, Albrecht U, Diepgen TL. Educational and dermatological aspects of secondary individual prevention in healthcare workers. Contact Dermatitis. 2006;54(5):254–60.
14. Wulfhorst B, Bock M, Gediga G, Skudlik C, Allmers H, John SM. Sustainability of an interdisciplinary secondary prevention program for hairdressers. Int Arch Occup Environ Health. 2010;83(2):165–71.
15. Apfelbacher CJ, Soder S, Diepgen TL, Weisshaar E. The impact of measures for secondary individual prevention of work-related skin diseases in health care workers: 1-year follow-up study. Contact Dermatitis. 2009;60(3):144–9.
16. Matterne U, Apfelbacher CJ, Soder S, Diepgen TL, Weisshaar E. Health-related quality of life in health care workers with work-related skin diseases. Contact Dermatitis. 2009;61(3):145–51.

Methods for Testing Irritation Potential

22

Michal Wen Sheue Ong, F. Anthony Simion, and Howard I. Maibach

Contents

M.W.S. Ong, BSc, MBBS (✉) • H.I. Maibach, M.D.
Department of Dermatology, University of California, San Francisco, 90 Medical Center Way, Surge 110, San Francisco, CA, USA
e-mail: michalong@gmail.com; maibachh@derm.ucsf.edu

F.A. Simion, Ph.D.
KAO Brands Co., 2535 Spring Grove Ave., Cincinnati, OH, USA
e-mail: tony.simion@kaobrands.com

22.1 Introduction

Skin irritation, the response to noxious chemicals, trauma, or other insults from the environment, is common and unpleasant. This can take many forms, both visible and sensory. The mechanisms by which skin irritation is produced can vary greatly. To develop optimal strategies to prevent or ameliorate the different forms of irritation, better mechanistic understanding of irritation is needed. This is best achieved by examining each form of irritation separately in a model system.

22.2 Theoretical Models of Irritation

Theoretical, in vitro, and in vivo models have been developed to assess many distinct forms of irritation. As they all affect the same substrate, the skin, they frequently have common characteristics.

Two theoretical models help us better understand how the skin reacts to a variety of irritants. The model of irritation proposed by Malten suggests that visible irritation occurs when the intensity of the insult exceeds a threshold [1]. A single large insult (a) or a series of small ones (b) that cumulatively exceed the threshold can cause observable clinical signs (Fig. 22.1). As the skin repairs itself, the intensity is reduced, eventually falling below the threshold, and the clinical signs disappear.

A. Alikhan et al. (eds.), *Textbook of Hand Eczema*,
DOI 10.1007/978-3-642-39546-8_22, © Springer-Verlag Berlin Heidelberg 2014

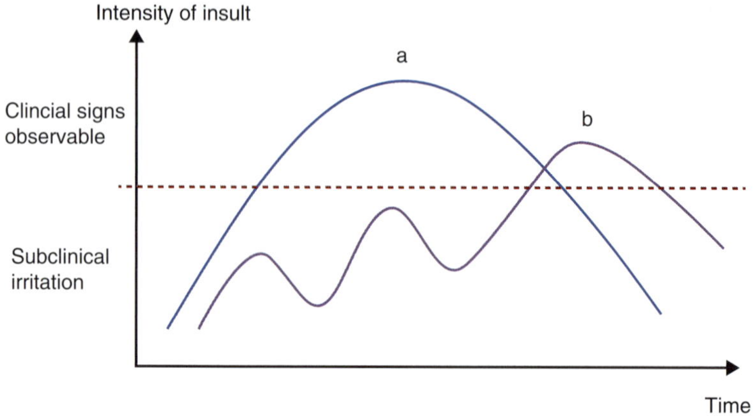

Fig. 22.1 Malten theory of irritation (Modified from [54] with kind permission from Springer Science and Business Media)

For normal skin

Method	Skin Strata Affected	Observable	Instrumental	Sensory
Brief Wash Normal washes	Surface	No	Conductance	Feels soft, tight and dry
Exaggerated Wash Short wash (10 seconds) Leave lather on skin Repeat up to 4 times a day for several days	Stratum Corneum	Dryness	Conductance Sticky tape stain Image analysis Photography	Feels dry, looks dry and itches
Prolonged Wash Longer wash (>1 minute) Immediate rinse Repeat up to 4 times a day for several days. **Closed Patch Test** Occlusive patching on responsive subjects for >24 hours	Surface to Dermis	Erythema Dryness	TEWL* Colorimeter Laser Doppler Conductance	Feels dry, stings, and looks red

*TEWL: Trans-epidermal Water Loss

Increased Treatment Intensity

Fig. 22.2 Type of skin response to a cleanser is a function of treatment intensity (Modified from [54] with kind permission from Springer Science and Business Media)

One key implication from this model is that the skin can respond before clinical signs are apparent. This is the basis of "invisible dermatoses" proposed by Kligman [2]. He demonstrated that the skin might be damaged at the histological level, even though nothing is visible at the surface. For instance, in photobiology, half the minimal dose of UV required to produce erythema (1/2 MED) causes cell death in the epidermis (i.e., produces "sunburn" cells). Another example is patching the skin with 0.5 % sodium lauryl sulfate (SLS) for 24 h. In many subjects, erythema was not observed, nor were there any histological changes apparent in hematoxylin-eosin stained sections. However, thin sections showed much epidermal damage, with swollen keratinocytes and edematous intercellular spaces [2].

This also explains why damaged or compromised skin is more responsive. It already has a significant but subclinical level of damage, thus requiring a smaller insult to produce a visible sign of irritation. This is supported by a study conducted by Freeman and Maibach that showed an elevated transepidermal water loss (TEWL) response to a second SLS patch (applied to the same site as a first 2 weeks before), even though the TEWL rate had apparently returned to baseline in the intervening time [3]. This model suggests that different forms of irritation have different thresholds. Therefore, a mild insult may produce only a few, mild forms of irritation, whereas with a greater insult, the threshold for more forms of irritation is surpassed, so they, too, arc expressed.

The second model relates skin strata to the type and degree of irritation (Fig. 22.2). Each strata produces irritation characteristic of that level; for instance, the stratum corneum and the upper epidermis can produce sensory irritation and dryness. Erythema, which involves increased blood flow, requires dermal involvement.

If the stratum corneum is damaged, then the irritants can penetrate to lower strata and produce a more intense irritation than is expected. This is the basis of the enhanced response of compromised skin.

22.3 Initial Effects of Surfactants on Skin

Surfactants and other irritants initially interact with the stratum corneum. Thus, in normal skin it is the stratum corneum and the structures within the upper epidermis that initially respond to chemical irritants. These responses can take different forms, including:

- Sensory irritation
- Damage to the surface corneocytes
- Super-hydration of the stratum corneum

However, as the exposure to the irritant becomes exaggerated (such as increased intensity, increased duration, or damage to the stratum corneum), the lower skin structures will become involved and other signs of irritation will appear.

22.3.1 Sensory Irritation

Exposure to many chemicals or products can produced unwanted sensations such as dryness, stinging, itching, or skin burning. These sensations can occur even in the absence of visible signs of irritation. Epidemiological studies indicate that half of the adverse reactions caused by personal care products fall into this category [4]. There are many mechanisms by which such sensations are produced. Some personal care products such as sunscreens and lactic acid-containing lotions cause facial stinging in a responsive subpopulation of consumers. Placing a 10 % lactic acid solution on the face can identify these individuals while the individual is sweating [5]. The responsiveness of panelists can be increased by facial washing with soap and decreased by repeated applications of a good moisturizer. This suggests that the skin of lactic acid "stingers" is somewhat damaged, although the mechanism by which stinging is produced is inadequately understood.

Exposure to capsaicin, the active component in chili peppers, can produce a burning sensation. Green and colleagues have measured this phenomenon using a labeled magnitude scale and have shown that although there is a large person-to-person variation in response, there is good reproducibility of the measurements within individuals [6]. The relative sensitivities to other chemical irritants such as lactic acid (stinging) and ethanol may be different in different individuals.

The mechanisms by which these sensory irritations are produced are unclear. There appear to be several sensory mediators, such as histamine and substance P. Indeed, intradermal injections of histamine can induce itching in many subjects [7].

As the unmyelinated C fibers appear to play an important role in the detection of chemical irritancy via the sensations of itching and stinging, it is likely that histamine stimulates them. These fibers can also detect heat and cold. It has been hypothesized that stimulation of a few fibers results in the perception of itching. As more of the fibers are stimulated, the signal is interpreted as stinging. The response of the C fiber can be blocked. Maibach and his colleagues have shown that a variety of anti-irritants, such as menthol and anesthetics, can modify the ability of the C fibers to detect heat and cold, itching, and stinging [8].

Sensory irritation can frequently be detected before clinical signs can be observed. Simion et al. showed that in an exaggerated forearm wash test panelists could detect differences between soap and a milder synthetic detergent bar before a trained observer could visually differentiate the products [9]. This is consistent with the results of the epidemiological study by DeGroot et al.; they reported that many people experience sensory irritation in the absence of visible signs and discontinue use of that product before visible irritation appears.

22.3.2 Squamometry

Any short-term exposure of the skin surface to surfactants can damage the surface corneocytes. Two things happen as a result. First, the corneocyte sheet begins to break into smaller sheets and individual cells. Second, these cells will take up hydrophilic stains more readily than undamaged corneocytes. Both processes can be assessed. Whether sheets of corneocytes are present can be determined by visual inspection under a light microscope. Dye uptake is readily quantified by colorimetric assessment. This is the basis of both squamometry and corneosurfometry. Corneosurfometry is an in vitro approach in which the corneocytes are harvested first using an adhesive tape then exposed to surfactants. Squamometry involves treating the skin first then harvesting the corneocytes with adhesive tape and dyeing them.

Paye and Cartiaux utilized squamometry to assess the effects of cleansing products in a manner that resembles normal usage. Paye and Cartiaux showed that daily usage of dishwashing liquids combined with a 5-min soak for four consecutive days at normal usage concentrations (0.25 %) would give the same level of skin damage as the highly exaggerated Frosch-Kligman soap chamber test (occlusive patching for 24 h with a 2.25 % solution of the dishwashing liquid, followed by 6-h occlusive patches on the next four consecutive days) [10].

Piérard et al. extended this methodology beyond surfactant-induced irritation. They showed squamometry was extremely sensitive in its ability to detect the effects of a fabric softener in reducing the degree of skin surface damage caused by repeated rubbing with wet towels. In this study, squamometry was more discriminating than a visual observer, TEWL, or capacitance [11].

Squamometry can also be used to assess moisturizer efficacy. Effective moisturizers can stimulate the desquamation of damaged surface corneocytes. This results in the reduced dye uptake as measured by a lower C* value (Fig. 22.3). Polyol-based moisturizers are more effective than those without polyols at reducing C* value and enhancing skin conductance. This suggests that the polyol-containing moisturizers are more effective at removing damaged aggregates of corneocytes otherwise known as dry skin scales or flakes.

22.3.3 Super-Hydration of Stratum Corneum

Short-term (minutes) exposure of the stratum corneum to aqueous solutions of anionic surfactants causes it to swell. Wilhelm et al. showed that this swelling is related to the primary irritation potential of the surfactant [12]. When examined in an *ex vivo* model, Rhein et al. speculated the hydrophobic tails of the surfactants binding to the stratum corneum caused the swelling [13]. The negatively charged head groups would then repel each other. This would have two effects – first, it enables the small hydrophilic molecules such as the natural moisturizing factors (NMFs) to leach out, resulting in the skin's reduced ability to hold moisture; second, the bound surfactants are not readily desorbed. As they remain in the upper stratum corneum, they damage the skin. Imokawa et al. proposed that surfactant binding to the skin is a major cause of skin roughness and perceived tightness [14, 15].

Note that nonionic and cationic surfactants do not cause the stratum corneum to swell; yet cationic surfactants can be just as irritating as their anionic analogs.

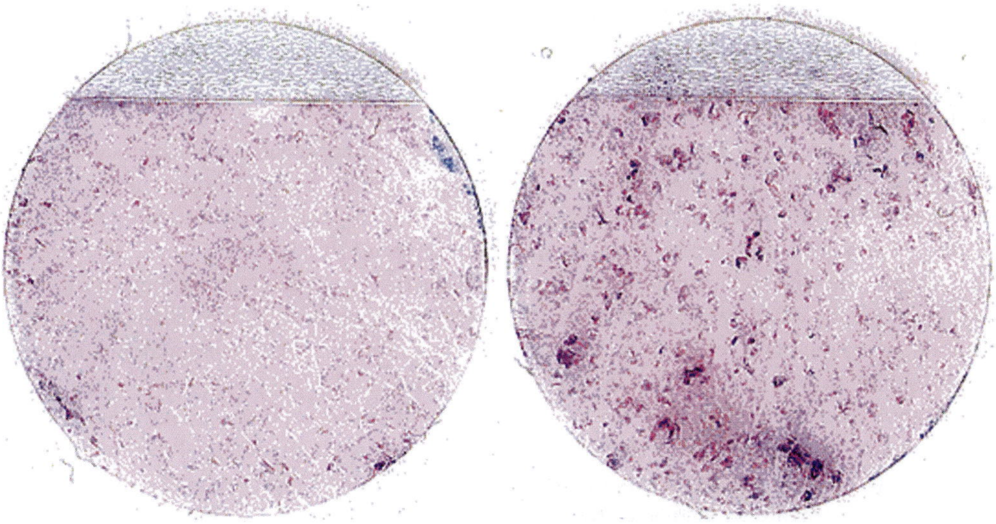

Fig. 22.3 Reduced dye uptake in specimen with moisturizer treatment compared to specimen without moisturizer treatment. Modified from [54] with kind permission from Springer Science and Business Media

22.4 Role of Skin Condition on the Irritant Response

The condition of the skin is a crucial factor in the type and intensity of the response to a set insult. Skin on different parts of the body will react with different intensities to the same stimulus. Cua et al. showed that the thigh was the most responsive anatomical site to SLS exposure, whereas the palms were least responsive. TEWL was a more sensitive measure of damage than visual scoring [16].

Although there are many ways of measuring irritant response to stimuli, the basis for these differences in responsiveness is unclear. These differences may be related to the ease at which molecules can diffuse through the stratum corneum or the size of corneocyte. Rougier et al. demonstrated that there was a correlation between the skin's permeability to water exiting and the absorption of hydrophobic molecules such as benzoic acid, acetyl salicylic acid, and caffeine [17]. The correlation coefficient (R) ranged from 0.92 down to 0.72. This may be a function of corneocyte size. The idea that the skin's permeability to irritants is related to its responsiveness is not only intuitively reasonable but is supported by experimental data, especially for ionic irritants. For instance:

1. Pre-damaging the stratum corneum by immersing the skin in dilute surfactant solutions increases the erythema induced by subsequent patching with SLS [18].
2. Pre-damaging the skin by physically abrading the stratum corneum with a needle significantly decreases the threshold concentration of Triton X-100, formalin, or nickel ions required to elicit irritation. This scarification procedure has much less effect on the skin's responsiveness to hydrophobic irritants such as lauric or benzoic acids [19].
3. Panelists who had a stronger than average vasodilation response due to the percutaneous penetration of methyl nicotinate also had a stronger irritant response to SLS [20].
4. Skin responds more strongly to patching with SLS in the winter, than in the summer [21]. The basal level of TEWL is higher in the winter, indicating the stratum corneum barrier is more permeable (i.e., damaged).
5. Agner showed that patients with atopic dermatitis, where the stratum corneum barrier is compromised (basal TEWL rate is higher), show a stronger TEWL response to SLS-induced irritation than non-atopic controls [22].
6. Pinnagoda et al., extending Agner's observation to a non-atopic population, showed that

the baseline TEWL (TEWL measurements made prior to the 0.5 % SLS on day 1) is a better indicator of an individual's susceptibility to weak irritants than having a high TEWL value, following a single 24-h patch test [23].

7. Simion et al. showed that the stratum corneum is more readily damaged than the dermis, as it is the initial point of contact between the surfactant and skin, and they proposed that evaporimetry is an effective way to measure stratum corneum damage [24]. In the skin strata model, shown in Fig. 22.2, damage to the stratum corneum implies that the irritants can penetrate more deeply into the skin and produce more intense forms of irritation than if the stratum corneum were intact.

22.5 Models for Assessing Skin Irritation

22.5.1 Closed Patch Testing for Assessing Hazard

Closed patch testing is used to assess the overall dermal primary irritation potential (toxicological hazard) of chemicals including surfactants and other products. The Draize test in rabbits has been used as the standard, especially for regulatory assessments.

However, there are experimental data that question how predictive rabbit skin is of human skin's response. Phillips et al. assessed the primary irritation potential (hazard) of chemicals in human volunteers by occlusive patching for up to 21 consecutive days (i.e., the cumulative irritation test) [25]. They found that while the Draize test could differentiate strong irritants from chemicals that were not irritating to humans, it was not effective at comparing materials of mild and moderate irritation potential. More refined comparative human models are required.

For cosmetic ingredients and products, Burger and Bowman reduced the original 21-day cumulative irritation test to only 14 days. They demonstrated that the relative magnitude of irritation does not change between 14 and 21 days. Reducing study duration greatly reduces the risk of tape reactions. Inclusion of positive and negative controls (0.1 % SLS and a blank, respectively) can be used to standardize the results between studies.

Another, approach for product safety assessment is the Maibach-Marzulli Human Repeated Insult Patch Test (HRIPT) where test patches are replaced three times a week. The erythema produced is recorded when patches are replaced. In this procedure, 100 panelists or more are occlusively patched continually for almost 3 weeks.

A 4-h human exposure test has been developed to assess irritation potential (or hazard) [26]. Volunteers are patched occlusively with test material and a standard solution (positive control – 20 % SLS aqueous solution) for up to 4 h. At specified times, the test site is checked to determine if erythema is induced. Once this occurs, that particular chemical is removed from the test site. The response is then statistically compared with the positive control. As European Regulations defined the 20 % SLS solution as an irritant (R38), materials that produce a response that is not statistically different than that produced by 20 % SLS solution are also regarded as irritants.

Companies are interested in the primary irritation potential of cosmetics and cleansers, both as a measure of consumer acceptability in the marketplace and as the basis of commercial claims support. Since the intrinsic "hazard" of these products is similar, they are difficult to differentiate using those tests designed to assess intrinsic hazard. Instead, the sensitivity of the test must be increased and focused on the type of response expected.

One example of a high-resolution test is the soap chamber method developed by Frosch and Kligman [27]. This requires a panel of people with "sensitive" skin – defined as a person who will give a strong erythema reaction (>1.5 on a 0–4 scale) when patched overnight with either 1 % SLS or 5 % soap. Panelists are then occlusively patched for 24 h with 5–8 % soap solution (in-use concentration). This is followed by a series of four 6-h patches on subsequent days. The skin is evaluated for erythema and dryness (scaling and fissures) 3 days after the application of the last patch. This method differentiated soap bars from a synthetic detergent based on sodium cocoyl isethionate (Dove™), the latter inducing less primary irritation (erythema) and dryness. Dove™ and soap are frequently used as the mild and irritating controls, respectively, to ensure adequate test sensitivity. This methodology has also been applied to differentiate the irritation potential of dishwashing liquids.

A modified soap chamber test was developed to decrease testing time without reducing the ability to differentiate between soap and synthetic detergent bars based on irritation potential only [28]. This methodology involves a single 24-h exposure only – day 1 of the Frosch-Kligman soap chamber test. Erythema is assessed by a trained observer and by use of a colorimeter, and stratum corneum barrier damage is measured as the increase in TEWL rate using an evaporimeter. To differentiate between products that are milder than Dove™, exposure time may be increased to two consecutive days of patching. This closed patch test only produces dryness if there is sufficient irritation and then only several days after patching is completed. Dryness produced by this method is a result of the primary irritation – perhaps part of the repair response. In subjects with darker skin tones, especially Fitzpatrick types IV, V, and VI, hyperpigmentation is also a major response to primary dermal irritation [29].

Skin responses in the closed patch test depend on climate and season. Agner and Serup showed that during the summer, the erythema and TEWL responses to SLS are greatly diminished. This emphasizes the importance of running mild and irritating controls, to ensure that the test has sufficient discriminating power. If the soap and syndet bar cannot be distinguished, other null results should be strongly questioned.

Patch testing is an assessment of hazard. It takes no account of the way the product is used or of other factors that may modify the amount of irritation induced. To develop a better understanding of the type and severity of irritation produced in normal usage, alternative approaches such as open application and exaggerated use tests were developed.

22.5.2 Exaggerated Usage Tests

Intuitively, we understand that the closer a clinical test mimics the way it is used by consumers, the more predictive of in-use problems such as irritation it will be. This has led to development of exaggerated wash tests for personal cleansers and immersion testing for dishwashing liquids.

For personal cleansers, the physical nature of a product, such as lubricity or the presence of abrasive beads, and the method or tool used for product application will greatly influence the level of irritation experienced by consumers. For dishwashing liquids, chemical composition, dosage, and water temperature are key determinants of irritation potential. For catamenial products, the friction between the skin and the products contribute the overall irritating potential.

22.5.2.1 Exaggerated Wash Tests

Initially Frosch used an exaggerated half-face wash method to distinguish soap and synthetic detergent based cleansing bars. After 2-min washes twice a day for 4–5 days, Dove™ was demonstrated milder than Zest™ or Ivory™ soap based on lower observable erythema and panelist self-assessed tightness and stinging.

Since then, two types of exaggerated arm wash studies have been developed. Strube, Sharko, and their colleagues at Unilever™ have developed methods that focus on irritation (erythema and increased TEWL rates) as the primary endpoints to differentiate between products. These methods are characterized by longer periods (minutes) of washing the skin. In contrast, the methods developed by Lukacovik, Ertel, and their colleagues at Procter and Gamble™ focus on skin dryness as the primary endpoint. These methods are characterized by short washes (seconds), after which the lather remains on the skin more than a minute before it is rinsed away.

Arm Wash Methods: Using Irritation as the Primary Endpoint

The antecubital flex test developed by Strube et al. uses repeated washes with an abrasive applicator to damage the stratum corneum and produce erythema in the fold of the elbow [30]. The erythema is evaluated by a trained observer and can be measured instrumentally using a colorimeter (e.g., a chromameter). Measuring increases in TEWL rates using an evaporimeter assesses stratum corneum barrier damage. The flex test is relatively sensitive to product differences as it is able to distinguish between soap bars that have about 10 % of the soap replaced with a milder synthetic detergent such as sodium cocoyl isethionate. The soap chamber test was not able to differentiate between these bars. The irritation response to the products in the flex test does not vary greatly with season. This is an advantage over closed patch testing (see above) and the arm wash method of Lukacovic et al. [31], where the response is reduced in the summer.

As the test is aggressive, effects of damage to the outer stratum corneum are readily overwhelmed and dryness is not observed. The flex test has been criticized for being unnecessarily traumatic and very dependent on the roughness of the accessory (e.g., sponge) that is used to apply the product to the skin [32].

Sharko et al. developed a method to detect differences in both dryness and primary irritation (erythema and TEWL rates) induced by a soap and Dove™, a synthetic detergent bar, after four and half days of twice-daily treatment [33]. For smaller product differences, Sharko, Nicoll, and their colleagues showed that this method could distinguish between mild cleansing products and a low level of sodium cocoyl isethionate based on erythema and TEWL rates, but not on observed dryness scores [34]. The reason for this greater discriminatory power for primary irritation rather than dryness is uncertain. Lather is applied to the volar forearms by rubbing with gloved hands for 1 min or more, several times daily. The increased rubbing may slightly damage the stratum corneum, enabling the surfactants to penetrate more readily. Thus, irritation rather than drying potential is the main basis for differentiating between products. Furthermore, the rubbing may mechanically remove the scaling of upper stratum corneum, so flaking is less apparent.

Washing Studies Using Dryness as the Primary Endpoint

In the method developed by Lukacovic et al., lather is applied to the forearms with a towel or muslin cloth for 10 s and remains there for an additional 90 s. The surfactant remains on the surface of the skin and primarily damages the outer stratum corneum. This leads to visible dryness and skin roughness. Without the additional abrasion, little surfactant penetrates into the viable epidermis and primary irritation is not induced. Hence, soap and mild syndet bars are differentiated based on observable dryness and tactile softness. When the differences between products are large, erythema can be observed as well. This methodology produces lower responses than that of Sharko et al. and appears to differentiate products more on their ability to induce dryness, rather than on irritation potential. It is, however, sensitive to prevailing weather conditions, especially humidity level. Increasing the number of wash cycles each day may overcome this limitation.

In the past, the number of samples that could be tested simultaneously was limited. Original published reports focused on running a single product on each arm. In contrast, the soap chamber test could evaluate eight samples simultaneously on the same panelist. Two approaches have been described to overcome this limitation, especially for less exaggerated methods that use dryness rather than primary irritation (observed in closed patch tests) as the key endpoint.

Ertel et al. described modifications to the original method (where only single product running on each arm) that allowed up to eight products to be tested simultaneously, four on each leg [35]. Alternatively, using a statistical method (e.g., meta-analysis) can be used to estimate the difference in mildness of a product and it can be cost-effective.

22.5.2.2 Use Testing

A major cause of irritation in both the home and the work place is repeated exposure to dilute detergent solutions used for dishwashing and housekeeping (i.e., wet work). Epidemiological studies indicate that occupations that involve much hand washing (e.g., nursing, hairdressing, bartending, and kitchen work) have a significantly higher incidence of hand irritation than the general population [36, 37]. Therefore, it is important to be able to model these effects in vivo. Three approaches are described in the following section: immersion testing, repeated hand washing, and open application tests.

Immersion Testing

To fully assess the in-use effects of the dishwashing liquids, a realistic exposure immersion testing should be used. Repeated short-term (15–30 min) immersions of the hands and/or forearms are used to assess primary irritation and dryness [38, 39]. Paye et al. showed that two products that could be differentiated in a Frosch-Kligman soap chamber test could also be differentiated in a hand immersion test – if the dominant and nondominant hands are assessed separately. The products could also be differentiated using bioengineering methods such as skin conductance and squamometry [40]. Interestingly, the dominant hand was observed to have a lower conductance at baseline than the nondominant hand.

Similarly Grammer-West et al. showed that the closed patch (soap chamber) test is able to differentiate the primary irritation potential of anionic and nonionic surfactant-based dishwashing liquids [41]. This enables a formulator to screen up to eight samples at one time, making formula optimization based on irritation potential more efficient. The method of usage or applicator does not usually play a significant role in the amount of irritation produced in an in-use situation. However, the intensity of skin effects is dependent on the products' compositions, concentration, and temperature [42], as well as the reactivity of the subjects' skin.

Repeated Hand Washing

Repeated hand washing with soap has been used to generate skin dryness [42]. Initially, dryness and surface corneocyte damage are produced. This can be assessed by a trained observer, by conductance measurements, and by squamometry. With more washings, erythema and stratum corneum barrier damage (measured by TEWL) are produced [43]. However, this method is more frequently used to assess the efficacy of moisturizers to prevent dryness than to compare the ability of different surfactants to elicit it.

Open Application Tests

Repeated exposure of a small test site to surfactant-based cleansers or other cosmetics can produce irritation even when the skin is left open to the environment (i.e., not occluded). This has been used as a diagnostic tool in identifying products or ingredients that have caused adverse reactions (Repeated Open Application Test, or ROAT) [44]. It has also been used predictively and as a test model. Wigger-Albert, Elsner, and their colleagues have used the repeated irritation test to elicit dryness and stratum corneum barrier damage and to assess the ability of protective (barrier) creams to inhibit the irritation [45].

In two related papers, Wilhelm et al. compared the response of different surfactants to induce irritation and dryness in open and closed patch testing [12, 46]. They showed that closed patch testing produced more erythema rather than the dryness observed in open patch exposure. In open patching the response was observed at a higher surfactant concentration – 7.5 % compared with 0.5 % in occlusive patches. Furthermore, in occlusive patches the anionic surfactant SLS gave stronger stratum corneum barrier disruption, as measured by TEWL, and dryness, as measured by conductance. However, the erythema response was similar with observer and colorimeter measurements.

Behind-the-Knee Test

Farage developed a method called behind-the-knee (BTK) test to include other irritant factors [47–49]. This method not only demonstrates the potential of chemical irritation from substrates/products, but also illustrates that mechanical irritation could contribute to the overall irritation potential. In this test protocol, samples are applied to the back of the knee using an elastic band, allowing panelists to carry on with their daily activities. Movements during these activities help generate friction between the test sample and the skin. This adds the element of mechanical irritation to patch testing. The main advantage of this method is that two products can be tested on the same panelist at the same point in time. Compared to other standard patch tests, BTK testing consistently showed higher irritation levels with reproducible results. Although this test was developed to test catamenial products, the author suggests that it has potential for evaluating textiles, facial tissues, baby and adult diapers, and laundry products, because mechanical irritation may contribute to the overall irritation potentials [50].

22.6 Models for Measuring the Moisturizing Potential of Cleansers

Previously, most evaluations of cleanser effects on the skin have been to assess primary irritation or drying potential. Such studies start with the skin in good condition and the extent by which parameters such as erythema and dryness worsen is evaluated. Moisturization potential has the implication that skin condition is improved. Therefore, a different experimental design is required. Such studies incorporate aspects of moisturizer efficacy testing, especially with regard to:

- Starting with dry skin, to enable improvement to be observed
- Use of moisturizer endpoints, such as assessments of skin dryness and skin hydration, together with
- Application methods that reflect how the cleansing products are used

Ideally the application method should not greatly affect dry skin, especially by removing it. Thus, the method initially described by Lukakovic et al. in 1988 is probably the most appropriate method. Methods that involve rubbing for a longer time (e.g., the flex wash or the volar forearm wash test) have the potential to remove skin flakes, resulting in a loss of sensitivity.

22.6.1 Testing on Dry Skin

To demonstrate that the cleanser delivers a benefit to the skin, the skin must start out in poor condition. As with moisturizer efficacy studies, the skin should be dry at baseline (dryness score of 2 or more on a 0–4 scale). It is best to run the test on a body site that readily shows skin dryness, such as the lower legs or the dorsal aspect of the forearms. The former has sufficient area to enable multiple products (and a non-product control) to be tested simultaneously. Using a within-subject design enables potentially large person-to-person variations to be eliminated. There are three main ways to produce dry skin:

1. Rely on cold weather frequently occurring during the winter to produce dryness.
2. Selecting people that have a predisposition to dry skin. As people age they exhibit more dry skin, especially on the extremities.
3. Pre-wash their test area with a drying cleanser.

Combining the first and second methods is probably the best approach. Relying on the weather alone can be risky, as a few warm, humid days will significantly reduce the level of dryness observed.

Giving the panelists a drying soap bar for regular cleansing has two great disadvantages. Firstly, the soap bar may interfere with the effects of the moisturizing cleanser, and consumers do not use two cleansing products on the same body sites. Secondly, Ertel et al. suggested that artificially drying out the skin with soap reduces the response compared with naturally dry skin. The basis of this is unclear, but it contrasts with the enhanced irritation response observed when subclinically or mildly irritated skin is exposed to an irritant.

22.6.2 Measuring the Clinical Effects of Moisturizing Cleansers on the Skin

Based on the approaches used to assess moisturizer efficacy, the two main parameters to assess the moisturizing potential of cleansing products are skin dryness and skin hydration.

It is advisable to use multiple methods for assessing efficacy, as each individual method has potential shortcomings. The use of a panopoly of methods will yield a fuller assessment of skin condition.

22.6.2.1 Skin Dryness

Traditionally, a trained observer using an ordinal scale has evaluated skin dryness. However, this approach has two major drawbacks. Firstly, it is dependent on the evaluator – great care must be taken to ensure reproducibility between evaluators, between studies, and between different testing laboratories. In this setting, a standardized photographic scale is helpful. Secondly, there are many factors that can reduce the appearance of dryness without any benefit to the skin. These include short-term humidity, and occlusive lotions that matte the dry skin flake down without removing them. These problems can be overcome by using an adhesive tape to sample the skin's surface; an example is DeSquame™ tape (CuDerm Inc., Dallas, TX, USA). The tape is pressed onto the skin's surface and then removed. The greater the scaling, the more skin flakes are removed by the tape. These can be quantified by using an analog scale or by image analysis [51]. The tape will remove the flakes even if they are matted down or obscured by hydration.

The use of DeSquame™ tape has been expanded to assess the damage to surface corneocytes (i.e., squamometry).

22.6.2.2 Conductance and Capacitance

Conductance and/or capacitance are frequently used to measure skin hydration. This approach has been supported empirically by Morrison and Scala [52], who showed a strong correlation between dryness and reduction in skin conductance (measured by a Skicon 200™) and capacitance (measured by a Nova™ dermal phase meter). There are two explanations of how skin conductance measures dryness. First, as the skin becomes drier, the concentration of water in the stratum corneum is reduced. As water is a good conductor compared with the more hydrophobic stratum corneum, a reduction in water activity will reduce conductance. Another possible mechanism by which dryness reduces conductance is that as scales develop, air pockets are formed in the damaged stratum corneum. Because air is a poor conductor, this scaling also results in reduced conductance. Clearly these two mechanisms are not mutually exclusive and may occur simultaneously.

Note that residues left on the skin's surface may modify conductance in the absence of dryness. For instance, petrolatum, silicones, and mineral oil are good insulators and can reduce conductance even as they moisturize the skin. Conductance data should be evaluated based on the product's composition and an understanding of which ingredients may remain on the skin after rinsing.

22.7 Bioengineering Measurements of Skin Condition

The last 30 years have seen a great expansion in the number and sophistication of bioengineering instruments to assess skin condition. These instruments provide a quantitative assessment of a single characteristic of the skin. Based on our knowledge of skin physiology and irritation processes, bioengineering instruments are used as a measure of irritation. Like all metrics, bioengineering methods can be misleading when used inappropriately. Though they provide objective responses that can be reduced to a single number or series of numbers, each measurement can be affected by parameters that have nothing to do with skin irritation. For instance, an evaporimeter measures water loss from the skin's surface, but cannot differentiate water loss due to sweating from that due to disruption of the stratum corneum. Thus, the environmental temperature must be kept below that causing most panelists to sweat (70 °F).

For most bioengineering methods, environmental and experimental conditions must be tightly controlled and the data carefully interpreted. To help with this, guidelines for many instrumental methods, such as TEWL, have been published and should be followed [53]. Table 22.1 shows the bioengineering methods most frequently used to measure irritation.

Table 22.1 Bioengineering instruments used to assess skin irritation

Skin characteristic	Interpretation	Issues	Instrumentation
TEWL[a]	Measure of stratum corneum barrier integrity/damage	Measures water regardless of source (e.g., sweat)	Evaporimeter
		Must use in temperature- and humidity-controlled environment	DermaLab TEWL[a] probe
			Tewameter
Skin color/redness	Erythema		Chromameter
			Erythema meter
			Dermaspectrometer
Blood flow	Irritation increases blood flow in the superficial dermis	Due to laser, cannot be used near eyes	Laser Doppler Velocimeter
Desquamation Index	Skin dryness (scaling/flaking)	Reproducible sampling of the skin	DeSquame tape
			Image analysis
Skin conductance/capacitance	Skin hydration	Materials that change dielectric of skin will effect reading	Skicon 200
			DermaLab
			Nova meter
Stained DeSquame (squamometry)	Skin surface integrity	Reproducible sampling of the skin	DeSquame tape Polymultichrome stain
		High levels of damage can disintegrate cells and cause loss of dye	Chromameter

Modified from [54] with kind permission from Springer Science and Business Media
[a]*TEWL* transepidermal water loss

References

1. Malten KE. Thoughts on irritant contact dermatitis. Contact Dermatitis. 1981;7:238–47.
2. Kligman AM. The invisible dermatoses. Arch Dermatol. 1991;127:1375–82.
3. Freeman S, Maibach H. Study of irritant contact dermatitis produced by repeat patch test with sodium lauryl sulfate and assessed by visual methods, transepidermal water loss, and laser Doppler velocimetry. J Am Acad Dermatol. 1988;19:496–502.
4. Degroot AC, Nater JP, Vanderlende R, Rijcken B. Adverse-effects of cosmetics and toiletries – a retrospective study in the general-population. Int J Cosmet Sci. 1987;9:255–9.
5. Frosch P. A method for appraising the stinging capacity of topically applied substances. J Soc Cosmet Chem. 1977;28:197–209.
6. Green B, Bluth J. Measuring the chemosensory irritability of human skin. J Toxicol Cutan Ocul. 1995;14:23–48.
7. Yosipovitch G, Maibach HI. Effect of topical pramoxine on experimentally induced pruritus in humans. J Am Acad Dermatol. 1997;37:278–80.
8. Leopold CS, Maibach HI. Percutaneous penetration of local anesthetic bases: pharmacodynamic measurements. J Invest Dermatol. 1999;113:304–7.
9. Simion FA, Rhein LD, Morrison BM, Scala D, Salko DM, Kligman AM, Grove GL. Self-perceived sensory responses to soap and synthetic detergent bars correlate with clinical signs of irritation. J Am Acad Dermatol. 1995;32:205–11.
10. Paye M, Cartiaux Y. Squamometry: a tool to move from exaggerated to more and more realistic application conditions for comparing the skin compatibility of surfactant-based products. Int J Cosmet Sci. 1999;21:59–68.
11. Piérard G, Arrese J, Rodríguez C. Effects of softened and unsoftened fabrics on sensitive skin. Contact Dermatitis. 1994;30:286–91.
12. Wilhelm KP, Cua AB, Wolff HH, Maibach HI. Surfactant-induced stratum-corneum hydration in-vivo – prediction of the irritation potential of anionic surfactants. J Invest Dermatol. 1993;101:310–5.
13. Rhein L, Robbins C. Surfactant structure effects on swelling of isolated human stratum corneum. J Soc Cosmet Chem. 1986;37:125–39.
14. Imokawa G, Mishima Y. Cumulative effect of surfactants on cutaneous horny layers: adsorption onto human keratin layers in vivo. Contact Dermatitis. 1979;5:357–66.
15. Kawai M, Imokawa G. The induction of skin tightness by surfactants. J Soc Cosmet Chem. 1984;35:147–56.
16. Cua AB, Wilhelm KP, Maibach HI. Cutaneous sodium lauryl sulfate irritation potential – Age and regional variability. Br J Dermatol. 1990;123:607–13.
17. Rougier A, Lotte C, Maibach HI. In vivo relationship between percutaneous absorption and transepidermal water loss. In: Bronaugh RL, Maibach HI, editors. Topical absorption of dermatological products. New York: CRC Press; 2002. p. 108–20.

18. Allenby CF, Basketter DA, Dickens A, Barnes EG, Brough HC. An arm immersion model of compromised skin (I). Influence on irritation reactions. Contact Dermatitis. 1993;28:84–8.
19. Frosch PJ, Kligman AM. The chamber-scarification test for irritancy. Contact Dermatitis. 1976;2: 314–24.
20. Berardesca E, Cespa M, Farinelli N, Rabbiosi G, Maibach H. In vivo transcutaneous penetration of nicotinates and sensitive skin. Contact Dermatitis. 1991;25:35–8.
21. Agner T, Serup J. Seasonal-variation of skin resistance to irritants. Br J Dermatol. 1989;121:323–8.
22. Agner T. Susceptibility of atopic dermatitis patients to irritant dermatitis caused by sodium lauryl sulphate. Acta Derm Venereol. 1991;71:296–300.
23. Pinnagoda J, Tupker RA, Coenraads PJ, Nater JP. Prediction of susceptibility to an irritant response by transepidermal water loss. Contact Dermatitis. 1989;20:341–6.
24. Simon F, Rhein L, Grove G. Sequential order of skin responses to surfactants during a soap chamber test. Contact Dermatitis. 1991;25:242–9.
25. Phillips L, Steinberg M, Maibach HI, Akers WA. A comparison of rabbit and human skin response to certain irritants. Toxicol Appl Pharmacol. 1972;21: 369–82.
26. Robinson M, McFadden J, Basketter D. Validity and ethics of the human 4-h patch test as an alternative method to assess acute skin irritation potential. Contact Dermatitis. 2001;45:1–12.
27. Frosch PJ, Kligman AM. The soap chamber test. A new method for assessing the irritancy of soaps. J Am Acad Dermatol. 1979;1:35–41.
28. Babulak SW, Rhein LD, Scala DD, Simion FA, Grove GL. Quantitation of erythema in a soap chamber test using a Minolta chroma (reflectance) meter: comparison of instrumental results with visual assessments. J Soc Cosmet Chem. 1986;37:475–9.
29. Morrison B, Babulak SW, Scala D, Simion FA, Woo-Ming G, Gyening I, Kenney JA, Kligman AM. Evaluation of the response of African-American skin to facial cleansing products using a soap chamber test. 51st American Academy of Dermatology annual meeting, San Francisco; 1992.
30. Strube DD, Koontz SW, Murahata R, Theiler RF. The flex wash test: a method for evaluating the clinical mildness of cleansing products. J Soc Cosmet Chem. 2012;40:297–306.
31. Lukacovic MF, Dunlap FE, Michaels SE, Visscher MO, Watson DD. Forearm wash test to evaluate the clinical mildness of cleansing products. J Soc Cosmet Chem. 1988;39:355–66.
32. Keswick BH, Ertel KD, Visscher MO. Comparison of exaggerated and normal use techniques for assessing the mildness of personal cleansers. J Soc Cosmet Chem. 1992;43:187–93.
33. Sharko P, Murahata R, Leyden J. Arm wash with instrumental evaluation: a sensitive technique for differentiating the irritation potential of personal washing products. J Dermatol Clin Eval Soc. 1991;2: 19–27.
34. Nicoll G, Murahata R, Grove G, Barrows J, Sharko P. The relative sensitivity of two arm-wash test methods for evaluating the mildness of personal washing products. J Soc Cosmet Chem. 1995;46:129–40.
35. Ertel KD, Neumann PB, Hartwig PM, Rains GY, Keswick BH. Leg wash protocol to assess the skin moisturization potential of personal cleansing products. Int J Cosmet Sci. 1999;21:383–97.
36. Halkier-Sorensen L. Notified occupational skin diseases in Denmark. Contact Dermatitis. 1996;35:1–44.
37. Wall LM, Gebauer KA. Occupational skin disease in Western Australia. Contact Dermatitis. 1991;24: 101–9.
38. Kooyman D, Snyder FH. Tests for mildness of soap. Arch Dermatol. 1942;46:846–55.
39. Justice J, Travers J, Vinson L. The correlation between animal tests and human tests in assessing product mildness. Proc Sci Sect Toilet Goods Assoc. 1961;35:12–7.
40. Paye M, Gomes G, Zerweck C, Pierard GE, Grove GL. A hand immersion test under laboratory controlled usage conditions: the need for sensitive and controlled assessment methods. Contact Dermatitis. 1999;40:133–8.
41. Grammer-West N, Fitzpatrick J, Jackson R, Horton H, Damiano M. Comparison of the irritancy of hand dishwashing liquids with modified patch testing methods. J Am Acad Dermatol. 1996;35:258–60.
42. Clarys P, Manou I, Barel AO. Influence of temperature on irritation in the hand/forearm immersion test. Contact Dermatitis. 1997;36:240–3.
43. Simion F, Babulak SW, Morrison B Jr, Rhein L. Experimental method for soap-induced dryness in the absence of erythema. American Academy of Dermatology, 50th annual meeting, 1991
44. Hannuksela M, Salo H. The repeated open application test (ROAT). Contact Dermatitis. 1986;14:221–7.
45. Wigger-Alberti W, Krebs A, Elsner P. Experimental irritant contact dermatitis due to cumulative epicutaneous exposure to sodium lauryl sulphate and toluene: single and concurrent application. Br J Dermatol. 2000;143:551–6.
46. Wilhelm KP, Freitag G, Wolff HH. Surfactant-induced skin irritation and skin repair – evaluation of a cumulative human irritation model by noninvasive techniques. J Am Acad Dermatol. 1994;31:981–7.
47. Farage MA, Gilpin DA, Enane NA, Baldwin S. Development of a new test for mechanical irritation: behind the knee as a test site. Skin Res Technol. 2001;7:193–203.
48. Farage MA, Meyer S, Walter D. Development of a sensitive test method to evaluate mechanical irritation potential on mucosal skin. Skin Res Technol. 2004;10:85–95.
49. Farage MA, Meyer S, Walter D. Evaluation of modifications of the traditional patch test in assessing the chemical irritation potential of feminine hygiene products. Skin Res Technol. 2004;10:73–84.

50. Farage MA. The behind-the-knee test: an efficient model for evaluating mechanical and chemical irritation. Skin Res Technol. 2006;12:73–82.
51. Schatz H, Kligman AM, Manning S, Stoudemayer T. Quantification of dry (xerotic) skin by image-analysis of scales removed by adhesive disks (D-squames). J Soc Cosmet Chem. 1993;44:53–63.
52. Morrison B, Scala D. Comparison of instrumental measurements of skin hydration. J Toxicol Cutan Ocul. 1996;15:305–14.
53. Elsner P. Bioengineering of the Skin. Skin Biomechanics: CRC Press. 2002;5:296.
54. Simion FA, Maibach HI. In vivo models of skin irritation. In: Irritant dermatitis. 1st ed. Berlin/London: Springer; 2005. p. 562.

23

Acute Irritancy Testing for Predicting Increased Susceptibility to Irritant Contact Dermatitis in Atopic Individuals

Irena Angelova-Fischer, Swen Malte John, and Sanja Kezic

Contents

I. Angelova-Fischer, M.D., Ph.D. (✉)
Department of Dermatology, University of Lübeck, Ratzeburger Allee 160, Lübeck 23538, Germany
e-mail: irena.angelova-fischer@uk-sh.de

S.M. John, M.D.
Department of Dermatology, Environmental Medicine and Health Theory, University of Osnabrueck, Sedanstr. 115, Osnabrueck 49069, Germany
e-mail: sjohn@uos.de

S. Kezic, Ph.D.
Coronel Institute of Occupational Health, Academic Medical Center, Meibergdreef 9, Amsterdam AZ 1105, The Netherlands
e-mail: s.kezic@amc.uva.nl

23.1 Background

Atopic dermatitis is a relapsing and intensely pruritic inflammatory skin disease that results from a complex interplay of genetic, immunologic and environmental factors. Epidemiological data provide evidence that atopic dermatitis confers an increased risk for development of chronic irritant dermatitis and raise the question whether experimentally-induced challenge may predict the enhanced susceptibility to irritant damage in atopic skin [1, 2]. In the present chapter, we summarize the scientific knowledge derived from the acute irritant exposure studies in atopic individuals that have been published so far, with respect to the type of applied irritant, test conditions and measured endpoints.

23.2 Acute Irritancy Testing with Sodium Lauryl Sulfate

Exposure to the anionic surfactant sodium lauryl sulfate (SLS) is an established experimental model for the *in vivo* study of skin irritation. The clinical manifestations and histopathological findings after single or repetitive SLS-induced damage to the skin barrier have been characterized in detail and are known to be dependent on the purity, concentration and mode of exposure among other factors [3–9]. The outcomes of SLS challenge in atopic dermatitis patients in acute stage and during remission have been extensively studied and show considerable variations.

A. Alikhan et al. (eds.), *Textbook of Hand Eczema*,
DOI 10.1007/978-3-642-39546-8_23, © Springer-Verlag Berlin Heidelberg 2014

Basketter et al. [10] investigated the irritant response after single patch test exposure to 0.5 %, 1.0 %, 5.0 %, and 20 % SLS applied for 24 h, 8 h, 4 h and 2 h, respectively, on the back of atopic dermatitis patients without active eczema lesions in the test area at the time of irritant challenge and healthy aged-matched controls. Comparison of the irritant reactivity assessed by visual grading, transepidermal water loss (TEWL), erythema and blood flow measured 15 min, 24 h, 48 h and 72 h after removal of the test chambers showed no significant differences between the groups at any observation time point. In agreement with these findings, evaluation of the skin response after a single 23-hour patch test application of 0.5 % SLS in 205 metalworker trainees performed by Stolz et al. [11] showed no correlation between the skin atopy score [12] and the post-exposure TEWL values.

Analysis of the outcomes of a 48-hour patch test challenge with 0.5 % SLS, dependent on the presence or absence of eczematous lesions, performed by Löffler and Effendy [13], found significantly higher post-irritation TEWL values in patients with inflammatory lesions at the time of exposure, suggesting that the skin irritant susceptibility might be influenced by disease activity. Atopic dermatitis severity and activity have been shown to modify the epidermal barrier function [14–17] and patients with active disease were reported to have increased baseline TEWL values at uninvolved skin sites with respect to patients without skin lesions at the time of evaluation [18]. As baseline TEWL is considered an indicator for the skin irritant susceptibility [19–22], the higher pre-exposure TEWL values in the group of patients with clinical manifestations of eczema at the time of testing might explain the observations of Löffler and Effendy.

Increased skin reactivity after experimentally induced SLS challenge in atopic dermatitis patients was first reported by van der Valk et al. [23]. Sixty-nine patients with different types of eczema without skin lesions at the time of investigation and 34 controls were exposed to 2 % SLS solution in a large Finn chamber for 48 h, among other irritants. The eczema group included patients with atopic dermatitis, allergic or irritant contact dermatitis, dyshidrotic dermatitis or unclassified eczema based on the history, clinical manifestations and immediate skin and patch tests. The control panel consisted of healthy volunteers as well as patients with skin diseases other than eczema. Comparison of the differences in post-exposure TEWL values among the eczema subgroups, measured immediately after removal of the test chamber and 24 h later, showed significantly higher TEWL in the patients with atopic dermatitis compared to those with irritant contact dermatitis.

Agner [24] observed a similar reactivity pattern after patch test challenge in 28 atopic dermatitis patients exposed to 0.5 % aqueous solution of SLS for 24 h. In addition to the more pronounced atopic skin response assessed by visual scoring and bioengineering measurements, the findings of the study supported the evidence for a correlation between the baseline and post-exposure TEWL values. In agreement with these results, Tabata et al. [25] found a greater and longer lasting increase in TEWL after 24-hour patch test exposure to 1 % SLS in atopic patients than in controls. Enhanced responses to acute irritancy testing have been further reported by Cowley et al. [26], who investigated the dose–response after challenge with SLS concentrations ranging from 0.125 % to 4 % in patients with atopic dermatitis, seborrheic dermatitis and healthy controls. The results of the study showed significant differences in the lowest SLS concentration inducing erythema and increase in the blood flux, measured by laser Doppler flow meter, between the group of atopic patients and the healthy controls.

Increased skin reactivity after acute irritation with SLS has also been documented in studies investigating the effects of combined exposure to irritants and allergens in atopic skin. Seidenari et al. [27] observed a more pronounced decrease in the superficial echogenicity of the skin in atopic patients exposed to 5 % SLS for 30 min under occlusion compared to nickel-sensitized controls without atopy. Similarly, Löffler et al. [28] investigated the endpoints of single and concurrent patch test application of 0.5 % SLS and aeroallergens in atopic dermatitis patients sensitized to house dust mite, cat dander, birch or grass pollen compared to healthy non-sensitized controls and reported higher post-irritation TEWL values in the atopic dermatitis group.

The factors that contribute to the reported differences after acute SLS-induced irritation in atopic skin remain unknown. Comparison across studies is hampered by variations in the exposure conditions, such as duration, applied SLS concentration and measured effect parameters. In addition to the external factors, the outcomes of acute irritancy testing may be influenced by intrinsic factors, other than atopic dermatitis, that modify the epidermal barrier properties and inflammatory skin response [1, 29–37]. Furthermore, even though independent studies in various occupational settings provide evidence that atopic dermatitis is a significant risk factor for development of irritant dermatitis and hand eczema [1, 38–44], the results of experimentally induced SLS irritation suggest that short-term patch test exposure to a single irritant may not adequately reflect the mechanisms involved in cumulative irritation and, consequently, may not predict the outcomes of repeated subthreshold damage to the skin barrier [8, 9, 45].

23.3 Sodium Hydroxide Exposure Tests

Sodium hydroxide (NaOH) has been extensively used for the study of skin irritation in health and disease. Predictive testing with NaOH was introduced by Burckhardt, who aimed to establish a screening procedure that could predict the individual susceptibility to skin irritation induced by chemicals [46]. The original method developed in 1947 as "alkali resistance test" was based on repeated exposures to 0.5 N NaOH under glass blocks for 10 min and the endpoint was defined as the time until vesicles and erosions became manifest. Further development of the test procedure was the introduction of nitrazine yellow to facilitate the recognition of eroded sites [47]. Subsequent modifications aimed to standardize and improve the reliability of the test for use in experimental studies and individual risk assessment in occupational dermatology [48–51].

The relationship between the irritant reactivity after NaOH challenge and skin atopy defined by the Erlanger atopy score [12] has been investigated by Stolz et al. [11], who exposed 205 metalworker trainees, as previously mentioned, to 0.1 mL of a 0.2 mol/L aqueous solution of the irritant applied for 5 min on the volar surface of the forearm in a modified alkali resistance test. The results of the study showed a poor correlation between the atopy score and the increase in TEWL measured 5–10 min after the irritants had been removed. These observations are partly in contrast to the findings of another study of patients with a history of clinically resolved, in most cases, occupational irritant contact dermatitis using a swift modified alkali resistance test (SMART; 52). The test is based on a 0.5 M NaOH challenge for 2 × 10 min with intermediate TEWL measurements and clinical assessment; an adjacent area exposed to 0.9 % NaCl serves as control (Fig. 23.1). The test procedure has been validated in two cohorts with a total of 1,111 individuals with previous occupational dermatitis [51–53]. Comparing the skin reactivity to NaOH on the forearm and the back of the dominant hand simultaneously (Differential Irritation Test, DIT), the authors confirmed that in general the back of the hand is relatively robust to 0.5 M NaOH irritation, although this is less pronounced in atopics. The test was indicative of atopic skin disposition as evidenced by the almost fivefold increased odds for a positive clinical reaction to NaOH (OR 4.8, 95 % CI: 3.0–7.8) when performed on the volar forearm and threefold increased odds on the back of the hand (OR 3.1, 95 % CI: 1.8–5.5). Furthermore, the results of the study [51] suggest that ambient meteorological conditions such as absolute humidity and temperature on the day of patch testing influence the outcomes of NaOH irritation, the impact being even more pronounced in atopic individuals. Taken together, these findings may contribute to explain the controversies with regard to the published outcomes and predictive value of acute irritancy testing.

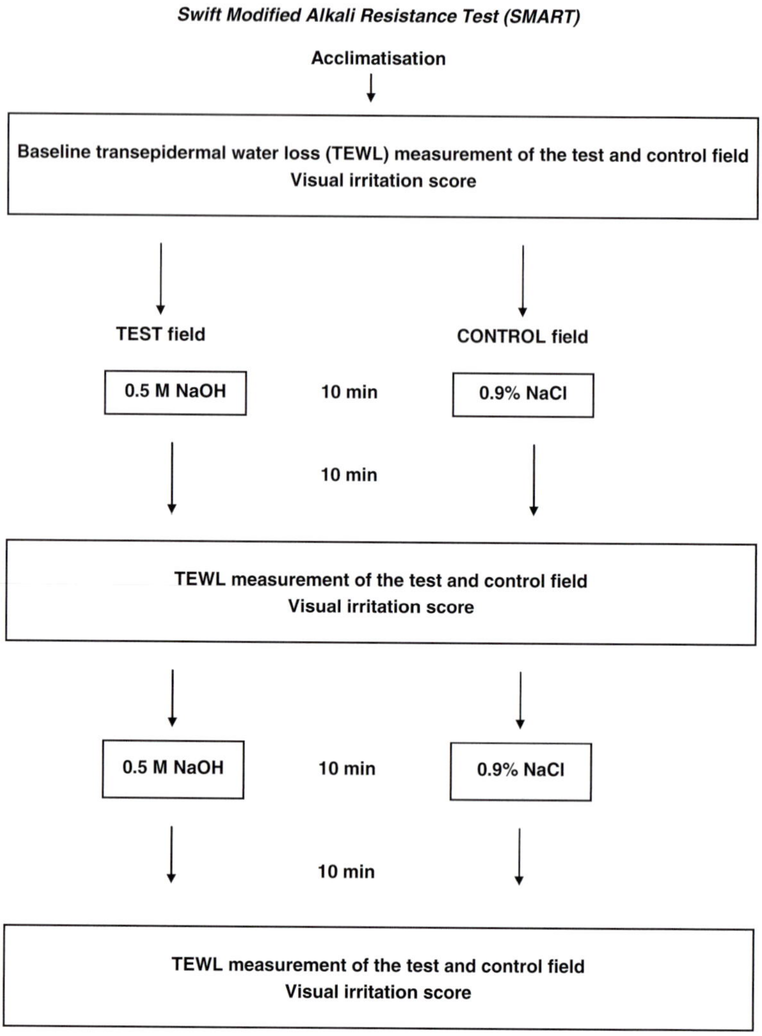

Fig. 23.1 Swift Modified Alkali Resistance Test (SMART) procedure. Test site: mid-volar forearm; the results may be compared to the same challenge performed on the back of the hand (Differential Irritation Test, or DIT)

23.4 Exposure to Other Irritants

Few published studies assess the skin reactivity in atopic dermatitis after acute irritancy testing with surfactants other than SLS, dimethyl sulfoxide (DMSO), benzalkonium chloride, propylene and hexylene glycol, coco trimethyl ammonium chloride and hydrochloric acid [54–56].

Van der Valk et al. [23] compared the irritant response in patients with different types of eczema, non-eczematous skin diseases, and healthy controls after 48-hour patch test application of eight different surfactants, including SLS. The increase in TEWL after exposure to cocobetaine, ceteareth-12, cocamidopropylbetaine, and polysorbate-60 revealed significant differences between the subgroups of patients with atopic and irritant dermatitis, whereas no differences in the skin response to sodium laurate, sodium stearate or potassium soap were found.

Santucci et al. [57] investigated the influence of pre-existing dermatitis on patch test challenge with a panel of surfactants (disodium laureth sulfosuccinate, potassium cocoate, potassium oleate, zinc coleth sulfate, sodium myreth sulfate, and sodium cocoamphoacetate) found in marketed products compared to standard irritants such as 1 % SLS, 1 % benzalkonium chloride, and 10 % DMSO. The tested irritants were applied for 2 days under occlusion to the skin of the upper back of 40 healthy nonatopic volunteers and 40 patients with manifest atopic dermatitis among 480 patients with different skin diseases including psoriasis, eczema, urticaria or generalized pruritus and the reaction was assessed 1 h after removal of the chamber by visual grading. Based on the number of positive responses, no evidence for increased susceptibility to irritant damage in the patients with atopic dermatitis was found. The assessment of the irritant response in the study, however, relied on a single reading shortly after removal of the patch and the time point the scoring was performed might have influenced the outcomes as well as contributed to the differences to earlier exposure tests with benzalkonium chloride or DMSO in atopic skin [1, 58].

The endpoints of different application modes of a commercially available detergent in atopic dermatitis patients free of inflammatory lesions at the time of irritant exposure and healthy controls were studied by Hannuksela and Hannuksela [59]. The visual assessment and instrumental measurement of erythema and TEWL after 48-hour patch test challenge revealed no significant differences between the groups.

23.5 Irritant Challenge Studies in Atopic Dermatitis Carriers of Filaggrin Gene Loss-of-Function Mutations

The irritant-challenge responses in relation to atopic dermatitis and filaggrin gene (*FLG*) mutations carrier state have been investigated in two studies showing similar results. Jungerstedt et al. [60] compared the outcomes of a 24-hour patch test application of 1 % SLS in 27 atopic dermatitis patients subdivided into *FLG* mutation carriers or wild type based on genotyping for R501X and 2282del4 loss-of-function variants and found no statistically significant differences between the groups with regard to the post-irritation delta TEWL and erythema values. These observations have been confirmed and extended in another study [61] that monitored the clinical severity, barrier impairment and recovery after 1 % SLS exposure

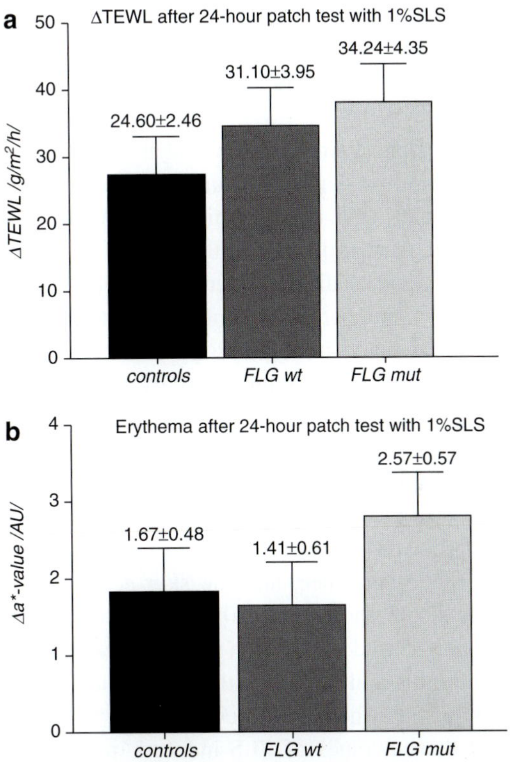

Fig. 23.2 Transepidermal water loss (**a**) and erythema (**b**) after 24-hour patch test challenge with 1 % sodium lauryl sulfate (SLS) in atopic dermatitis carriers of the prevalent European R501X, 2282del4, R2447X or S3247X loss-of-function filaggrin gene mutations (*FLG mut*) noncarriers (*FLG wt*) and healthy controls. Mean ± SEM; **Δ** value = post-exposure value – baseline value, level of significance <0.05. *TEWL* – transepidermal water loss

under the same conditions in atopic dermatitis patients homozygous, heterozygous, or compound heterozygous for the prevalent R501X, 2282del4, R2447X and S3247X European *FLG* mutations compared to non-carriers and healthy controls. Though compared to baseline, 3 h after removal of the chamber filaggrin-related eczema was characterized by a more pronounced TEWL and a*-value increase than non-filaggrin eczema or the healthy controls, the differences among the groups were not significant (Fig. 23.2). Furthermore, repeated measurements of TEWL and erythema every 24 h up to 72 h post-irritation showed no significant differences in the rate of barrier recovery between the atopic *FLG* mutation carriers and non-carriers or mutation carriers and controls.

23.6 Acute Irritancy Testing in Atopic Individuals Without Dermatitis

Independent studies provide evidence for comparable baseline skin barrier function parameters in individuals with allergic rhinitis and/or asthma without dermatitis and healthy nonatopic controls. Irritant-challenge experiments, even though limited in number, show conflicting results.

Based on visual scoring, Nassif et al. [62] reported a lower irritant reactivity threshold in patients with allergic rhinitis without atopic skin manifestations after 48-hour exposure to serial dilutions of SLS ranging from 0.0625 % to 4.0 %. In contrast to these findings, Seidenari et al. [63, 64] showed no differences in post-exposure TEWL, capacitance, and the skin echogenicity after single short-term (30 min) application of 0.5 % SLS under occlusion in patients with allergic rhinitis and asthma without AD and healthy controls. Furthermore, they provided evidence that the outcomes of SLS-induced irritation in patients with respiratory atopy are consistent independent of whether the skin was challenged in a symptom-free or active stage of disease. Comparison of the post-exposure TEWL values after 48-hour patch test irritation with 0.5 % SLS performed by Löffler and Effendy [65] confirmed these observations by showing similar skin responses in individuals with allergic airway disease without dermatitis and healthy nonatopic controls.

Independent of the endpoints, the current understanding of the skin reactivity in individuals with allergic rhinitis or asthma without dermatitis relies entirely on single irritant-challenge experiments with SLS, whereas the outcomes of cumulative irritation or exposure to other primary irritants have not been systematically studied.

Conclusion

Though the scientific knowledge generated from epidemiological and occupational risk assessment studies provides strong evidence for the positive association of atopic dermatitis with enhanced irritant susceptibility, the acute irritant exposure studies with model irritants in atopic skin published so far show conflicting results. Compared to the inconsistent findings after SLS-induced irritation, the swift modified alkali resistance test (SMART) may provide advantages, as shown by the positive association of the atopic skin disposition to pronounced clinical responses and barrier function impairment after NaOH challenge. Thus far, there is limited knowledge on the endpoints of acute irritancy testing in atopic dermatitis *FLG* loss-of-function mutation carriers. Whereas the published reports suggest no *FLG*-dependent differences in the outcomes, the findings are based on a small number of patients and refer to 24-hour patch test with 1 % SLS that may not necessarily predict the skin response to other chemically unrelated irritants. The skin reactivity after patch test exposure to SLS in individuals with allergic rhinitis and/or asthma without dermatitis is considered to be independent of disease activity and similar to the irritant-induced response in healthy skin.

References

1. Seidenari S, Giusti F. Atopy. In: Chew AL, Maibach HI, editors. Irritant dermatitis. Berlin: Springer; 2006. p. 185–97.
2. Visser MJ, Landeck L, Campbell LE, McLean WH, Weidinger S, Calkoen F, et al. Impact of loss-of-function mutations in the filaggrin gene and atopic dermatitis on the development of occupational irritant contact dermatitis. Br J Dermatol. 2013;168:326–32.
3. Tupker RA, Willis C, Berardesca E, Lee CH, Fartasch M, Agner T, et al. Guidelines on sodium lauryl sulfate (SLS) exposure tests. Contact Dermatitis. 1997;37:53–69.
4. Lee CH, Maibach HI. Sodium lauryl sulfate. In: Chew AL, Maibach HI, editors. Irritant dermatitis. Berlin: Springer; 2006. p. 257–67.
5. Aramaki J, Loffler C, Kawana S, Effendy I, Happle R, Löffler H, et al. Irritant patch testing with sodium lauryl sulphate: interrelation between concentration and exposure time. Br J Dermatol. 2001;145:704–8.
6. Agner T, Serup J, Handlos V, Batsberg W. Different skin irritation abilities of different qualities of sodium lauryl sulphate. Contact Dermatitis. 1989;21:184–8.
7. Agner T, Fullerton A, Broby-Johansen U, Batsberg W. Irritant patch testing: penetration of SLS into human skin. Skin Pharmacol. 1990;3:213–7.

8. De Jongh CM, Verberk MM, Withagen CE, Jacobs JJ, Kezic S, Rustemeyer T. Stratum corneum cytokines and skin irritation response to sodium lauryl sulfate. Contact Dermatitis. 2006;54:325–33.
9. De Jongh CM, Lutter R, Verberk M, Kezic S. Differential cytokine expression in skin after single and repeated irritation by sodium lauryl sulphate. Exp Dermatol. 2007;16:1032–40.
10. Basketter D, Miettinen J, Lahti A. Acute irritant reactivity to sodium lauryl sulfate in atopics and non-atopics. Contact Dermatitis. 1998;38:253–7.
11. Stolz R, Hinnen U, Elsner P. An evaluation of the relationship between "atopic skin" and skin irritability in metalworker trainees. Contact Dermatitis. 1997;36:281–4.
12. Diepgen TL, Fartasch M, Horstein OP. Evaluation and relevance of atopic basic and minor features in patients with atopic dermatitis and in the general population. Acta Dermatol Venereol. 1989;144:50–4.
13. Löffler H, Effendy I. Skin susceptibility of atopic individuals. Contact Dermatitis. 1999;40:239–42.
14. Aalto-Korte K. Improvement of skin barrier function during treatment of atopic dermatitis. J Am Acad Dermatol. 1995;33:969–72.
15. Angelova-Fischer I, Bauer A, Hipler UC, Petrov I, Kazandjieva J, Bruckner T, et al. The objective severity assessment of atopic dermatitis (OSAAD) score: validity, reliability and sensitivity in adult patients with atopic dermatitis. Br J Dermatol. 2005;153:767–73.
16. Holm EA, Wulf HC, Thomassen L, Jemec GBE. Assessment of atopic eczema: clinical scoring and non-invasive measurements. Br J Dermatol. 2007;157:674–80.
17. Holm EA, Wulf HC, Thomassen L, Jemec GBE. Instrumental assessment of atopic eczema: validation of transepidermal water loss, stratum corneum hydration, erythema, scaling and edema. J Am Acad Dermatol. 2006;55:772–80.
18. Seidenari S, Giusti G. Objective assessment of the skin of children affected by atopic dermatitis: a study on pH, capacitance and TEWL in eczematous and clinically uninvolved skin. Acta Dermatol Venereol. 1995;75:429–33.
19. Murahata R, Crove DM, Roheim JR. The use of transepidermal water loss to measure and predict the irritation response to surfactants. Int J Cosmet Sci. 1986;8:225–31.
20. Pinnagoda J, Tupker R, Coenraads P, Nater J. Prediction of susceptibility to an irritant response by transepidermal water loss. Contact Dermatitis. 1989;20:341–6.
21. Tupker R, Pinnagoda J, Nater J. The transient and cumulative effect of sodium lauryl sulphate on the epidermal barrier assessed by transepidermal water loss: inter-individual variation. Acta Dermatol Venereol. 1990;70:1–5.
22. Tupker R, Pinnagoda J, Coenraads P, Nater J. Susceptibility to irritants: role of barrier function, skin dryness and history of atopic dermatitis. Br J Dermatol. 1990;123:199–205.
23. Van der Valk P, Nater J, Bleumink E. Vulnerability of the skin to surfactants in different groups of eczema patients and controls as measured by water vapour loss. Clin Exp Dermatol. 1985;10:98–103.
24. Agner T. Susceptibility of atopic dermatitis patients to irritant dermatitis caused by sodium lauryl sulphate. Acta Dermatol Venereol. 1991;71:296–300.
25. Tabata N, Tagami H, Kligman AM. A twenty-four hour occlusive exposure to 1% sodium lauryl sulfate induces a unique histopathologic inflammatory response in the xerotic skin of atopic dermatitis patients. Acta Derm Venereol. 1998;78:244–7.
26. Cowley NC, Farr PM. A dose-response study of irritant reactions to sodium lauryl sulphate in patients with seborrhoeic dermatitis and atopic eczema. Acta Dermatol Venereol. 1992;72:432–5.
27. Seidenari S. Reactivity to nickel sulfate at sodium lauryl sulfate pretreated skin sites is higher in atopics: an echographic evaluation by means of image analysis performed on 20 MHz B-scan recordings. Acta Dermatol Venereol. 1994;74:245–9.
28. Löffler H, Steffes A, Happle R, Effendy I. Allergy and irritation: an adverse association in patients with atopic eczema. Acta Dermatol Venereol. 2003;83: 328–31.
29. Willis CM. Variability in responsiveness to irritants: thoughts on possible underlying mechanisms. Contact Dermatitis. 2002;47:267–71.
30. Fluhr JW, Darlenski R, Angelova-Fischer I, Tsankov N, Basketter D. Skin irritation and sensitization: mechanisms and new approaches for risk assessment. Skin Pharmacol Physiol. 2008;21:124–35.
31. Allen MH, Wakelin SH, Holloway D, Lisby S, Baadsgaard O, Barker JN, et al. Association of TNFA gene polymorphism at position -308 with susceptibility to irritant contact dermatitis. Immunogenetics. 2000;51:201–5.
32. De Jongh CM, Khrenova L, Kezic S, Rustemeyer T, Verberk MM, John SM. Polymorphisms in the interleukin-1 gene influence the stratum corneum interleukin-1 alpha concentration in uninvolved skin of patients with chronic irritant contact dermatitis. Contact Dermatitis. 2008;58:263–8.
33. De Jongh CM, John SM, Bruynzeel DP, Calkoen F, van Dijk FJ, Khrenova L, et al. Cytokine gene polymorphisms and susceptibility to chronic irritant contact dermatitis. Contact Dermatitis. 2008;58:269–77.
34. Landeck L, Visser M, Kezic S, John SM. IL-1A 889 C/T gene polymorphism in irritant contact dermatitis. J Eur Acad Dermatol Venereol. 2013;27:1040–3.
35. Landeck L, Visser M, Kezic S, John SM. Impact of TNF-α polymorphisms on irritant contact dermatitis. Contact Dermatitis. 2012;66:221–7.
36. Jakasa I, De Jongh CM, Verberk MM, Bos JD, Kezic S. Percutaneous penetration of sodium lauryl sulfate is increased in uninvolved skin of patients with atopic dermatitis compared with control subjects. Br J Dermatol. 2006;155:104–9.
37. De Jongh CM, Jakasa I, Verberk MM, Kezic S. Variation in barrier impairment and inflammation of human skin as determined by sodium lauryl sulphate penetration rate. Br J Dermatol. 2005;154:651–7.

38. Dickel H, Bruckner T, Schmidt A, Diepgen T. Impact of atopic skin diathesis on occupational skin disease incidence in a working population. J Invest Dermatol. 2003;121:37–40.
39. Lammintausta K, Kalimo K. Atopy and hand dermatitis in hospital wet work. Contact Dermatitis. 1981;7:301–8.
40. Meding B, Swanbeck G. Predictive factors for hand eczema. Contact Dermatitis. 1990;23:154–61.
41. Kristensen O. A prospective study of the development of hand eczema in an automobile manufacturing industry. Contact Dermatitis. 1992;26:341–5.
42. Rystedt I. Work-related hand eczema in atopics. Contact Dermatitis. 1985;12:164–71.
43. Bauer A, Bartsch R, Stadeler M, Schneider W, Grieshaber R, Wollina U, et al. Development of occupational skin disease during vocational training in baker and confectioner apprentices: a follow-up study. Contact Dermatitis. 1998;39:307–11.
44. Berndt U, Hinnen U, Iliev D, Elsner P. Role of atopy score and of single atopic features as risk factors for the development of hand eczema in trainee metal workers. Br J Dermatol. 1999;140:922–4.
45. Koopman DG, Kezic S, Verberk MM. Skin reaction and recovery: a repeated sodium lauryl sulphate patch test vs. a 24-h patch test and tape stripping. Br J Dermatol. 2004;150:493–9.
46. Burckhardt W. Neue Untersuchungen über die Alkaliempfindlichkeit der Haut. Dermatologica. 1947;94:8–96.
47. Locher G. Permeabilitätsprüfung der Haut Ekzemkranker und Hautgesunder für den neuen Indikator Nitrazingelb Geigy, Modifizierung der Alkaliresistenzprobe, pH-Verlauf in der Tiefe des stratum corneum. Dermatologica. 1962;124:159–82.
48. Kolbe L, Kligman AM, Stoudemayer T. The sodium hydroxide erosion assay: a revision of the alkali resistance test. Arch Dermatol Res. 1998;290:382–7.
49. Ummenhofer B. Zur Methodik der Alkaliresistenzprüfung. Dermatosen. 1980;28:104–9.
50. Wilhelm KP, Pasche F, Surber C, Maibach HI. Sodium hydroxide-induced subclinical irritation. A test for evaluating stratum corneum barrier function. Acta Dermatol Venereol. 1990;70:463–7.
51. John SM, Uter W. Meteorological influence on NaOH-irritation varies with body site. Arch Dermatol Res. 2005;296:320–6.
52. John SM. Klinische und experimentelle Untersuchungen zur Diagnostik in der Berufsdermatologie. Konzeption einer wissenschaftlich begründeten Qualitätssicherung in der sozialmedizinischen Begutachtung. In: Schwanitz HJ, editor. Studien zur Prävention in Allergologie, Berufs- und Umweltdermatologie (ABU4). Universitätsverlag Rasch Osnabrück; 2001.
53. John SM, Schwanitz HJ. Functional skin testing: the SMART procedures. In: Chew AL, Maibach HI, editors. Irritant dermatitis. Berlin/Heidelberg: Springer; 2006. p. 211–21.
54. Gallacher G, Maibach HI. Is atopic dermatitis a predisposing factor for experimental acute irritant contact dermatitis? Contact Dermatitis. 1998;38:1–4.
55. Kinnunen T, Hannuksela M. Skin reaction to hexylene glycol. Contact Dermatitis. 1989;21:154–8.
56. Basketter D, Blaikie L, Reynolds F. The impact of atopic status on a predictive human test of skin irritation potential. Contact Dermatitis. 1996;35:33–9.
57. Santucci B, Cannistraci C, Lesnoni I, Ferraro M, Rocco MGDE, Dell'Anna L, et al. Cutaneous response to irritants. Contact Dermatitis. 2003;48:69–73.
58. Goh CL. Comparing skin irritancy in atopics and non-atopics to sodium lauryl sulphate and benzalkonium chloride using TEWL measurements. Environ Dermatol. 1997;4:30–2.
59. Hannuksela A, Hannuksela M. Irritant effects of a detergent in a wash, chamber and repeated open application tests. Contact Dermatitis. 1996;34:134–7.
60. Jungersted JM, Scheer H, Mempel M, Baurecht H, Cifuentes L, Høgh JK, et al. Stratum corneum lipids, skin barrier function and filaggrin mutations in patients with atopic eczema. Allergy. 2010;65:911–8.
61. Angelova-Fischer I, Mannheimer AC, Hinder A, Ruether A, Franke A, Neubert RH, et al. Distinct barrier integrity phenotypes in filaggrin-related atopic eczema following sequential tape stripping and lipid profiling. Exp Dermatol. 2011;20:351–6.
62. Nassif A, Chan S, Storrs F, Hanifin J. Abnormal skin irritancy in atopic dermatitis and in atopy without dermatitis. Arch Dermatol. 1994;130:1402–7.
63. Seidenari S, Belletti B, Schiavi ME. Skin reactivity to sodium lauryl sulphate in patients with respiratory atopy. J Am Acad Dermatol. 1996;35:47–52.
64. Seidenari S, Conti A. No increased skin reactivity in subjects with allergic rhinitis during the active phase of the disease. Acta Derm Venereol. 2000; |80:192–5.
65. Löffler H, Effendy I. Skin susceptibility of atopic individuals. Contact Dermatitis. 1999;40:239–42.

Patch Testing in Hand Eczema

24

Ali Alikhan and Prof.Howard I. Maibach

Contents

A. Alikhan, M.D. (✉)
Department of Dermatology, Mayo Clinic, 200 1st St SW, Rochester, MN 55905, USA
e-mail: alialikhan1@yahoo.com

P.H.I. Maibach, M.D.
Department of Dermatology, University of California, San Francisco, 90 Medical Center Way, Surge 110, San Francisco, CA 94143-0989, USA
e-mail: maibach@derm.ucsf.edu

24.1 Introduction

First described in the late nineteenth century, patch testing remains the most sensitive and specific test for diagnosis of allergic contact dermatitis (ACD). Previous chapters have discussed differential diagnosis for hand eczema, as well as differentiating irritant from allergic contact dermatitis of the hands. Therefore, this chapter focuses primarily on patch testing, itself.

24.2 Evaluation for Patch Testing

As previously discussed, hand dermatitis can arise from exogenous, endogenous (e.g., atopic dermatitis), and both exogenous and endogenous causes [1]. The exogenous causes include irritant contact dermatitis, ACD, contact urticaria, and *Tinea manuum* [2].

Investigative tools in hand eczema include detailed history and physical exam, patch testing, prick testing, potassium hydroxide (KOH) testing of scales, and potentially IgE blood level. Furthermore, patch testing results may be bolstered by semi-open tests and repeat open application tests.

Once the decision has been made to pursue patch testing, it is imperative to determine what the patient is coming into contact with on a regular,

This chapter was adapted and modified with permission from Lachapelle J-M, Maibach HI. Patch testing and prick testing: a practical guide. Official publication of the ICDRG. Berlin, Heidelberg: Springer; 2012.

A. Alikhan et al. (eds.), *Textbook of Hand Eczema*,
DOI 10.1007/978-3-642-39546-8_24, © Springer-Verlag Berlin Heidelberg 2014

and even a sporadic, basis. The clinician should always ask detailed questions about the patient's profession, hobbies, and activities at home (e.g., wet work, food preparation). This history can help determine what compounds should be included in the patch testing (i.e., special series); in certain cases, the patient may bring products to which they are exposed for patch testing (e.g., topical medications, gloves, skin care products).

Furthermore, the patient's medication list must be examined for any systemic immunomodulators, as these can alter the patch test reaction (e.g., corticosteroids in higher doses). An opinion paper published by Fowler et al. serves as a good reference when encountering these cases, though much remains to be learned [3].

Note that when allergic contact dermatitis is not the primary cause of the hand eczema, it may be an exacerbating factor, and patch testing should be considered in all cases of chronic hand eczema. Interestingly, a population-based study of 270 individuals found positive patch test reactions in 31.3 % of those with hand eczema versus 17.6 % of those without hand eczema [4].

24.3 Patch Testing Procedure

For a detailed discussion of patch testing methodology, please read *Patch Testing and Prick Testing* by Lachapelle and Maibach [2].

There is no single, correct protocol to perform patch testing, and the process can vary from country-to-country and office-to-office [5]. It can last from 4 to 7 days, and potentially longer with certain special series (e.g., metals) [5].

Prior to patch testing, the procedure should be discussed in detail with the patient, including potential side effects (e.g., "angry back," test reaction, hyperpigmentation) [2], caring for the patch test site, and cost of the procedure (i.e., patient may need to contact their insurance provider).

24.3.1 Patch Test Units

Most patch testing is performed with chambers, though non-chamber tests are available. For a detailed discussion on the various chamber and non-chamber brands, please read Chap. 3 of *Patch Testing and Prick Testing* by Lachapelle and Maibach [2]. Finn Chambers (SmartPractice, Phoenix, USA), currently the most popular chamber brand worldwide, are made of aluminum (optional polypropylene coating if patient has an allergy to aluminum), provide good occlusion, and come as loose chambers (in which the physician would select an overlying tape) or come premounted as larger test strips on Scanpor Tape (SmartPractice, Phoenix, USA).

Test substances, typically applied in petrolatum, are placed in the chambers, which are then placed on the patient's back in strips, and secured. Of note, semisolid-based substances can be applied directly on the chamber (usually ≈ 20 mg), while liquids should be applied to a filter-paper disk placed in the chamber. A test strip should be applied from below and pressure placed upwards to remove excess air pouches. After the chambers and tape are applied to the back, the physician should press each chamber containing a semisolid gently and rub the tape, particularly on the corners to increase adherence [2]. Additional tape can be placed at the margins or on the entire surface of the patches if adherence is an issue.

24.3.2 Allergens

Allergens are available for purchase from several companies worldwide. A detailed list of these companies can be found in Appendix C of *Patch Testing and Prick Testing* by Lachapelle and Maibach [2]. It is important to be aware of the vehicle in which an allergen is dispersed – most allergens come in white petrolatum, but a few come in aqueous solutions (e.g., formaldehyde, ammonium thioglycolate). It is also important to select an appropriate allergen concentration (generally, the highest concentration that does not cause irritation in a large group of patients). Finally, allergens should be stored appropriately, usually in a cool dark place.

24.3.3 Application

An important principle is that patches be applied to clear (devoid of lesions or rashes), intact skin. The preferred test site is the upper back; the outer upper arm may be acceptable but is not preferred. If the test site is hairy, it is recommended that the patient clip these areas 1–2 days prior to testing. Patients must be advised to avoid (1) wetting the test site, (2) exercising excessively so as to loosen the patches, and (3) irradiating the test site during the entire testing period.

The order and location of allergens should be recorded on a document in the patient's chart. Furthermore, it is useful to demarcate the patch test sites on the patient's back (a marker with either visible ink or fluorescent ink can be used). At our institution, we do not mark each allergen, but rather all four corners of each test strip; a reading plate (which is provided with the Finn Chamber on Scanpor Tape) is then used to determine positive and negative reactions for each strip.

24.3.4 Reading Time

In standard patch testing, the allergens are left on the skin for 2 days (48 h), and the first reading is performed 15–30 min after the strips are removed. Further readings are performed at 3, 4, and 7 days after initiation of patching (i.e., 1, 2, and 5 days after removal of allergens).

Conventional patch test readings, however, are typically performed on day 2 (48 h) and day 4 (96 h) after the allergens are placed. A second reading at day 4 rather than day 3 appears to result in fewer false negatives, as some allergens react later than others [2]. Patients should return to clinic if any of the areas become positive after this period, which can occasionally occur (see below). This "conventional" reading schedule is performed at the first author's institution and seems to work well [6].

The initial reading at day 2 is not considered important unless the reaction persists into subsequent days. Some allergens (e.g., neomycin, corticosteroid) are "late reactors" and may not react until day 5, day 7, or later.

24.3.5 Scoring

Scoring patch test reactions usually involves grading reactions based on degree of erythema, infiltration, and vesiculation. There is no single correct scoring system [7, 8], but it is important to develop guidelines in one's institution and adhere to these guidelines. What to do in special circumstances such as the "edge" or "ring" effect, questionable reactions, and pustular reactions should also be discussed.

24.3.6 Reactions to Testing

The physician should be aware of irritant patch test reactions. These include erythematous reactions, purpuric reactions (e.g., cobalt chloride, para-phenylenediamine), "soap or shampoo effect" reactions, blistering reactions, pustular reactions, and necrotic reactions. Excited skin syndrome ("angry back") occurs when a strongly positive reaction results in regional skin hyperreactivity in which other patch sites appear reactive – sequential retesting should performed for allergens in question [2].

Adverse reactions can occur in patch testing, including but not limited to "angry back," Koebner phenomenon, dyspigmentation, and bacterial infections. Table 3.5 in *Patch Testing and Prick Testing* by Lachapelle and Maibach [2] summarizes some of these adverse reactions.

False-positive and false-negative reactions can occur; tips to avoid these are thoughtfully summarized on Tables 3.3 and 3.4 of *Patch Testing and Prick Testing* by Lachapelle and Maibach [2]. Rarely, patients can develop "active sensitization" from patch testing; para-phenylenediamine is an occasional example of this phenomenon.

24.3.7 Other Issues

Special considerations for patch testing in regard to various ethnic populations (e.g., fluorescent marking pens) and different climatic environments (e.g., tropical vs. temperate climates) are discussed in greater detail in Chap. 3 of *Patch Testing and Prick Testing* by Lachapelle and Maibach [2].

24.4 T.R.U.E. (Thin-Layer Rapid Use Epicutaneous) Test

The T.R.U.E. test system is a convenient, all-in-one, reproducible [9], ready-to-use patch test system that improves upon issues with variations in allergen application and dispersion onto skin [10]. Allergens are incorporated in hydrophilic gels, which are coated on an impermeable polyester sheet; the allergen-gel preparation is dried into a film. The system comes in panels of 12 allergens that are stored in an airtight, opaque aluminum pouch; once the pouch is opened and the protective backing is removed, the panel can be placed on the patient's back and secured with surgical tape (provided). Perspiration and transepidermal water loss rehydrate the gel, which causes release of the allergens onto the skin. Currently, there are 36 allergens (three strips of 12 allergens each) available for T.R.U.E. testing.

Due to the consistent structure of the strip and uniformity of the allergen content and dose, the T.R.U.E. test potentially provides a higher level of standardization than traditional patch testing. While the T.R.U.E. test is far more convenient and easier to use than traditional patch testing, limitations include cost and limited number of allergens. Similar to standard patch testing, reactions can be checked at 48 h and at 72–96 h. The reader can learn more about the T.R.U.E. test system, as well as the various allergens currently available, at http://www.truetest.com.

24.5 Additional Testing Procedures

Open test, semi-open test, and repeated open application test are various methods to determine if a particular product that the patient is in contact with may be causing an allergic reaction. These tests are typically cheaper and more convenient than patch testing, but are not as specific or detailed. A full discussion can be found in Chap. 7 of *Patch Testing and Prick Testing* by Lachapelle and Maibach [2].

Suspicion of photoallergic reactions (not typically isolated to the hands) requires photopatch testing; this is explained in greater depth in Chap. 5 of *Patch Testing and Prick Testing* by Lachapelle and Maibach [2].

24.6 Allergens of Special Significance

Depending on geographic location, there are various baseline series of allergens [5]. Using a baseline series in patch testing has advantages (e.g., includes most common allergens in environment, provides a more complete "checkup") and disadvantages (e.g., physician may not obtain an appropriate detailed history to determine if non-baseline allergens could be culprits). Of note, the ICDRG recently published a revised international minimal baseline series for international use, taking into account various national and continental baseline series [11]. Special series should also be considered based on history; a list of various special series can be found in Appendix A of *Patch Testing and Prick Testing* by Lachapelle and Maibach [2].

Unfortunately, there is no specific series for hand eczema, but certain allergens have been identified as noteworthy culprits in ACD of the hands. It is also important to note that hand dermatitis has been associated with polysensitization in patients with and without atopic dermatitis [12, 13].

Table 24.1 summarizes the top three allergens in several international studies examining patch test results in adult hand eczema patients. Fortunately, many are components of various international baseline series. Notable allergens include metals (nickel sulfate, potassium dichromate, cobalt chloride), rubber allergens, and cosmetic ingredients (fragrance, para-phenylenediamine). A systematic review of fragrance allergy in hand eczema by Heydorn et al. elaborates on this common, and sometimes frustrating, association [25].

In a study of 799 hand eczema patients, Hald et al. found that certain allergens correlate with

Table 24.1 Three most common allergens in various international studies of patch testing results in adult hand eczema patients

Author, year	Country of origin	No. subjects	Top 3 allergens											
			Potassium dichromate	Nickel sulfate	Fragrance mix	Thimerosal	Para-phenylenediamine	Cobalt chloride	Thiuram mix	Quaternium-15	Formaldehyde	Black rubber mix	Colophony	Rubber mix[30]
Handa et al. 2012 [14]	India	100	1	3	2									
Suman et al. 2003 [15]	India	100	2	1				3						
Kishore et al. 2005 [16][a]	India	50	1	2										
Laxmisha et al. 2008 [1]	India	36	1									3	2	
Vani et al. 2005 [17]	India	50	1 (tie)	1	3									
Veien et al. 2008 [18]	Denmark	425		1	2			3						
Lerbaek et al. 2007 [4]	Denmark	185		1	3	2								
Duarte et al. 1998 [19]	Brazil	250	2 (tie)	1					2 (tie)					
Templet et al. 2004 [20]	USA	1,034							3	1	2			
Li et al. 2002 [21]	China	105			3		2							1
Ni et al. 2011 [22]	China	366		2	3		1							
Magina et al. 2003 [23]	Brazil	714	2	1		3								
Murphy et al. 2003 [24]	UK	200		2	1			3						

[a]Only the top two most common allergens were given

more severe symptoms, namely, formaldehyde, methyldibromo glutaronitrile, sesquiterpene lactone mix, nickel sulfate, and potassium dichromate [26]. Furthermore, chromate was associated with a poor prognosis. Further studies may help solidify these findings.

A Spanish study of pediatric hand eczema patients demonstrated positive testing in 52 of 111 (46.8 %) [13]. The most common allergens were nickel, methylchloroisothiazolinone/methylisothiazolinone, fragrance mix I, *Myroxylon pereirae*, and cobalt chloride. Furthermore, current or past relevance was present in over 80 % (62/76) of positive reactions; the authors recommended patch testing in all pediatric patients with chronic hand eczema. Nonetheless, an older Norwegian study found less striking results in regard to contact allergy in pediatric hand eczema patients [27].

Patch testing for hand eczema in specific professions has also yielded interesting results. A study of 536 Finnish hospital workers with hand eczema found that nickel was the most common allergen (49), followed by fragrances (30) and cobalt (23) [28]. A much smaller study of 44 nurses patch tested for hand eczema demonstrated allergies to nickel sulfate (10), fragrance mix (7), natural rubber latex (3), and thiuram mix (2), among others; it was felt that certain allergens (e.g., natural rubber latex) were more work related than others (e.g., nickel sulfate) [29].

Positivity to nickel should prompt a discussion regarding an oral provocation test [30, 31]. Several studies indicate a possible association between nickel allergy and recurrent vesicular hand eczema; furthermore, oral intake of nickel may correlate with vesicular hand eczema in nickel-sensitive patients [32]. Reduction in nickel-rich foods and possibly use of medications that bind nickel (see Chap. 39) may improve this type of hand dermatitis. A similar phenomenon may be seen in balsam-sensitive patients to spices [33, 34].

24.7 Interpretation of Patch Test Results and Counseling

Once patch testing is completed, it is up to the physician and patient to determine the significance (relevance) of positive reactions. A detailed clinical history regarding occupational exposure, homework, and hobbies, along with use of cosmetics, toiletries, topical medicaments, and even protective wear (e.g., gloves) is warranted. Furthermore, a discussion about which allergens are positive and where these allergens may be encountered (workplace, home, hobbies) is crucial.

The patient can also bring in products from their home or workplace (e.g., data sheets for occupational exposures) to see if these contain the allergen(s) in question [35]. In certain cases, the physician may need to contact the product manufacturer in order to obtain full ingredients and/or particular chemicals for further patch testing. In extreme cases, the physician may need to make a workplace visit to identify any possible source of exposure in the patient's environment. Special chemical analysis and allergen isolation of particular products in the workplace may be warranted to determine exposure [2].

Even when a patient has a positive reaction to a substance and the substance is in his/her environment, the physician should still explore whether a temporal relationship exists, and whether the exposure and the clinical pattern of the dermatitis correlate with each other. Maibach and Lachapelle further explain the concept of clinical relevance in patch testing (as well as additional investigations) in Chap. 8 of *Patch Testing and Prick Testing* [2]. Several relevance algorithms are available to help guide the practitioner in determining the significance of positive patch testing [36–38].

The Contact Allergen Replacement Database (C.A.R.D) [39] and Contact Allergen Management Program (C.A.M.P.; from the American Contact Dermatitis Society) are two online programs in which physicians can enter their patients' allergens into a database, which then creates a list of safe topical products and topical medicaments. These programs empower patients by developing a list of safe cosmetics, toiletries, and medicaments (e.g., shampoos, soaps, detergents) that they use without fear of developing dermatitis.

The concept of cross-sensitization should also be considered when counseling patients. When a patient is sensitized to one allergen, they may also be sensitized to chemically similar substances (e.g., azo compounds in patients with para-phenylenediamine allergies).

Chemical spot tests are also available to help patients avoid certain allergenic products (e.g., dimethylglyoxime for nickel, disodium-1-nitoso-2-naphthol-3,6-disulfonate for cobalt, and diphenylcarbazide for chromium) [2].

24.8 Follow-Up in Patch Test Positive Patients

Unfortunately, in many cases follow-up with hand eczema patients is suboptimal. A Swedish survey study demonstrated that 39 % of patients remembered the correct name of diagnosed allergens 1 year after patch testing, compared with 26 % 5 years after patch testing and only 17 % 10 years after patch testing [40]. Males and those with more diagnosed allergens were significantly less likely to remember their allergens.

Ideally, hand eczema patients are followed closely (at short intervals at first, and then longer intervals once disease is in remission or stable) to reinforce day-to-day management. Continually discussing the importance of emollient and barrier creams, minimizing hand washing and direct contact with irritating and allergenic substances, and what to do in case of flare-ups (e.g., short course of topical corticosteroids) are an essential component of treatment. In patients who have had positive (relevant) patch test results, the offending allergens should be discussed at each appointment, as well as how the patient is avoiding these.

It may useful to periodically retest patients with positive (and negative) patch tests – it is possible that an individual could become less reactive to a substance over time or, conversely, develop new sensitivities. An interesting study comparing T.R.U.E. test results from 1997 to 1998 to those from 2005 to 2006 in 274 individuals (of which 185 had hand eczema) demonstrated that 74 % (64 of 87 positive reactions) were reproduced at the second testing [4].

Periodically, new allergen information sheets and printouts from the C.A.R.D. or C.A.M.P. databases are helpful to keep the patient up-to-date about what products they can safely use.

Conclusion

Remember that multiple types of hand eczema may occur concurrently. Positive patch testing, even if relevant, and subsequent avoidance may not entirely resolve hand eczema if there are other causative factors. Furthermore, avoidance of allergens may be extremely difficult in certain cases.

References

1. Laxmisha C, Kumar S, Nath AK, Thappa DM. Patch testing in hand eczema at a tertiary care center. Indian J Dermatol Venereol Leprol. 2008;74:498–9.
2. Lachapelle J-M, Maibach HI. Patch testing and prick testing: a practical guide. Official publication of the ICDRG. Berlin: Springer; 2012.
3. Fowler Jr JF, Maibach HI, Zirwas M, Taylor JS, Dekoven JG, Sasseville D, et al. Effects of immunomodulatory agents on patch testing: expert opinion 2012. Dermatitis. 2012;23:301–3.
4. Lerbaek A, Kyvik KO, Menne T, Agner T. Retesting with the TRUE test in a population-based twin cohort with hand eczema – allergies and persistence in an 8-year follow-up study. Contact Dermatitis. 2007;57:248–52.
5. Cheng LS, Alikhan A, Maibach HI. Compilation of international standards for patch testing methodology and allergens. Dermatitis. 2009;20:257–60.
6. Wetter DA, Davis MD, Yiannias JA, Cheng JF, Connolly SM, el-Azhary RA, et al. Patch test results from the mayo clinic contact dermatitis group, 1998–2000. J Am Acad Dermatol. 2005;53:416–21.
7. Wilkinson DS, Fregert S, Magnusson B, Bandmann HJ, Calnan CD, Cronin E, et al. Terminology of contact dermatitis. Acta Derm Venereol. 1970;50:287–92.
8. Menne T, White I. Standardization in contact dermatitis. Contact Dermatitis. 2008;58:321.
9. Ale SI, Maibach HI. Reproducibility of patch test results: a concurrent right-versus-left study using TRUE test. Contact Dermatitis. 2004;50:304–12.
10. Fischer T, Maibach HI. Easier patch testing with TRUE test. J Am Acad Dermatol. 1989;20:447–53.
11. Alikhan A, Cheng LS, Ale I, Andersen KE, Bruze M, Eun HC, et al. Revised minimal baseline series of the international contact dermatitis research group: evidence-based approach. Dermatitis. 2011;22:121–2.
12. Carlsen BC, Andersen KE, Menne T, Johansen JD. Sites of dermatitis in a patch test population: hand dermatitis is associated with polysensitization. Br J Dermatol. 2009;161:808–13.
13. Toledo F, Garcia-Bravo B, Fernandez-Redondo V, De la Cuadra J, Gimenez-Arnau AM, Borrego L, et al. Patch testing in children with hand eczema. A 5-year multicentre study in Spain. Contact Dermatitis. 2011;65:213–9.
14. Handa S, Kaur I, Gupta T, Jindal R. Hand eczema: correlation of morphologic patterns, atopy, contact

sensitization and disease severity. Indian J Dermatol Venereol Leprol. 2012;78:153–8.
15. Suman M, Reddy BS. Pattern of contact sensitivity in Indian patients with hand eczema. J Dermatol. 2003;30:649–54.
16. Kishore NB, Belliappa AD, Shetty NJ, Sukumar D, Ravi S. Hand eczema – clinical patterns and role of patch testing. Indian J Dermatol Venereol Leprol. 2005;71:207–8.
17. Vani G, Rao AG, Gowri V, Lakshmi TS. Allergic contact dermatitis of the hands and/or feet–common sensitizers. Contact Dermatitis. 2005;52:50–2.
18. Veien NK, Hattel T, Laurberg G. Hand eczema: causes, course, and prognosis I. Contact Dermatitis. 2008;58:330–4.
19. Duarte I, Terumi Nakano J, Lazzarini R. Hand eczema: evaluation of 250 patients. Am J Contact Dermat. 1998;9:216–23.
20. Templet JT, Hall S, Belsito DV. Etiology of hand dermatitis among patients referred for patch testing. Dermatitis. 2004;15:25–32.
21. Li LF, Wang J. Contact hypersensitivity in hand dermatitis. Contact Dermatitis. 2002;47:206–9.
22. Ni C, Dou X, Chen J, Zhu X, Liu L. Contact sensitization in Chinese patients with hand eczema. Dermatitis. 2011;22:211–5.
23. Magina S, Barros MA, Ferreira JA, Mesquita-Guimaraes J. Atopy, nickel sensitivity, occupation, and clinical patterns in different types of hand dermatitis. Am J Contact Dermat. 2003;14:63–8.
24. Murphy R, Gawkrodger DJ. Contact allergens in 200 patients with hand dermatitis. Contact Dermatitis. 2003;48:227–8.
25. Heydorn S, Johansen JD, Andersen KE, Bruze M, Svedman C, White IR, et al. Fragrance allergy in patients with hand eczema – a clinical study. Contact Dermatitis. 2003;48:317–23.
26. Hald M, Agner T, Blands J, Ravn H, Johansen JD. Allergens associated with severe symptoms of hand eczema and a poor prognosis. Contact Dermatitis. 2009;61:101–8.
27. Dotterud LK, Falk ES. Contact allergy in relation to hand eczema and atopic diseases in north Norwegian schoolchildren. Acta Paediatr. 1995;84:402–6.
28. Lammintausta K, Kalimo K, Havu VK. Occurrence of contact allergy and hand eczemas in hospital wet work. Contact Dermatitis. 1982;8:84–90.
29. Strauss RM, Gawkrodger DJ. Occupational contact dermatitis in nurses with hand eczema. Contact Dermatitis. 2001;44:293–6.
30. Veien NK, Hattel T, Justesen O, Norholm A. Oral challenge with nickel and cobalt in patients with positive patch tests to nickel and/or cobalt. Acta Derm Venereol. 1987;67:321–5.
31. Veien NK, Menne T. Nickel contact allergy and a nickel-restricted diet. Semin Dermatol. 1990;9:197–205.
32. Nielsen GD, Jepsen LV, Jorgensen PJ, Grandjean P, Brandrup F. Nickel-sensitive patients with vesicular hand eczema: oral challenge with a diet naturally high in nickel. Br J Dermatol. 1990;122:299–308.
33. Veien NK, Hattel T, Justesen O, Norholm A. Dietary restrictions in the treatment of adult patients with eczema. Contact Dermatitis. 1987;17:223–8.
34. Veien NK, Hattel T, Justesen O, Norholm N. Oral challenge with balsam of Peru. Contact Dermatitis. 1985;12:104–7.
35. Menne T, Johansen JD, Sommerlund M, Veien NK. Hand eczema guidelines based on the Danish guidelines for the diagnosis and treatment of hand eczema. Contact Dermatitis. 2011;65:3–12.
36. Hostynek JJ, Maibach HI. Thresholds of elicitation depend on induction conditions. Could low level exposure induce sub-clinical allergic states that are only elicited under the severe conditions of clinical diagnosis? Food Chem Toxicol. 2004;42:1859–65.
37. Lachapelle JM. A proposed relevance scoring system for positive allergic patch test reactions: practical implications and limitations. Contact Dermatitis. 1997;36:39–43.
38. Marrakchi S, Maibach HI. What is occupational contact dermatitis? An operational definition. Dermatol Clin. 1994;12:477–84.
39. Kist JM, el-Azhary RA, Hentz JG, Yiannias JA. The contact allergen replacement database and treatment of allergic contact dermatitis. Arch Dermatol. 2004;140:1448–50.
40. Jamil WN, Erikssohn I, Lindberg M. How well is the outcome of patch testing remembered by the patients? A 10-year follow-up of testing with the Swedish baseline series at the department of dermatology in Orebro, Sweden. Contact Dermatitis. 2012;66:215–20.

Prick Testing in Hand Eczema

25

Marléne A.I. Isaksson and Laura Malinauskiene

Contents

M.A.I. Isaksson, M.D., Ph.D. (✉)
Department of Occupational and Environmental Dermatology, Lund University, Skåne University Hospital, Jan Waldenströms Gata 18 Ingang 73, Plan 5, Malmö, SE 20502, Sweden
e-mail: marlene.isaksson@skane.se

L. Malinauskiene, M.D.
Allergologist and Clinical Immunologist, Allergy Center, Vilnius University Antakalnio Hospital, Antakalnio 124, Vilnius, 10200, Lithuania
e-mail: laura.malinauskiene@med.lu.se

25.1 Introduction

The skin prick test (SPT) is the most widely used test for detecting immunoglobulin E (IgE)-mediated hypersensitivity caused by food, inhalant, venom, or drug allergens. This technique is simple to perform, gives rapid results, and is relatively painless. It is possible to perform tests with several allergens during the patient's first visit, and the risk of a systemic reaction during testing is much smaller than using other techniques in vivo (e.g., intradermal testing). Besides, the SPT is inexpensive and can also be performed with nonstandardized allergens [1].

Blackley was the first to introduce allergy skin tests in 1873 in the form of scarification. The SPT was described by Lewis and Grant in 1924 and modified by Pepys in 1975 [2]. Skin prick tests are still performed by this method described by Pepys, and it is also the current reference method [3, 4]. The U.S. Joint Council of Allergy, Asthma and Immunology and the European Academy of Allergy and Clinical Immunology recommend the SPT as the primary test for diagnosis of IgE-mediated allergic disease [3, 4].

25.2 Mechanisms of Skin Prick Tests

The pathogenesis of the positive SPT represents a type I hypersensitivity reaction, mediated by allergen-specific IgE in a previously sensitized individual [5]. Skin challenge involves allergen

A. Alikhan et al. (eds.), *Textbook of Hand Eczema*,
DOI 10.1007/978-3-642-39546-8_25, © Springer-Verlag Berlin Heidelberg 2014

penetration through the epidermis, IgE binding on mast cells, their degranulation, and subsequent release of histamine and other vasoactive substances such as prostaglandins, leukotrienes, and kinins.

Many of the protein allergens have not been identified yet. The same substance can induce different clinical pictures by distinct mechanisms [6]. For example, curcumin, a potential cause of immediate and delayed allergic reactions, has also been reported as a cause of nonimmunological contact urticaria in a woman exposed to this spice powder at work [7].

Some allergens can induce a combination of type I and type IV hypersensitivity. For example, it is suggested that protein contact dermatitis is an eczematous IgE-mediated reaction to proteins.

Anaphylaxis after skin exposure with the eliciting allergen has been reported and is called "contact anaphylaxis"; it often starts as contact urticaria [6]. Very rarely, a protein contact dermatitis may present with anaphylactic symptoms as described by Willi et al. regarding chicory [8].

It is important to remember that the SPT measures sensitization and not clinical disease. Therefore, a positive SPT should always be correlated to the patient's case history, including exposure to the suspected allergen [9].

25.3 Technique

The performance of SPT is described in detail in the position papers of the European Academy of Allergy and Clinical Immunology [4].

The tip of the ordinary blood lancet (or a fine disposable needle) is inserted at an angle of 60–70° into the superficial layer of the skin through a drop of test solution placed on the skin. Then, the tip is gently lifted to allow the test solution to penetrate. Since 1979, new devices for SPT were introduced, such as the plastic Morrow-Brown needle (Stallerpoint, Stallergenes, Antony, Hauts-de-Seine, France) [10, 11]. These devices usually have a 1-mm long tip and shoulders preventing further penetration and should be pressed at 90° to the skin surface through a drop of test solution. Then the test device is pulled out, and the extract may be wiped off immediately [5]. Prick tests with these devices can decrease SPT variability [4]. It is important to use a different sterile needle or test device for each test [3].

The type of device used for SPT significantly influences results. A head-to-head prospective comparative study of eight skin test devices found that there are statistically significant differences among virtually all devices tested [12]. It is important to note that different devices also have differences in the recommended technique of application, so it would be advisable that technicians undergo some type of training before using a given device.

Recently, four SPT devices were investigated in terms of the sensitivity, reproducibility, and acceptability of SPT. In terms of sensitivity, the IV needle (100 %) and metal lancets (96–98 %) were superior ($p < 0.01$) to plastic SPT devices. Metal needles and/or lancets also were the best tolerated by the patients [13].

25.4 Performance of Skin Prick Tests

It is recommended to perform SPT on the volar surface of the forearm or on the back [5]. Some authors recommend the skin to be cleaned with disinfectant before skin tests are performed. It is, however, important that the skin be dry where the skin tests are to be done. The test sites should be marked and placed at least 3 cm apart to avoid overlapping of reactions and influence of strong reactions on slightly positive or negative tests. Tests should not be placed within 5 cm from the wrist and 3 cm from the elbow, as these places are the least and the most reactive parts of the volar side of the forearm [5].

Reactivity to both allergen and histamine varies between different parts of the skin surface. For SPT, the back was found more reactive than the forearm, but not for all test substances [1].

SPT should be carried on normal skin that has apparently never before been the site of dermatitis. If negative, some authors suggest testing on previously affected skin or on eczematous skin if the area to be tested shows only light erythema, so that a positive reaction may be noted [14].

25.5 Control Solutions

For SPT, negative and positive control solutions must be used in parallel with the allergen tests in order to evaluate nonspecific reactions caused by the trauma of the skin induced by test devices and to find out the normal reactivity of the skin [5, 15].

Histamine dihydrochloride 10 mg/mL is recommended for use as a positive control for the SPT [1, 3]. Some clinics use codeine phosphate 9 %, which shows aptitude for mast cell degranulation [16]. 0.9 % sodium chloride (or 50 % glycerinated human serum albumin-saline) is routinely used as a negative control and should be applied at the same time as the allergens.

25.6 Allergens

Standardized and nonstandardized allergens can be used for the SPT. If raw or dry material is suspected, using 0.9 % sodium chloride is normally sufficient for dissolving it (e.g., flour), because most allergens that give rise to type I reactions are water soluble. Liquids can be used as such after appropriate dilution, but when you have a solid object that is suspected to have caused an immediate reaction, you can make an extract to test with. Ultrasonic bath extracts are used in the Malmö department to test with the SPT technique, if necessary [17].

According to our experience, we cut or divide a specimen into 1–2 cm or smaller pieces (depending on how big a specimen we have) and put them into a glass jar with a diameter of 6 cm to which up to 150 mL of the solvent (e.g., 0.9 % saline solution, ethanol, or acetone) is added. It is important to cover the specimen with the solution. We use mainly acetone as a solvent for preparation of the extracts because it can dissolve both polar and nonpolar compounds. The glass jar is put in an ultrasonic bath for 5 min. Thereafter, the pieces of the specimen are removed and the solvent is evaporated in the fume cupboard or by using a rotary evaporator. To the dry residue in the glass jar, 1 mL of the solvent (e.g., 0.9 % sodium chloride) is added, and this solution with the dissolved residue then constitutes the stock solution for testing. Any solvent suitable for prick testing may be used for the stock solution, and usually the same solvent as for the extraction is used. The stock solution can be tested as is or together with dilutions made from it [17]. The extraction procedure using an ultrasonic bath means an improved technique to get more standardized extracts from the same kind of products.

When there has been a systemic presentation of the allergic reaction (e.g., anaphylaxis) or when such a reaction is suspected to occur, it is advisable to begin testing with an extremely diluted allergen solution to minimize allergen exposure. You can make a serial dilution of the suspected allergen in a suitable vehicle and start testing with the very lowest concentration. If the SPT is negative, incremental doses of the allergen in the vehicle are prick tested up to the dose you wish to investigate. When testing with nonstandardized substances and having a positive reaction, control tests should be assessed on at least 20 persons to avoid false-positive interpretations [1, 16].

The quality of the allergen extracts used in the SPT influences the results. Some food allergens rapidly lose their antigenic properties, and the corresponding extracts sometimes have no allergenic activity [5].

25.7 Complications of the SPT

Life-threatening reactions have been documented during skin tests, although the safety of the SPT is well established [1, 16]. Analysis of fatal reactions from 1990 to 2001 showed no instances of near-fatal or life-threatening reactions to inhalant prick or puncture tests [18]. Immediate systemic reactions are more common with intradermal tests than prick or puncture skin tests. Therefore, caution is advised, especially when testing certain occupational substances or in patients with systemic symptoms (such as anaphylaxis) [18, 19]. The SPT should be performed only where resuscitation equipment and trained personnel are available [1, 3, 4].

25.8 Influence of Skin Diseases and Drug Treatment on SPT

Skin tests should not be performed on anatomical locations with eczema/dermatitis or obvious dermographism. Neurological disorders as well as infectious disease (e.g., leprosy) can lead to false-negative SPTs [20].

Short-acting H_1 antihistamines should be discontinued at least 3 days prior to the SPT [3, 20]. Corticosteroids in doses equivalent to 30 mg of prednisone/prednisolone per day for 1 week do not reduce the response to the SPT, and it was shown that low-dose oral glucocorticoids (less than 10 mg of prednisolone per day) for a long period did not influence results of the SPT [21]. Topical application of potent corticosteroid ointments suppressed the SPT response markedly [22]. Thus, the SPT should not be performed on skin areas treated with topical corticosteroids in the preceding week (Table 25.1).

Some authors suggest that nonsteroidal anti-inflammatory drugs also should be avoided because of false-negative SPT results, especially when testing in contact urticaria [14].

25.9 Reading Time of Skin Prick Tests

Test sites should be inspected and reactions recorded after 15 min [5]. It is recommended to reevaluate test sites after 25–30 min, because in some patients reactions take longer to develop. The largest reaction is recorded [5].

25.10 Recording and Evaluation of Skin Prick Test Results

For recording purposes, the contours of the wheal (and erythema) should be outlined with a fine filter-tip or ball-point pen, and the con-

Table 25.1 Inhibitory effect of various treatments on skin prick tests[a]

Treatment	Degree	Duration	Clinical significance
Intranasal			
H_1-antihistamine			None
Oral			
H_1-antihistamine	++++	2–7 days	Yes
H_2-antihistamine	0 to +		None
Imipramines	++++	Up to 21 days	Yes
Phenothiazines	+ to ++	Up to 10 days	Yes
Corticosteroids			
Systemic short term	0		None
Systemic long term	Possible		None
Inhaled	0		None
Topical skin	+ to ++	Up to 7 days	Yes
Dopamine	+		None
Clonidine	++		None
Montelukast	0		None
Specific Immunotherapy	0 to ++		None
UV light treatment, *systemic depending on light source, most intensive with PUVA*	+++	Up to 4 weeks	Yes

0 to ++++, strength of the inhibitory action on SPT result

[a]Reprinted from Bousquet et al. [20], with permission from John Wiley and Sons

Table 25.2 Example of the evaluation of the positive skin prick test reaction to allergen and histamine

SPT solution	How to measure positive reaction	D	d	D+d/2	Ratio to histamine
Allergen	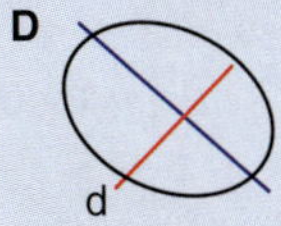	12	10	11	11/5 = 2.2
Histamine	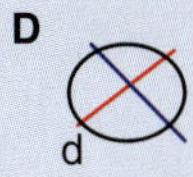	5	5	5	

D largest diameter (mm), *d* perpendicular to D diameter in its center (mm)
Ratio to histamine: allergen (D+d)/2
Histamine (D+d)/2

Table 25.3 Grading systems for the skin prick test with histamine as a reference[a]

Grade or class	*Wheal size*
0	No discernible wheal
1+	<½ Histamine diameter
2+	>½ Histamine, but <histamine diameter
3+	Equal size of histamine wheal
4+	> Histamine diameter, but <2 x diameter
5+	>2 × Histamine diameter
Grade	*% of the area of the wheal induced by histamine reference*
–	Same size as negative reference
1+	25
2+	50
3+	100
4+	200

[a]Table created with data from [3, 4]

tours transferred by means of a translucent tape to a record sheet (Table 25.2). The size of the skin reaction should be recorded as the mean of the longest and the midpoint orthogonal diameters [4].

Most studies on the SPT have used only the wheal and not the erythema reaction for evaluation of the response [1]. The wheal induced by the trauma of the needle and the negative control solution is often 0 but may be discernible up to 2.5 mm in diameter in patients without obvious dermographism. Therefore, wheals <3 mm in mean diameter should be regarded as negative, and only wheals equal to or bigger than 3 mm in diameter should be regarded as positive [1] (Table 25.3).

Table 25.4 Common errors in the skin prick testing[a]

1. Tests are placed too close together (<2 cm), and overlapping reactions cannot be separated visually
2. Induction of bleeding, leading possibly to false-positive results
3. Insufficient penetration of skin by puncture device (more frequently with plastic ones), leading to false-negative results
4. Spreading of allergen solutions during the test or when the solution is wiped away

[a]Reprinted from Bousquet et al. [20], with permission from John Wiley and Sons

Other methods, such as the laser Doppler technique for determining the blood flow in the wheal and erythema and ultrasound for estimating the area, thickness, and volume of the wheal, can be used for scientific purposes [23, 24].

It is recommended that one performs the SPT in duplicate in order to estimate the reproducibility of the SPT, because single negative tests (5 %) will be obtained in clearly sensitive patients even by skilled technicians, and the risk for false-negative tests due to technical problems is high in patients with low skin sensitivity [25]. For scientific purposes, even quadruplicate tests with each test solution are recommended [5]. For the SPT, a coefficient of variation less than 40 % (ideally 20 %) based on area or 20 % (ideally 10 %) based on mean diameter is recommended [26, 27], but variation about 15–20 % based on area and 7–10 % based on mean diameter can be reached by skilled technicians [5]. A few common errors that can occur while performing SPT are outlined in Table 25.4.

25.11 Modifications of the Skin Prick Tests

25.11.1 Prick-Prick Test

The prick-prick test is used when the suspected allergen is confined in a solid material. This material may be a food item, rubber item, plant material, soft wood, and so forth. It is performed in the following way: The same lancet is used to prick the food item or another potential allergenic product/substance and immediately after is used to prick of the skin of the patient. The skin response is evaluated and recorded in the same way as in the SPT. The negative and positive controls should be performed, and the response should be related to the histamine SPT.

Some allergens, especially food allergens, are not available as well-characterized, freeze-dried allergen preparations with known allergenic composition. Therefore, fresh fruits, meat, nuts, and so forth can be used for testing according to the prick-prick method [1] (Fig. 25.1). Fresh food extracts give a stronger, more sensitive response than commercial extracts [28]. Some food allergens are destroyed in a few minutes by oxidation, making standardization difficult. Few researchers have demonstrated the superiority of the SPT with fresh foods [29–31].

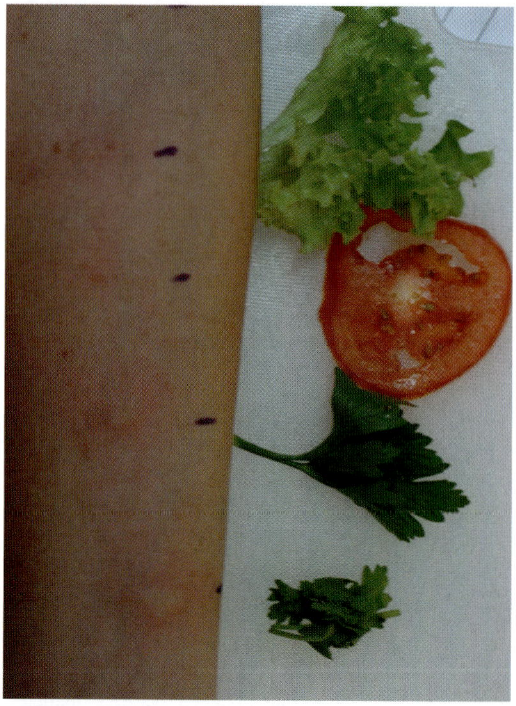

Fig. 25.1 Positive skin prick-prick tests performed with fresh foods (Courtesy of C. Tillman)

Rancé et al. compared the SPT using fresh foods and commercial extracts and looked at correlations obtained with oral challenge of the allergens in question [28]. They found that SPTs were positive in 40 % of cases with commercial extracts and in 81.3 % with fresh foods. The overall concordance between a positive prick test and a positive challenge was 58.8 % with commercial extracts and 91.7 % with fresh foods. These results indicate that fresh foods may be more effective for detecting sensitivity to food allergens [28].

Food extracts may not contain all relevant allergens, partly because some of the allergens could be destroyed during preparation and testing with such preparations will result in false-negative reactions. It is generally recommended that fresh foods should be tested in the same state that caused the reaction (e.g., cooked, if the reaction was caused by a cooked product), as some allergens may also be created during heating. Vester et al., investigating occupational food-related hand dermatoses, also concluded that the SPT with fresh foods is more beneficial and effective than when using food extracts, when patients suspected of having contact urticaria are tested. They suggested that a baseline SPT series, used in everyday practice, must include high-allergenic foods, which patients are likely to react to, and the food series should, therefore, continuously be renewed, and testing with fresh foods provided most frequently by the patients should be carried out [32]. Some authors suggest that if the SPT on normal, previously affected, or currently eczematous skin is negative, the suspected contactant should be rubbed gently into a small scratch [14].

25.11.2 Open Tests and Closed Tests

Sometimes one may start with an "open test" of the suspected allergen/product in question if the history of the patient gives an indication of an anaphylactic nature or other hazardous extracutaneous reaction. For a liquid solution, a drop is placed on a 1 × 1-cm area on the volar skin of the forearm, and the reaction is read after 15–20 min. If the product is solid, a minute amount of the product is placed on the volar skin of the forearm without occlusion. Sometimes the object has to be secured with a small piece of tape in order not to fall off the arm. When the open test is negative, you may continue with the "closed test" or the "chamber test." You may also try testing the substance on damaged or eczematous skin, which may give a vesicular reaction [33]. The closed test is performed in the same way as the open test, but the test site is covered with a plastic chamber secured with a tape. If negative, the procedure may be repeated on damaged skin before a SPT is performed. The time of reading is the same as for the open test. Positive and negative control solutions are used, and the reaction equal or greater than that from histamine is usually clinically significant.

25.11.2.1 Indications

The Contact Urticaria Syndrome

The contact urticaria syndrome comprises a heterogeneous group of immediate contact inflammatory reactions that usually appear within minutes after contact with eliciting substances. Systemic involvement (as bronchial asthma, rhinoconjunctivitis, gastrointestinal dysfunction, or even anaphylaxis) can also be present. It was defined in 1975 by Maibach and Johnson [34].

Protein Contact Dermatitis

In 1976, Hjorth and Roed-Petersen in Denmark described hand and forearm eczema of several kitchen workers in whom high-molecular-weight proteins were suspected as allergens. They named the condition "protein contact dermatitis" [35]. In 1983, Veien and colleagues defined specific criteria for its diagnosis, which include a chronic or recurrent dermatitis caused by contact with high-molecular-weight proteins in foods, an immediate itching urticarial eruption that occurs within 30 min of contact, positive prick/or scratch testing with the suspected causative substance, and patch test results that are often negative [36].

The pathogenesis of protein contact dermatitis is not entirely understood. Recent investigations show that it is a combination of immediate (type I) and delayed (type IV) hypersensitivity. Approximately 50 % of cases are associated with atopy [37]. The reasons for this are unclear. It is possible that the immune mechanisms in atopic dermatitis and protein contact dermatitis are similar. Probably high-molecular-weight proteins in foods are more likely to penetrate the epidermis and cause sensitization if the epidermis is damaged, perhaps due to atopic dermatitis or other kinds of eczema, particularly of the hands [37] (Fig. 25.2). In most cases described, patients have had professions in which irritant contact dermatitis is very common, and this may be a prerequisite for protein contact dermatitis.

Eczematous Reactions to Ingested Food in Atopic Eczema

Food has been discussed as a controversial trigger factor of atopic eczema (AE) for many years, and there is a certain degree of disagreement between dermatologists and allergists regarding it. Although food is more frequently related to AE in children, some studies have shown that severe adult AE may be worsened by ingested foods (especially due to cross-reactivity to pollens) as well [38–40]. The position paper of the European Academy of Allergy and Clinical Immunology proposed a diagnostic algorithm to elucidate the role of food allergens for eczematous reactions in AE [41]. No single parameter can prove the clinical relevance of a sensitizing food in patients with AE. If there is a history of the immediate food reactions in patients suffering from AE, SPT and/or determining food-specific IgE in vitro is recommended. Since specific IgE, SPT, and the history sometimes do not correlate with clinical observations, double-blind, oral food challenges are necessary to show the clinical relevance of the findings.

If there is persistent, moderate-to-severe AE and no history of immediate reactions to food and thus no suspected eczematous reactions to food, screening tests (in vitro or SPT) to detect specific sensitizations against common food allergens (especially those associated with pollen) are still recommended.

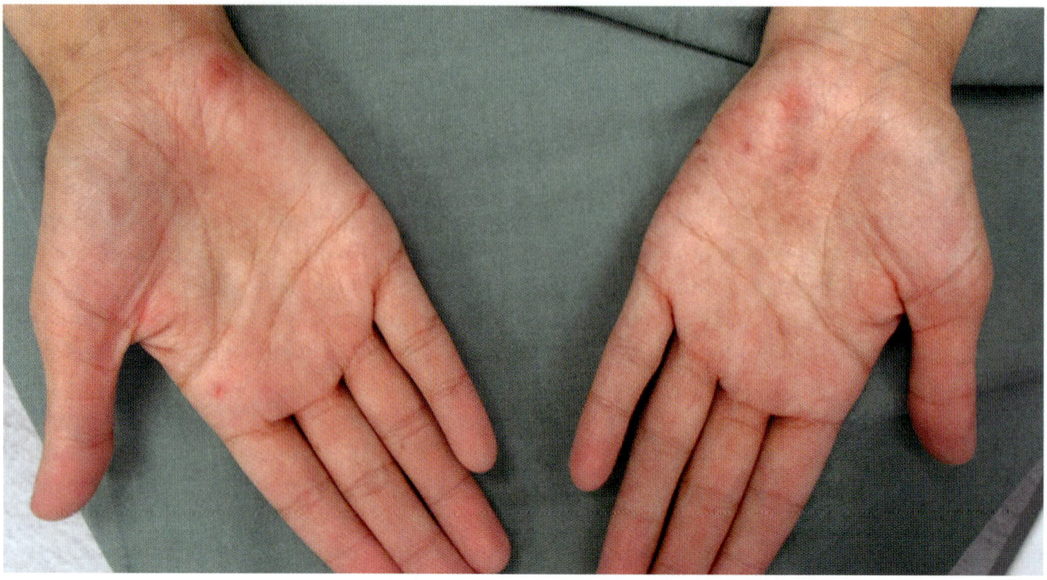

Fig. 25.2 Protein contact dermatitis caused by chapatti flour in an atopic patient

In case of a mono-sensitization or very strong sensitization to one food, a specific diagnostic elimination diet and subsequent oral food challenge should be performed. The same procedure is recommended if food is suspected by patients or parents as trigger factor of persistent AE (although no immediate reactions are known) [41]. It should be stressed that although AE can manifest as hand eczema only, especially in adults, it is very unlikely that ingested food would be the culprit in case hand eczema alone is present and no manifestation of AE in the other skin sites could be seen.

Evaluation of Atopy

Atopic status may be evaluated from a skin test reaction to aeroallergens, taking into account other prerequisites of atopy. This procedure is done in many countries by dermatologists (e.g., in Finland). The position statement of the European Academy of Allergy and Clinical Immunology proposed the following definition of atopy: "Atopy is a personal or familial tendency to produce IgE antibodies in response to low doses of allergens, usually proteins, and to develop typical symptoms such as asthma, rhino-conjunctivitis, or eczema/dermatitis" [42].

Thus, a positive SPT alone is not sufficient to detect atopy, but in connection with inheritance trait and typical presentation, it may be used as an objective sign of atopy.

High-Risk Occupations for Occupational Contact Urticaria and Protein Contact Dermatitis

There are some occupations in which workers are at increased risk of developing occupational contact urticaria on their hands and protein contact dermatitis presenting as hand eczema. Health care workers, food handlers, and hairdressers are such professions [43]. Health care workers are exposed to latex from natural rubber gloves and chlorhexidine in disinfectants for the hands (Fig. 25.3) [44]. Food handlers such as cooks, kitchen personnel, caterers, bakers, butchers, and some shop assistants are exposed to a multitude of foodstuffs containing proteinaceous material, such as fruits, vegetables, spices, plants, grains, enzymes, and animals [33]. Chapatti was the cause of protein contact dermatitis in a Pakistani woman who cooked for her family every night [45]. Hairdressers are exposed to ammonium persulfate in hairdressing bleach [43]. Atopy is also a significant risk factor [43], and in the aforementioned professions, irritant contact dermatitis is also very common and may be a prerequisite for protein contact dermatitis.

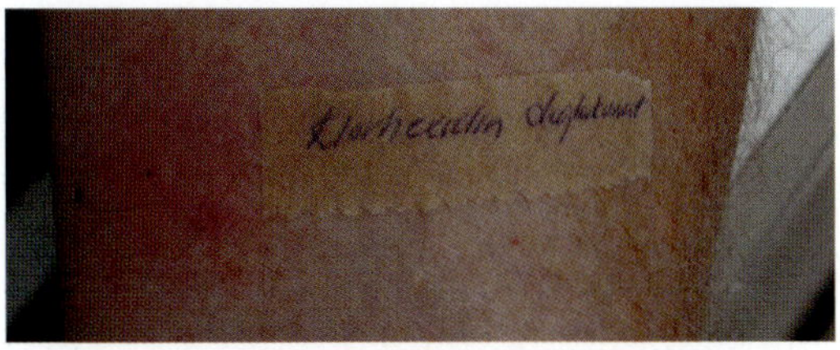

Fig. 25.3 Positive skin prick test reaction with chlorhexidine digluconate (Courtesy of M. Hindsén)

Conclusion

The SPT is recommended as the method to test for immediate-type hypersensitivity. In dermatology practice, it could be used to assess the etiology of the contact urticaria syndrome, protein contact dermatitis, and to evaluate possible triggers of persistent, moderate-to-severe atopic eczema. It could be a useful tool to evaluate the atopic status of a patient. Skin prick tests are easy to perform, and they are relatively inexpensive. For dermatological diagnostic work-up, testing with nonstandardized allergens or extracts from suspected objects may be very valuable.

The SPT measures sensitization and not the clinical disease, so a positive SPT should always be correlated to the case history, taking into account the exposure. In short, the SPT should be part of the routine investigation of patients with hand eczema in high-risk occupations for occupational contact urticaria, especially if there is a history of atopy and exposure to urticants.

References

1. Dreborg S. Skin testing. The safety of skin tests and the information obtained from using different methods and concentrations of allergen. Allergy. 1993;48(7):473–5.
2. Pepys J, Roth A, Carroll KB. RAST, skin and nasal tests and the history in grass pollen allergy. Clin Allergy. 1975;5(4):431–42.
3. Cox L, Nelson H, Lockey R, Calabria C, Chacko T, Finegold I, et al. Allergen immunotherapy: a practice parameter third update. J Allergy Clin Immunol. 2011;127(1):1–55.
4. European Academy of Allergy and Clinical Immunology. Position paper: immunotherapy. Allergy. 1993;48(1):9–35.
5. Dreborg S. The skin prick test in the diagnosis of atopic allergy. J Am Acad Dermatol. 1989;21(4):820–1.
6. Amaro C, Goossens A. Immunological occupational contact urticaria and contact dermatitis from proteins: a review. Contact Dermatitis. 2008;58(2):67–75.
7. Liddle M, Hull C, Liu C, Powell D. Contact urticaria from curcumin. Dermatitis. 2006;17(4):196–7.
8. Willi R, Pfab F, Huss-Marp J, Buters JT, Zilker T, Behrendt H, et al. Contact anaphylaxis and protein contact dermatitis in a cook handling chicory leaves. Contact Dermatitis. 2009;60(4):226–7.
9. Bindslev-Jensen C. Skin tests for immediate hypersensitivity. In: Johansen JD, Frosch PJ, Lepoittevin J-P, editors. Contact dermatitis. 5th ed. Berlin: Springer; 2011. p. 511–7.
10. Brown HM, Su S, Thantrey N. Prick testing for allergens standardized by using a precision needle. Clin Allergy. 1981;11(1):95–8.
11. Osterballe O, Weeke B. A new lancet for skin prick testing. Allergy. 1979;34(4):209–12.
12. Carr WW, Martin B, Howard RS, Cox L, Borish L. Comparison of test devices for skin prick testing. J Allergy Clin Immunol. 2005;116(2):341–6.
13. Masse MS, Granger Vallee A, Chiriac A, Dhivert-Donnadieu H, Bousquet-Rouanet L, Bousquet PJ, et al. Comparison of five techniques of skin prick tests used routinely in Europe. Allergy. 2011;66(11):1415–9.
14. Rietschel R, Fowler Jr JF. Contact urticaria. In: Rietschel R, Fowler Jr JF, editors. Fisher's contact dermatitis. 5th ed. Philadelphia: Lippincott Williams & Wilkins; 2001. p. 581–604.
15. Malling HJ. Skin prick testing and the use of histamine references. Allergy. 1984;39(8):596–601.
16. Lachapelle J-M, Maibach HI. Patch testing and prick testing. A practical guide. Official publication of the ICDRG. 3rd ed. Berlin: Springer; 2003.
17. Bruze M, Trulsson L, Bendsöe N. Patch testing with ultrasonic bath extracts. Am J Contact Dermat. 1992;3:133–7.
18. Gimenez-Arnau A, Maurer M, De La Cuadra J, Maibach H. Immediate contact skin reactions, an update of contact urticaria, contact urticaria syndrome and protein contact dermatitis – "a never ending story.". Eur J Dermatol. 2010;20(5):552–62.
19. Cox L, Williams B, Sicherer S, Oppenheimer J, Sher L, Hamilton R, et al. Pearls and pitfalls of allergy diagnostic testing: report from the American College of Allergy, Asthma and Immunology/American Academy of Allergy, Asthma and Immunology Specific IgE Test Task Force. Ann Allergy Asthma Immunol. 2008;101(6):580–92.
20. Bousquet J, Heinzerling L, Bachert C, Papadopoulos NG, Bousquet PJ, Burney PG, et al. Practical guide to skin prick tests in allergy to aeroallergens. Allergy. 2012;67(1):18–24.
21. Des Roches A, Paradis L, Bougeard YH, Godard P, Bousquet J, Chanez P. Long-term oral corticosteroid therapy does not alter the results of immediate-type allergy skin prick tests. J Allergy Clin Immunol. 1996;98(3):522–7.

22. Pipkorn U, Hammarlund A, Enerback L. Prolonged treatment with topical glucocorticoids results in an inhibition of the allergen-induced weal-and-flare response and a reduction in skin mast cell numbers and histamine content. Clin Exp Allergy. 1989;19(1):19–25.
23. Diameter SJ. Thickness, area, and volume of skin-prick histamine weals. Measurement of skin thickness by 15 MHz A-mode ultrasound. Allergy. 1984;39(5):359–64.
24. Serup J, Staberg B. Quantification of weal reactions with laser Doppler flowmetry. Comparative blood flow measurements of the oedematous centre and the perilesional flare of skin-prick histamine weals. Allergy. 1985;40(4):233–7.
25. Dreborg S, Basomba A, Belin L, Durham S, Einarsson R, Eriksson NE, et al. Biological equilibration of allergen preparations: methodological aspects and reproducibility. Clin Allergy. 1987;17(6):537–50.
26. Malling HJ. Reproducibility of skin sensitivity using a quantitative skin prick test. Allergy. 1985;40(6):400–4.
27. Taudorf E, Malling HJ, Laursen LC, Lanner A, Weeke B. Reproducibility of histamine skin prick test. Inter- and intravariation using histamine dihydrochloride 1, 5, and 10 mg/ml. Allergy. 1985;40(6):344–9.
28. Rancé F, Juchet A, Bremont F, Dutau G. Correlations between skin prick tests using commercial extracts and fresh foods, specific IgE, and food challenges. Allergy. 1997;52(10):1031–5.
29. Norgaard A, Skov PS, Bindslev-Jensen C. Egg and milk allergy in adults: comparison between fresh foods and commercial allergen extracts in skin prick test and histamine release from basophils. Clin Exp Allergy. 1992;22(10):940–7.
30. Ortolani C, Ispano M, Pastorello EA, Ansaloni R, Magri GC. Comparison of results of skin prick tests (with fresh foods and commercial food extracts) and RAST in 100 patients with oral allergy syndrome. J Allergy Clin Immunol. 1989;83(3):683–90.
31. Rosen JP, Selcow JE, Mendelson LM, Grodofsky MP, Factor JM, Sampson HA. Skin testing with natural foods in patients suspected of having food allergies: is it a necessity? J Allergy Clin Immunol. 1994;93(6):1068–70.
32. Vester L, Thyssen JP, Menne T, Johansen JD. Occupational food-related hand dermatoses seen over a 10-year period. Contact Dermatitis. 2012;66(5):264–70.
33. Goossens A, Amaro C. Protein contact dermatitis. In: Johansen JD, Frosch PJ, Lepoittevin J-P, editors. Contact dermatitis. 5th ed. Berlin: Springer; 2011. p. 407–13.
34. Maibach HI, Johnson HL. Contact urticaria syndrome. Contact urticaria to diethyltoluamide (immediate-type hypersensitivity). Arch Dermatol. 1975;111(6):726–30.
35. Hjorth N, Roed-Petersen J. Occupational protein contact dermatitis in food handlers. Contact Dermatitis. 1976;2(1):28–42.
36. Veien NK, Hattel T, Justesen O, Nørholm A. Causes of eczema in the food industry. Derm Beruf Umwelt. 1983;31(3):84–6.
37. Levin C, Warshaw E. Protein contact dermatitis: allergens, pathogenesis, and management. Dermatitis. 2008;19(5):241–51.
38. Reekers R, Busche M, Wittmann M, Kapp A, Werfel T. Birch pollen-related foods trigger atopic dermatitis in patients with specific cutaneous T-cell responses to birch pollen antigens. J Allergy Clin Immunol. 1999;104(2):466–72.
39. Werfel T, Ahlers G, Schmidt P, Boeker M, Kapp A, Neumann C. Milk-responsive atopic dermatitis is associated with a casein-specific lymphocyte response in adolescent and adult patients. J Allergy Clin Immunol. 1997;99(1):124–33.
40. Worm M, Forschner K, Lee HH, Roehr CC, Edenharter G, Niggemann B, et al. Frequency of atopic dermatitis and relevance of food allergy in adults in Germany. Acta Derm Venereol. 2006;86(2):119–22.
41. Werfel T, Ballmer-Weber B, Eigenmann PA, Niggemann B, Rance F, Turjanmaa K, et al. Eczematous reactions to food in atopic eczema: position paper of the EAACI and GA2LEN. Allergy. 2007;62(7):723–8.
42. Johansson SG, Hourihane JO, Bousquet J, Bruijnzeel-Koomen C, Dreborg S, Haahtela T, et al. A revised nomenclature for allergy. An EAACI position statement from the EAACI nomenclature task force. Allergy. 2001;56(9):813–24.
43. Williams JD, Lee AY, Matheson MC, Frowen KE, Noonan AM, Nixon RL. Occupational contact urticaria: Australian data. Br J Dermatol. 2008;159(1):125–31.
44. Nagendran V, Wicking J, Ekbote A, Onyekwe T, Garvey LH. IgE-mediated chlorhexidine allergy: a new occupational hazard? Occup Med (Lond). 2009;59(4):270–2.
45. Malinauskiene L, Isaksson M. Protein contact dermatitis caused by allergy to Chapatti flour. Acta Derm Venereol. 2013;93(1):91–93. doi:10.2340/00015555-1365.
46. Haustein U. Anaphylactic shock and contact urticaria after patch test with professional allergens. Allerg Immunol (Leipz). 1976;22(4):349–52.

Prevention of Hand Eczema: Barrier Creams and Emollients

26

Sibylle Schliemann and Peter Elsner

Contents

S. Schliemann, M.D. (✉) • P. Elsner, M.D.
Department of Dermatology, University Hospital Jena, Erfurter Str. 35, Jena 07743, Germany
e-mail: schliemann@derma-jena.de; elsner@derma-jena.de

26.1 Introduction

Hand eczema is the most frequent manifestation of occupational skin disease. Therefore, prevention measures play an important role in reducing the incidence and prevalence of irritant and allergic hand dermatitis. Apart from elimination of cutaneous exposure to hazardous substances and the use of gloves or protective clothing, barrier creams (BCs) are one of the classical means of skin protection against irritant chemicals from the environment [1]. BCs as topical preparations cannot replace protective gloves but can add to protection of the hands in situations where gloves are unfeasible.

26.2 Definitions and Terms

The term "barrier cream" refers to the designated purpose of preparations to be applied prior and during procedures that bear a potential harmful impact on the epidermal skin barrier. "Barrier cream" permits a didactic, albeit somehow artificial, distinction from the more general definition of moisturizers that may be used as postexposure or everyday skin care products to maintain the skin "in a healthy condition." Other terms, such as "skin protection product" or "protective cream," are synonymously in use both in scientific literature and in marketing. The term "protective cream" is considered most accurate by many, since it does not insinuate a specific physical mode of action [2]. However, "barrier

A. Alikhan et al. (eds.), *Textbook of Hand Eczema*,
DOI 10.1007/978-3-642-39546-8_26, © Springer-Verlag Berlin Heidelberg 2014

cream" is a catchy and widespread expression and will therefore be used further on in this chapter. Emollients are topical preparations that increase or help to passively maintain the moisture of the stratum corneum by occluding the skin surface. One example is petrolatum.

BCs cannot be definitely distinguished from moisturizers or emollients on the basis of their galenical composition, since they share common characteristics [3] (see also Chap. 27). For this reason, they are sometimes addressed altogether as moisturizers [4]. However, compared to moisturizers intended to actively increase the stratum corneum water content, BCs are designed for a different purpose and meant as preexposure preparations. Their linguistic distinction is therefore useful in terms of their intended effects and areas of application [1].

Regarding their composition, certain ingredients are discussed controversially. Urea or propylene glycol, for example, may potentially enhance the penetration of irritants and allergens into the skin barrier [5]. Therefore, some authors recommend avoiding these ingredients in BCs at workplaces [6]. There are, however, examples of prework products on the market that do contain urea. Manufacturers in Europe have also started to eliminate fragrances from prework products because of the common problem of fragrance allergy, particularly in the context of hand dermatitis [7–9]. This development occurs on the background of an ongoing discussion regarding the labeling of 26 supposedly allergenic fragrances, the so-called 26 allergens rule (Article 1 (10) of Directive 2003/15/EC) [10], in cosmetic products in Europe [11]. The composition of a BC designated to be used in a certain occupational environment is, therefore, not trivial and should be carefully formulated by the manufacturer.

In theory, BCs are designed to diminish the irritant impact of the known key factors of skin irritation that are related to wet work, namely, hand washing and exposure to hot water or detergents and other mild irritants. In addition, BCs may facilitate the removal of sticky oils, greases, and resins from the skin surface, thus decreasing the need to use abrasives and waterless cleansers. This claim appears plausible but has never been investigated systematically in scientific trials. In the context of prevention of occupational hand dermatitis, apart from BCs, the so-called 3-step occupational skin protection concept also includes skin cleansers and skin care products [12, 13]. While BCs shall be used prior to and in between exposures at workplaces, mild skin cleansers are intended to remove irritants and allergens from the skin surface in the sense of decontamination. They may help to reduce the irritant burden by replacing unnecessarily aggressive cleansing products. Subsequent use of skin care products after work supports the natural skin barrier regeneration. The 3-step concept is easy to understand and well accepted by workers [14], has a high compliance [15], and is altogether considered very practicable. Therefore, many manufacturers follow the 3-step model when formulating their products.

26.3 Efficacy and Intended Application Areas

Although BCs are one of the common measures to prevent irritant contact dermatitis (ICD), their actual benefit at the workplace has been subject to debate [12], due to a relative scarcity of randomized, controlled trials, especially under daily working conditions. However, in the past years, several experimental and interventional trials have been performed with respect to the efficacy of the various preventive measures. The best results in terms of barrier integrity maintenance were achieved by the combination of both prework skin protection and postexposure skin care as indicated by some experimental studies [16, 17]. Meanwhile the principal benefit of the 3-step concept has also been confirmed in intervention studies at workplaces, where the combination of both skin protection and post-expositional skin care again was superior to either one of these elements alone [18, 19]. Despite emerging evidence from randomized, controlled trials that the combined strategies do actually work under workplace conditions, the relative value of BCs compared to after-work moisturizers is not yet definitively clarified and depends on the respective preparations. The question raised by some whether distinguishing between the pre- and postexposure creams is necessary is still ongoing [12].

BCs may aim at certain occupational exposures and irritant groups. Examples of different types of irritants are hydrophilic ones, on the one hand, such as detergents and weakly acidic or alkaline aqueous solutions. Cutting fluids are typically aqueous alkaline irritants. On the other hand, lipophilic substances, such as oils, fats, and organic solvents, have to be considered. BCs may offer protection against some, but not necessarily all, irritants, even within the group of water-soluble irritants (unpublished observation). It is therefore necessary that the products undergo efficacy testing with respect to the intended exposures and claims prior to marketing, thus ensuring efficacy and enabling better product selection for consumers. This requirement has already been introduced into national guidelines in Germany [20]. Currently, various in vitro and in vivo tests are used by manufacturers for claim support. However, many of them are not considered to be close enough to real working situations [12]. Repetitive exposure to wet work and mild irritants, which is the predominant pattern at workplaces that leads to cumulative irritation, cannot be mimicked by test models using single exposures, whether they be performed as in vitro, ex vivo, or with the help of artificial skin models. Consequently, screening in vitro or ex vivo efficacy tests should be confirmed by repetitive in vivo exposure models. Cumulative patch tests, repetitive washing procedures with sodium lauryl sulfate (SLS), and other tests have been presented and summarized [1, 21]. Standardized and validated efficacy test models using appropriate positive and negative controls are nevertheless lacking at present.

26.4 Mechanism of Action

The mechanisms of BC action are still largely unknown. Several years ago, the prevailing opinion was that BCs are effective by shielding the skin from harmful substances in a physical way, thus preventing penetration into the epidermal barrier. It was a logical conclusion to recommend that lipophilic emulsions (w/o emulsions) should be used against hydrophilic irritants, such as detergents, weak acids and alkalis, and metal-working fluids. In contrast, hydrophilic ointments (w/o emulsions) were postulated to be used against lipophilic irritants, such as oils, varnishes, and organic solvents. Currently, this principle has to be judged as outdated, according to studies that demonstrated failure of particular BCs against specific lipophilic and hydrophilic model irritants [22, 23]. Most likely, the action may at least be a variable combination of shielding and effects on physiological barrier strengthening – for example, by stimulation of barrier repair (see Chap. 27) – depending on the specific preparation. These effects may depend on the ointment base rather than on any potential "active" ingredients.

Some ingredients, such as natural or synthetic tanning substances, zinc oxide, talcum, perfluoropolyethers, chelating agents, and other substances that can bind metal ions or reduce their penetration through the skin, are nonetheless claimed to have special protective properties. Tannin is supposed to harden the skin in order to increase the mechanical resistance of the skin surface against microtrauma. Tannins cause a local decrease of perspiration [24] by denaturation of keratin proteins in the stratum corneum which affects the sweat pores. Aluminum chlorohydrate is also used for reduction of perspiration by reversibly blocking eccrine sweat excretion. Both tanning agents and aluminum chlorohydrate are, therefore, used in products that are recommended against wet work and while wearing gloves. Some chelating agents are claimed to protect against sensitizing substances [25].

26.5 Appropriate Application and Educational Aspects

In order to be effective, BCs have to be applied frequently enough and in sufficient amounts. Some studies document that the acceptance of BCs is poor on the level of primary prevention, especially in men compared to women. It is increasing among subjects with a past or present history of hand eczema [15]. Although BCs are intended to be used on healthy skin, these products are broadly used on the level of secondary and even tertiary prevention of occupational skin diseases, when eczema has already developed.

Due to insufficient acceptance and knowledge, it can be assumed that BCs are often used in deficient doses. It is, therefore, necessary to train subjects carefully. Education may take place on an individual basis or in group seminars (reviewed in [26] and in Chap. 42). Educational programs for apprentice hairdressers, health care workers, and bakers that include information about appropriate usage of BCs have been proven to be successful with respect to reduced prevalence of developing hand dermatitis [27–29]. Training should be performed with regard to appropriate coverage of problem areas such as the interdigital, wrist, and fingertip regions. Usage of the fluorescence technique is a simple method to monitor self-application [30]. It is also useful to ask the individual whether the designated product is judged to be pleasant (after applying the BC under supervision). If not, an alternative product should be offered. Subsequently, the subjects should have opportunity to provide feedback about their experiences and practicability after testing the selected product for a period of time. In many cases, further encouragement will be necessary until the preparation is used on a regular basis throughout the day (personal experience).

From a scientific point of view, there are still many open questions to be addressed in experimental and clinical trials with respect to the function and appropriate usage of BCs (e.g., appropriate frequencies and quantities of application). Some manufacturers recommend reapplication of their products every 3–4 h. Some also recommend how much of their product should be applied (e.g., 1–2 mL). Experimental evidence for the recommended doses is lacking. In a recent pilot study, it was found that nurses applied a low mean dose of 0.97 mg/cm^2 (SD+/− 0.6) on the hands [31]. The amounts used in other sectors might differ broadly. It can be assumed that the benefit of BCs is positively correlated to the amounts applied. A positive dose-dependent efficacy was confirmed in a recent trial. Three BCs showed partial efficacy when applied in low doses (2 mg/cm^2); however, better efficacy was confirmed with tenfold dose [32]. These findings also have implications for industry, since it appears reasonable to perform efficacy tests with the doses that are actually achieved at workplaces. Systematic investigation of this subject is still lacking.

26.6 Limitations of Barrier Creams

It should be noted that BCs do not offer protection against strong irritants or corrosive agents. In addition, the use of BCs against contact allergens is very limited. They cannot prevent the elicitation of contact dermatitis in already sensitized individuals, and it has not been proven whether they can reduce the risk of sensitization. There are, however, single products on the market with a protective claim against certain problem allergens such as poison ivy [33].

In some instances, BCs were not only found to fail but to actually aggravate the irritation instead of offering protection. This was especially the case for organic solvents [34–36]. The mechanisms of skin damage caused by solvents seem to be substantially different from water-soluble irritants, due to their ability to penetrate intact skin [37]. In a recent experimental study with BCs marketed to protect against lipophilic irritants, two out of six products aggravated skin irritation induced by two different organic solvents [23]. The use of BCs when handling solvents should therefore be regarded with caution, as long as substantiated efficacy proofs are not available.

26.7 Emollients and Moisturizers

Emollients are designed to smoothen the skin and to increase the water content indirectly by creating an occlusive film on the skin surface, thereby trapping the water in the upper layers of the stratum corneum, while moisturizers are designed to actively increase the water content of the skin [38]. Emollients and moisturizers are used in postexposure skin care products that are designed to counteract the damaging effects of irritants. On many occasions, "emollients" and "moisturizers" are used as synonyms. Humectants are compounds of moisturizers, such as urea, lactic acid, glycerine, sorbitol, or modern substances such as hyaluronic acid and mucopolysaccharides. They increase hydration, binding water at the skin surface by retaining large amounts of water relative to their weight. Close to 200 compounds are used for skin hydration, but hydration and improved dryness do not always lead to a better barrier function. For example, 15 % glycolic acid has been shown to improve xerosis on the legs but also to increase transepidermal water loss, as well as susceptibility to externally applied irritants [39].

The exact mechanism of action of moisturizers and emollients is still unknown, but there is accumulated efficacy data regarding their occlusive properties, lipid content, and pH. Taken together, the amount of data is increasing that moisturizers are capable of both preventing and treating ICD [1, 4]. The various ingredients and potential mechanisms of moisturizers are reviewed elsewhere (see Chap. 27).

References

1. Zhai H, Maibach HI. Protection from irritants. Curr Probl Dermatol. 2007;34:47–57.
2. Kresken J, Klotz A. Occupational skin-protection products – a review. Int Arch Occup Environ Health. 2003;76(5):355–8.
3. Loden M, Wiren K, Smerud K, Meland N, Honnas H, Mork G, et al. Treatment with a barrier-strengthening moisturizer prevents relapse of hand-eczema. An open, randomized, prospective, parallel group study. Acta Derm Venereol. 2010;90(6):602–6.
4. Yokota M, Maibach HI. Moisturizer effect on irritant dermatitis: an overview. Contact Dermatitis. 2006;55(2):65–72.
5. Drexler H. Skin protection and percutaneous absorption of chemical hazards. Int Arch Occup Environ Health. 2003;76(5):359–61.
6. Schliemann S. Limitations of skin protection. Curr Probl Dermatol. 2007;34:171–7.
7. Buckley DA, Rycroft RJ, White IR, McFadden JP. Fragrance as an occupational allergen. Occup Med (Lond). 2002;52(1):13–6.
8. Heydorn S, Menne T, Johansen JD. Fragrance allergy and hand eczema – a review. Contact Dermatitis. 2003;48(2):59–66.
9. Uter W, Schnuch A, Geier J, Pfahlberg A, Gefeller O. Association between occupation and contact allergy to the fragrance mix: a multifactorial analysis of national surveillance data. Occup Environ Med. 2001;58(6):392–8.
10. Article 1. Directive 2003/15/EC of the European Parliament and of the Council of 27 February 2003. Official Journal of the European Union. 11.3.2203
11. Klaschka U. The hazard communication of fragrance allergens must be improved. Integr Environ Assess Manag. 2013;9(3):358–62; [Epub ahead of print].
12. Kutting B, Drexler H. Effectiveness of skin protection creams as a preventive measure in occupational dermatitis: a critical update according to criteria of evidence-based medicine. Int Arch Occup Environ Health. 2003;76(4):253–9.
13. Wigger-Alberti W, Elsner P. Preventive measures in contact dermatitis. Clin Dermatol. 1997;15(4):661–5.
14. Elsner P, Wigger-Alberti W. Skin-conditioning products in occupational dermatology. Int Arch Occup Environ Health. 2003;76(5):351–4.
15. Kutting B, Weistenhofer W, Baumeister T, Uter W, Drexler H. Current acceptance and implementation of preventive strategies for occupational hand eczema in 1355 metalworkers in Germany. Br J Dermatol. 2009;161(2):390–6.
16. Berndt U, Gabard B, Schliemann-Willers S, Wigger-Alberti W, Zitterbart D, Elsner P. Integrated skin protection from workplace irritants: a new model for efficacy assessment. Exog Dermatol. 2002;1:45–8.
17. Antonov D, Kleesz P, Elsner P, Schliemann S. Impact of glove occlusion on cumulative skin irritation with or without hand cleanser – comparison in an experimental repeated irritation model. Contact Dermatitis. 2013;68(5):293–9 [Epub ahead of print].
18. Kutting B, Baumeister T, Weistenhofer W, Pfahlberg A, Uter W, Drexler H. Effectiveness of skin protection measures in prevention of occupational hand eczema: results of a prospective randomized controlled trial over a follow-up period of 1 year. Br J Dermatol. 2010;162(2):362–70.
19. Winker R, Salameh B, Stolkovich S, Nikl M, Barth A, Ponocny E, et al. Effectiveness of skin protection creams in the prevention of occupational dermatitis: results of a randomized, controlled trial. Int Arch Occup Environ Health. 2009;82(5):653–62.
20. Fartasch M, Diepgen TL, Drexler H, Elsner P, Fluhr JW, John SM, et al. Berufliche Hautmittel AWMF-Leitlinien-Register Nr.013/056. 2008. Available from: http://www.awmf.org/leitlinien/aktuelle-leitlinien/ll-liste/deutsche-dermatologische-gesellschaft-ddg.html
21. Zhai H, Willard P, Maibach HI. Evaluating skin-protective materials against contact irritants and allergens. An in vivo screening human model. Contact Dermatitis. 1998;38(3):155–8.
22. Frosch PJ, Kurte A. Efficacy of skin barrier creams (IV). The repetitive irritation test (RIT) with a set of 4

standard irritants. Contact Dermatitis. 1994;31(3):161–8.
23. Schliemann S, Kleesz P, Elsner P. Protective creams fail to prevent solvent-induced cumulative skin irritation. Results of a randomised double-blind study. In preparation contact dermatitis. 2013 jul 11 doi:10.MMcod.12103 (epub ahead of print).
24. Jepsen JR, Sparre Jorgensen A, Kyst A. Hand protection for car-painters. Contact Dermatitis. 1985;13(5):317–20.
25. Romaguera C, Grimalt F, Vilaplana J, Carreras E. Formulation of a barrier cream against chromate. Contact Dermatitis. 1985;13(2):49–52.
26. Seyfarth F, Schliemann S, Antonov D, Elsner P. Teaching interventions in contact dermatitis. Dermatitis. 2011;22(1):8–15.
27. Bauer A, Bartsch R, Hersmann C, Stadeler M, Kelterer D, Schneider W, et al. Occupational hand dermatitis in food industry apprentices: results of a 3-year follow-up cohort study. Int Arch Occup Environ Health. 2001;74(6):437–42.
28. Loffler H, Bruckner T, Diepgen T, Effendy I. Primary prevention in health care employees: a prospective intervention study with a 3-year training period. Contact Dermatitis. 2006;54(4):202–9.
29. Schwanitz HJ, Riehl U, Schlesinger T, Bock M, Skudlik C, Wulfhorst B. Skin care management: educational aspects. Int Arch Occup Environ Health. 2003;76(5):374–81.
30. Wigger-Alberti W, Maraffio B, Wernli M, Elsner P. Training workers at risk for occupational contact dermatitis in the application of protective creams: efficacy of a fluorescence technique. Dermatology. 1997;195(2):129–33.
31. Schliemann S, Petri M, Elsner P. How much skin protection cream is actually applied in the workplace? Determination of dose per skin surface area in nurses. Contact Dermatitis. 2012;67(4):229–33.
32. Schliemann S, Petri M, Elsner P. Preventing irritant contact dermatitis by protective creams: influence of the application dose. Contact Dermatitis. 2013 jul 11. doi:10.MMcod.12104 (Epub ahead of print).
33. Schalock PC, Zug KA. Protection from occupational allergens. Curr Probl Dermatol. 2007;34:58–75.
34. Goh CL. Cutting oil dermatitis on guinea pig skin (I). Cutting oil dermatitis and barrier cream. Contact Dermatitis. 1991;24(1):16–21.
35. Schliemann-Willers S, Wigger-Alberti W, Elsner P. Efficacy of a new class of perfluoropolyethers in the prevention of irritant contact dermatitis. Acta Derm Venereol. 2001;81(6):392–4.
36. Wigger-Alberti W, Rougier A, Richard A, Elsner P. Efficacy of protective creams in a modified repeated irritation test. Methodological aspects. Acta Derm Venereol. 1998;78(4):270–3.
37. Rowse DH, Emmett EA. Solvents and the skin. Clin Occup Environ Med. 2004;4(4):657–730. vi.
38. Gabard B. Testing the efficacy of moisturizers. In: Elsner P, Berardesca E, Maibach HI, editors. Bioengineering of the skin: water and the stratum corneum. Boca Raton: CRC Press; 1994. p. 147–67.
39. Loden M. The clinical benefit of moisturizers. J Eur Acad Dermatol Venereol. 2005;19(6):672–88. quiz 86–7.

27 Moisturizers in the Prevention and Treatment of Hand Eczema

Marie Lodén

Contents

M. Lodén, Ms Pharm Sci, Dr Med Sci
Research and Development, Eviderm Institute, Bergshamra Allé 9, Solna 17077, Sweden
e-mail: marie.loden@eviderm.se

27.1 Introduction

The hands are vulnerable parts of the body and are constantly exposed to a number of bad and good chemicals. The combination of various bad cumulative interacting factors, such as wet work, contact allergy (especially nickel), or frictional irritancy with genetic predisposition, such as atopic dermatitis, increases the risks for hand eczema [1]. Around half of the hand eczema cases develop into a chronic disease, and symptoms may persist for many years or recur after disease-free intervals [2, 3]. The 1-year prevalence is around 10 %, and the lifetime prevalence around 20 % [1, 4, 5]. In adults with moderate and severe atopic dermatitis in childhood, the prevalence has been reported as 25–41 %, respectively [6]. Atopic dermatitis associated with null mutations within the gene encoding the key epidermal protein filaggrin (*fil*ament-*aggr*egating prote*in*) is particularly associated with an earlier onset and higher persistence of hand eczema and dryness [7–9]. In addition, psychological stress has been shown experimentally to retard recovery of the permeability barrier in humans [10].

A wide range of approaches is available for the management of hand eczema (Fig. 27.1). The first choice is reduction of provocative agents. Anti-inflammatory treatments include topical corticosteroids, phototherapy, and chemotherapy [11]. Moisturizing creams or emollients are important treatment adjuncts, both in the acute phase and to prevent the eczema. The products

A. Alikhan et al. (eds.), *Textbook of Hand Eczema*,
DOI 10.1007/978-3-642-39546-8_27, © Springer-Verlag Berlin Heidelberg 2014

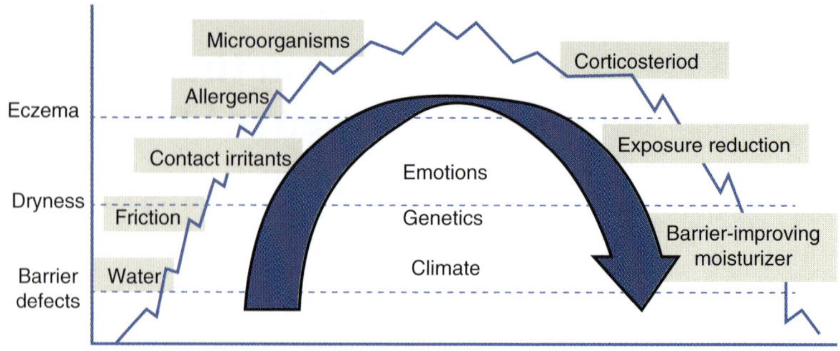

Fig. 27.1 Hand eczema is a common and multifactorial condition in which several factors contribute to the disease development

that not only diminish dryness symptoms but also repair the skin barrier or prevent barrier dysfunction appear most promising [12–17]. Moisturizers usually contain substances considered to be actives (e.g., humectants, ceramides, essential fatty acids, vitamins, and herbal extracts) and substances considered to be excipients (e.g., emulsifiers, antioxidants, preservatives).

However, moisturizers have different effects on the skin, and some may even worsen the skin. More rigorous data and controlled studies on the effectiveness of moisturizers have therefore been requested [18]. So far, the links between the abnormality and the composition of the moisturizer remain largely unexplored, and it may be a matter of trial and error to find the most suitable formulation for an individual. Today the best product for an individual may be the one they prefer because they will use it regularly. The majority of moisturizers on the market are regulated as cosmetics. However, according to medical regulation in most countries, only pharmaceuticals and medical devices can be recommended for treatment of skin diseases [19].

27.2 Chemicals in Moisturizers

27.2.1 Definitions and Structures

The term "emollient" is defined as (from the Latin derivation) a material designed to soften the skin – that is, a material that "smooths" the surface to the touch and makes it look smoother to the eye. The term "moisturizer" is often used synonymously with emollient, but the term implies the addition of water to the skin. Therefore, moisturizers usually contain humectants to enhance the water-binding capacity of the stratum corneum. Irrespective of their possible humectant content, the term "moisturizer" is used in this chapter.

Large differences exist in the composition and function of moisturizing creams. Knowledge about the interplay between ingredients is fundamental to develop a stable and cosmetically attractive product with preferred impact on the skin. The smell, greasiness, and stickiness of some products can be difficult to accept.

Creams are the most common types of delivery system used for moisturizers. In its simplest form they are two-phase systems (emulsion) containing two immiscible liquids – oil and water (Fig. 27.2). Usually the oil is dispersed in the water phase in the form of microscopic or submicroscopic droplets. Such oil-in-water (O/W) emulsions are more common than water-in-oil (W/O) emulsions. The ratio between oil and water is important, as well as the type of oil and the amount and type of other ingredients. Typically the oil content is about 15–30 %. The droplet size is often between 1 and 100 μm, which gives white formulations. Emulsifiers embed the droplets and provide stability. Emulsifiers combine both hydrophilic and lipophilic components in one molecule and turn their nonpolar hydrocarbon end into the oil phase and their polar end into the water phase.

Ointments are a single-phase system, in which hydrophilic ointments are preparations that are miscible with water, in contrast to hydrophobic ointments, which are not miscible with water. When large amounts of finely dispersed solids are incorporated in ointments, they are called

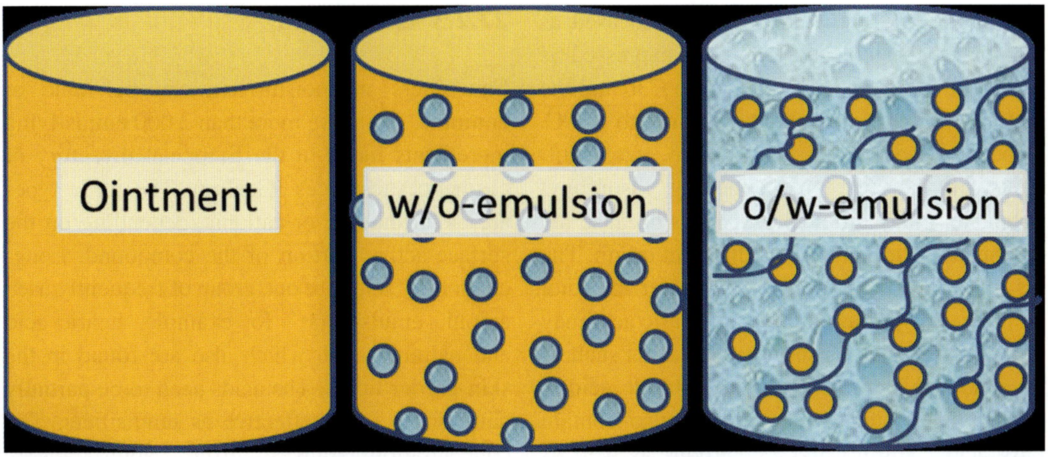

Fig. 27.2 The composition and the organization of the ingredients determine the cosmetic properties and the functional characteristics of the topical products. Ointments and water-in-oil (w/o) emulsions are greasier and less easy to rinse off than oil-in-water (o/w) emulsions

pastes (e.g., zinc pastes). Gels are hydrophilic or hydrophobic liquids that are gelled by means of suitable gelling agents.

27.2.2 Oils, Fats, and Lipid Materials in Moisturizers

Topical formulation terminology does not always have a distinct definition of the words oils, fats, and lipids. Oils (liquid) and fats (solid) are typically mixtures of triglyceride bulk storage material produced by plants and animals. Mineral oils and silicon oils are other types of semisolid materials with oily properties. Mineral oils are hydrocarbons derived from petroleum, whereas silicons originate from silica found in sand, quartz, and granites. The properties of silicons are derived from their molecular structure in addition to the characteristics of the organic group joined to the silica. Lipids can be defined as substances biochemically or functionally related to fatty acids. Skin lipids consist mainly of ceramides, cholesterol, and fatty acids, and such lipids can also be used in creams to provide stability of the emulsion.

Common fats in moisturizers are mono-, di-, and triglycerides; waxes; long-chain esters; fatty acids; lanolin; and mineral oils. There is a large variety of fatty acids among the glycerides, with the saturated fatty stearic acid, the monounsaturated oleic acid, and the polyunsaturated linoleic acid being the most abundant fatty acids.

Vegetable oils and fats (triglycerides) are derived from a variety of vegetable sources, of which palm oil, soybean oil, rapeseed oil, and sunflower seed oil are the most important ones. The latter three are liquid oils with a high degree of unsaturation, as they have high levels of linoleic (C18:2) and linolenic acids (C18:3). The number and distribution of double bonds over the carbon chain are important features of oils. The fatty acid profile is typical for oils and influences its characteristics with respect to stability, skin feel, and effects on the skin. The degree of unsaturation influences the ease of handling, and those with a higher degree of unsaturation are more easily oxidized. The unsaturation of soybean, rapeseed, and sunflower oil restricts their use in skin care, as they are difficult to stabilize against oxidation. Oxidation is increased by the presence of heat, light, metals, and oxygen.

Esters are also a popular and versatile group of emollients, owing to the availability of a large number of ingredients with large differences in properties. This versatility can be used by the formulator to bring various functions to the moisturizer, influencing stability, aesthetics, skin feel, and delivery of actives. Simple esters can be defined as esters of monohydric alcohols with acids with only one acid group. When used as emollients, the molecular weights, expressed as carbon numbers, range from C16 to C36 and the melting points from about −30 up to 40°C. Depending on the starting material, two emollients with the same INCI name (e.g., "isopropyl palmitate") may differ in properties because the "palmitate" part may have a different origin. The acid used for production of this ester may not be pure, and various amounts of stearic acid may be present as well as shorter fatty acids such as myristic and lauric acid. If the palmitic acid is derived from animal fats, it may also contain fatty acids with 15 and 17 carbons as well as branched fatty acids.

Waxes may be classified into animal, vegetable, and mineral type. The most commonly used animal wax is lanolin. Lanolin (from the Latin *lana* for wool and *oleum* for oil) is secreted by the sebaceous glands of the sheep. Unlike human sebum, lanolin contains no triglycerides but does contain a complex mixture of esters, diesters, and hydroxy esters of high molecular weight lanolin alcohols and lanolin acids. Beeswax is a complicated mixture of hydrocarbons, esters, and fatty acids. A typical example of a vegetable-derived wax is carnauba, which is obtained from the leaves of the carnauba palm tree.

Mineral oils are derived from petroleum. The two most important materials are liquid paraffin (also called mineral oil and paraffinum liquidum) and petrolatum, consisting of complex combinations of hydrocarbons. Depending on the distribution of the molecular weight, materials with different viscosity are obtained. Physicochemically, petrolatum is an oleogel, an oil-based, lipophilic, gel stabilized by network-forming crystals of high-melting hydrocarbons. During the refining process, the hydrocarbon material is hydrogenated to create oxidation-resistant molecules throughout, from the liquid to the solid waxes. This gives a long shelf life to the products. Petrolatum has been used in topical formulations since its discovery by Robert A. Chesebrough in 1872 [20]. Liquid mineral oils or paraffin oils are chemically similar to petrolatum but do not contain the high-melting waxes that give petrolatum its consistency.

27.2.3 Emulsifiers

Emulsifiers in moisturizers can be ionic or nonionic. There are more than 2,000 emulsifying ingredients listed in the European inventory of cosmetic substances (CosIng). The ionic types are either anionic or cationic, depending on the surface-active portion of the compound. Long-chain fatty acids are one group of frequently used anionic emulsifiers – for example, stearic acid and palmitic acid, which also are found in the skin-barrier lipids. The acids need to be partially neutralized to be effective as emulsifiers. The concentration ranges from approximately 1–10 %. Fatty acids with a chain length of 14–22 carbons are also found in the epidermal tissue. Cholesterol is another component of the lipid bilayer, which is also found as an emulsifier (nonionic) in moisturizers. Nonionic emulsifiers depend primarily upon hydroxyl groups and ether linkages (from polyhydric alcohol anhydrides and polyoxyethylene chains) to create the hydrophilic action.

The effects of emulsifiers on skin-barrier properties are not well described, but nonionic emulsifiers are expected to be less irritating than ionics, although nonionics also interact with the skin-barrier function and induce changes in TEWL [21].

27.2.4 Hydrating Substances

There are more than 800 humectants in the European cosmetics inventory of ingredients. The majority of humectants used in moisturizers are low molecular weight substances with water-attracting properties. A few high molecular weight substances are also used (e.g., polymers such as hyaluronic acid). Humectants differ in water-binding capacity as well as in their ability to penetrate and influence the degree of skin hydration.

Glycerol is probably the most commonly used humectant. Glycerol has been suggested to ameliorate dry flaky skin by facilitating the digestion of the superficial desmosomes in subjects with dry skin [22]. Glycerol also modulates the phase behavior of stratum corneum lipids in vitro and prevents crystallization of their lamellar structures at low relative humidity [23]. In dry skin the proportion of lipids in the solid state may be increased, and glycerol may then help to maintain the lipids in a liquid crystalline state at low relative humidity [23, 24].

In sebaceous gland-deficient mice, dryness has been found to be linked to reduced levels of glycerol, due to the primary source for glycerol – triglycerides [25]. This type of dryness may also be applicable to clinical situations in which sebaceous glands are absent or involuted, such as in prepubertal children showing eczematous patches that disappear with the onset of sebaceous gland activity. Moreover, xerosis on the distal extremities of aged skin and in patients receiving systemic isotretinoin for treatment of acne has been suggested to be linked to glycerol depletion due to lower sebaceous gland activity [25].

Propylene glycol and butylene glycol are other frequently used alcohols with humectant properties. Propylene glycol is often used as a solvent and vehicle for substances unstable or insoluble in water and is regarded as a penetration enhancer. Moisturizers containing high concentrations (>20 %) of propylene glycol are used for the treatment of dry skin, especially when microorganisms are considered important triggering factors for the inflammation. Propylene glycol is used as inhibitor of fermentation and mold growth.

Panthenol is another alcohol that is converted in tissues to D-pantothenic acid (vitamin B_5), a component of coenzyme A in the body. The substance can be isolated from various living creatures, hence, its name (pantothen is Greek for "everywhere") [26]. Panthenol is found in topical treatments for sunburn and for wound healing (ulcers, burns, bedsores, and excoriations) [26, 27]. Topically applied panthenol penetrates the skin and is transformed into pantothenic acid [26, 28].

PCA is the cosmetic ingredient term used for the cyclic organic compound known as 2-pyrrolidone-5-carboxylic acid (also pidolic acid). The sodium salt is a naturally occurring humectant in the stratum corneum corresponding to approximately 2 % by weight in the stratum corneum [29]. PCA belongs to a faction of low molecular weight humectants that are termed "natural moisturizing factor" (NMF) [30]. Natural moisturizing factor is derived from filaggrin, and mutations in the gene have been identified as the major predisposing factor for atopic eczema and skin dryness [8, 9]. Defects in the filaggrin gene are also linked to the cytokine cascade and the formation of the cornified envelope of corneocytes [31, 32]. Treatment of solvent-damaged guinea pig footpad corneum with humectant solutions shows that the water held by the corneum decreases in the following order: sodium PCA > sodium lactate > glycerol > sorbitol [33].

Alpha hydroxy acids (AHAs) are another important group of humectants. An AHA is an organic carboxylic acid in which there is a hydroxy group at the two, or alpha (α), position of the carbon chain. Formulations containing an AHA have an acidic pH in the absence of any inorganic alkali or organic base. Lactic acid, glycolic acid, and tartaric acid belong to AHA. Lactic acid is a part of NMF and has been used in topical preparations for several decades because of its buffering properties and water-binding capacity [33]. Lactic acid has also been suggested to stimulate ceramide synthesis and improve skin-barrier function [34, 35]. The concentrations used for treatment dry skin disorders have ranged up to 12 % [36].

Urea is another physiological NMF. Solutions containing 20 % urea have been proposed to reduce experimentally induced itching [37]. Urea is used as a 10 % cream for the treatment of hyperkeratotic skin disorders [20, 38] and in lower concentrations for the treatment of less severe dryness.

27.2.5 Botanical Substances

A number of herbal products and extracts have been used in topical formulations since historical times and are part of dermatology practice [39]. Herbs are identified in Latin by their Linnaean

Table 27.1 Examples of differences in the nomenclature of the same ingredient used in topical formulation depending on, for example, regulatory status and geographical region

Cosmetic ingredients named according to the nomenclature in the European Union	Other names, e.g., in cosmetics in the United States, medical devices
Aqua	Water
Arachis hypogaea oil	Peanut oil
Butyrospermum parkii oil	Shea oil
Cera alba	Beeswax
Citrus bergamia	Citrus aurantium bergamia fruit oil
Cocos nucifera oil	Coconut oil
Elaeis guineensis kernel oil	Palm kernel oil
Helianthus annuus seed oil	Sunflower seed oil
Lanolin alcohol	Wool alcohols
Melaleuca alternifolia leaf oil	Tea tree oil
Olea europaea fruit oil	Olive oil, Olivae oleum
Paraffinum liquidum	Mineral oil
Persea gratissima oil	Avocado oil
Ricinus communis oil	Castor oil
Sesamum indicum seed oil	Sesame oil
Triticum vulgare germ oil	Wheat germ oil

description, where every entity is given two names. This binominal system was introduced by the Swedish naturalist Carl Linnaeus in the eighteenth century. Botanical substances used in cosmetics in Europe are ingredient-labelled with their Latin name, which may be different than the name used in, for example, cosmetics in the United States (Table 27.1).

There are many pitfalls in using herbs. The right species must be chosen, and the time of harvest, the method of preparation, and the stability of the actives have to be determined, making it hard to judge the quality of the treatment. The rationale for the inclusion of herbal extracts in moisturizers may not always be based upon controlled studies or evidence-based meta-analyses of clinical trials [39]. Instead, herbal extracts may be added for marketing reasons to nurture consumer interest in the perceived benefits of "natural ingredients" on the skin.

Aloe vera might be one of the most widely found natural materials in moisturizers. There are more than 300 species of aloe plants; aloe vera is now referred to by taxonomists as *Aloe barbadensis* [40]. The different species of aloe have different chemical compositions, and many investigations of the constituents found do not report the species studied [40]. Much of the consumer perception about the efficacy of aloe is anecdotal. Healing of burns and skin ulcers and antibacterial and anti-inflammatory properties are proposed effects, but evidence to support its use is not convincing [40]. Several studies of the efficacy of aloe vera components have shown conflicting results, and clinical investigations that incorporate vehicle controls are considered necessary [40].

Oatmeal baths for soothing rashes have been part of nursing practice for decades [39]. Oatmeal is processed oats (*Avena sativa*).

Allantoin is the synthesized active from the comfrey root (*Symphytum officinale*), known as aluminum dihydroxy allantoinate. It is suggested to be a keratolytic agent and is frequently used in moisturizers for the healing of dry skin. Controlled studies confirming the efficacy are lacking.

Bioflavonoids, plant-derived polyphenols, are becoming increasingly popular in topical products owing to their antioxidant properties. Normal skin contains several antioxidants, such as ascorbic acid, vitamin E, ubiquinol, and uric acid. During oxidative stress, the levels in the skin are affected, and topical treatment with antioxidants is suggested to be beneficial to the skin. For example, red tomato (*Lycopersicum esculentum*) contains an unsaturated, open-chain carotenoid with protective effects against UV-radiation [41].

27.2.6 Preservatives, Antioxidants, and Chelators

Preservatives are included in formulations to kill or inhibit the growth of microorganisms inadvertently introduced during use or manufacturing. Contaminating organisms may be either pathogens or nonpathogens. The ideal preservative must have a broad spectrum of activity; it must be safe to use; it should be stable in the product; and it should not affect the physical properties of the product [42].

No single preservative meets all these requirements, and usually a combination of substances is used. In Europe, 58 preservatives are approved for use in cosmetics. Ethanol and propylene glycol may enhance the effect of the preservatives.

Products without preservatives have to rely on low water activity (e.g., high concentrations of alcohols [20]), low pH, and/or other agents that are not classified as preservatives, such as essential oils, in order to withstand contamination. Such restrictions may induce other types of inconveniences, such as bad cosmetic properties, risks for other adverse reactions, or insufficient preservation. Caprylyl glycol and ethylhexylglycerin are examples of substances used to replace preservatives, where case reports on allergy exist [43–45].

Antioxidants inhibit oxidation of ingredients by reacting with free radicals and blocking the chain reaction. Typical antioxidants are tocopherols (vitamin E), butylated hydroxytoluene (BHT), and alkyl gallates [20]. Reducing agents, such as ascorbic acid, may also act by reacting with free radicals, as well as oxidize more readily than the ingredients they are intended to protect.

Edetic acid (EDTA), citric acid, and tartaric acid and their salts enhance the efficacy of antioxidants by reacting with heavy-metal ions and "removing" the ions from the solution [20]. The stability of the EDTA-metal complex depends on the metal ion involved and also on the pH. The calcium chelate is relatively weak, and EDTA will preferentially chelate heavy metals, such as iron, copper, and lead [20]. EDTA has been noticed to increase the rate of cell dissociation ex vivo, probably due to capturing of calcium, which is known to regulate the dissociation [46]. Mixtures of magnesium and calcium salts have been found to accelerate the barrier recovery in tape-stripped mice [47].

27.3 Compliance and Surface Effects

Application of moisturizer changes the surface friction [48] and smooths the skin when the spaces between partially desquamated skin flakes are filled [49, 50].

After being applied to the skin, the ingredients can stay on the surface, be absorbed into the skin, be metabolized, or disappear from the body by evaporation, sloughing off, or by contact with other materials. Approximately 50 % of applied creams remain on the surface 8 h after application [51]. Transfer of the actives to surrounding surfaces appears to be easier from creams and ointments than from lotions and tinctures [52]. However, oil-in-water emulsions are usually not water resistant and are easily rinsed away upon exposure to water.

Treatment adherence is a challenge with topical products. Patients can receive conflicting advice, leading to frustration, noncompliance, and difficulty in following an effective routine [53]. The appearance of the product [54] and the container can enhance the amount applied. For example, jars promote the use of larger quantities compared to tubes [55]. The distribution of the product has also been found to vary over the treated region [56]. In addition, distribution within the treated area is dependent on the type of vehicle [57]. A thick ointment (with a low water percentage) was equally distributed in the center and periphery of the treated area, whereas formulations with lower viscosity and more volatile ingredients (e.g., creams) were less evenly spread on the skin [57].

After covering the surface with a moisturizer, the produced layer of nonvolatile constituents will reduce the loss of water from the skin [58]. The degree of reduction of TEWL depends on the amount applied and the types of lipids in the formulation. Approximately 50 % reduction in TEWL is observed after application of a thick and greasy layer of petrolatum (3 mg/cm^2) to normal skin [59], whereas ordinary moisturizers provide a much smaller decrease in TEWL [60].

27.4 Prework Creams

Prework creams, so-called barrier-creams, should be applied at the start of work or after rest breaks. Such creams are designed to be effective on the surface of the skin. However, the term "barrier-cream" can be misleading, giving rise to a perception that these agents form a physical barrier to protect skin and are a substitute for wearing gloves or other protective equipment.

A systematic review reveals that there is mixed evidence for the effectiveness of prework creams [61]. In fact, evidence from animal studies indicates that they are very limited in forming a true barrier. While some are effective in preventing irritant contact dermatitis or allergic contact dermatitis for specific allergens, there are limitations in the extent to which this finding can be generalized. Other limitations include a well-recognized failure of users to apply them properly [62], uncertainty about penetration for many substances [63], and difficulty for workers in recognizing when the creams wear off during a shift. However, one potential advantage with prework creams is that they make it easier to wash off contaminants and allow milder cleansing agents to be used. Therefore, they can play a useful role in an overall skin management program.

27.5 Moisturizers in Experimental Models of Dryness

In experimental models of dryness, moisturizers have been found to reduce susceptibility to irritants [64] and to promote normalization of the skin-barrier function [65–70]. In one study the subjects were asked to wash their upper arms with a liquid detergent and apply eight different moisturizers for comparative purposes after each wash in the first week to one upper arm and twice daily without wash in the second week. Evaluation of skin blood flow and TEWL concluded that the regular use of emollients reduced irritant dermatitis from this detergent [64]. In another study on sodium lauryl sulfate (SLS)-irritated human skin using a hand-immersion test, it was found that a moisturizer was effective in preventing the development of irritant contact dermatitis and also accelerated skin-barrier repair, judged by measurement of TEWL and electrical capacitance, and it improved the clinical signs, which were observed on the control hand [71]. A moisturizer was also reported to speed healing in hand-immersion and SLS-patch tests [72].

The percentages of lipids in creams have been suggested to influence the recovery of skin-barrier function, as the level of lipids in creams was found to correlate with the recovery in one study [66]. In another double-blind, randomized study mimicking a work situation, the regular use of detergents and emollients in a wash test showed that three of five tested moisturizers were more effective in increasing epidermal hydration, and one moisturizer out of five led to a significant reduction in TEWL [73]. However, there were no comments on the composition in the publication. The aforementioned studies support the view that moisturizers are different and that regular application of certain compositions will give protection against repeated exposure to irritants.

Studies on ingredients show that petrolatum is absorbed into delipidized stratum corneum and decreases TEWL [74]. Canola oil and its unsaponifiable-enriched fraction are also found to be superior in reducing the degree of acute irritation than a number of other oils [75]. Application of structural lipids from stratum corneum has also been suggested to be more efficient than other type of lipids to correct hydration and scaling disorders [69, 76–79]. Complete mixtures of ceramide, fatty acid and cholesterol, or pure cholesterol have been shown to allow normal barrier recovery in acetone-treated murine skin, while two-component mixtures of fatty acid plus ceramide, cholesterol plus fatty acid, or cholesterol plus ceramide have been reported to delay barrier recovery [69]. Cholesterol as the dominant lipid has also been found to accelerate barrier recovery in tape-stripped, aged human skin [75]. However, in SLS-damaged human skin, no acceleration of barrier recovery was detected after treatment with a ceramide in different emulsions [80]. Neither did a moisturizer consisting of ceramide-3, cholesterol, and fatty acids (so-called skin-identical lipids) in a petrolatum-rich emulsion show superiority to pure petrolatum in human skin, damaged by SLS, and tape strippings [77]. Hence, the absorption of ceramides and the superiority of certain lipid mixtures to other lipids remain to be proven in randomized and controlled studies on humans, since no evidence of such effects in humans appears to exist [77, 80, 81]. Furthermore, polyunsaturated fatty acids in oils have been suggested to be transformed into "putative" anti-inflammatory products in the epidermis [82]. It has also been shown that small hydrophobic compounds, such as free fatty acids and certain oxysterols, are recognized by nuclear hormone receptors. Oxidation of long-chain fatty acids has been linked to the activity of peroxisome proliferating activated receptor (PPARα (alpha)) [83]. Cutaneous inflammation as it occurs in irritant contact dermatitis is reduced by the PPARα (alpha)-agonist linoleic acid in mice [84]. Moreover, activators of liver X receptors display anti-inflammatory activity in both irritant and allergic models of dermatitis [85].

Not only lipids but also nonionic emulsifiers have been found to influence TEWL in irritated skin [21]. In addition, humectants such as glycerin [65] and dexpanthenol [86] enhance skin-barrier repair in chemically irritated human skin. Another substance that has received positive scientific attention is nicotinamide (vitamin B_3). Topical application of nicotinamide has been reported to increase the level of barrier lipids while decreasing TEWL [87]. It also seems that glycerin acts synergistically with lipids and reduces xerosis more rapidly than expected from results on skin dryness [88].

27.6 Moisturizers: Field and Patient Studies

One of the first clinical studies on hand eczema was published 1943 [89]. Two hundred and twenty-five hospital personnel were given two jars of cream, one with 3 % urea and one without urea, and were requested to use one on each hand. Both the investigators and the patients found that patches of slight dermatitis improved and that the skin became softer, smoother, and even whiter with the urea cream [89]. Two preparations containing 10 % urea were also found to be efficient in a double-blind, bilateral study on hand eczema [90]. Both investigators and patients expressed preference for the cream containing multisterols, phospholipids, and fatty diols (pH of about 6) to the other cream containing betaine and lactic acid (pH about 3). In another clinical study on cracked, chapped hands from wet work, the effect from a 10 % urea cream was not reported to be superior to that of a pharmacopoeia aqueous cream [91].

In a 2-month clinical study on mild to moderate hand eczema in adult males and females ($n=30$), the results showed that twice-daily use of emollients was useful in the therapy of hand dermatitis [81]. However, no superiority of the ceramide cream to the ordinary petrolatum emollient was observed [81].

In patients, one might expect the impaired skin-barrier function to improve in association with a reduction in the clinical signs of dryness. However, the composition of the moisturizer determines whether the treatment strengthens or deteriorates the skin-barrier function. For example, one field study indicated a positive effect on skin hydration from the use of a lipid-rich moisturizer in 55 cleaners and kitchen assistants exposed to water and detergents, but no reduction in TEWL was noted [92].

In another prospective study on metal workers, it was shown that an after-work moisturizer appeared to reduce the incidence of irritant dermatitis, but did not reduce the elevated TEWL caused by exposure to cutting oil [93].

In a randomized, controlled intervention study, a high-fat, petrolatum-based moisturizer was studied along with protective gloves and a regular moisturizer in wet-work occupations (gut cleaners in Danish swine slaughterhouses). The results showed a significant reduction in eczema frequency in the intervention group compared to the control group. The best protective means was achieved with gloves alone or in combination with inner gloves and moisturizer. The high-fat cream could not replace gloves. Information and discussions were found to also be important in the reduction of skin problems [94].

A prospective, randomized, four-tailed controlled pilot trial compared the effect of skin protection cream before work and skin care alone without protection cream or in combination with cleansing against a control group (only cleansing). A total of 1,006 workers from the building industry and the timber industry were recruited, and out of these 485 workers were examined longitudinally for at least three time points over 1 year. The main finding in the study was that skin protection creams alone have less effect on the skin barrier in workers in the building and timber industries than skin care alone or skin care in combination with skin protection [95].

In a similar study 1,020 male metalworkers were recruited for a 12-month prospective intervention study with four arms: skin care (after work), skin protection creams (before or during working hours but complete avoidance of postexposure skin care), both combined, and control group (i.e., no recommendation). Both hands were examined using a quantitative skin score, and a standardized personal interview was performed three times. The change of the objective skin score from baseline to 12 months was used as primary outcome measure. The largest (significant) improvement was noted in the skin care plus skin protection group, followed by skin protection alone as second best. A significant deterioration was found in the control group. Therefore, the compliance to follow the skin protection regimen, especially the use of skin protection creams, should be enhanced [96].

Moisturizers are also suggested to be a vital part of the management when the skin is under control [18, 53]. One 5 % urea-containing moisturizer has repeatedly been shown to improve skin-barrier function in dry atopic skin [97, 98] as well as in normal skin [13]. In a clinical study on controlled hand eczema, the use of this barrier-strengthening cream (5 % urea) was shown to delay the relapse of eczema in 53 randomized patients [99]. The median time to relapse was 20 days in the moisturizer group compared with 2 days in the control group (no medicated or non-medicated preparations were allowed). Eczema relapsed in 90 % of the patients within 26 weeks. No difference in severity was noted between the groups at relapse. Hence, the application of the moisturizer prolonged the disease-free interval in patients with controlled hand eczema. This urea moisturizer has also been found to prevent relapse of flares in patients with controlled atopic eczema [100].

Moisturizers are also frequently used in combination with corticosteroids to reduce the need for corticosteroids. As corticosteroids are known to weaken the permeability barrier and increase skin sensitivity [101–104], the addition of moisturizer treatment might be a good strategy. In a randomized, double-blind clinical study on hand eczema, a barrier-strengthening urea moisturizer was noted to enhance the efficacy of the corticosteroid treatment in moderate hand eczema [105]. Once-daily application of a strong corticosteroid (betamethasone valerate in the evening) combined with a morning application of the moisturizer was more effective than twice-daily application of the corticosteroid. The concomitant use of a barrier-strengthening moisturizer may thus potentially counteract the barrier-weakening effects from corticosteroids and further prolong the disease-free intervals, already noted from intermittent treatment with topical corticosteroids [106]. Repairing an abnormal skin-barrier function and preventing barrier dysfunction are important strategies for reducing the risk of eczema [12].

27.7 Negative Effects from Moisturizers

Positive effects from the use of moisturizers cannot always be granted. Held et al. in 1999 [14] and 2001 [107] reported that a lipid-rich moisturizer, which improved stratum corneum hydration, increased skin susceptibility to contact irritants. In these studies, a 4-week treatment of normal skin with moisturizer three times a day increased susceptibility to SLS as demonstrated by a significantly higher TEWL on the treated forearm compared with the untreated forearm. Also, the sensitivity to nickel was increased by the use of a lipid-rich cream [15]. The results suggest that long-term treatment with moisturizers on normal skin may not necessarily offer any protection against irritants or allergens but instead increased skin susceptibility. The authors suggested that increasing the hydration level of the stratum corneum progressively may reduce its barrier efficiency and allow the permeation of noxious substances into the skin with greater ease.

Moisturizers are usually free from strong irritants, but repeated exposure of sensitive areas to mildly irritating preparations may cause dermatitis. For example, frequent immersion of the skin in water is counterproductive as far as the moisturization is concerned. [108, 109] In addition, a classic hydrophilic ointment contains the well-known irritant SLS as a co-emulsifier [20]. Also fatty acids that are sometimes found in moisturizers as emulsifiers can influence skin-barrier properties [21, 110]. Nonionic emulsifiers are the preferred stabilizers for emulsions owing to their mildness, but TEWL measurements indicate that some of them may also produce invisible barrier damage in normal skin [21]. Furthermore, nonionic polyethylene glycol emulsifiers are susceptible to oxidation, inducing formation of peroxides and aldehydes [111].

Moisturizers may also contain sensitizing ingredients [112]; fragrances and preservatives are the ones most frequently used in topical formulations. Almost all moisturizers in the supermarket contain fragrances, and over 100 fragrance ingredients have been identified as allergens [113]. However, careful use of fragrances may not induce skin allergy [114–116]. The advantage with fragrances is that they may increase the adherence to the treatment. A relationship between hand eczema and fragrance contact allergy has been found in some studies based on patients investigated for contact allergy [117]. However, hand eczema is a multifactorial disease, and the clinical significance of fragrance contact allergy in (severe) chronic hand eczema has not been not fully elucidated.

Preservatives also have good and bad properties. Preservatives facilitate the development of cosmetically appealing moisturizers. Badly preserved emollients have been found to be contaminated with microorganisms, such as *S. aureus* [118]. The severity and persistence of both atopic and hand eczema has been associated with *S. aureus* colonization [119, 120]. Aggravation of eczema and dermal infections have also been linked to the use of a contaminated emollient [121].

Humectants, emulsifiers, and oils hardly ever cause contact allergy [113]. Lanolins are sometimes proposed to be a frequent cause of contact allergy, but this is believed to be due to inappropriate testing conditions leading to false-positive reactions [113]. Adverse reactions to herbal extracts are rare, probably owing to the trivial amounts present in the finished product. However, virtually all herbal remedies can cause allergic reactions, and several can be responsible for photosensitization [122]. For example, aloe vera, black cumin oil, chamomile, Chinese herbal mixture, olive oil, tea tree oil, and Inula helenium have been reported to be able to cause allergic contact dermatitis [122].

27.8 Conclusion: The Future

Studies support the prevention effects of moisturizers against irritants and outbreak of hand eczema. The protective effects of moisturizers may, however, not be broad spectrum, and products with different constituents may be specifically more effective against different skin irritants and in different individuals. A number of practical factors might also limit clinical efficacy in the workplace, including compliance, availability, interaction with other substances, and removal by washing.

The first-generation moisturizers were occlusive emollients based on petrolatum to reduce TEWL and to allow the epidermis heal itself. The second-generation moisturizers contained humectants to bind water and lipids for temporary barrier improvement. Today's "regular" moisturizers offer occlusive and humectant activity. The future products have occlusive and humectants properties and will contain ingredients for stimulating barrier repair for different dry syndromes. However, more evidence on their effectiveness compared to no treatment and compared to a reference or placebo is needed.

References

1. Meding B, Swanbeck G. Occupational hand eczema in an industrial city. Contact Dermatitis. 1990;22(1):13–23.
2. Meding B, Wrangsjo K, Jarvholm B. Fifteen-year follow-up of hand eczema: persistence and consequences. Br J Dermatol. 2005;152(5):975–80.

3. Halkier-Sorensen L. Occupational skin diseases. Contact Dermatitis. 1996;35(1 Suppl):1–120.
4. Meding B, Swanbeck G. Prevalence of hand eczema in an industrial city. Br J Dermatol. 1987;116(5):627–34.
5. Bryld LE, Agner T, Kyvik KO, Brøndsted L, Hindsberger C, Menné T. Hand eczema in twins: a questionnaire investigation. Br J Dermatol. 2000;142(2):298–305.
6. Rystedt I. Long-term follow-up in atopic dermatitis. Acta Derm Venereol Suppl (Stockh). 1985;114:117–20.
7. Thyssen JP, Carlsen BC, Menné T, Linneberg A, Nielsen NH, Meldgaard M, et al. Filaggrin null mutations increase the risk and persistence of hand eczema in subjects with atopic dermatitis: results from a general population study. Br J Dermatol. 2010;163(1):115–20.
8. Palmer CN, Irvine AD, Terron-Kwiatkowski A, Zhao Y, Liao H, Lee SP, et al. Common loss-of-function variants of the epidermal barrier protein filaggrin are a major predisposing factor for atopic dermatitis. Nat Genet. 2006;38(4):441–6.
9. Weidinger S, Illig T, Baurecht H, Irvine AD, Rodriguez E, Diaz-Lacava A, et al. Loss-of-function variations within the filaggrin gene predispose for atopic dermatitis with allergic sensitizations. J Allergy Clin Immunol. 2006;118(1):214–9.
10. Garg A, Chren MM, Sands LP, Matsui MS, Marenus KD, Feingold KR, et al. Psychological stress perturbs epidermal permeability barrier homeostasis: implications for the pathogenesis of stress-associated skin disorders. Arch Dermatol. 2001;137(1):53–9.
11. English J, Aldridge R, Gawkrodger DJ, Kownacki S, Statham B, White JM, et al. Consensus statement on the management of chronic hand eczema. Clin Exp Dermatol. 2009;34(7):761–9.
12. Elias PM, Hatano F, Williams ML. Basis for the barrier abnormality in atopic dermatitis: outside-inside-outside pathogenic mechanisms. J Allergy Clin Immunol. 2008;121(6):1337–43.
13. Buraczewska I, Berne B, Lindberg M, Törmä H, Lodén M. Changes in skin barrier function following long-term treatment with moisturizers, a randomized controlled trial. Br J Dermatol. 2007;156(3):492–8.
14. Held E, Sveinsdottir S, Agner T. Effect of long-term use of moisturizer on skin hydration, barrier function and susceptibility to irritants. Acta Derm Venereol. 1999;79(1):49–51.
15. Zachariae C, Held E, Johansen JD, Menné T, Agner T. Effect of a moisturizer on skin susceptibility to NiCl2. Acta Derm Venereol. 2003;83(2):93–7.
16. Vilaplana J, Coll J, Trullás C, Azón A, Pelejero C. Clinical and non-invasive evaluation of 12 % ammonium lactate emulsion for the treatment of dry skin in atopic and non-atopic subjects. Acta Derm Venereol (Stockh). 1992;72:28–33.
17. Held E, Sveinsdottir S, Agner T. Effect of long-term use of moisturizers on skin hydration, barrier function and susceptibility to irritants. Acta DermVenereol (Stockh). 1999;79:49–51.
18. Hoare C, Li Wan Po A, Williams H. Systematic review of treatments for atopic eczema. Health Technol Assess. 2000;4(37):1–191.
19. Sörensen A, Landvall P, Lodén M. Moisturizers as cosmetics, medicines, or medical device? The regulatory demands in the European Union. In: Lodén M, Maibach HI, editors. Treatment of dry skin syndrome. The art and science of moisturizers. Berlin/Heidelberg: Springer; 2012. p. 3–16.
20. Kibbe AW. Handbook of pharmaceutical excipients. 3rd ed. London: Pharmaceutical Press; 2000.
21. Barany E, Lindberg M, Lodén M. Unexpected skin barrier influence from nonionic emulsifiers. Int J Pharm. 2000;195(1–2):189–95.
22. Rawlings AV, Harding C, Watkinson A, Banks J, Ackerman C, Sabin R. The effect of glycerol and humidity on desmosome degradation in stratum corneum. Arch Dermatol Res. 1995;287:457–64.
23. Froebe CL, Simion A, Ohlmeyer H, Rhein LD, Mattai J, Cagan RH, et al. Prevention of stratum corneum lipid phase transitions in vitro by glycerol – an alternative mechanism for skin moisturization. J Soc Cosmet Chem. 1990;41:51–65.
24. Mattai J, Froebe CL, Rhein D, et al. Prevention of model stratum corneum lipid phase transitions in vitro by cosmetic additives – differential scanning calorimetry, optical microscopy, and water evaporation studies. J Soc Cosmet Chem. 1993;44:89–100.
25. Fluhr JW, Mao-Qiang M, Brown BE, Wertz PW, Crumrine D, Sundberg JP, et al. Glycerol regulates stratum corneum hydration in sebaceous gland deficient (asebia) mice. J Invest Dermatol. 2003;120(5):728–37.
26. Schmid-Grendelmeier P, Wyss M, Elsner P. Contact allergy to dexpanthenol. A report of seven cases and review of the literature. Dermatosen. 1995;43:175–8.
27. Reynolds JEF. Martindale: the extra pharmacopoeia. 13th ed. London: The Pharmaceutical Press; 1993.
28. Anonymous. Final report on the safety assessment of panthenol and pantothenic acid. J Am Coll Toxicol. 1987;6:139–163.
29. Laden K. Natural moisturization factors in skin. Am Perfum Cosmet. 1967;82:77–9.
30. Jacobi OK. Moisture regulation in the skin. Drug Cosmet Ind. 1959;84:732–812.
31. Rawlings AV, Harding CR. Moisturization and skin barrier function. Dermatol Ther. 2004;17 Suppl 1:43–8.
32. Candi E, Schmidt R, Melino G. The cornified envelope: a model of cell death in the skin. Nat Rev Mol Cell Biol. 2005;6(4):328–40.
33. Middleton J. Development of a skin cream designed to reduce dry and flaky skin. J Soc Cosmet Chem. 1974;25:519–34.
34. Rawlings AV, Davies A, Carlomusto M, Pillai S, Zhang K, Kosturko R, et al. Effect of lactic acid isomers on keratinocyte ceramide synthesis, stratum corneum lipid levels and stratum corneum barrier function. Arch Dermatol Res. 1996;288:383–90.
35. Berardesca E, Distante F, Vignoli GP, Oresajo C, Green B. Alpha hydroxyacids modulate stratum corneum barrier function. Br J Dermatol. 1997;137(6):934–8.
36. Wehr R, Krochmal L, Bagatell F, Ragsdale W. A controlled two-center study of lactate 12 % lotion and

a petrolatum-based cream in patients with xerosis. Cutis. 1986;37:205–9.
37. Swanbeck G, Rajka G. Antipruritic effect of urea solutions. Acta Derm Venereol (Stockholm). 1970; 50:225–7.
38. Rosten M. The treatment of ichthyosis and hyperkeratotic conditions with urea. Aust J Derm. 1970;11:142–4.
39. Dattner AM. From medical herbalism to phytotherapy in dermatology: back to the future. Dermatol Ther. 2003;16(2):106–13.
40. Shelton RM. Aloe vera. Its chemical and therapeutic properties. Int J Dermatol. 1991;30:679–83.
41. Andreassi M, Stanghellini E, Ettorre A, Di Stefano A, Andreassi L. Antioxidant activity of topically applied lycopene. J Eur Acad Dermatol Venereol. 2004;18(1):52–5.
42. Godfrey D. Preservation of moisturisers. In: Loden M, Maibach HI, editors. Treatment of dry skin syndrome. The art and science of moisturizers. Berlin: Springer; 2012. p. 355–66.
43. Linsen G, Goossens A. Allergic contact dermatitis from ethylhexylglycerin. Contact Dermatitis. 2002;47(3):169.
44. Mortz CG, Otkjaer A, Andersen KE. Allergic contact dermatitis to ethylhexylglycerin and pentylene glycol. Contact Dermatitis. 2009;61(3):180.
45. Stausbol-Gron B, Andersen KE. Allergic contact dermatitis to ethylhexylglycerin in a cream. Contact Dermatitis. 2007;57(3):193–4.
46. Lundstrom A, Egelrud T. Cell shedding from human plantar skin in vitro: evidence of its dependence on endogenous proteolysis. J Invest Dermatol. 1988;91(4):340–3.
47. Denda M, Katagiri C, Hirao T, Maruyama N, Takahashi M. Some magnesium salts and a mixture of magnesium and calcium salts accelerate skin barrier recovery. Arch Dermatol Res. 1999;291(10):560–3.
48. Lodén M, Olsson H, Skare L, Axéll T. Instrumental and sensory evaluation of the frictional response of the skin following a single application of five moisturizing creams. J Soc Cosmet Chem. 1992;43:13–20.
49. Nicholls S, King CS, Marks R. Short term effects of emollients and a bath oil on the stratum corneum. J Soc Cosmet Chem. 1978;29:617–24.
50. Garber CA, Nightingale CT. Characterizing cosmetic effects and skin morphology by scanning electron microscopy. J Soc Cosmet Chem. 1976;27: 509–31.
51. Rhodes LE, Diffey BL. Fluorescence spectroscopy: a rapid, noninvasive method for measurement of skin surface thickness of topical agents. Br J Dermatol. 1997;136(1):12–7.
52. Johnson R, Nusbaum BP, Horwitz SN, Frost P. Transfer of topically applied tetracycline in various vehicles. Arch Dermatol. 1983;119(8):660–3.
53. Holden C, English J, Hoare C, Jordan A, Kownacki S, Turnbull R, et al. Advised best practice for the use of emollients in eczema and other dry skin conditions. J Dermatolog Treat. 2002;13(3):103–6.
54. Loden M, Buraczewska I, Halvarsson K. Facial antiwrinkle cream: influence of product presentation on effectiveness: a randomized and controlled study. Skin Res Technol. 2007;13(2):189–94.
55. Lynfield YL, Schechter BA. Choosing and using a vehicle. J Am Acad Dermatol. 1984;10:56–9.
56. Schlagel CA, Sanborn EC. The weights of topical preparations required for total and partial body inunction. J Invest Dermatol. 1964;42:253–6.
57. Ivens UI, Steinkjer B, Serup J, Tetens V. Ointment is evenly spread on the skin, in contrast to creams and solutions. Br J Dermatol. 2001;145(2):264–7.
58. Lodén M, Lindberg M. The influence of a single application of different moisturizers on the skin capacitance. Acta Derm Venereol. 1991;71(1):79–82.
59. Lodén M. The increase in skin hydration after application of emollients with different amounts of lipids. Acta Derm Venereol. 1992;72(5):327–30.
60. Buraczewska I, Brostrom U, Loden M. Artificial reduction in transepidermal water loss improves skin barrier function. Br J Dermatol. 2007;157(1): 82–6.
61. Saary J, Qureshi R, Palda V, DeKoven J, Pratt M, Skotnicki-Grant S, et al. A systematic review of contact dermatitis treatment and prevention. J Am Acad Dermatol. 2005;53(5):845.
62. Kelterer D, Fluhr JW, Elsner P. Application of protective creams: use of a fluorescence-based training system decreases unprotected areas on the hands. Contact Dermatitis. 2003;49(3):159–60.
63. Kresken J, Klotz A. Occupational skin-protection products–a review. Int Arch Occup Environ Health. 2003;76(5):355–8.
64. Hannuksela A, Kinnunen T. Moisturizers prevent irritant dermatitis. Acta Derm Venereol. 1992;72(1):42–4.
65. Fluhr JW, Gloor M, Lehmann L, Lazzerini S, Distante F, Berardesca E. Glycerol accelerates recovery of barrier function in vivo. Acta Derm Venereol. 1999;79(6):418–21.
66. Held E, Lund H, Agner T. Effect of different moisturizers on SLS-irritated human skin. Contact Dermatitis. 2001;44:229–34.
67. Lodén M. Barrier recovery and influence of irritant stimuli in skin treated with a moisturizing cream. Contact Dermatitis. 1997;36(5):256–60.
68. Kucharekova M, Schalkwijk J, Van De Kerkhof PC, Van De Valk PG. Effect of a lipid-rich emollient containing ceramide 3 in experimentally induced skin barrier dysfunction. Contact Dermatitis. 2002;46:331–8.
69. Man MQ, Feingold KR, Elias PM. Exogenous lipids influence permeability barrier recovery in acetone-treated murine skin. Arch Dermatol. 1993;129(6): 728–38.
70. Mortz CG, Andersen KE, Halkier-Sørensen L. The efficacy of different moisturizers on barrier recovery in hairless mice evaluated by non-invasive bioengineering methods. A model to select the potentially most effective product. Contact Dermatitis. 1997;36:297–310.

71. Ramsing DW, Agner T. Preventive and therapeutic effects of a moisturizer. An experimental study of human skin. Acta Derm Venereol. 1997;77(5): 335–7.
72. Held E, Agner T. Comparison between 2 test models in evaluating the effect of a moisturizer on irritated human skin. Contact Dermatitis. 1999;40(5):261–8.
73. Williams C, Wilkinson SM, McShane P, Lewis J, Pennington D, Pierce S, et al. A double-blind, randomized study to assess the effectiveness of different moisturizers in preventing dermatitis induced by hand washing to simulate healthcare use. Br J Dermatol. 2010;162(5):1088–92.
74. Ghadially R, Halkier-Sorensen L, Elias PM. Effects of petrolatum on stratum corneum structure and function. J Am Acad Dermatol. 1992;26(3 Pt 2):387–96.
75. Zettersten EM, Ghadially R, Feingold KR, Crumrine D, Elias PM. Optimal ratios of topical stratum corneum lipids improve barrier recovery in chronologically aged skin. J Am Acad Dermatol. 1997;37:403–8.
76. Imokawa G, Akasaki S, Hattori M, Yoshizuka N. Selective recovery of deranged water-holding properties by stratum corneum lipids. J Invest Dermatol. 1986;87(6):758 61.
77. Lodén M, Barany E. Skin-identical lipids versus petrolatum in the treatment of tape-stripped and detergent-perturbed human skin. Acta Derm Venereol. 2000;80(6):412–5.
78. Chamlin SL, Kao J, Frieden IJ, Sheu MY, Fowler AJ, Fluhr JW, et al. Ceramide-dominant barrier repair lipids alleviate childhood atopic dermatitis: changes in barrier function provide a sensitive indicator of disease activity. J Am Acad Dermatol. 2002;47(2):198–208.
79. Man MM, Feingold KR, Thornfeldt CR, Elias PM. Optimization of physiological lipid mixtures for barrier repair. J Invest Dermatol. 1996;106(5): 1096–101.
80. De Paepe K, Derde MP, Roseeuw D, Rogiers V. Incorporation of ceramide 3B in dermatocosmetic emulsions: effect of the transepidermal water loss of sodium lauryl sulphate-damaged skin. J Eur Acad Dermatol Venereol. 2000;14:272–9.
81. Kucharekova M, Van De Kerkhof PC, Van Der Valk PG. A randomized comparison of an emollient containing skin-related lipids with a petrolatum-based emollient as adjunct in the treatment of chronic hand dermatitis. Contact Dermatitis. 2003;48(6):293–9.
82. Miller CC, Tang W, Ziboh VA, Fletcher MP. Dietary supplementation with ethyl ester concentrates of fish oil (n-3) and borage oil (n-6) polyunsaturated fatty acids induces epidermal generation of local putative anti-inflammatory metabolites. J Invest Dermatol. 1991;96:98–103.
83. Schurer NY. Implementation of fatty acid carriers to skin irritation and the epidermal barrier. Contact Dermatitis. 2002;47(4):199–205.
84. Sheu MY, Fowler AJ, Kao J, Schmuth M, Schoonjans K, Auwerx J, et al. Topical peroxisome proliferator activated receptor-alpha activators reduce inflammation in irritant and allergic contact dermatitis models. J Invest Dermatol. 2002;118(1):94–101.
85. Fowler AJ, Sheu MY, Schmuth M, Kao J, Fluhr JW, Rhein L, et al. Liver X receptor activators display anti-inflammatory activity in irritant and allergic contact dermatitis models: liver-X-receptor-specific inhibition of inflammation and primary cytokine production. J Invest Dermatol. 2003;120(2):246–55.
86. Proksch E, Nissen HP. Dexpanthenol enhances skin barrier repair and reduces inflammation after sodium lauryl sulphate-induced irritation. J Dermatol Treat. 2002;13:173–8.
87. Tanno O, Ota Y, Kitamura N, Katsube T, Inoue S. Nicotinamide increases biosynthesis of ceramides as well as other stratum corneum lipids to improve the epidermal permeability barrier. Br J Dermatol. 2000;143(3):524–31.
88. Summers RS, Summers B, Chandar P, Feinberg C, Gursky R, Rawlings AV. The effect of lipids, with and without humectant, on skin xerosis. J Soc Cosmet Chem. 1996;47:27–39.
89. Rattner H. Use of urea in hand creams. Arch Dermatol Syph. 1943;48:47–9.
90. Fredriksson T, Gip L. Urea creams in the treatment of dry skin and hand dermatitis. Int J Dermatol. 1975;32:442–4.
91. Baillie ATK, et al. General Practitioner Research Group. Carbamide in hyperkeratosis. Report No 179. The Practitioner. 1973; 294–6.
92. Halkier-Sorensen L, Thestrup-Pedersen K. The efficacy of a moisturizer (Locobase) among cleaners and kitchen assistants during everyday exposure to water and detergents. Contact Dermatitis. 1993;29(5):266–71.
93. Goh CL, Gan SL. Efficacies of a barrier cream and an afterwork emollient cream against cutting fluid dermatitis in metalworkers: a prospective study. Contact Dermatitis. 1994;31(3):176–80.
94. Mygind K, Sell L, Flyvholm MA, Jepsen KF. High-fat petrolatum-based moisturizers and prevention of work-related skin problems in wet-work occupations. Contact Dermatitis. 2006;54(1):35–41.
95. Winker R, Salameh B, Stolkovich S, Nikl M, Barth A, Ponocny E, et al. Effectiveness of skin protection creams in the prevention of occupational dermatitis: results of a randomized, controlled trial. Int Arch Occup Environ Health. 2009;82(5):653–62.
96. Kutting B, Baumeister T, Weistenhöfer W, Pfahlberg A, Uter W, Drexler H. Effectiveness of skin protection measures in prevention of occupational hand eczema: results of a prospective randomized controlled trial over a follow-up period of 1 year. Br J Dermatol. 2010;162(2):362–70.
97. Andersson A-C, Lindberg M, Lodén M. The effect of two urea-containing creams on dry, eczematous skin in atopic patients. I. Expert, patient and instrumental evaluation. J Dermatol Treat. 1999;10:165–9.
98. Lodén M, Andersson A-C, Lindberg M. Improvement in skin barrier function in patients with atopic dermatitis after treatment with a moisturizing cream (Canoderm®). Br J Dermatol. 1999;140:264–7.
99. Loden M, Wirén K, Smerud K, Meland N, Hønnås H, Mørk G, et al. Treatment with a barrier-strengthening moisturizer prevents relapse of hand-eczema. An open, randomized, prospective, parallel group study. Acta Derm Venereol. 2010;90(6):602–6.

100. Wirén K, Nohlgård C, Nyberg F, Holm L, Svensson M, Johannesson A, et al. Treatment with a barrier-strengthening moisturizing cream delays relapse of atopic dermatitis: a prospective and randomized controlled clinical trial. J Eur Acad Dermatol Venereol. 2009;23(11):1267–72.
101. Demerjian M, Choi EH, Man MQ, Chang S, Elias PM, Feingold KR. Activators of PPARs and LXR decrease the adverse effects of exogenous glucocorticoids on the epidermis. Exp Dermatol. 2009;18(7):643–9.
102. Jensen JM, Pfeiffer S, Witt M, Bräutigam M, Neumann C, Weichenthal M, et al. Different effects of pimecrolimus and betamethasone on the skin barrier in patients with atopic dermatitis. J Allergy Clin Immunol. 2009;124(3 Suppl 2):R19–28.
103. Kao JS, Fluhr JW, Man MQ, Fowler AJ, Hachem JP, Crumrine D, et al. Short-term glucocorticoid treatment compromises both permeability barrier homeostasis and stratum corneum integrity: inhibition of epidermal lipid synthesis accounts for functional abnormalities. J Invest Dermatol. 2003;120(3):456–64.
104. Kolbe L, Kligman AM, Schreiner V, Stoudemayer T. Corticosteroid-induced atrophy and barrier impairment measured by non-invasive methods in human skin. Skin Res Technol. 2001;7(2):73–7.
105. Loden M, Wirén K, Smerud KT, Meland N, Hønnås H, Mørk G, et al. The effect of a corticosteroid cream and a barrier-strengthening moisturizer in hand eczema. A double-blind, randomized, prospective, parallel group clinical trial. J Eur Acad Dermatol Venereol. 2012;26(5):597–601.
106. Veien NK, Olholm Larsen P, Thestrup-Pedersen K, Schou G. Long-term, intermittent treatment of chronic hand eczema with mometasone furoate. Br J Dermatol. 1999;140(5):882–6.
107. Held E. So moisturizers may cause trouble! Int J Dermatol. 2001;40(1):12–3.
108. Blank IH. Factors which influence the water content of the stratum corneum. J Invest Dermatol. 1952;18:433–40.
109. Tsai TF, Maibach HI. How irritant is water? An overview. Contact Dermatitis. 1999;41(6):311–4.
110. Aungst BJ. The influence of fatty acids and fatty alcohols on skin permeability. In: Lodén M, Maibach HI, editors. Dry skin and moisturizers: chemistry and function. Boca Raton: CRC Press; 2000. p. 299–325.
111. Donbrow M, Azaz E, Pillersdorf A. Autoxidation of polysorbates. J Pharm Sci. 1978;67:1676–81.
112. Travassos AR, Goossens A. Potential allergens in moisturizing creams. In: Lodén M, Maibach HI, editors. Treatment of dry skin syndrome. The art and science of moisturizers. Berlin: Springer; 2012. p. 341–54.
113. De Groot AC. Sensitizing substances. In: Lodén M, Maibach HI, editors. Dry skin and moisturizers: chemistry and function. Boca Raton: CRC Press; 2000. p. 403–11.
114. Barany E, Lodén M. Content of fragrance mix ingredients and customer complaints of cosmetic products. Am J Contact Dermat. 2000;11(2):74–9.
115. Jansson T, Lodén M. Strategy to decrease the risk of adverse effects of fragrance ingredients in cosmetic products. Am J Contact Dermat. 2001;12(3):166–9.
116. Api AM, Basketter DA, Cadby PA, Cano MF, Ellis G, Gerberick GF, et al. Dermal sensitization quantitative risk assessment (QRA) for fragrance ingredients. Regul Toxicol Pharmacol. 2008;52(1):3–23.
117. Buckley DA, Rycroft RJ, White IR, McFadden JP. Contact allergy to individual fragrance mix constituents in relation to primary site of dermatitis. Contact Dermatitis. 2000;43(5):304–5.
118. Lundov MD, Johansen JD, Zachariae C, Moesby L. Creams used by hand eczema patients are often contaminated with Staphylococcus aureus. Acta Derm Venereol. 2012;92(4):441–2.
119. Nilsson EJ, Henning CG, Magnusson J. Topical corticosteroids and Staphylococcus aureus in atopic dermatitis. J Am Acad Dermatol. 1992;27(1):29–34.
120. Haslund P, Bangsgaard N, Jarløv JO, Skov L, Skov R, Agner T. Staphylococcus aureus and hand eczema severity. Br J Dermatol. 2009;161(4):772–7.
121. Carr J, et al. Contamination of emollient creams and ointments with Staphylococcus aureus in children with atopic eczema. Br J Dermatol. 2008;159 Suppl 1:114.
122. Ernst E. Adverse effects of herbal drugs in dermatology. Br J Dermatol. 2000;143(5):923–9.

28 Protective Gloves

Curtis P. Hamann, Kim M. Sullivan,
and Peggy Wright

Contents

C.P. Hamann, M.D. (✉) • K.M. Sullivan, B.A.
SmartPractice, 3400 E. McDowell Rd,
Phoenix, AZ 85008, USA
e-mail: hamann@smarthealth.com;
sullivan@smarthealth.com

P. Wright
Contracted with SmartPractice, 1438 Stanford
Avenue, St. Paul, MN 55105, USA
e-mail: mwright1438@comcast.net

28.1 Introduction

Gloves can protect the hands from chemical, biological, mechanical, thermal, and electrical hazards, which may occur in occupational settings, at home, and through hobbies, sports, and recreation. In addition to protecting the hands of the user, gloves also minimize pathogen or toxin exposure (e.g., between health care worker and patient or patient to patient) and protect products (e.g., circuit boards, food) from skin contact. When avoidance of a hazard(s) is not possible, proper use of personal protective equipment (PPE), including gloves, is essential. To be truly effective, any protective glove – its material, physical properties, and quality – must be suitable for its intended use and not create or exacerbate hand eczema.

28.2 Materials: Medical and Utility Gloves

The manufacture of rubber gloves – and, to a lesser extent, plastic, leather, and textile gloves – requires additives that remain in the glove in sufficient quantities to cause or exacerbate irritant or allergic reactions in some individuals. Consequently, individuals must understand the physical properties and antigenic nature of the glove choices, the prospective hazard(s), and their own allergy profile to select the appropriate glove.

A. Alikhan et al. (eds.), *Textbook of Hand Eczema*,
DOI 10.1007/978-3-642-39546-8_28, © Springer-Verlag Berlin Heidelberg 2014

28.2.1 Rubber (Natural and Synthetic)

Rubber is made up of large molecules comprised of thousands of carbon atoms arranged in long stringlike chains in repeating sequences. Because of this molecular arrangement, rubber is classified as a polymer. The most common rubber polymers used today in glove manufacturing are isoprene, butadiene, chloroprene, and acrylonitrile. Rubber provides electrical resistance, gas impermeability, resistance to water and various chemicals, abrasion resistance, and elasticity, making it a good material for protective gloves. All rubber gloves (natural or synthetic) require vulcanization to cross-link the polymer chains and, therefore, require compounding with multiple chemicals known to cause irritant or allergic dermatitis.

28.2.1.1 Natural Rubber: Latex

Natural rubber latex (NRL) is a milklike liquid found in numerous plants, but primarily from the *Hevea brasiliensis* tree. It contains about 35 % natural polymeric rubber in the *cis* form of its 1,4-isoprene monomer. This rubber precursor molecule is synthesized within the cytoplasm of the laticifer cells of the tree and exists in the raw latex as long chains. NRL gloves are often the material of choice in medical and other occupational environments because of their exceptional flexibility, strength, elasticity, temperature resistance, and low cost. NRL resists abrasions from grinding and polishing and protects hands from most water-based solutions of acids, alkalis, salts, and ketones. NRL proteins have been reported to cause type I and type IV hypersensitivity. As with all rubber (natural or synthetic), type IV reactions to residual processing chemicals are possible and require user caution. NRL is susceptible to oxidation. The following steps are necessary to preserve the physical properties and shelf life of NRL gloves during storage: (1) maintain a temperature under 25°C, (2) provide a relative humidity low enough that condensation does not occur, and (3) protection from sunlight, fluorescent light, ionized radiation (x-ray equipment), and ozone (instrument asepsis, electrical equipment, air purification).

28.2.1.2 Synthetic Rubber: Nitrile

Nitrile or acrylonitrile butadiene rubber (NBR) is a synthetic alternative to NRL gloves. NBR provides users with good sensitivity and dexterity; however, NBR is less elastic than NRL [1]. Delivering good performance under heavy use, the material provides protection, even during prolonged exposure to substances that cause other gloves to deteriorate. NBR offers good resistance to chlorinated solvents, oils, greases, acids, caustics, and alcohols, although this resistance varies with the acrylonitrile content. NBR gives poor protection, however, against strong oxidizing agents, aromatic solvents, ketones, and acrylates. Generally, the material has good tensile strength and resistance to puncture; however, higher levels of strength require reinforcing agents. Although they provide good puncture resistance, NBR gloves are more prone to complete failure once a hole or tear is initiated. As with all rubbers, NBR must be vulcanized; therefore, delayed reactions to the processing chemicals may occur. Many NRL glove users switch to synthetic rubbers owing to concern about "latex allergy," only to find that they are really allergic to an accelerator or other chemical that is the same or similar to those in the NRL product. The synthetic rubbers do not, however, contain the NRL proteins; therefore, they are a good choice for those individuals with an NRL protein sensitivity.

Recent studies have compared the protective value of NBR, chloroprene, and barrier-laminate gloves and of NBR and NRL gloves against pesticides and have determined that the NBR gloves tested provided a higher level of protection [2]. Caution should be exercised when expanding this conclusion to include all NBR gloves in other chemical-exposure situations.

28.2.1.3 Synthetic Rubber: Chloroprene

Chloroprene (CR) (neoprene) is a synthetic rubber that is pliable, provides good dexterity, and is tear resistant [1]. CR has demonstrated resistance to hydraulic fluids, gasoline, alcohols, organic acids, alkalis, oils, and fats and may also provide enhanced chemical and wear resistance compared to natural or other synthetic rubbers in some situations. A 2003 study tested the permeability of seven brands of surgical gloves to seven chemicals commonly used in hospitals. The gloves offering the best protection were CR gloves and a thick, double-layered NRL glove with a polymeric hydrogel inner coating and an inner glove. The research indicated that permeation resistance depended on both the brand of glove and the chemical tested. CR is sometimes blended with NRL to improve resistance to oil, ozone, and weathering [3]. As with NBR, CR is a synthetic rubber and must be vulcanized. Delayed reactions to the processing chemicals are well documented.

28.2.2 Plastic

Vinyl or polyvinyl chloride (PVC) is an alternative to rubber gloves, especially in situations in which there is concern about NRL protein allergies. The material's low cost makes the gloves popular in some environments, such as in health care, food service, and cleaning. Thin, single-use PVC examination gloves offer poor resistance to solvents and chemical exposure and are intended for short-term wear. PVC gloves provide similar control and tactile sensitivity compared to rubber gloves; however, they do not have the same elastic qualities that impact fit and feel. Manufacturers can alter the modulus and stretch properties to create enhanced softness, flexibility, and elasticity with plasticizers. Some of these plasticizers contain phthalates that have been restricted in specific end uses owing to health and environmental concerns. Phthalate-free gloves are now available. Both irritant and allergic reactions have also been reported to occur with PVC gloves [4–6].

28.2.3 Other Polymers, Leathers, and Textiles

Manufacturers make protective gloves from a variety of other rubbers (Tables 28.1 and 28.2).

These materials all possess different strengths and weaknesses and may be options for some users and workplaces. When selecting any protective glove, it is essential that the hazard(s) be fully assessed.

28.2.3.1 Leather

Leather gloves are comfortable because the material breathes, absorbs humidity, is durable, permits dexterity, is resistant to heat, and gives mild abrasion protection. Manufacturers make leather from cowhide, pigskin, goatskin, deerskin, elkskin, and bison leather, all of which may be chromium or vegetable tanned. Chromium-tanned leather gloves can cause contact dermatitis [14]. Occlusive coverage of the hands fosters increased perspiration, which can increase release of chromium from the leather in sufficient amounts to induce contact allergy. The rubber underliner often used with leather gloves also can cause contact allergy. When individuals wear rubber gloves, they also often use *glove powder*, a cooling, frictionless powder that aids donning and absorbs moisture and perspiration. *Glove powder* is usually a talc that incorporates fragrance and preservatives and, therefore, may also be a source of contact irritant reactions.

28.2.3.2 Textiles

Manufacturers use many fibers in woven or knitted textile gloves – cotton, viscose, nylon, and polyester as well as Kevlar, Nomex, and carbon fiber. Textile gloves are pliable and cheaper than leather gloves and are machine washable. They can be partially or totally coated with rubber (NBR or butyl) or plastic materials to improve protection, grip, or dexterity. Totally coated gloves may be suitable for handling water and liquid chemicals. Potential users should check with the manufacturer to determine the gloves' effectiveness for use with specific chemicals or under specific environmental conditions.

28.2.3.3 Specialty Gloves

Manufacturers have developed specialized gloves, such as metal-mesh gloves, that typically consist of welded, nickel-plated brass, or stainless steel. Metal-mesh gloves have the potential to create problems in nickel-allergic users; however, some manufacturers wrap metal meshes in polyester and coat them with PVC.

Table 28.1 Synthetic rubber glove materials

Glove type	Pros	Cons
Butyl rubber (IIR) [1, 7]	Extreme resistance to moisture, oxidation, and corrosive chemicals	Difficult to manufacture, requiring more active accelerators during manufacture, including chemicals such as thiuram sulfides that can cause type IV allergic contact dermatitis
	Impermeability to gases	Not as resilient as NRL and other synthetics
	Enhanced thermal stability	Poor performance against aliphatic and aromatic hydrocarbons and halogenated solvents
	Resistance to abrasion	
	Flexibility at low temperatures	
	Protection against many chemicals, such as peroxide, rocket fuels, highly corrosive acids (nitric, sulfuric, and hydrofluoric acids and red-fuming nitric acid), strong bases, alcohols, aldehydes, ketones, esters, and nitro compounds	
Ethylene propylene rubber (copolymers [EPDM] or terpolymers [EPR]) [1, 8, 9]	Good tensile properties	Only fair resistance to aliphatic and aromatic hydrocarbons, such as mineral oils, gasoline, and fuels
	Good resistance to heat, low temperatures, oxidation, and ozone	Frequent combination with polyethylene, polypropylene, or other thermoplastic resins to make thermoplastic elastomers, causing varying degrees of heat and oil resistance and elasticity
	Resistance to electricity	
	Protection against chemicals and polar solvents, such as water, acids, alkalis, phosphate esters, and many ketones and alcohols	
Fluoro rubber (FPM) [10]	Very good resistance to heat and cold	Inflexibility at low temperatures
	Resistant to aging and ozone	Sensitivity to the effect of amines, organic acids, and polar solvents
	Low permeability to gas	
Chloroprene (CR) [1, 7, 11]	Resistant to chemicals, atmospheric degradation, oils, and fats, and tears	Numerous compounds with a broad range of physical properties
Neoprene, which DuPont developed in 1931, became the generic name for polymers of the monomer chloroprene	Good elastomeric properties, being pliable and providing finger dexterity	Expensive
	Protection against hydraulic fluids, gasoline, alcohols, organic acids, and alkalis	Poor tear propagation resistance
	Better chemical and wear resistance and a better grip than NRL	
	Manufacturers sometimes blend chloroprene with NRL to improve the product's resistance to oil, ozone, and weathering	
Nitrile or acrylonitrile butadiene rubber (NBR) [1, 7]	Good sensitivity and dexterity	Resistance to chemicals, oils, and body fat varies with the acrylonitrile content
	Good resistance to chemicals, oils, and body fat	Less elastic than NRL
	Good tensile strength	Necessity of reinforcing agents for high strength
	Protection against chlorinated solvents, such as trichloroethylene and perchloroethylene; oils; greases; acids; caustics; and alcohols	Poor protection against strong oxidizing agents, aromatic solvents, ketones, and acrylates
	Good performance under heavy use, even during prolonged exposure to substances that cause other gloves to deteriorate	Poor tear propagation resistance

Table 28.1 (continued)

Glove type	Pros	Cons
Polybutadiene rubber (BR) [1, 9]	Superior resistance to abrasion when blended with NRL or SBR	Relatively low gum tensile strength unless manufactured with reinforcing fillers (usually done)
	Resilience	
	Flexibility at low temperatures	
	Resistance to cracking due to its ozone resistance	
Polyisoprene rubber (IR) [1]	Qualities similar to NRL, without the sensitizing proteins	An expensive option
	Good tack, high tensile strength (depending on the compounding), and good hot tear properties	Poor aging
Silicone rubber (VMQ) [1, 10]	Little change when exposed to extreme temperatures	Sensitivity to hot water and steam
	Resistant to aging and ozone	Poor protection against fuels
	Good electrical insulation	
	Excellent protection against corrosion and solvents	
	Moderate protection against oil	
Thermoplastic elastomers (TPEs) [1]	High tensile strength	Dependency of a particular TPE's properties on the formulations and the solvents that the manufacturer uses
A class of copolymers or a physical mix of polymers, usually a plastic and a rubber	Superior to NRL in resistance to abrasion, cracking, and oxidation	Manufacture with solvents, causing poor resistance to similar solvents or chemicals
	Few ingredients compared with the numerous potentially allergenic chemicals that other rubbers contain	
	Manufacture without vulcanization with its use of antigenic materials	
Types of TPE		
Styrene-butadiene rubber (SBR) [1, 10]	Moderate tear strength	Use of dithiocarbamates, a sensitizer, as an anti-degradant, possibly causing type IV allergic contact dermatitis
	Better resistance to abrasion and aging than NRL	Staining for some SBRs in the presence of copper and other metals
		Low resistance to heat
		Fair to poor resistance to oils, greases, and fuels
Styrene-ethylene-butylene-styrene rubber (SEBS) [1]	Excellent resistance to aging and high temperatures	

28.3 Hazards

28.3.1 Chemical

The skin of the hands is an important route by which poisonous and carcinogenic chemicals can enter the body in amounts sufficient to evoke adverse effects. Researchers estimate that 70–75 % of all contact dermatitis and 80–95 % of occupational dermatitis will impair the worker's hands [15–17]. Although biological and physical causes contribute to the incidence of skin disease, chemical exposure is responsible for 80–90 % [18]. Examples of such chemicals found in the work environment include pesticides, herbicides, aromatic nitro and amino compounds, phenols, polyurethanes, hydrocarbons (*m*-xylene, polychlorinated biphenyls), epoxy resins, acrylates,

Table 28.2 Plastic glove materials

Glove type	Pros	Cons
Vinyl (polyvinyl chloride [PVC]) [1, 11]	Cost-effective alternative to rubber gloves, making the gloves popular in some environments, such as in food service and cleaning	Poor resistance to solvents and chemicals
	Similar control and sensitivity compared to rubber gloves	Use of a high proportion of plasticizing oils, some of which contain phthalates that regulators have restricted in specific end uses due to health and environmental concerns, to create softness, flexibility, and elasticity
	Rigidity or flexibility depending on the manufacturing process	Lower strength and protection than rubber gloves for the less expensive versions
Polyethylene (PE) [1, 12]	Flexibility	Lower elasticity
	Protection from organic vapors, dusts, and mists	Seams
	Good chemical resistance	Poor fit/poor dexterity
	Low extractables/particulates (lower particulate gloves are required in some clean room settings)	Stiff
		Poor electrical properties
Polyurethane (PU) [1, 11]	High toughness and elasticity	An expensive option
	Low levels of antigenic chemicals	Rigidity or extreme elasticity depending on the polymer used
	Resistance to tears and abrasion	
Polyvinyl alcohol (PVA) [13]	Good resistance to alcohol	Poor protection against water or water-based solutions being a water-soluble plastic used for dip-coating textile gloves
	Protection against methylene chloride, toluene, 1,1,1-trichloroethane, and trichloroethylene	

and organic and inorganic cyano compounds. These chemicals may have allergenic, irritant, toxic, or even teratogenic and carcinogenic effects [19–21]. Additionally, chemical substances, such as strong alkalis and acids, certain organic solvents, metal salts, and gases have the potential to cause chemical burns leading to ulcerations, even with minimal exposure [22] (Table 28.3).

Glove materials vary greatly in their resistance to chemicals, as do different formulations of the same glove material. For example, not all NRL gloves provide the same measure of barrier protection against the same chemicals [24]. The permeability of a glove's polymer to chemicals, and therefore the gloves protective capabilities, depends on many factors, including:

- Type and concentration of the chemical(s)
- Interaction with multiple chemicals
- Duration of exposure
- Interaction between chemical(s) and the glove's material
- Impact of simultaneous mechanical hazards
- Glove's base polymer
- Glove's formulation (plasticizers, fillers, stabilizers, pigments, degree of cross-linking)
- Glove's physical properties
- Barrier integrity (holes, defects, oxidation, etc.)

During exposure, a chemical's molecules can enter and migrate through the glove. This migration can occur with no visible change in the material, often leaving the user unaware that the chemical has permeated the glove [25]. This chemical migration can take place even if the glove has no pinholes, tears, or defects. Therefore, safe use requires an examination of the gloves breakthrough time, permeation rate, and degradation potential (Table 28.4).

28.3.1.1 Health Care Settings

In health care settings, acrylates, disinfectants, and cytotoxic drugs can permeate or degrade gloves. Examination gloves do not provide

Table 28.3 Glove materials available for chemical resistance[a]

Group of chemicals	Recommended glove material[b,c]
Aldehydes	Chloroprene rubber (CR), glutaraldehyde only Nitrile rubber (NBR), formaldehyde only Flouropropylene (FPM), formaldehyde and glutaraldehyde only
Aliphatic hydrocarbons	Nitrile rubber (NBR) Polyvinyl alcohol (PVA), cyclohexane excluded Flouropropylene (FPM)
Alkalis	Butyl rubber (IIR) Natural rubber latex (NRL), potassium hydroxide (up to 70 %) and sodium hydroxide (70+ %) only Chloroprene rubber (CR), potassium hydroxide (up to 70 %) and sodium hydroxide (70+ %) only Nitrile rubber (NBR) Polyvinyl chloride (PVC), potassium hydroxide (up to 70 %) and sodium hydroxide (70+ %) only Flouropropylene (FPM), potassium hydroxide (up to 70 %) only
Amines	Butyl rubber (IIR), butylamine and triethylamine excluded Chloroprene rubber (CR), ethanolamine only Nitrile rubber (NBR), aniline and ethylamine excluded Flouropropylene (FPM), aniline and ethylamine excluded
Aromatic hydrocarbons	Nitrile rubber (NBR), benzene, toluene, and xylene excluded Polyvinyl alcohol (PVA), ethyl benzene excluded Flouropropylene (FPM), benzene excluded
Esters/glycols	Butyl rubber (IIR), ethylene glycol, methyl acetate, and isobutyl acrylate only Flouropropylene (FPM), ethylene glycol only
Halogenated hydrocarbons	Butyl rubber (IIR), polychlorinated biphenyls (PCBs) only Chloroprene rubber (CR), polychlorinated biphenyls (PCBs) only Polyvinyl alcohol (PVA) Flouropropylene (FPM), methyl chloride and halothane excluded
Inorganic acids	Butyl rubber (IIR), chromic acid (up to 70 %), hydrochloric acid (up to 37 %), phosphoric acid (up to 70+ %), and sulfuric acid (up to 70+ %) only Natural rubber latex (NRL), perchloric acid (up to 70 %) and phosphoric acid (up to 70+ %) only Chloroprene rubber (CR), perchloric acid (up to 70 %) and phosphoric acid (up to 70+ %) only Nitrile rubber (NBR), perchloric acid (up to 70 %) and phosphoric acid (up to 70+ %) only Polyvinyl chloride (PVC), perchloric acid (up to 70 %) and phosphoric acid (up to 70+ %) only Flouropropylene (FPM), chromic acid (up to 70 %), nitric acid (up to 70+%), perchloric acid (up to 70 %), and phosphoric acid (up to 70+ %) only
Organic acids	Butyl rubber (IIR), maleic acid excluded Natural rubber latex (NRL), lactic acid and oxalic acid only Chloroprene rubber (CR), lactic acid and oxalic acid only Nitrile rubber (NBR), lactic acid and oxalic acid only Polyvinyl chloride (PVC), oxalic acid only

[a]This table provides general information regarding chemical groupings and potential choices of glove materials but does not represent specific selection criteria regarding the chemical resistance of a type of glove. Created with data from [12, 13, 23]

[b]The table includes recommendations reflecting the gloves that best fit the category for intended use. Those gloves and other gloves may meet requirements for use with other chemicals under certain conditions, such as use for less than 4 h

[c]Laminated plastic materials of folio type or Teflon are suitable for protection against most chemicals

Table 28.4 Chemical resistance criteria

Breakthrough time	Usually expressed in minutes, this rating indicates the time that it takes from the initial chemical exposure of the glove's surface to the first detection of the chemical on the other side of the glove's wall
	These times indicate how long a user can expect a glove to provide effective permeation resistance when totally immersed in the tested chemical [12, 26]
	The permeation rate evaluates the time it takes for a chemical to pass through the glove's (intact) material without going through pores or visible openings
Permeation rate	The permeation rate represents the highest *flow rate* recorded for a chemical with respect to its permeation of a glove's material during 6–8 h of testing [12]
	Many chemicals permeate gloves without visibly affecting the materials and thus gain access to the skin often unbeknownst to the user
	If a chemical permeates through the glove, it may cause adverse effects to the skin, or it can be absorbed through the skin and cause exposure effects elsewhere in the body [21]
	Even chemicals that are considered "harmless" can damage the skin if the exposure is frequent or prolonged. It is crucial to be aware that chemical permeation through disposable gloves can sometimes be efficient and rapid [27]
Degradation	This characteristic evaluates the change in a glove's physical properties with chemical contact
	The material may disintegrate or become stiff or brittle due to exposure to chemicals. Alternatively, the materials may become softer and weaker, expand to several times their initial size, and even melt or dissolve
	A change in the physical properties of a glove's material can quickly impair the glove's permeation resistance to microorganisms [28]

adequate protection against many cytotoxic drugs and are primarily intended to provide short-term protection from biological transmission, not chemical or mechanical hazards. A glove's thickness is also a consideration but is not the only factor in assessing a glove's protection capabilities.

Acrylates

Methyl methacrylate used in orthopedic surgery is the best-known chemical against which rubber surgical gloves fail to offer protection [29, 30]. In a 2000 in vitro study of five different brands/types of NBR and NRL gloves, Munksgaard found in general that NBR gloves protected against skin contamination from methacrylates longer than NRL gloves, in the absence of solvents. Dilution of the methacrylates in organic solvents reduced or removed that advantage [31]. A 2009 study compared and measured time for methyl methacrylate monomer (MMA) to permeate NRL, PVC examination gloves, and industrial CR gloves. Both NRL and PVC clinical gloves became permeable quickly. CR industrial gloves remained impervious for 25 min. Clinicians participating in the study were advised by the researchers of the toxic effects of MMA and the limitations of examination gloves as a chemical barrier [27].

Disinfectants

The use of disinfectants and sterilants is important in many occupational settings, and researchers have performed several chemical-permeation studies comparing multiple brands of single-use examination, surgical, and utility gloves [32–34]. These studies described permeation tests against glutaraldehyde, ethanol, isopropanol, chlorhexidine digluconate, hydrogen peroxide, peracetic acid, p-chloro-m-cresol, and formaldehyde and indicated varied results depending on the material, glove type (examination, surgical, utility), and testing methodology.

In 1992, Mellstrom et al. tested isopropanol, ethanol, p-chloro-m-cresol, and glutaraldehyde on the material structure and protective effect of NRL and PVC examination gloves and polyethylene utility gloves for 10, 30, and 60 min. Isopropanol permeated both NRL and PVC (<10 min.). Breakthrough times for the different brands of polyethylene varied and ranged from 4 to 240 min. Ethanol permeated NRL and PVC gloves at a much lower rate. The p-chloro-m-cresol and glutaraldehyde did not permeate any of the gloves within 60 min. Isopropanol had a destructive effect on both NRL and PVC [25]. In 2000, Connor and Xiang also studied the effect of isopropyl alcohol on the permeation of NRL and NBR gloves exposed to antineoplastic agents (cancer chemotherapy drugs, cytotoxic drugs), including carmustine, cyclophosphamide, fluorouracil, doxorubicin, thiotepa, and cisplatin. The researchers evaluated the gloves against the antineoplastic agents after exposing them to 70 % isopropyl alcohol for 0.5, 1, and 5 min. The researchers concluded that disinfecting with 70 % isopropyl alcohol did not affect the integrity of the NRL and NBR gloves [35].

Jordan et al. (1996) tested the permeability of six gloves with various glutaraldehyde formulations. The NBR (utility), butyl rubber (utility), styrene–butadiene-block polymer (surgical), and polyethylene(utility) gloves were each impermeable for at least 4 h to 2 % and 3.4 % glutaraldehyde. The two NRL examination gloves showed breakthrough at 45 min. When double-gloving with the NRL gloves, breakthrough time increased to 3–4 h. With 50 % glutaraldehyde, only the butyl- and NBR-rubber utility gloves were impermeable for extended periods. The surgical glove had breakthrough at 1 h, and the polyethylene and the two NRL examination gloves had breakthrough at less than 1 h [36].

In 2000, Monticello et al. evaluated six types of glove materials, comparing thickness measurements for resistance to permeation by a 7.5 % hydrogen peroxide. Both the PVC and NRL examination gloves at 4.5-mm thickness provided less than 30 min of protection, while the thicker NRL glove (16.5 mm) lasted for 8 h without any detectable penetration. CR (15 mm) and NBR butyl rubber (18 mm) gloves both provided protection throughout the 8 h test period [34].

Cytotoxic Drugs

Researchers have also shown that examination gloves do not provide adequate protection against many cytotoxic drugs; thus, they have examined surgical gloves and industrial gloves to identify which of these gloves acts as an adequate barrier to these agents. In 1984, Connor et al. tested the permeability of both single- and double-thickness NRL (surgical and utility) and PVC (utility-0.20 mm and 0.35 mm) gloves for 5–90 min. A double thickness of all gloves (especially the thicker PVC) reduced the amount of drug permeation. The researchers concluded that both single and double thickness of NRL and PVC gloves offered limited protection against carmustine. NRL surgical gloves were slightly less permeable [37]. Dolezalová et al. assessed the permeation of cisplatin, cyclophosphamide, doxorubicin, 5-fluorouracil, and paclitaxel through PVC, NRL, and NBR gloves. Their simulated, time-dependent permeation experiments showed that only the NBR gloves provided good protection [38]. In 1999, Singleton and Connor evaluated permeability of carmustine, etoposide, and paclitaxel in 13 brands of chemotherapy (thicker) gloves and one brand of examination glove. Of the 14 glove types tested, 11 were NRL, and three were NBR. All 14 gloves were impermeable to carmustine at 2 h. Only two (NRL chemotherapy) of the 14 gloves were impermeable to all three drugs. The remaining 12 gloves all demonstrated permeation within 2 h. Thirteen gloves tested for paclitaxel permeability were impermeable at 2 h [39].

28.3.1.2 Other Work Settings

Manufacturers use acrylates in production of glues, paints, lacquers, varnishes, printing inks, artificial nails, bone cement, insulin pump plates (glues), transcutaneous electrical nerve stimulators, disposable electrosurgical grounding plates (glues), spectacle frames, hearing aids, electron microscopy embedding medium, and many other products, resulting in sensitization of workers in many different fields [40, 41]. Other studies have examined the relationship between sensitization to particular chemicals and the use of gloves in other occupations, such as hairdressers [42], workers in swine slaughterhouses [43], cleaners [44], leather workers [45], and automechanics/machinists [46]. Owing to the complexity of selecting the appropriate gloves against chemical exposure, it is essential that these decisions be based on an understanding of the task involved, properties of the chemical(s), glove-material formulation, and the physical properties of the glove to ensure adequate protection (Table 28.5).

Table 28.5 Occupational exposure to chemicals commonly causing contact dermatitis

Occupation	Chemicals
Agricultural workers	Pesticides, weed killers, oils, solvents
Cleaners/janitorial workers	Solvents, detergents, cleaning agents, water
Construction workers	Epoxy resins, metals, cement, glues, paints, lacquers, varnishes
Cosmetologists/hairdressers	Water, shampoos, dyes, bleaching products, chemicals for permanents
Food service workers	Proteins in fruits, vegetables, and grains; water
Health care workers (medicine, dentistry, veterinary science)	Preservatives, disinfectants, topical medications, acrylates, metals, antineoplastics, water
Maintenance workers	Solvents, oils, paint, epoxy resins, degreasers, cement, tar
Mechanics/engineering	Metalworking fluids, oils, solvents, degreasers, adhesives, cement, etc.
Painters	Paints, solvents, primers
Printers/lithographers	Processing chemicals, inks, plate-cleaning solvents, adhesives

28.3.2 Biological

Biological hazards refer to organisms or the organic substances they produce that are detrimental to human health, including parasites, viruses, bacteria, fungi, and proteins. Contact with these microorganisms poses a risk of infection or allergic reaction. Although the skin offers natural protection against external threats, it is often inadequate, especially if a person has a compromised dermal barrier. Therefore, safe handling of biological materials requires protective gloves that minimize the risk of contamination and protect workers.

Individuals in many occupations come into contact with biological hazards, including workers in health care, agriculture, forestry, fishing, and food preparation. The list of biological causes of occupationally related dermatoses includes, but is not limited to, the following allergens:

- Animal-derived allergens (cow dander, wool fats, or alcohols)
- Enzymes (papain, fungal cellulase)
- Plants (poison ivy, oak, NRL, or Compositae)
- Woods
- Foods (shrimp, beef, garlic, mango)

28.3.3 Mechanical

Injuries from mechanical and physical hazards include damage from friction and pressure, impacts, cuts, lacerations, abrasions, burns, vibration, animal bites, and repetitive strain [47]. Often protective gloves must protect users not only from chemical and biological exposures but also against mechanical hazards including cuts, tears, needlesticks, and abrasion. In health care, single-use disposable gloves do not offer a high degree of protection against physical and mechanical hazards, and thicker utility gloves may be a better choice for certain tasks. The use of two pairs of gloves (double-gloving), underliners, and gloves impregnated with disinfectants are also strategies used to address these multiple hazards [48].

Leather comes in multiple styles and thicknesses with varied protective capabilities. For greater protection, users sometimes add disposable, chemically resistant, multilayered plastic gloves as inner gloves. Reinforcement of leather gloves using steel staples or studs improves their cut resistance.

Plastic and rubber coatings improve the cut resistance of textile gloves, also ensuring a slip-resistant grip. In some textile gloves, tough filaments, such as high-tenacity polymers or even fine steel wires, form part of the fabric's structure. Materials providing mechanical-hazard protection may include Kevlar (para-aramid fiber), NRL, NBR, or PVC on a fabric liner.

28.3.4 Thermal and Electrical

Both heat and cold can damage skin, and manufacturers make thermally protective gloves from aluminized leathers or fibers, Kevlar, leather, or cotton. Electrical hazards require specially designed insulating gloves that most often are rubber, and, generally, users wear glove liners against the skin to improve fit and decrease friction between the hand and the glove. Workers also often wear leather glove protectors over the rubber gloves to provide mechanical protection against cuts, abrasion, and punctures.

Conclusion

Chemical, biological, mechanical, thermal, and electrical hazards pose threats to individuals at home, in workplaces, and through hobbies, sports, or recreation. Gloves can provide protection against some threats, but their use also entails problems, including use of materials that can cause irritant or allergic contact dermatitis. Each glove user must consider the unique requirement of the environment and the hazard(s) as well as his or her health history, allergic profile, and dermal condition to ensure appropriate protection.

References

1. Hamann CP, Sullivan KM. Natural rubber latex hypersensitivities. In: Charlesworth E, editor. Cutaneous allergy. Cambridge: Blackwell Scientific; 1996. p. 155–208.
2. Guo C, Stone J, Stahr HM, Shelley M. Effects of exposure time, material type, and granular pesticide on glove contamination. Arch Environ Contam Toxicol. 2001;41(4):529–36.
3. Makela EA, Vainiotalo S, Peltonen K. The permeability of surgical gloves to seven chemicals commonly used in hospitals. Ann Occup Hyg. 2003;47(4):313–23.
4. Aalto-Korte K, Alanko K, Henriks-Eckerman ML, Estlander T, Jolanki R. Allergic contact dermatitis from bisphenol A in PVC gloves. Contact Dermatitis. 2003;49(4):202–5.
5. Ponten A. Formaldehyde in reusable protective gloves. Contact Dermatitis. 2006;54(5):268–71.
6. Sowa J, Kobayashi H, Tsuruta D, Sugawara K, Ishii M. Allergic contact dermatitis due to adipic polyester in vinyl chloride gloves. Contact Dermatitis. 2005;53(4):243–4.
7. US Department of Labor. Personal protective equipment. Occupational Safety and Health Administration (OSHA)0 2003;OSHA 3151-12R.
8. Shell Chemical Company. Synthetic rubbers. 2012. www.shell.com/static/chemicals/downloads/products_services/ethylene_product_stewardship_manual.pdf. Accessed 6 Aug 2012.
9. Gesamtverband der Deutschen Versicherungswirtschaft e.V.(GDV). Synthetic Rubber: Transport Information Service. Berlin: 2012. http://www.tis-gdv.de/tis_e/ware/kautschuk/synthesekautschuk/synthesekautschuk.htm. Accessed 6 Aug 2012.
10. Stöffl Rudolf. Elastomer properties. 2012. www.stoeffl.at/download/elastomers-properties.pdf. Accessed 5 Aug 2012.
11. Satra Technology. Protective gloves-part 1: the correct materials. 2012. www.satra.co.uk/spotlight/article_view.php?id=383
12. Ansell Healthcare. Chemical Resistance Guide: Permeation & Degradation Data. 2012. www.ansellpro.com/download/Ansell_8thEditionChemicalResistanceGuide.pdf. Accessed 6 Aug 2012.
13. Boman A, Estlander T, Wahlberg JE. Protective gloves for occupational use. 2nd ed. Boca Raton: CRC Press; 2005.
14. Thyssen JP, Jensen P, Carlsen BC, Engkilde K, Menne T, Johansen JD. The prevalence of chromium allergy in Denmark is currently increasing as a result of leather exposure. Br J Dermatol. 2009;161(6):1288–93.
15. Clark SC, Zirwas MJ. Management of occupational dermatitis. Dermatol Clin. 2009;27(3):365.
16. Adams RM. Occupational skin disease. 3rd ed. Philadelphia: WB Saunders; 1999.
17. Thyssen JP, Johansen JD, Linneberg A, Menne T. The epidemiology of hand eczema in the general population prevalence and main findings. Contact Dermatitis. 2010;62(2):75–87.
18. DeCraecker W, Roskams N, Op de Beek R. Occupational skin diseases and dermal exposure in the European Union (EU-25): policy and practice overview. Belgium: European Agency for Safety and Health at Work; 2012. Report No.: European Risk Observatory Report.
19. Feldmann RJ, Maibach HI. Percutaneous penetration of some pesticides and herbicides in man. Toxicol Appl Pharmacol. 1974;28:126.
20. Riihimaki V. How workplace chemical enter the body. Oslo: International Labour Office, Geneva and Scandinavian Science Publisher; 1997.
21. Andersen KE. Systemic toxicity from percutaneous absorption of industrial chemicals. In: Adams RM, editor. Occupational skin disease. 2nd ed. Philadelphia: WB Saunders; 1990. p. 73.
22. Lammintausta K, Maibach HI. Contact dermatitis due to irritants. Occupational skin disease. 2nd ed. Philadelphia: WB Saunders; 1990.
23. Forsberg K, Keith LH. Chemical protective clothing permeation and degradation compendium. Boca Raton: Lewis Publishers, CRC Press; 1993.
24. Oztan M, Pekiner BD, Can A. Permeability of latex gloves after exposure to 6 chemical agents. Quintessence Int. 2007;38(9):537–43.
25. Mellstrom G, Lindberg M, Boman AS. Permeation and destructive effects of disinfectants on protective gloves. Contact Dermatitis. 1992;26(3):163–70.
26. Nielsen JB, Sorensen JA. Glove material, reservoir formation, and dose affect glove permeation and

subsequent skin penetration. Sci Total Environ. 2012;417–418:87–91.
27. Thomas S, Padmanabhan TV. Methyl methacrylate permeability of dental and industrial gloves. NY State Dent J. 2009;75(4):40–2.
28. Klein RC, Party E, Gershey EL. Virus penetration of examination gloves. Biotechniques. 1990;9(2):196–9.
29. Fisher AA. Paresthesia of fingers accompanying dermatitis due to methyl methacrylate bone cement. Contact Dermatitis. 1979;5:56–7.
30. Lonnroth EC, Wellendorf H, Ruyter E. Permeability of different types of medical protective gloves to acrylic monomers. Eur J Oral Sci. 2003;111(5):440–6.
31. Munksgaard EC. Permeability of protective gloves by HEMA and TEGDMA in the presence of solvents. Acta Odontol Scand. 2000;58(2):57–62.
32. Leinster P, Baum JM, Baxter PJ. An assessment of exposure to glutaraldehyde in hospitals: typical exposure levels and recommended control measures. Br J Ind Med. 1993;50:107–11.
33. Makela EA, Vainiotalo S, Peltonen K. Permeation of 70 % isopropyl alcohol through surgical gloves: comparison of the standard methods ASTM F739 and EN 374. Ann Occup Hyg. 2003;47(4):305–12.
34. Monticello MV, Gaber DJ. Glove resistance to permeation by a 7.5 % hydrogen peroxide sterilizing and disinfecting solution. Am J Infect Control. 1999;27(4):364–6.
35. Connor TH, Xiang Q. The effect of isopropyl alcohol on the permeation of gloves exposed to antineoplastic agents. J Oncol Pharm Pract. 2000;6(3):109–14.
36. Jordan SLP, Stowers MF, Trawick EG, Theis AB. Glutaraldehyde permeation: choosing the proper glove. Am J Infect Control. 1996;24(2):67–9.
37. Connor TH, Laidlaw JL, Theiss JC, Anderson RW, Matney TS. Permeability of latex and polyvinyl chloride gloves to carmustine. Am J Hosp Pharm. 1984;41(4):676–9.
38. Dolezalová L, Odráska P, Gorná L, Prudilová M, Vejpustková R, Bláha L. Evaporation of selected cytotoxic drugs and permeation of protective gloves – research into the occupational risks of health care personnel handling hazardous cytotoxic drugs (CYTO project). Klin Oncol. 2009;22(5):218–22.
39. Singleton LC, Connor TH. An evaluation of the permeability of chemotherapy gloves to three cancer chemotherapy drugs. Singleton. 1999;26(9):1491–6.
40. Surakka J, Lindh T, Rosn G, Fischer T. Workers' dermal exposure to UV-curable acrylates in the furniture and parquet industry. Ann Occup Hyg. 2000;44(8): 635–44.
41. Sasseville D. Acrylates in contact dermatitis. Dermatitis. 2012;23(1):6–16.
42. Lysdal SH, Johansen JD, Flyvholm MA, Sosted H. A quantification of occupational skin exposures and the use of protective gloves among hairdressers in Denmark. Contact Dermatitis. 2012;66(6):323–34.
43. Mygind K, Sell L, Flyvholm MA, Jepsen KF. High-fat petrolatum-based moisturizers and prevention of work-related skin problems in wet-work occupations. Contact Dermatitis. 2006;54(1):35–41.
44. Jungbauer FHW, van der Harst JJ, Schuttelaar ML, Groothoff JW, Coenraads PJ. Characteristics of wet work in the cleaning industry. Contact Dermatitis. 2004;51(3):131–4.
45. Hansen MB, Rydin S, Menne T, Duus JJ. Quantitative aspects of contact allergy to chromium and exposure to chrome-tanned leather. Contact Dermatitis. 2002;47(3):127–34.
46. Donovan JCH, Kudla I, Holness LD. Hand dermatitis in auto mechanics and machinists. Dermatitis. 2007;18(3):143–9.
47. Kwok T, Arrandale V, Skotnicki-Grant S. Repeated mechanical trauma to the hands: the use of anti-impaction gloves for treatment and return to work. Dermatitis. 2009;20(5):278–83.
48. Laine T, Aarnio P. How often does glove perforation occur in surgery? Comparison between single gloves and a double-gloving system. Am J Surg. 2001;181(6):564–6.

How to Manage Hand Eczema in a Wet Work Setting

29

Britta Wulfhorst, Annika Wilke, Christoph Skudlik, and Swen Malte John

Contents

B. Wulfhorst, Ph.D.
Faculty of Human Sciences, Department of Educational Sciences, MSH Medical School Hamburg University of Applied Sciences and Medical, Am Kaiserkai 1, 20457, Hamburg, Germany
e-mail: wulfhorst@uos.de

A. Wilke • C. Skudlik, M.D. • S.M. John, M.D. (✉)
Department of Dermatology, Environmental Medicine and Health Theory, University of Osnabrueck, Sedanstr 115, Osnabrueck, 49090, Germany
e-mail: awilke@uos.de; christoph.skudlik@uos.de; sjohn@uos.de

29.1 Introduction

In many industrialized countries, occupational skin diseases (OSD), of which hand eczema (HE) comprises about 90 % of cases, are the most frequent occupational diseases, with a high socioeconomic burden for society as well as for the affected individual [1–4]. The point prevalence of HE in the general population is 9.7 %, and the incidence rate is 5.5–8.8 per 1,000 person years [5].

The European Risk Observatory report entitled "Occupational Skin Diseases (OSD) and Dermal Exposure in the EU (EU-25)," published in 2008 by the European Agency for Safety and Health at Work, lists skin diseases as the second most common occupational health problem in Europe. Occupational skin diseases are considered to represent "one of the most important emerging risks related to the exposure to chemical, physical and biological risk factors" [6]. The percentage of skin diseases among all occupational diseases is calculated at 7 %. Furthermore, the report points out the high economic costs of these diseases, now calculated to be exceeding 5 billion euros per year in the EU [6, 7].

In the European Risk Observatory Report EN8 from 2009, the problem of OSD, mainly HE, is once again presented as an urgent issue. Besides dealing with skin irritants as the cause of skin diseases, the report also gives special attention to operational structures. Also mentioned is the particular need for action regarding implementation of worker protection systems in small- and

A. Alikhan et al. (eds.), *Textbook of Hand Eczema*,
DOI 10.1007/978-3-642-39546-8_29, © Springer-Verlag Berlin Heidelberg 2014

medium-sized enterprises (SMEs), whose workers have a significantly higher risk for developing OSD when handling skin-damaging substances:

> SMEs have particular difficulty in implementing complex technical legislation as they often have only limited technical expertise and often lack of dedicated OSH (Occupational Safety and Health) professionals. Simple guidance is therefore needed to assist in the process of risk assessment and control. [8]

In addition, this report highlights an urgent need for provision of information regarding risk awareness. According to the report, employees and employers consider the risks of sudden chemical accidents to be serious, while the chronic and long-term effects of skin-damaging substances are drastically underestimated. Furthermore, "SMEs lack the knowledge required to identify chemical risks and to choose and implement preventive measures for workers against hazardous substances" [8].

Accordingly, the National Institute for Occupational Safety and Health (NIOSH) states that in the United States skin disease accounts for nearly 25 % of all occupational injuries for which workers' compensation claims are filed (www.cdc.gov/niosh). NIOSH comments, "Skin diseases of occupational origin outnumber all other work-incurred illnesses. Early recognition and preventive measures can effectively reduce the incidence of occupational dermatoses in the United States" [9].

In Germany in 2011, OSD (mainly HE) constituted 35.2 % ($N=25{,}056$) of all notifications of occupational diseases to the statutory accident insurance [10].

Risk factors for development have been identified by epidemiologic studies that underline the necessity of implementation of evidence-based management programs to prevent HE in occupational settings as well as to manage HE on secondary and tertiary prevention levels [11–13]. The most important external risk factor for the development of HE is a wet work setting (see Chap. 8). Employees in wet work settings are at a high risk of acquiring occupational HE [14].

There is no international classification for "wet work settings." The German occupational health and safety legislation defined it as follows: Work settings in which the employees (1) spend more than 2 h of the daily work time (daily shift) in wet environments, or (2) spend a corresponding amount of time wearing water-impermeable gloves, or (3) must frequently clean their hands (>20 × daily). If this definition for wet work is met, a set of rules on information to the employees, screening, physical examination time limits, and so forth come into force [15–17].

29.2 Wet-Work Professions

A complete list of wet-work professions will not be presented here. Some typical professions at high risk for HE are described in other chapters in this book (e.g., hairdressers, in Chap. 15; metalworkers, in Chap. 16; dentists, in Chap. 17; hospital and medical industry employees, in Chap. 18; construction industry workers, in Chap. 20; workers in janitorial and related industries, in Chap. 21).

Skudlik et al. [18] recently reported about inpatients, severely affected by OSD, participating in a nationwide interdisciplinary tertiary rehabilitation program. Of 1,788 patients seen in five centers throughout Germany, most were from the areas of "healthcare" (29.4 %) or "metal" (27.4 %). Other frequent professional areas were the hairdressing (10.1 %), building (8.8 %), food handling (6.2 %), cleaning (4.5 %), and chemical (3.5 %) industries. In this study, it was found that in all occupational groups wet work was the most frequent occupational hazard. The criteria for wet work settings – "2 h or more of wet work a day" – were met particularly often by hairdressers (96.7 %), followed by the "cleaning" group (91.4 %), the "food-handlers" group (87.4 %), and the "healthcare" group (82.1 %) (Fig. 29.1). The proportion of "cleaning the hands during work" varied between the occupational groups, as did the proportion of "soiling the hands during work." In the construction workers group, Skudlik et al. [18] found the highest proportion of 2 h or more a day of soiling of the hands at work, whereas in the food group, 41.4 % reported that they washed their hands 10–20 times daily and 27.0 % more than 20 times daily.

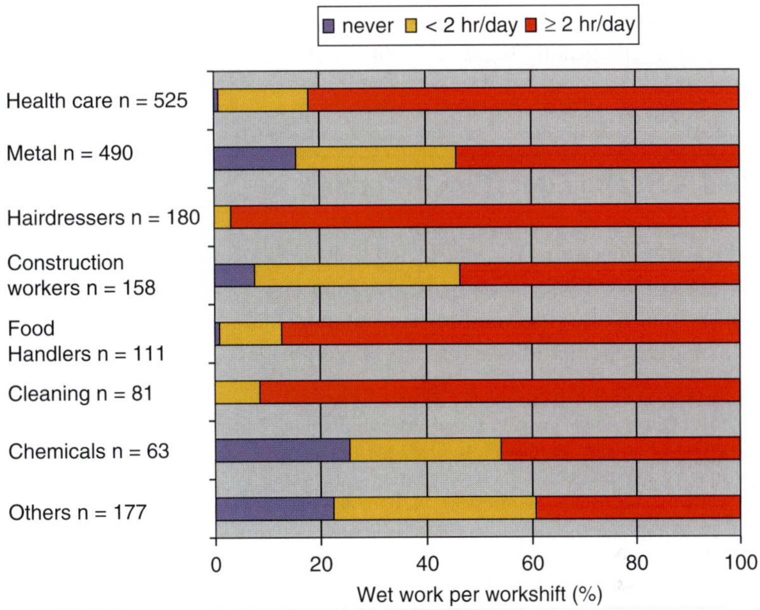

Fig. 29.1 Proportion of wet work in different occupations, $N=1788$ (Reprinted with permission from Skudlik et al. [18]. Copyright © 2011 John Wiley & Sons A/S)

29.3 Prevention Levels and Interdisciplinary Approaches to Managing Hand Eczema in Wet Work Settings

In recent years, a number of intervention studies to prevent HE in high-risk professions have been published. Most of the studies have produced fair-quality evidence that prevention is effective [18–34]. This fair-quality evidence and the degree of transferability are based on various methodological approaches, the great diversity of workplace settings with largely varying exposure profiles, and different outcome variables. There is a demand for more high-quality studies to develop best-practice models for disseminating information, treatment and management of workers in high-risk professions, a common risk and susceptibility assessment, evidence-based standards of personal protective measures, set up of databases and public Internet information platforms, and so forth [7, 12, 35].

Most intervention studies pointed out a lack of information about personal skin protection in affected (and unaffected) workers, which appears to be uniform to basically all at-risk professions. This finding underlines a future task for prevention to improve on workers' education. In this context, multidisciplinary approaches seem most promising [36]. Thus, further research particularly has to focus on work-related educational activities, including longitudinal studies assessing effectiveness by return to work and course of disease as outcome variables. Furthermore, the strategies of HE prevention need to be further clarified; however, as yet, there already is a range of some evidence-based recommendations [1, 13, 23, 37, 38].

HE education programs within skin protection schemes are part of complex interventions that are difficult to evaluate because of problems in identifying and separately assessing the effect of the various components. To demonstrate links between outcomes and patient education program components, there is a need for more trials that combine process and outcome evaluation. Programs to date have relied too heavily on the provision of medical information to patients. Programs that also aim to improve disease management, self-efficacy, and other determinants of health behavior should be included. Program components need to be clearly described and the rationale for their use justified in trial reports. This will produce an evidence base to clarify the role educational programs can play in improving outcomes and enable the development of more effective programs [7, 39]. An open question is, for instance, whether health education may reduce the likelihood of allergic sensitization/HE in at-risk professions (e.g., by improved skin protection).

29.4 Health Education Programs

Educational measures for unaffected individuals (primary prevention) and patient education (secondary and tertiary prevention) are components of skin protection/HE management programs:

> A skin protection program is a series of practical instructions about skin care aimed at a well-defined group of people. In relation to OSD the program may be directed at a certain occupation (i.e., wet workers, mechanics, hairdressers, etc.), or at a certain workplace. It is necessary that the skin protection program is an integrated part of an educational program, which should provide information on healthy and diseased skin, lead to early recognition of skin symptoms, and give the employees prerequisites to understand evidence-based recommendations regarding skin-protective procedures. Ideally, an educational program should improve knowledge about skin care, followed by a change in behavior of skin protection and a decrease in clinical symptoms. Recommendations given in a skin protection program should be evidence-based, as far as this is available. [1]

Generally, health education was shown to be an effective tool in the primary, secondary, and tertiary prevention of skin disorders [2, 12, 35, 36] and will be discussed in the following sections.

29.5 Management of Hand Eczema: Primary Prevention Level

Primary prevention aims at avoiding HE in healthy individuals employed in wet work settings. In most countries, there are detailed legal regulations providing the background for primary prevention at workplaces.

Primary prevention should focus on the following levels [7]:

1. Workplace-related risk-reduction strategies, such as:
    - Elimination or substitution of harmful exposures (e.g., substituting glyceryl monothioglycolate in the hairdressing trade [40] and natural rubber latex gloves in the health sector [20] or adding ferrous sulfate to cement to inhibit the formation of potentially sensitizing chromium VI; see Chap. 20)
    - Technical measures (e.g., "no touch" techniques in cleaning by using specific leverage systems, encapsulation of cooling fluids in the metal industry, splash guards, dust-absorbing systems, ventilation, automation) [37] and changing work organization (e.g., equal distribution of wet work among all employees, introducing breaks to avoid the continuous wearing of gloves)
2. Worker-related risk-reduction strategies, such as:
    - Identification of susceptible individuals (e.g., by dermatological preemployment counseling; recent observations have helped to define risk populations more precisely, including genetic risk factors) [41, 42]. To such risk groups targeted, preventive measures and education should be specifically made accessible at an early stage of their career (personalized prevention).
    - Continuous health surveillance.
    - Optimizing personal skin protection (gloves, protective creams, after-work creams; see Chaps. 26, 27, and 28).
    - Education and training, including curricula in vocational schools (see Chap. 42).
    - Prevention campaigns (e.g., "healthy skin @ work/europrevention"; see below).

As pointed out, primary HE prevention will chiefly be directed towards risk groups, particularly people in hazardous professions, and only secondarily to the general population, but it will also include the dissemination of medical knowledge in terms of health promotion and health education (see Chap. 42). As the EU has defined occupational skin diseases a top-priority health problem [6], the European Academy of Dermatology and Venereology (EADV) in 2009 started a pan-European awareness campaign: "europrevention / healthy skin @work" (Slogan: "Your skin. The most important 2 m^2 of your life."). This is a joint scientific effort for the individual and society as a whole to encourage the development of common health and safety policies to reduce OSD prevalence, stimulate further research, and put science into practice. Prevention of OSD should be ascribed a higher priority in the affected industries, as every employee is entitled to a safe working environment. Presently, in various European countries, national activities in the realm of the EADV campaign are taking place, directed at the public and involving political decision makers. In Germany, this dermatological campaign is supported by the Ministry of Labour, the statutory employers' liability insurance (DGUV), and the occupational physicians. Since the start of the campaign in 2009, official figures of notifications of OSD have risen by 30 % (now 35.2 % of all notifications of occupational diseases). Obviously, this does not reflect a rise in OSD incidence but a reduction in underreporting. Official figures show that affected workers now see their dermatologists earlier, resulting in a 40 % reduction of costs for retraining associated with a reduction of job losses (comparison 2006 vs. 2011; source [10]).

Furthermore, recent EADV campaign activities in the WHO and in the EU Parliament/EU Commission underlined the epidemiological importance of OSD, the disease burden, as well as the need for accurate coding of OSD in the forthcoming ICD 11 and improved workers' education. The campaign also has taken a successful initiative regarding the EU Clinical Trials Directive and national drug laws that jeopardized workers' health by restrictions to patch testing in some EU countries.

Also, in the realm of these activities, substantial progress has been made concerning the high-risk OSD profession of hairdressing. The sectoral social dialogue represented by different European employers' and workers' associations under the EU commissioner of employment has reached a European consensus called "European framework agreement on the prevention of health risks in the hairdressing sector." To implement the regulations of the abovementioned framework, SafeHair was initiated by the University of Osnabrück in cooperation with the European Employees Association (UNI Europa Hair & Beauty), the European Employers Association (Coiffure EU), and national partners in France, Denmark, Belgium, Slovenia, Malta, and Germany. The European Commission has granted funding for two unprecedented research projects (SafeHair 1.0 and 2.0) from 2009 to 2012. The overall objectives were the reduction of HE by supporting transfer of knowledge, networking between different countries, the harmonization of national structures, and the dialogue and implementation process of evidence-based prevention measures. Specifically, the project focused on the formulation of action recommendations for the implementation of the sectoral agreement ("Declaration of Dresden") and on the development of an evaluation questionnaire (EvaHair) to assess the state-of-the-art before and after the implementation process to objectify the success of new measures (acting as a surveillance instrument). It aims at preventing HE by defining common standards of safety and health in the top high-risk profession for HE, which is hairdressing. It includes implementing teaching syllabi for apprentices and masters courses in order to make adequate skin protection and skin care a habit in this trade. This is the first European Commission initiative in the field of HE prevention in at-risk professions. Similar initiatives for other branches at risk may follow. The basis for a scientifically guided consensus on the importance of prevention in the hairdressing trade among all stakeholders, including the European hairdressers,' employers,' and workers' associations, as well as suppliers and safety engineers, has been established. SafeHair 2.0 has focused on the development of a "SafeHair Skin&Beauty Toolbox," a multi-language tool for teaching and learning about skin-protective measures in hairdressing. This virtual toolbox can be used in all European and other countries where English is spoken, educating hairdressers in prevention of skin diseases (www.safehair.eu).

The project underlines that trades affected by HE are increasingly becoming aware of the disease burden and that education and training in occupational safety and health offer the solution.

29.6 Management of HE: Secondary Prevention Level

Target groups of secondary prevention are individuals with initial signs of HE. Secondary prevention aims at early disease detection, thereby increasing opportunities for interventions to prevent HE chronification or progression of symptoms. Secondary prevention requires accurate medical diagnostics and treatment, teaching and education, psychological understanding, and an improvement of working conditions [43].

In Germany, due to specificities in the social insurance system in the last decade, specific prevention concepts aiming chiefly at early detection of HE but including all levels of prevention could be scientifically developed, implemented, and evaluated. This work has meanwhile formed the basis for a nationwide systematic approach to HE by the respective statutory employers' liability insurance bodies, the so-called multistep intervention approach ("Verfahren Haut" DGUV). This approach offers quick preventive help for all severity grades of HE for every employee regardless of profession, including dermatological outpatient and, if needed in severe cases, inpatient therapy, skin protection seminars, and a multidisciplinary intervention with one focus on teaching and systematic follow-up [44]. As was recently suggested, the experience gained may be helpful to further establish complex prevention strategies in other countries with different insurance systems and work environments, too [45]. Obviously, regardless of the social insurance systems, relevant costs to society will always have to be covered if HE prevention is neglected – let alone the impact on the affected individuals.

In the classical HE high-risk profession of hairdressing, the first extensive preventive experience was gained; an almost tenfold reduction of HE was observed due to a systematic preventive program [46, 47]. Similar observations were obtained in geriatric nursing, as well as in other parts of the health sector [21, 24, 29, 31]; this explains why, in the last 15 years, the expenses for HE keep dropping in these branches. Interestingly, there was a greater than 70 % cost reduction for occupational rehabilitation after job loss due to HE in the German health and hairdressing sector over the last decade. We need more health economic studies to encourage the development of health and safety policies even in industries where HE, in spite of its prevalence and economic burden, is not yet considered a high priority.

The question of how accident or health insurers are informed that an employee has developed HE is of vital importance for early intervention. In Germany, even if there is only a slight suspicion that HE may be work related, a dermatologist's report (Hautarztbericht) is filed with the respective employer's liability insurance institution [48, 49]. This report requires the consent of the person concerned. It is based on a detailed examination, including patch tests and atopy screening. It also includes recommendations concerning therapy, personal skin protection, and after-work skin care. Once the insurer has been notified, it will – if an occupational cause is likely – usually commission the reporting dermatologist to follow up the patient with regular consultations and provide all required treatments for a consecutive 6 months period. In an attempt to handle potential occupational dermatoses as quickly and non-bureaucratically as possible, this so-called dermatologist's procedure was recently updated, and the dermatologist's compensation has been increased. For the purposes of optimal early intervention, rapid medical treatment following completion of the report and documentation of progress at close intervals are now required as a rule. In doing so, rapid enforcement of an insured person's legal claim to prevention measures for purposes of preserving employment shall be guaranteed; the follow-up period of 6 months can be extended, if necessary. Additionally, multidisciplinary skin protection seminars are offered to affected employees.

These recent initiatives show that the insurer's administrations have widely accepted that these low-threshold preventive measures eventually save money; and it also demonstrates appreciation for the important role of dermatologists in the field of prevention.

For quality management, the operational effectiveness of the aforementioned comprehensive scheme of secondary prevention measures has recently been analyzed in a randomized quota sample with 1 year follow-up, defining its effectiveness [49].

Wilke et al. [50] evaluated the long-term effectiveness of secondary prevention in geriatric nurses. Geriatric nurses with occupational hand eczema ($n = 102$) participated in an interdisciplinary prevention program; also, affected geriatric nurses in the control group ($n = 107$) were medically treated by local dermatologists only. Data on job continuation, skin lesions, and skin protection behavior were obtained by standardized questionnaires 6 years after intervention and were compared with baseline values and data from a 3 month follow-up. 6 years after intervention, 65.3 % in the intervention group have continued with their job in comparison to 56.8 % in the control group, and 6.9 % of the intervention group and 13.6 % of the control group had given up work because of occupational HE. The skin status improved in both cohorts. The data indicated a lower frequency of skin lesions and morphological signs in the intervention group, underlining sustainability of HE prevention.

In another study by Wilke et al. [51] on long-term effectiveness (sustainability) of an interdisciplinary secondary prevention program, similar results were observed: 5 years after participation in a program that has combined educational and dermatological interventions, the outcomes "job continuation," "skin condition," "skin protection behavior," and "disease management" were evaluated. Results showed the program has been most successful in patients suffering from milder forms of HE, and there was less success in patients with severe HE. The results showed a significant reduction in the frequency of "hand washing" but no measurable change in the use of skin care products. The authors conclude that the intervention showed sustainable long-term effects. Regarding the results, they claim that early detection and reporting of HE are of utmost importance for the effectiveness of secondary prevention.

For hairdressers, Wulfhorst et al. [52] have shown the long-term effectiveness of secondary prevention regarding the possibility to remain in a job despite having OSD. An intervention group comprising 215 hairdressers suffering from OSD was followed up 5 years after participation in a combined dermatological and educational prevention program with an education and counseling scheme, as well as an intervention in the respective hairdressers' shops in comparison to a control group ($N = 85$). After 5 years, 58.7 % of the intervention group remained at work versus 29.1 % of the control group. In the intervention group, 12.8 % had stopped work because of HE versus 27.3 % in the control group ($p < 0.001$).

Furthermore, it was shown that the intervention program led to an increased and sustained knowledge of HE and more adequate prevention at the workplace in the intervention group [53].

29.7 Management of HE: Tertiary Prevention Level

The German stepwise procedure of handling OSDs (description see below) offers interdisciplinary integrated (inpatient/outpatient) rehabilitation measures (tertiary individual prevention [TIP]) for severe HE.

For those cases of severe HE, in which the abovementioned secondary prevention measures are not successful, inpatient prevention measures have been developed (tertiary individual prevention, or TIP). TIP includes 2–3 weeks of dermatological diagnostics and treatment, as well as health education and psychological counseling and ergotherapeutic exercises for use tests of adequate skin protection methods, counseling by the case manager of the statutory insurance institutions, and involvement of the employer's occupational physician. The local dermatologist follows up the case of each patient at close intervals for another 3 weeks (Fig. 29.2). This outpatient treatment, as well as the sick leave reimbursement, is also being covered by the employer's liability insurance bodies ("Osnabrueck Model," [44]).

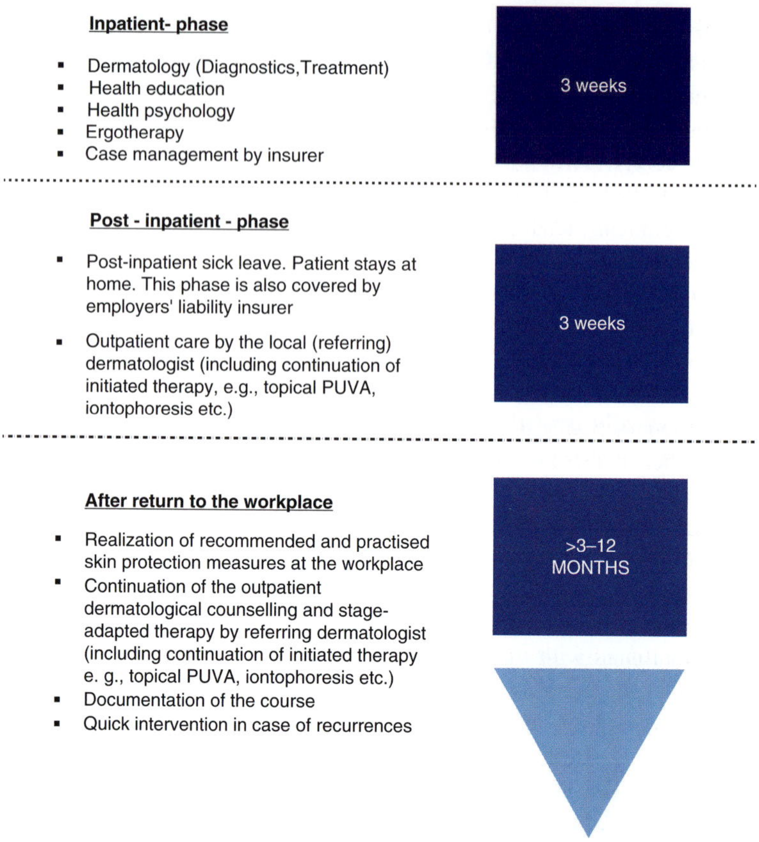

Fig. 29.2 Flow chart of TIP (Osnabrueck Model) (Reprinted with permission from Wulfhorst et al. [7])

In 2005, a nationwide prospective cohort multicenter study was started in order to evaluate TIP. One thousand seven hundred and eighty-eight patients with severe HE were treated and educated in five clinics with follow-up before and 4 weeks after return to work. During the inpatient phase, there was a significant improvement in the severity of HE (Osnabrueck Hand Eczema Severity Index, $p<0.001$) and in the quality of life (Dermatology Life Quality Index, $p<0.001$). These effects were largely sustained during the outpatient follow-up phase and in the 4 weeks after return to work. Among all patients, 89.4 % used topical steroids before TIP, including 52.5 % using high-grade topical steroids; 93.2 % of the patients were able to refrain from using topical steroids before returning to work. As a result of TIP, return to work was possible for 1,587 patients (88.8 %) [18]. The recently published 12 month follow-up reaffirmed a sustained significant reduction in the severity of OSD, in the use of topical corticosteroids, and regarding the days of absence from work because of OSD. Quality of life was significantly improved, and 87.4 % had been able to remain in the workforce in the observation period. More than 75 % of the workers who reentered work did not suffer any more from HE-related sick leave in the year after the measure [30].

These results underline that targeted prevention, even in recalcitrant cases of HE, has a pivotal role regarding the sustainable reduction of the personal and public burden of HE. We may have to reconsider our current recommendations given to seemingly “hopeless” cases of HE.

29.8 Evidence of Hand Eczema Management Systems

In the last 10 years, there have been some reviews on evidence of various treatments, the prevention of hand dermatitis in general, and the effectiveness of educational programs in particular. Saary et al. [54] found – focusing on topical treatment of HE – that a limited number of interventions effectively prevent or treat irritant and allergic contact dermatitis.

Moore et al. [55] have proven the effectiveness of clinical management of atopic eczema. Their conclusion is that the most effective way to manage atopic eczema is to provide adequate time for education and demonstration of intervention. This management procedure resulted in greater adherence to intervention and increased patient satisfaction with care.

Another review by Cahill et al. [56] included 15 studies. Improved patient knowledge and early diagnosis were found to be associated with improved prognosis.

Van Gils et al. [35] conclude on the basis of their review that there is moderate evidence for the effectiveness of skin care education and skin protection measures in reducing occurrence and improving adherence to therapy. There is a low level of evidence for the effect in improving clinical outcomes. The authors recommend including skin care education and skin protection measures in the training of people who (will) work in wet-work or high-risk occupations.

Smedley et al. [11], on behalf of the Dermatitis Guideline Development Group, published systematic review informed evidence-based guidelines for the management of occupational dermatitis, with a particular focus on healthcare workers. They pointed out that only 11 from 1677 identified papers met the quality standard (SIGN grading ++ or +). Main results for evidence-based recommendations for the management of hand eczema were as follows:

- Using alcohol gel for hand decontamination is less damaging to skin than antiseptics or soap (limited evidence).
- Conditioning creams improve dermatitis, but are not more effective than their inactive vehicle (small body of evidence).
- Workplace skin care programs improve dermatitis (small inconsistent body of evidence) [11].

In conclusion, the authors summarize:

> Healthcare workers should seek early treatment for dermatitis and should be advised about the risk of bacterial colonization. Work adjustments should be considered for those with severe or acute dermatitis who work with patients at high risk of hospital-acquired infection. Healthcare workers with dermatitis should follow skin care programs, and use alcohol gel where appropriate for hand decontamination. [11]

To evaluate the effect of a secondary prevention program with education on skin care and individual counseling ($N=123$) versus treatment as usual ($N=132$) in healthcare workers with HE, Ibler et al. [36] have performed a randomized, observer-blinded parallel group superiority clinical trial in three hospitals in Denmark. The authors found that the investigated secondary prevention program for HE improved severity and quality of life and had a positive effect on self-evaluated severity and skin-protective behavior by hand washings and wearing of protective gloves.

English et al. [12] stated that "the management of chronic hand eczema is often inadequate. There are currently no evidence-based guidelines specifically for the management of chronic hand eczema, and evidence for established treatments for hand eczema is not of sufficient quality to guide clinical practice." As a result of a panel (dermatologists and a general practitioner) discussion in which published data were discussed, English et al. [12] and Nicholsen et al. [13] prepared guidelines for the care of contact dermatitis. These guidelines include recommendations for the management of dermatitis at all potentially affected sites (details of treatment and diagnostics are not discussed here; see Chaps. 24, 25, 30, 31, 32, 33, 34, 35, 36, 37, 38, and 39). English et al. suggest that referred patients should have their management reviewed:

> This should include patient education (to achieve realistic expectations from treatment); detailed tailored information; a detailed history and assessment of hand eczema; and assessment of treatment prescribed, the response to it and adherence. [12]

Furthermore, the authors state that management strategies include a skin education program, lifestyle changes, and the use of emollients, barrier creams, and soap substitutes [12].

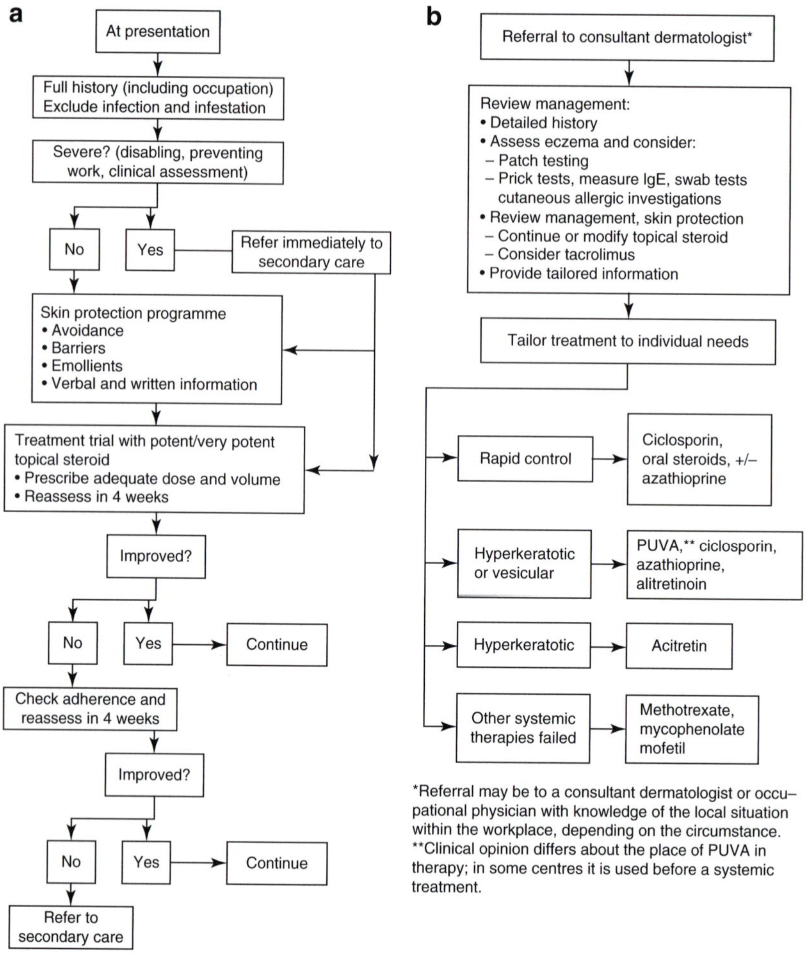

Fig. 29.3 Algorithm for the management of chronic hand eczema in (**a**) primary and (**b**) secondary care (Reprinted with permission from English et al. [12]. Copyright © 2009 The Author(s). Journal compilation © 2009 British Association of Dermatologists)

The recommendations for management of the guidelines are summarized in a treatment algorithm, which is shown in Fig. 29.3.

Conclusion

- Adequate management of hand eczema (HE) in a wet work setting can help severely affected persons stay on the job.
- HE management should focus on reducing the multifactorial risk factors.
- HE management in wet work settings should be based on integrated, multidisciplinary approaches.
- Contents of management are effective skin education programs, lifestyle changes, and the use of adequate skin protection products (e.g., gloves, emollients, barrier creams, and cleansing products).
- On the level of primary prevention, preemployment counseling and screenings of workers in high-risk professions should be performed regularly ("personalized prevention").
- The aim is to offer targeted specific preventive intervention measures and knowledge dissemination to susceptible individuals at an early stage.
- On the level of secondary and tertiary prevention, evidence-based treatments along existing guidelines are mandatory.
- Further investigations should focus on the health economical impact of preventive approaches in evidence-based patient management concepts.

References

1. Agner T, Held E. Skin protection programs. Contact Dermatitis. 2002;47:253–6.
2. Brown T. Strategies for prevention: occupational contact dermatitis. Occup Med (Lond). 2004;54:450–7.
3. Moberg C, Alderling M, Meding B. Hand eczema and quality of life: a population-based study. Br J Dermatol. 2009;161:397–403.
4. Skudlik C, Wulfhorst B, Gediga G, Bock M, Allmers H, John SM. Tertiary individual prevention of occupational skin diseases: a decade's experience with recalcitrant occupational dermatitis. Int Arch Occup Environ Health. 2008;81:1059–64.
5. Diepgen TL, Andersen KE, Brandao FM, Bruze M, Bruynzeel DP, Frosch P, et al. Hand eczema classification: a cross-sectional, multicentre study of the aetiology and morphology of hand eczema. Br J Dermatol. 2009;160:353–8.
6. De Craecker W, Roskams N, Op de Beek R (European Agency for Safety and Health at Work). Occupational skin diseases and dermal exposure in the European Union (EU-25): policy and practice overview. Belgium: European Risk Observatory Report; 2008. Available from: http://osha.europa.eu/en/publications/reports/TE7007049ENC_skin_diseases (March 2013)
7. Wulfhorst B, Bock M, Skudlik C, Wigger-Alberti W, John SM. Prevention of hand eczema: gloves, barrier creams and workers' education. In: Johansen JD, Frosch PJ, Lepoittevin J-P, editors. Contact dermatitis. Berlin/Heidelberg: Springer; 2011. p. 985–1011.
8. European Agency for Safety and Health at Work. European Risk Observatory Report EN8; 2009. http://osha.europa.eu/en/publications/reports/TE3008390ENC_chemical_risks
9. National Occupational Research Agenda. Developing dermal policy based on laboratory and field studies. A new National institute for occupational safety and health (NIOSH) research program in response to the National occupational research agenda (NORA). DHHS (NIOSH) Publication No. 2000–142. [www.cdc.gov/niosh/topics/skin/pdfs/NORADermal-2.pdf. Accessed 10 Aug 2009].
10. Deutsche Gesetzliche Unfallversicherung (DGUV) 2013. Available from: http://www.dguv.de
11. Smedley J, Williams S, Peel P, Pederssen K. Management of occupational dermatitis in healthcare workers: a systematic review. Occup Environ Med. 2012;69:276–9.
12. English J, Aldrigde R, Gawkrodger DJ, Kownacki S, Statham B, White JML, et al. Consensus statement on the management of chronic hand eczema. Clin Exp Dermatol. 2009;34:761–9.
13. Nicholson PJ, Llewellyn D, English JS. Evidence-based guidelines for the prevention, identification and management of occupational contact dermatitis and urticaria. Contact Dermatitis. 2010;63:177–86.
14. Held E, Mygind K, Wolff C, Gyntelberg F, Agner T. Prevention of work related skin problems: an intervention study in wet work employees. Occup Environ Med. 2002;59:556–61.
15. Flyvholm MA, Lindberg M. OEESC-2005 – summing up on the theme irritants and wet work. Contact Dermatitis. 2006;55:317–21.
16. TRGS 401 Gefährdung durch Hautkontakt Ermittlung – Beurteilung – Massnahmen Ausgabe: Juni 2008 zuletzt berichtigt GMBl. 2011 S. 172–175 (Nr. 9) [Joint Ministerial Gazette of the Federal Government Commissioner for Culture and Media, the Federal Ministry of Labour and Social Affairs, the Foreign Office, the Federal Ministry of the Interior, the Ministry of Finance, the Federal Ministry of Economics and Technology, the Federal Ministry of Food, Agriculture and Consumer Protection of the Federal Ministry for Family Affairs, Senior Citizens, Women and Youth, the Federal Ministry of Health, the Ministry of Transport, Building and Urban Development, the Federal Ministry for Environment, Nature Conservation and Nuclear Safety, the Federal Ministry of Education and Research, the Federal Ministry for Economic Cooperation and Development].
17. Wetzky U, Bock M, Wulfhorst B, John SM. Short- and long-term effects of single and repetitive glove occlusion on the epidermal barrier. Arch Dermatol Res. 2009;301:595–602.
18. Skudlik C, Weisshaar E, Scheidt R, Elsner P, Wulfhorst B, Schoenfeld M, et al. First results from the multicentre study "Rehabilitation of Occupational Skin Diseases – Optimisation and Quality Assurance of Inpatient Management (ROQ)". Contact Dermatitis. 2012;66:140–7.
19. Held E, Wolff C, Gyntelberg F, Agner T. Prevention of work-related skin problems in student auxiliary nurses: an intervention study. Contact Dermatitis. 2001;44:297–303.
20. Allmers H, Schmengler J, John SM. Decreasing incidence of occupational contact urticaria caused by natural rubber latex allergy in German healthcare workers. J Allergy Clin Immunol. 2004;114:347–51.
21. Schwanitz HJ, Riehl U, Schlesinger T, Bock M, Skudlik C, Wulfhorst B. Skin care management: educational aspects. Int Arch Occup Environ Health. 2003;76:374–81.
22. Löffler H, Bruckner T, Diepgen TL, Effendy I. Primary prevention in health care employees: a prospective intervention study with a 3-year training period. Contact Dermatitis. 2006;54:202–9.
23. Mygind K, Borg V, Flyvholm MA, Sell L, Jepsen KF. A study of the implementation process of an intervention to prevent work-related skin problems in wet-work occupations. Int Arch Occup Environ Health. 2006;79:66–74.
24. Schurer NY, Klippel U, Schwanitz HJ. Secondary individual prevention of hand dermatitis in geriatric nurses. Int Arch Occup Environ Health. 2005;78:149–57.
25. Held E, Agner T. The Danish experience: prevention of skin problems in wet work employees. In: Frosch PJ, Menné T, Lepoittevin J-P, editors. Contact dermatitis. Berlin/Heidelberg: Springer; 2006. p. 864–7.

26. Brown TP, Rushton L, Williams HC, English JS. Intervention implementation research: an exploratory study of reduction strategies for occupational contact dermatitis in the printing industry. Contact Dermatitis. 2007;56:16–20.
27. Bauer A, Kelterer D, Bartsch R, Stadeler M, Elsner P. Skin protection in the food industry. Curr Probl Dermatol. 2007;34:138–50.
28. Kaatz M, Ladermann R, Stadeler M, Fluhr JW, Elsner P, Bauer A. Recruitment strategies for a hand dermatitis prevention program in the food industry. Contact Dermatitis. 2008;59:165–70.
29. Weisshaar E, Radulescu M, Soder S, Apfelbacher CJ, Bock M, Grundmann JU, et al. Secondary individual prevention of occupational skin diseases in health care workers, cleaners and kitchen employees: aims, experiences and descriptive results. Int Arch Occup Environ Health. 2007;80:477–84.
30. Weisshaar E, Skudlik C, Scheidt R, Matterne U, Wulfhorst B, Schönfeld M, et al. Multicentre study "Rehabilitation of Occupational Skin Diseases – Optimisation and Quality Assurance of Inpatient Management (ROQ)" – results from 12-months follow-up. Contact Dermatitis. 2013;68:169–74.
31. Skudlik C, Dulon M, Wendeler D, John SM, Nienhaus A. Hand eczema in geriatric nurses in Germany – prevalence and risk factors. Contact Dermatitis. 2009;60:136–43.
32. Kütting B, Weistenhöfer W, Baumeister T, Uter W, Drexler H. Current acceptance and implementation of preventive strategies for occupational hand eczema in 1355 metalworkers in Germany. Br J Dermatol. 2009;161:390–6.
33. Attwa E, el-Laithy N. Contact dermatitis in car repair workers. J Eur Acad Dermatol Venereol. 2009;23:138–45.
34. Winker R, Salameh B, Stolkovich S, Nikl M, Barth A, Ponocny E, et al. Effectiveness of skin protection creams in the prevention of occupational dermatitis: results of a randomized, controlled trial. Int Arch Occup Environ Health. 2009;82:653–62.
35. van Gils RF, Boot CL, van Gils PF, Bruynzeel D, Coenraads PJ, van Mechelen W, et al. Effectiveness of prevention programs for hand dermatitis: a systematic review of the literature. Contact Dermatitis. 2011;64:63–72.
36. Ibler KI, Agner T, Hansen JL, Gluud C. The hand eczema trial (HET): design of a randomised clinical trial of the effect of classification and individual counselling versus no intervention among health-care workers with hand eczema. BMC Dermatol. 2010; 10:1–10.
37. English JS. Current concepts of irritant contact dermatitis. Occup Environ Med. 2004;61:722–6.
38. Bourke J, Coulson I, English J. Guidelines for the management of contact dermatitis: an update. Br J Dermatol. 2009;160:946–54.
39. Harris M, Smith BJ, Veale A. Patient education programs – can they improve outcomes in COPD? Int J Chron Obstruct Pulmon Dis. 2008;3:109–12.
40. Uter W, Geier J, Lessmann H, Schnuch A. Is contact allergy to glyceryl monothioglycolate still a problem in Germany? Contact Dermatitis. 2006;55:54–6.
41. de Jongh CM, John SM, Bruynzeel DP, Calkoen F, van Dijk FJH, Khrenova L, et al. Cytokine gene polymorphisms and susceptibility to chronic irritant contact dermatitis. Contact Dermatitis. 2008;58:269–77.
42. Li H, Dai Y, Huang H, Li L, Leng S, Cheng J, et al. HLA-B*1301 as a biomarker for genetic susceptibility to hypersensitivity dermatitis induced by trichloroethylene among workers in China. Environ Health Perspect. 2007;115:1553–6.
43. John SM. Occupational skin diseases: options for multidisciplinary networking in preventive medicine. GMS Ger Med Sci. 2008;6:Doc07. Available from: www.egms.de/en/gms/2008-6/000052.shtml
44. Skudlik C, Breuer K, Junger M, Allmers H, Brandenburg S, John SM. Optimal care of patients with occupational hand dermatitis: considerations of German occupational health insurance. Hautarzt. 2008;59:690–5.
45. Slodownik D, Lee A, Nixon R. Irritant contact dermatitis: a review. Australas J Dermatol. 2008;49:1–11.
46. Kuss O, Schmidt A, Diepgen TL. Impact of preventive strategies on trend of occupational skin disease in hairdressers: population based register study. BMJ. 2002;324:1422–3.
47. Nienhaus A, Rojahn K, Skudlik C, Wulfhorst B, Dulon M, Brandenburg S. Secondary individual prevention and rehabilitation in female hairdressers suffering from skin diseases. Gesundheitswesen. 2004;66:759–4.
48. John SM, Skudlik C, Römer W, Blome O, Brandenburg S, Diepgen TL, et al. Recommendation: dermatologist's procedure. Recommendations for quality assurance of the German Society of Dermatology (DDG) and the Task Force on Occupational and Environmental Dermatology (ABD). JDDG. 2007;5:1146–8.
49. Voss H, Gediga G, Gediga K, Maier B, Mentzel F, Skudlik C, John SM. Secondary prevention of occupational dermatoses: first systematic evaluation of optimized dermatologist's procedure and hierarchical multi-step-intervention. Accepted JDDG; 2013.
50. Wilke A, Gediga K, Weinhöppel U, John SM, Wulfhorst B. Long-term effectiveness of secondary prevention in geriatric nurses with occupational hand eczema: the challenge of a controlled study design. Contact Dermatitis. 2012;66:79–86.
51. Wilke A, Gediga G, Schlesinger T, John SM, Wulfhorst B. Sustainability of interdisciplinary secondary prevention in patients with occupational hand eczema: a 5-year follow-up survey. Contact Dermatitis. 2012;67:208–16.
52. Wulfhorst B, Bock M, Gediga G, Skudlik C, Allmers H, John SM. Sustainability of an interdisciplinary secondary prevention program for hair dressers. Int Arch Occup Environ Health. 2010;83:165–71.
53. Bregnhøj A, Menne T, Johansen JD, Soested H. Prevention of hand eczema among Danish hairdressing apprentices: an intervention study. Occup Environ Med. 2012;69:310–6.

54. Saary J, Qureshi R, Eng M, Palda V, DeKoven J, Pratt M, et al. A systematic review of contact dermatitis treatment and prevention. J Am Acad Dermatol. 2005;53:845–55.
55. Moore E, Williams A, Manias E, Varigos G. Nurse-led clinics reduce severity of childhood atopic eczema: a review of the literature. Br J Dermatol. 2006;155:1242–48.
56. Cahill J, Keegel T, Nixon R. The prognosis of occupational contact dermatitis in 2004. Contact Dermatitis. 2004;51:219–26.

Topical Treatment of Hand Eczema: Corticosteroids

30

Iris S. Ale and Howard I. Maibach

Contents

I.S. Ale, M.D. (✉)
Departments of Dermatology and Allergology, Universidad de la República del Uruguay, Avenida Italia s/n, Montevideo, PC 11600, Uruguay
e-mail: irisale@gmail.com

H.I. Maibach
Department of Dermatology School of Medicine, University of California in San Francisco, Surge 110, San Francisco, 0989, CA 94143-0989, USA
e-mail: maibach@derm.ucsf.edu

30.1 Introduction

Hand eczema (HE) is a common disorder that often adopts a chronic relapsing course, placing a considerable burden on both patients and society [1]. It has a point prevalence of 1–5 % among adults in the general population, and the 1-year prevalence is up to 10 % [2, 3]. The physical and psychological burden for patients is comparable to that for patients with other chronic diseases, such as multiple sclerosis and migraine, and even higher than that for patients with diabetes mellitus [4]. Also, HE is the most frequently recognized occupational skin disease in most countries. The incidence of notified occupation-related cases is estimated to be higher than 0.7 workers per 1,000 per year [5, 6].

Occupations with an increased risk of developing HE are often those that involve repeated and/or prolonged skin exposure to water, chemical irritants, and allergens (e.g., hairdressers, health-care workers, bakers, and print workers) [7].

30.2 General Management of Hand Eczema

Treatment of HE is based on the etiology, morphological features, and severity of the lesions, as well as the acute or chronic nature of the disease. Therefore, treatment must be tailored to the individual patient. Management strategy includes a skin-protection program consisting of education, lifestyle changes (i.e., avoidance of identified

A. Alikhan et al. (eds.), *Textbook of Hand Eczema*,
DOI 10.1007/978-3-642-39546-8_30, © Springer-Verlag Berlin Heidelberg 2014

allergens, irritants, wet work, and mechanical trauma), and the use of appropriate gloves, emollients, barrier creams, and soap substitutes. Skin-protection measures and emollients are essential regardless of the treatment chosen. Topical drug therapy includes corticosteroids, calcineurin inhibitors, and retinoids. Phototherapy and systemic therapies, alone or as a combination therapy, are mostly used for severe HE.

Treatment is often difficult and unsatisfactory for several reasons. HE is a multifaceted disease entity, encompassing a variety of morphological presentations and underlying pathophysiological processes. The most important causative factors are contact allergy and irritant exposure. In addition, atopic skin diathesis is thought to play a role in HE in up to 50 % of cases [8]. A comprehensive and thorough differential diagnosis constitutes an essential foundation for therapy. However, even if morphological subtypes and patterns of distribution may suggest causation, there are no pathognomonic clinical signs and symptoms that can unambiguously discriminate between the different types of HE, thus misleading the physician with respect to appropriate management. In addition, HE frequently has a multifactorial etiology, resulting from a combination of irritant, allergic, and endogenous factors acting concurrently [9].

Despite the magnitude of the problem, there is a lack of evidence-based data on therapeutic options for HE. A recent European Dermato-Epidemiology Network (EDEN) HE survey, revising therapeutic intervention studies for hand eczema from January 1977 to April 2003, identified only 31 randomized controlled trials (RCTs) involving a total of 1,200 participants. Most of the studies had poor quality and short follow-up. Only a small proportion of them had a duration greater than 4 months, which is indispensable to corroborate significant data such as duration and frequency of disease relapse [10]. A recent review of customarily prescribed treatments for hand eczema concluded that there was little evidence for advocating any one treatment over another [11]. Therefore, there are no clear-cut, evidence-based recommendations for treating HE patients, particularly those who do not respond to conventional therapy.

Some recent RCTs have evaluated the value of an integrated care program in the management of chronic HE. The integrated care, provided by a multidisciplinary team consisting of a dermatologist, a specialized nurse/physician assistant, and an occupational clinical physician, significantly improved the clinical severity score (HECSI) when compared with usual care[12].

Recommendations for a standardized approach to HE diagnosis and management, based on published data and expert opinion, have been recently generated by different groups in Germany [13], Great Britain [14], and Canada [15].

30.3 Topical Corticosteroids in the Treatment of Hand Eczema

Topical corticosteroids (TCs) are considered the first-line pharmacologic therapy of HE because of their anti-inflammatory, immunosuppressive, and antiproliferative activity, although there are only limited data from RCTs to substantiate their efficacy.

Considering data from clinical studies, expert panels, and working party consensus, it is possible to make some general statements concerning the use of TCs.

When prescribing TCs, it is important to consider the steroid potency (Table 30.1), delivery vehicle, frequency of administration, duration of treatment, and side effects. High-potency TCs are usually needed in the topical treatment of HE, especially for palmar skin and the skin around the nails. Strong TCs will provide a faster response at the beginning of therapy to gain control of the eczematous process, allowing the patient to taper to less potent TCs with a better therapeutic index as HE improves. Another strategy to taper the use of potent TCs is to reduce the frequency of application.

Limitation for the frequent or extended use of these drugs is the risk for skin atrophy and skin

Table 30.1 Relative potency of selected topical corticosteroids

Class	Drug
I: Superpotent	Betamethasone dipropionate 0.05 % ointment
	Clobetasol propionate 0.05 % cream or ointment
	Diflorasone diacetate 0.05 % ointment
	Halobetasol propionate 0.05 % cream or ointment
II: Potent	Amcinonide 0.1 % ointment
	Betamethasone dipropionate 0.05 % cream
	Desoximetasone 0.25 % cream, 0.05 % gel, 0.25 % ointment
	Fluocinonide 0.05 % cream, gel, ointment, or solution
	Halcinonide 0.1 % cream
	Mometasone furoate 0.1 % ointment
III: Upper mid-strength	Amcinonide 0.1 % cream or lotion
	Betamethasone dipropionate 0.05 % cream
	Betamethasone valerate ointment 0.1 %
	Desoximetasone 0.05 % cream
	Diflorasone diacetate 0.05 % cream
	Fluocinonide cream 0.05 %
	Fluticasone propionate ointment, 0.005 %
	Halcinonide 0.1 % solution
	Triamcinolone acetonide 0.1 % ointment
	Triamcinolone acetonide cream 0.5 %
IV: Mid-strength	Fluocinolone acetonide 0.025 % ointment
	Flurandrenolide 0.05 % ointment
	Betamethasone dipropionate 0.05 % lotion
	Mometasone furoate 0.1 % cream or lotion
	Triamcinolone acetonide 0.1 % cream
	Clocortolone pivalate 0.1 % cream
	Desoximetasone 0.05 % cream
V: Lower mid-strength	Betamethasone valerate 0.1 % cream
	Fluocinolone acetonide 0.025 % cream
	Flurandrenolide 0.05 % cream
	Fluticasone propionate 0.05 % cream
	Desonide 0.05 % ointment
	Hydrocortisone butyrate 0.1 % cream, ointment, or solution
	Hydrocortisone valerate 0.2 % cream or ointment
	Triamcinolone acetonide 0.1 % lotion or 0.025 % ointment
	Prednicarbate 0.1 % emollient cream
VI: Mild strength	Alclometasone dipropionate 0.05 % cream or ointment
	Betamethasone valerate 0.1 % lotion
	Desonide 0.05 % cream
	Fluocinolone acetonide 0.01 % cream or solution
	Flumethasone pivalate 0.03 % cream
	Triamcinolone acetonide 0.1 % cream
	Triamcinolone acetonide 0.025 % cream or lotion
VII: Least potent	Hydrocortisone 1 % or 2.5 % cream, 1 % or 2.5 % lotion, 1 % or 2.5 % ointment
	Hydrocortisone acetate 1 % or 2.5 % cream, 1 % or 2.5 % lotion, 1 % or 2.5 % ointment
	Pramoxine hydrochloride 1 %

barrier deterioration, especially in the dorsum of the hands. Therefore, the dosage and frequency of application of TCs should be limited to the smallest amount compatible with effective treatment.

Several well-controlled paired comparison studies demonstrated that once-daily treatment with TCs is just as effective as twice-daily treatment, especially for superpotent and potent agents [16]. In a double-blind 3-week comparison study of the efficacy of betamethasone dipropionate in the treatment of patients with corticosteroid-responsive dermatoses (63 patients with eczema and 34 patients with psoriasis), English et al. [17] found no differences between once-daily and twice-daily application for all parameters examined. Tharp compared the efficacy and safety of once- and twice-daily application of 0.05 % fluticasone propionate cream over a 28-day treatment period in 238 patients with moderate to severe eczema. There were no statistically significant differences between the once-daily and twice-daily application groups at day 8 and at the end of the 28-day treatment period, suggesting that once-daily application may be recommended for the treatment of moderate to severe eczema in most patients [18]. In another RCT, no statistical difference between once-daily and twice-daily treatment of HE with betamethasone-17,21-dipropionate cream 0.05 % was observed after 1 week [19]. In view of these findings, once-a-day application of TCs may be preferable, as it also offers distinct advantages over more frequent applications. For instance, the risk of developing tachyphylaxis and/or local or systemic adverse effects, which increase with excessive use, could be minimized; the cost of therapy halved; and patient compliance improved. Furthermore, studies in patients with HE demonstrated that long-term control can be achieved by intermittent treatment with TCs. Generally, potent TCs are used daily for approximately 1 month, followed by a maintenance treatment two or three times a week [20].

In a 30-week prospective, open-label, randomized trial, Veien and colleagues [21] compared the efficacy and safety of two different schedules for the treatment of HE with mometasone furoate, a medium-high-potency TC. One hundred and twenty patients with chronic HE were treated daily with mometasone furoate fatty cream until the dermatitis cleared or for a maximum of 9 weeks. Those whose HE had cleared were randomized to receive treatment with mometasone furoate three times per week or twice per week or with emollients only for up to 36 weeks. Recurrence rates after 36 weeks were 17 %, 32 %, and 74 %, respectively ($p=0.001$), suggesting that maintenance therapy can prevent recurrences.

Moller and colleagues [22] examined the long-term maintenance effects of two TCs, one of very strong potency (clobetasol propionate) and one of medium potency (fluprednidene acetate). Sixty-one patients were initially treated continuously on both hands for up to 3 weeks with clobetasol monotherapy, which produced healing in 90 % of cases (mean time to healing: 11 days). In a subsequent double-blind self-controlled, left-right randomized trial, the capacity of the two agents for keeping the dermatitis in remission was compared using an intermittent schedule of two applications a week. The protocol was followed by 46 patients, and the mean observation period was 138 days. Treatment with clobetasol kept 70 % of patients free from relapse compared to only 30 % with fluprednidene. Relapses occurred with clobetasol after a mean of 66 days; with fluprednidene, relapses occurred after 36 days. Side effects, which occurred with similar frequency with both drugs, were few and mild. The authors suggested that an intermittent schedule is advantageous when using TCs of high potency [22]. Short-term and intermittent use of potent TCs reduces the risk of local or systemic adverse effects, prevents tachyphylaxis, and enhances patient compliance. At the same time, abrupt discontinuation must be avoided to prevent rebound events. Upon improvement, the application of a less potent preparation and/or the alternate use of a moisturizer is recommended until the complete resolution of the lesions is achieved.

TCs should preferably be combined with a moisturizing, nonsteroidal topical therapy. Moisturizers are commonly used in conjunction with TCs, and this adjunctive therapy is considered to potentially affect the absorption of the applied corticosteroid and to provide a steroid-sparing effect. In a recent parallel, double-blind RCT on 44 patients with a recent relapse of hand eczema, Lodén et al. compared once- and twice-daily applications of a strong corticosteroid cream (betamethasone valerate 0.1 %) in addition to maintenance therapy with a moisturizer. The urea-containing moisturizer was applied regularly every day and also was used as a substitute for the corticosteroid cream in the once-a-day application regimen. The clinical assessment demonstrated a larger benefit from once-daily treatment compared with twice-daily treatment, especially in the group of patients with mild and moderate eczema at inclusion. The beneficial effect was believed to be due to the skin barrier-repairing effect of the moisturizer [23].

Bleeker et al. showed a significant improvement in symptom severity of subacute and chronic HE after 1 week of once-a-day treatment with either fluprednidene-21-acetate 0.1 % or betamethasone-17-valerate 0.1 % combined with use of the emollient Unguentum M (Almirall Ltd., Uxbridge, UK). No statistically significant differences were seen between the two treatments. The short observation period (3 weeks) did not allow one to ascertain the long-term effects of the two treatments [24]. Corticosteroids reduce the barrier lipid synthesis and the density of corneodesmosomes, which compromises both the cutaneous permeability barrier and the stratum corneum integrity [25–27].

Moisturizers may help to restore the normal moisturizing process of the skin, improving the permeability barrier homeostasis and preventing some of the adverse effects observed from TC treatment [28, 29]. Repairing an abnormal skin barrier function and preventing barrier dysfunction are among the most important strategies to prevent chronicity and reduce the risk of HE relapse [30, 31].

The vehicle through which the active steroid is delivered also plays an important effect in the skin barrier function and may influence the activity and percutaneous penetration of the corticosteroid. TCs are available in a variety of vehicles, including ointments, creams, lotions, gels, and, more recently, foams. The choice of the vehicle depends on morphology, severity, and eczema stage. Generally, ointments are more effective than creams or lotions, as their moisturizing ability and occlusive effect result in better penetration. However, the presence of particular excipients or special characteristics of the formulation can modify absorption, so this established belief may not always hold true. Also, preference studies reveal that patients often find application of ointments to be messy, raising concerns about proper adherence to treatment [32].

In acute eczema, lotions or nongreasy oil in water cream formulations may be preferred. Exudative inflammation responds well to lotions because of their drying effects. Creams usually have good moisturizing qualities, and their ability to vanish into the skin makes them cosmetically appealing. However, we should take into consideration that creams and lotions contain more preservatives than ointments, so the potential for irritant and allergic reactions is higher. Occasionally, in acute HE with a high degree of vesiculation and edema or in pompholyx, the penetration of the TCs is insufficient, and systemic corticosteroids must be used on a short-term basis.

The application method is also important. Application under occlusion enhances penetration, with up to 100 times more vasoconstriction observed if a polyethylene film is applied over the TC formulation than if no occlusion is used. Wet wraps or water soaks for 20 min prior to TC application also enhance absorption and appear to provide better results. Some authors advocate the "soak and smear" technique for dry and hyperkeratotic HE, where mid- to high-potency corticosteroid ointments are applied after thorough hydration of the hands with an emollient [33]. The hands must be soaked continuously in a pan of water for 20 min at night, and a corticosteroid ointment must be applied immediately, without drying the skin. After the skin is under control, the soaks at night can be stopped, and the ointment will be applied each night as required. Soaking will allow water to go into the skin and hydrate it. Smearing on the ointment will trap the water, increasing the penetration of the active agent.

30.4 Adverse Effects of Topical Corticosteroids

Corticosteroids are valuable in the short-term treatment of HE, but they may inhibit the stratum corneum repair, interfering with skin recovery in the long term. Local cutaneous reactions are more common than systemic side effects and are mainly due to the antiproliferative effects of these agents. The skin on the dorsum of the hands is prone to atrophy, and epidermal barrier damage is especially relevant. Other disadvantages of topical steroids include tachyphylaxis and, more rarely, adrenal suppression after systemic absorption [34].

Clinical experience suggests that intermittent dosing, alternating TCs with an emollient, may reduce the risk of adverse effects. In addition, as the epidermal barrier may be not fully restored upon discontinuation or tapering of the TCs, the concomitant use of a nonsteroidal topical therapy, such as phototherapy or a topical calcineurin inhibitor, is often required [35]. Looking for a useful treatment for chronic, relapsing dyshidrotic palmoplantar eczema, Schnopp et al. performed a randomized, observer-blinded, intraindividual comparison study of topical tacrolimus 0.1 % (FK506) versus mometasone furoate (0.1 %) ointment. Both agents demonstrated to be effective for the palmar lesions, and the authors deemed that treatment with tacrolimus offers the possibility for rotational therapy with mometasone furoate in long-standing cases of chronic dyshidrotic palmar eczema [36].

It is important to keep in mind that TCs may also be allergens. Consequently, the possibility of contact sensitization to the corticosteroid itself or other ingredients in the topical formulation should always be considered if the HE does not improve before attributing treatment failure to the disease itself [37, 38]. Patients with hand eczema that does not respond to topical steroids and good skin care should be referred for patch testing.

Conclusion

HE is a highly prevalent disorder, which in many patients is chronic, debilitating, and associated with impaired quality of life. Both endogenous and exogenous factors play a role in the development of the disease. A skin-protection program consisting of avoidance of irritants and allergens, the use of emollients, and TCs is a satisfactory and sufficient treatment for some patients, but many require supplementary intervention. The best way to manage these patients is not clear on the basis of the current level of evidence. Also, clear directions in the appropriate management of TCs are needed. Problems of tachyphylaxis, local side effects, systemic toxicity, patient compliance, and expense might be minimized by a more rational use of TCs.

Well-designed, randomized trials are necessary prerequisites to achieve optimal and successful management of HE.

References

1. Thyssen JP, Johansen JD, Linneberg A, Menné T. The epidemiology of hand eczema in the general population – prevalence and main findings. Contact Dermatitis. 2010;62(2):75–87.
2. Meding B, Jarvholm B. Hand eczema in Swedish adults – changes in prevalence between 1983 and 1996. J Invest Dermatol. 2002;118:719–23.
3. Montnémery P, Nihlén U, Löfdahal C, Nyberg P, Svensson A. Prevalence of hand eczema in an adult Swedish population and the relationship to risk occupation and smoking. Acta Derm Venereol. 2005;85:429–32.
4. Verhoeven EW, Kraaimaat FW, van de Kerkhof PC. Psychosocial well-being of patients with skin diseases in general practice. J Eur Acad Dermatol Venereol. 2007;21:662–8.

5. Diepgen TL. Occupational skin-disease data in Europe. Int Arch Occup Environ Health. 2003;76:331–8.
6. Dickel H, Bruckner T, Berhard-Klimt C, Koch T, Scheidt R, Diepgen TL. Surveillance scheme for occupational skin disease in the Saarland, FRG: first report from BKH-S. Contact Dermatitis. 2002;46:197–206.
7. Warshaw E, Lee G, Storrs FJ. Hand dermatitis: a review of clinical features, therapeutic options, and long-term outcomes. Am J Contact Dermat. 2003;14:119–37.
8. Coenraads PJ, Diepgen TL. Risk of hand eczema in employees with past or present atopic dermatitis. Int Arch Occup Environ Health. 1998;71(1):7–13.
9. Coenraads PJ. Hand eczema is common and multifactorial. J Invest Dermatol. 2007;127(7):1568–70.
10. Van Coevorden AM, Coenraads PJ, Svensson A, Bavinck JN, Diepgen TL, Naldi L, et al. European Dermato-Epidemiology Network (Eden). Overview of studies of treatments for hand eczema-the EDEN hand eczema survey. Br J Dermatol. 2004;151(2):446–51.
11. Coenraads PJ, van Coevorden AM, Diepgen TL. Hand eczema. In: Williams HC, Bigby M, Diepgen TL, Herxheimer A, Naldi L, Rzany B, editors. Evidence-based dermatology. London: BMJ Books; 2003. p. 132–43.
12. van Gils RF, Boot CR, Knol DL, Rustemeyer T, van Mechelen W, van der Valk PG, et al. The effectiveness of integrated care for patients with hand eczema: results of a randomized, controlled trial. Contact Dermatitis. 2012;66(4):197–204.
13. Diepgen TL, Elsner P, Schliemann S, Fartasch M, Köllner A, Skudlik C, et al. Guideline on the management of hand eczema ICD-10 Code: L20. L23. L24. L25. L30. J Dtsch Dermatol Ges. 2009;7 Suppl 3:S1–16.
14. English J, Aldridge R, Gawkrodger DJ, Kownacki S, Statham B, White JM, et al. Consensus statement on the management of chronic hand eczema. Clin Exp Dermatol. 2009;34:761–9.
15. Lynde C, Guenther L, Diepgen TL, Sasseville D, Poulin Y, Gulliver W, et al. Canadian hand dermatitis management guidelines. J Cutan Med Surg. 2010;14(6):267–84.
16. Lagos BR, Maibach HI. Frequency of application of topical corticosteroids: an overview. Br J Dermatol. 1998;139:763–6.
17. English JS, Bunker CB, Ruthven K. A double blind comparison of the efficacy of betamethasone dipropionate cream twice daily versus once daily in the treatment of steroid responsive dermatoses. Clin Exp Dermatol. 1989;14:32–4.
18. Tharp M. Comparison of twice daily and once daily administration of fluticasone propionate cream 0.05 % in the treatment of eczema. Cutis. 1996;57:19–26.
19. Gartner L, Tarras-Wahlberg C. A double-blind controlled evaluation of diproderm cream 0.05 % twice a day treatment in comparison with once a day treatment in eczema. J Int Med Res. 1984;12:59–61.
20. Drake LA, Dinehart SM, Farmer ER, Goltz RW, Graham GF, Hordinsky MK, et al. Guidelines/outcomes committee. Guidelines of care for the use of topical glucocorticosteroids. J Am Acad Dermatol. 1996;35:615–9.
21. Veien NK, Olholm Larsen P, Thestrup-Pedersen K, Schou G. Long-term, intermittent treatment of chronic hand eczema with mometasone furoate. Br J Dermatol. 1999;140(5):882–6.
22. Moller H, Svartholm H, Dahl G. Intermittent maintenance therapy in chronic hand eczema with clobetasol propionate and flupredniden acetate. Curr Med Res Opin. 1983;8:640–4.
23. Lodén M, Wirén K, Smerud KT, Meland N, Hønnås H, Mørk G, et al. The effect of a corticosteroid cream and a barrier-strengthening moisturizer in hand eczema. A double-blind, randomized, prospective, parallel group clinical trial. J Eur Acad Dermatol Venereol. 2012;26(5):597–601.
24. Bleeker J, Anagrius C, Iversen N, Stenberg B, Culberg Valentin K. Double-blind comparative study of Corticoderm cream + Unguentum Merck and Betnovate cream + Unguentum Merck in hand dermatitis. J Dermatol Treat. 1989;1:87–90.
25. Demerjian M, Choi EH, Man MQ, Chang S, Elias PM, Feingold KR. Activators of PPARs and LXR decrease the adverse effects of exogenous glucocorticoids on the epidermis. Exp Dermatol. 2009;18:643–9.
26. Kao JS, Fluhr JW, Man MQ, Fowler AJ, Hachem JP, Crumrine D, et al. Short-term glucocorticoid treatment compromises both permeability barrier homeostasis and stratum corneum integrity: inhibition of epidermal lipid synthesis accounts for functional abnormalities. J Invest Dermatol. 2003;120:456–64.
27. Kolbe L, Kligman AM, Schreiner V, Stoudemayer T. Corticosteroid induced atrophy and barrier impairment measured by non-invasive methods in human skin. Skin Res Technol. 2001;7:73–7.
28. Holden C, English J, Hoare C, Jordan A, Kownacki S, Turnbull R, et al. Advised best practice for the use of emollients in eczema and other dry skin conditions. J Dermatol Treat. 2002;13:103–6.
29. Watsky KL, Frieije L, Lenevue M-C, Wenck HA, Leffell DJ. Water-in oil emulsions as steroid-sparing adjunctive therapy in the treatment of psoriasis. Cutis. 1992;50:383–6.
30. Andersson A-C, Lindberg M, Lodén M. The effect of two urea containing creams on dry, eczematous skin in atopic patients. I. Expert, patient and instrumental evaluation. J Dermatol Treat. 1999;10:165–9.
31. Lodén M. Barrier recovery and influence of irritant stimuli in skin treated with a moisturizing cream. Contact Dermatitis. 1997;36:256–60.

32. Zivkovich AH, Feldman SR. Are ointments better than other vehicles for corticosteroid treatment of psoriasis? J Drugs Dermatol. 2009;8(6):570–2.
33. Gutman AB, Kligman AM, Sciacca J, James WD. Soak and smear: a standard technique revisited. Arch Dermatol. 2005;141:1556–9.
34. Hengge UR, Ruzicka T, Schwartz RA, Cork MJ. Adverse effects of topical glucocorticosteroids. J Am Acad Dermatol. 2006;54(1):1–15.
35. Norris DA. Mechanisms of action of topical therapies and the rationale for combination therapy. J Am Acad Dermatol. 2005;53(1 Suppl 1):S17–25.
36. Schnopp C, Remling R, Möhrenschlager M, Weigl L, Ring J, Abeck D. Topical tacrolimus (FK506) and mometasone furoate in treatment of dyshidrotic palmar eczema: a randomized, observer-blinded trial. J Am Acad Dermatol. 2002;46(1):73–7.
37. Baeck M, Goossens A. Immediate and delayed allergic hypersensitivity to corticosteroids: practical guidelines. Contact Dermatitis. 2012;66(1):38–45.
38. Coloe J, Zirwas MJ. Allergens in corticosteroid vehicles. Dermatitis. 2008;19(1):38–42.

Topical Treatment of Hand Eczema: Calcineurin Inhibitors

31

Alexandra Katsarou and Konstantina Papagiannaki

Contents

A. Katsarou, M.D., Ph.D. (✉) • K. Papagiannaki, M.D.
University of Athens School of Medicine,
Department of Dermatology, A. Sygros Hospital,
5 Dragoumi Street, Athens 16121, Greece
e-mail: alkats.duoa@yahoo.gr;
nantiapapagianaki@yahoo.gr

31.1 Introduction

Hand eczema is a common relapsing skin condition and among the most common of all occupational diseases [1]. The pathogenic mechanism of hand eczema is complicated because both endogenous and environmental factors are involved. Repeated irritant exposure is important to the development of hand eczema, and its etiology is often complex, with multiple factors (allergic, irritant, mechanical, physical) contributing to disease risk. Additionally, patients with hand eczema often have an atopic background [2].

The definition of etiologic and risk factors is necessary in order to correctly advise patients about prevention and treatment [3].

Irritant contact dermatitis is the most common etiology of hand eczema, but patients with hand eczema should be patch-tested [4]. Hand eczema in atopic patients usually takes a chronic course, and the role of occupation is very important [5].

Hand eczema may be a chronic condition [4], and management must consider the need for long-term treatment [6]. Skin protection and the frequent use of moisturizers are extremely important [7]. Topical corticosteroids are of primary importance in the treatment of hand eczema, and their use is very effective. However, the potentially chronic duration of the disease and the long-term use of topical corticosteroids can have local adverse effects on skin barrier function [8], especially cutaneous atrophy [9]. Additionally, topical formulations of cyclosporine proved to be ineffective, according to the study of Griffith and his colleagues [10].

A. Alikhan et al. (eds.), *Textbook of Hand Eczema*,
DOI 10.1007/978-3-642-39546-8_31, © Springer-Verlag Berlin Heidelberg 2014

Topical calcineurin inhibitors (TCIs) may represent a useful alternative to topical corticosteroids for the treatment of various inflammatory skin diseases. In addition to atopic dermatitis, their efficacy is demonstrated in contact dermatitis, hand eczema, flexural and facial psoriasis, vitiligo, and many other skin diseases.

Benefits are greatest in the treatment of face, head, neck, and other sensitive skin areas, because TCIs lack the atrophic potential of corticosteroids [11].

31.2 Tacrolimus in Contact Dermatitis and Hand Eczema

The first topical immunomodulator approved for human use, tacrolimus was originally used systemically to prevent allograft rejection in transplant patients. Its use has now extended into the topical treatment of various dermatologic diseases, especially atopic dermatitis [12]. Tacrolimus is a topical macrolactam immunosuppressant that inhibits T-lymphocyte activation by first binding to an intracellular protein FKBP-12. A complex of tacrolimus, FKBP-12, calcium, calmodulin, and calcineurin is then formed, and the phosphatase activity of calcineurin is inhibited. This prevents the dephosphorylation and translocation of the nuclear factor of activated T lymphocytes and eventually the production of lymphokines (IL-2, INF-γ). It also inhibits the transcription for genes that encode IL-3, IL-4, IL-5, GM-CSF, and TNF-α, all of which are involved in the early stages of T-cell activation. Additionally, tacrolimus has been shown to inhibit the release of preformed mediators from skin mast cells and basophils and to regulate the expression of FcεRI on Langerhans cells [13].

A number of surveys have been conducted in order to evaluate the efficacy of tacrolimus in treating atopic dermatitis and several other types of dermatitis [11, 14–17].

According to Fujii et al., topical tacrolimus demonstrated suppressive effects as potent as those of betamethasone valerate when used as a treatment to a rat's ear with chronic allergic contact dermatitis induced by repeated application of oxazolone [14].

Furthermore, another study that was conducted by Katsarou et al. demonstrated that tacrolimus ointment 0.1 % may be effective in the treatment of allergic contact eyelid dermatitis [15]. This study complies with Freeman's study, which showed that tacrolimus ointment 0.1 % may be a safe and effective nonsteroidal alternative in the treatment of moderate to severe eyelid dermatitis [16].

The efficacy of tacrolimus in the treatment of hand eczema has attracted the interest of many scientists who indicated that tacrolimus may be considered as a useful alternative as well as maintenance therapy for the long-term management of hand eczema.

A recent study has shown mometasone furoate 0.1 % and tacrolimus 0.1 % to be approximately equipotent in the treatment of dyshidrotic palmar eczema. In this study, 16 patients with moderate to severe chronic, relapsing dyshidrotic eczema were assigned to apply mometasone furoate 0.1 % twice daily on one side and tacrolimus 0.1 % ointment twice daily on the corresponding side. Treatment period was 4 weeks followed by a washout phase of 2 weeks. Both drugs were well tolerated [17]. Tacrolimus was shown to be equally effective to mometasone in chronic dyshidrotic eczema of the hands.

Furthermore, Lauerma et al. found that pretreatment with topical tacrolimus in concentrations ranging from 0.01 % to 0.1 % inhibited the elicitation of an allergic response within 5 days when compared with the placebo [18].

Saripalli et al. showed that tacrolimus 0.1 % appeared to be both safe and effective for the treatment of nickel-induced contact dermatitis, because, according to his study, 18 out of 19 volunteers had an improvement in total signs and symptoms with tacrolimus versus ten patients with vehicle [19]. Moreover, Belsito et al., in order to evaluate the tolerability and safety of 0.1 % tacrolimus ointment in a model of chronic allergic contact dermatitis, conducted a randomized, double-blind, vehicle-controlled, right-left arm comparative study. The results of their study proposed tacrolimus ointment to be well tolerated and significantly more effective than vehicle in treating chronically exposed nickel-induced allergic contact dermatitis [20].

According to Nakada et al., tacrolimus may be effective for allergic contact dermatitis patients who cannot avoid repeated allergen exposure, as it may not only reduce inflammation but also inhibit recurrences [21]. Thelmo and his colleagues demonstrated that a daily 8-week application of tacrolimus ointment to the areas of the hand and foot affected with eczema resulted in significant improvement in erythema, scaling, induration, fissuring, composite severity, and pruritus, except for vesiculation [22].

The efficacy of tacrolimus has been compared to the efficacy of corticosteroids and other agents as well.

Meingassner et al. studied the effects of 0.4 % and 0.04 % tacrolimus ointment in comparison with topical treatment with rapamycin, cyclosporine, dexamethasone, and clobetasol propionate solution prepared with ethanol and propylene glycol (3:7). Their study revealed that tacrolimus caused a pronounced inhibition of inflammatory skin reactions of hypersensitivity to dinitrofluorobenzene (DNFB), dexamethasone was less effective than clobetasol, and rapamycin and cyclosporine were inactive at concentrations of 1.2 % and 10 %, respectively [23].

In addition, Dunkan et al. showed that in vivo only tacrolimus suppressed T-cell infiltration and erythema, in comparison with cyclosporine and rapamycin, but did not have effects on keratinocyte growth, which the other agents inhibited [24].

Furthermore, Katsarou and her colleagues conducted a prospective randomized clinical study to compare the therapeutic results between tacrolimus 0.1 % and mometasone furoate topical treatment in allergic contact hand eczema. In this study, two groups were formed, each consisting of 15 individuals. Prior to clinical evaluation, both groups were treated twice daily for 3 days with clobetasol propionate 0.05 % cream. Afterwards, Group A used TAC ointment 0.1 % twice daily for a month and once daily for the following 2 months, and Group B used mometasone furoate ointment 0.1 % twice daily for the first week, once daily for 2 weeks, once daily three times per week for 2 weeks, and once daily two times per week until the 90th day of the study period (Fig. 31.1). This study indicates that FK

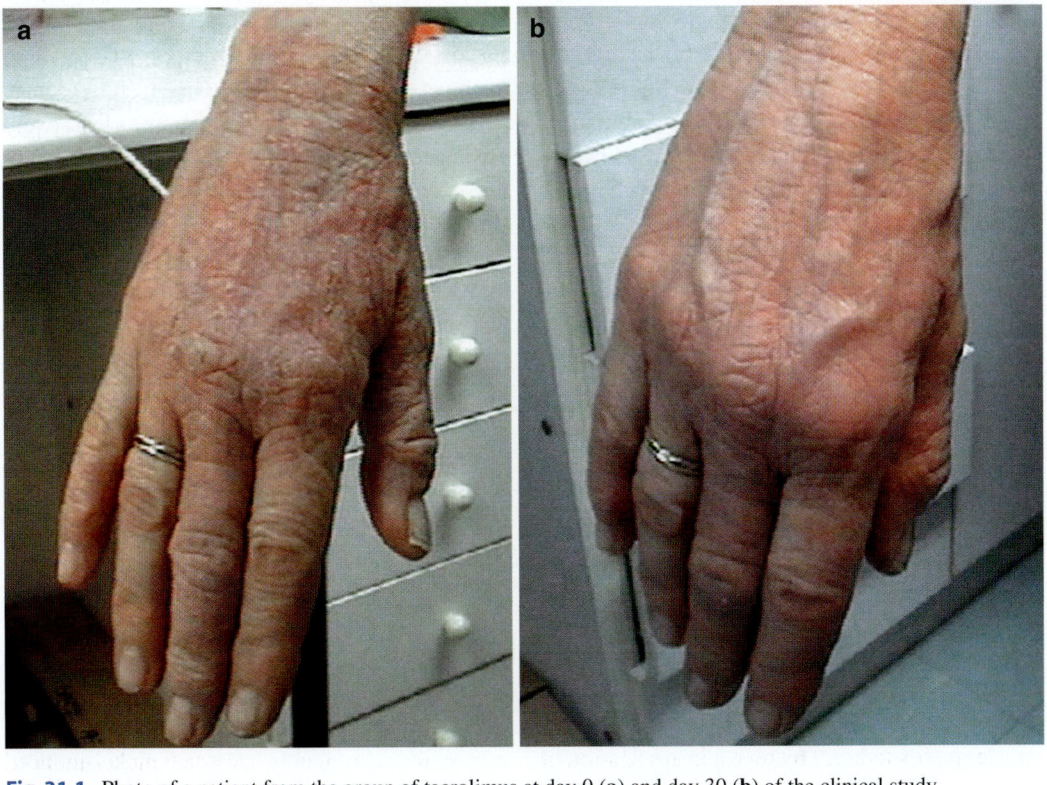

Fig. 31.1 Photo of a patient from the group of tacrolimus at day 0 (**a**) and day 30 (**b**) of the clinical study

506 (tacrolimus) is a promising alternative therapy for allergic contact hand dermatitis because it is effective from the first month of treatment, is well tolerated, and offers similar therapeutic results as topical corticosteroids [25]. Additionally, a previous clinical study demonstrated that topical tacrolimus 0.1 % ointment reverses nickel contact dermatitis elucidated by allergen challenge to a similar degree to mometasone furoate 0.1 % with greater suppression of late erythema [26].

31.3 Pimecrolimus in Contact Dermatitis and Hand Eczema

Pimecrolimus is the second member of the topical calcineurin inhibitors developed for the treatment of inflammatory skin diseases. Pimecrolimus inhibits the production and release of proinflammatory cytokines in T cells in vitro. This involves T-helper type-1 cell (TH1) as well as T-helper type-2 cell (TH2) cytokines, such as interleukin-2, interferon-γ, interleukin-4, interleukin-8, interleukin-10, and tumor necrosis factor-alpha (TNF-α) [27, 28]. Additionally, pimecrolimus may alter the function of activated mast cells and was found to inhibit the production of TNF-α and to prevent the release of preformed proinflammatory mediators, such as histamine, tryptase, and hexosaminidase, by degranulation from mast cells [27, 29, 30]. Pimecrolimus, in contrast to tacrolimus, seems to have a cell-selective mode of action and does not affect the proliferation and the production of cytokines/chemokines in B cells, keratinocytes, endothelial cells, Langerhans cells, or fibroblasts [27, 28, 31, 32]. Moreover, pimecrolimus has no effect on differentiation and maturation or the capacity of human and murine dendritic cells to activate T cells [33]. Because pimecrolimus selectively affects effector mechanisms of inflammation and does not impair the primary immune response, it appears to be advantageous when compared with cyclosporine or tacrolimus [34, 35]. Topical pimecrolimus as a 1 % cream proved to be highly effective, safe, and well tolerated in patients with atopic dermatitis [11, 23, 36–40].

A few studies have already been undertaken in order to estimate the efficacy of pimecrolimus in the treatment of dermatitis. The study of Mensing et al., which included 27 patients with periocular irritant dermatitis treated twice daily with pimecrolimus cream 1 % for 7 days, followed by one daily application for another 7 days, demonstrated that pimecrolimus is a very promising therapeutic option for periocular dermatitis [41]. This study is in accordance with Schurmeyer's study, which demonstrated the long-term efficacy of topical pimecrolimus, initially applied occlusively, in severe dyshidrosiform hand and foot eczema [42].

Amrol and his colleagues, who examined the effectiveness of pimecrolimus in the treatment of toxicodendron-induced allergic contact dermatitis in 12 patients, demonstrated that the application of pimecrolimus was ineffective [43].

A multicenter, randomized vehicle-controlled 3-week study was conducted in 29 patients with chronic hand eczema by Belsito and his colleagues. Patients were randomized to receive pimecrolimus 1 % cream or a corresponding vehicle cream twice a day for up to 3 weeks. The evening application was followed by occlusion for at least 6 h using vinyl gloves. Even though the investigator's global assessment (IGA) scores corresponding to "clear" or "almost clear" were greater in the pimecrolimus-treated group than in the vehicle-treated group, the results were of low statistical significance. It is worth mentioning that patients without palmar involvement responded to treatment better than those with palmar involvement [44]. According to a recent study of Hordinsky et al., topical treatment of mild to moderate chronic hand dermatitis with pimecrolimus 1 % cream did not prove to be significantly superior to treatment with vehicle concerning the signs of inflammation, but pruritus relief was significantly more pronounced in the pimecrolimus group [45].

Queille-Roussel et al. compared the effectiveness of pimecrolimus 0.2 % and 0.6 % creams with a vehicle and betamethasone-17-valerate 0.1 % cream. Their study included 66 adults with nickel contact dermatitis who were treated twice daily for up to 2 days. Both formulations of SDZ ASM 981 (pimecrolimus) were significantly more effective than the vehicle, and pimecrolimus 0.6 % cream was comparable with corticosteroid cream [36].

31.4 Tacrolimus Versus Pimecrolimus in Topical Absorption and Immunosuppression

While the structures of pimecrolimus and tacrolimus are similar, the structure of pimecrolimus possesses two different chemical group attachments by the replacement of a hydroxyl group with chloride and the propenyl side chain of tacrolimus with an ethyl side chain, resulting in its being 20 times more lipophilic than tacrolimus. Because of its structure, pimecrolimus has a higher affinity for the skin and a lower permeation potential through the skin, resulting in less percutaneous absorption and, therefore, a lower risk of systemic drug exposure and systemic side effects and weaker immunosuppressive capacity as compared with corticosteroids and tacrolimus [46]. Kembers et al. conducted a randomized, investigator-blinded study to compare the local tolerability, efficacy, formulation attribute, and safety of pimecrolimus 1 % cream with tacrolimus 0.03 % ointment in a population of pediatric patients with moderate atopic dermatitis. Even though there was no significant difference between the efficacy of the two TCIs, pimecrolimus seemed to provoke fewer and shorter-lasting topical side effects than tacrolimus. In this study, fewer patients reported erythema, irritation, and itching with pimecrolimus; in addition, fewer patients receiving pimecrolimus experienced local side effects for more than 30 min, in contrast to those who applied tacrolimus [47]. Bochelen et al. demonstrated that pimecrolimus has about a threefold lower inhibition potential of calcineurin than tacrolimus. According to his study, this may result in pimecrolimus being less effective at lower doses but may be as effective as tacrolimus at higher doses [48].

31.5 Contraindications and Adverse Events

TCIs are contraindicated in eroded ulcerous lesions and for patients with severe renal impairment or hyperkalemia, pregnancy, and those under ultraviolet therapy.

The most common adverse events associated with tacrolimus/pimecrolimus are skin burning and itching, which resolve quickly as the skin condition improves [37].

Since 2006, the TCIs have a black box warning of a possible risk of NMSC and lymphoma, and it is clarified that these drugs are recommended for use as second-line therapy for the short-term and noncontinuous treatment of atopic dermatitis in patients who do not respond adequately to topical corticosteroids or in whom they are contraindicated [38]. The hypothetical mechanism of carcinogenesis is based on the fact that TCIs directly affect keratinocytes, inhibiting DNA repair and reducing apoptosis in epidermal keratinocytes. In addition, when they are systemically absorbed, they lead to systemic immunosuppression and increased cancer risk. Until now, multiple studies have been conducted in order to measure the blood levels of the drugs in infants, children, and adults undergoing treatment with one of the TCIs. The systemic absorption rate was below the level of quantification or extremely low in more than 99 % of the patients, excluding any possibility of systemic absorption [37, 39, 40, 49–54]. A 3-week twice-daily application of pimecrolimus cream to pediatric patients, aged 4 months to 14 years, to at least 10 % of their total body surface area (BSA), led to blood concentrations of less than 1 ng/mL (81 %) [53]. According to Wen-Rou Wong et al., topical treatment with 0.03 % (for pediatric group) or 0.1 % (for the adult group) tacrolimus ointment for 4 weeks to at least 10 % of BSA led to blood concentrations less than 5 ng/mL [54]. Finally, according to a previous study by Thaci et al., even occlusive topical therapy with pimecrolimus results in low systemic absorption and is well tolerated and safe [55]. In summary, according to the latest knowledge, there is no scientific evidence of an increased risk of malignancy due to topical administration of calcineurin inhibitors [38].

It should be noted that a few cases of allergic contact dermatitis due to TCIs have been described in the literature. In 2010 Neczyporenko and colleagues described a case of contact allergic dermatitis to Elidel [56]. Furthermore, Andersen et al. had previously described a case of allergic contact dermatitis resulting from oleyl alcohol in Elidel cream, and Saitta et al. reported allergic contact dermatitis to pimecrolimus cream [57, 58]. In addition, other authors have described patients who are allergic to both creams [59].

Conclusion

TCIs and especially tacrolimus may be considered as a promising alternative therapy, as well as maintenance therapy, for the long-term management of hand eczema. More controlled studies are needed to confirm their efficacy and to assess local tolerability and long-term safety in the future.

References

1. Smit HA, Burdorf A, Coenraads PJ. Prevalence of hand dermatitis in different occupations. Int J Epidemiol. 1993;22(2):288–93.
2. Coenraads PJ, Diepgen TL. Risk for hand eczema in employers with past or present atopic dermatitis. Int Arch Occup Environ Health. 1998;71(1):7–13.
3. Johansen JD, Frosch PJ, Lepoittevin J-P, editors. Contact dermatitis. 5th ed. Berlin: Springer; 2011.
4. Meding B. Epidemiology of hand eczema in an industrial city. Acta Derm Venereol. 1990;153:1–43.
5. Svensson A. Hand eczema: an evaluation of the frequency of atopic background and the difference in clinical pattern between patients with and without atopic dermatitis. Acta Derm Venereol. 1988;68(6):509–13.
6. Diepgen TL, Agner T, Aberer W, Berth-Jones J, Cambazard F, Elsner P, et al. Management of chronic hand eczema. Contact Dermatitis. 2007;57(4): 203–10.
7. Menné T, Johansen JD, Sommezlund M, Veien N. Hand eczema guidelines based on the Danish guidelines for the diagnosis and treatment of hand eczema. Contact Dermatitis. 2011;65:3–12.
8. Cork MJ, Robinson DA, Vasilopoulos Y, Ferguson A, Moustafa M, MacGowan A, et al. New perspectives on epidermal barrier dysfunction in atopic dermatitis: gene-environment interactions. J Allergy Clin Immunol. 2006;118(1):3–21.
9. Epstein E. Hand dermatitis: practical management and current concepts. J Am Acad Dermatol. 1984;10:395–424.
10. Griffith CE, Powles AV, Baker BS, Fry L, Valdimarsson H. Topical cyclosporin and psoriasis. Lancet. 1987;1(8536):806.
11. Luger T, Paul C. Potential new indications of topical calcineurin inhibitors. Dermatology. 2007;215(1):45–54.
12. Goto T, Kino T, Hatanaka M. FK506: historical perspectives. Transplant Proc. 1991;23:2713–7.
13. Plosker GL, Foster RH. Tacrolimus: a further update of its pharmacology and therapeutic use in the management of organ transplantation. Drugs. 2000;59(2):323–89.
14. Fujii Y, Takeuchi H, Tanaka K, Sakuma S, Ohkubo Y, Mutoh S. Effects of FK506 (tacrolimus hydrate) in chronic oxazolone induced dermatitis in rats. Eur J Pharmacol. 2002;456(1–3):115–21.
15. Katsarou A, Armenaka M, Vosynioti V, Lagogianni E, Kalogeromitros D, Katsambas A. Tacrolimus ointment 0.1 % in the treatment of allergic contact eyelid dermatitis. J Eur Acad Dermatol Venereol. 2009;23(4):382–7.
16. Freeman AK, Serle J, VanVeldhuisen P, Lind L, Clarke J, Singer G, et al. Tacrolimus ointment in the treatment of eyelid dermatitis. Cutis. 2004;73(4):267–71.
17. Schnopp C, Remling R, Mohsenschlager M, Weigl L, Ring J, Abeck D. Topical tacrolimus (FK506) and mometasone furoate in treatment of dyshidrotic palmar eczema: a randomized observer blinded trial. J Am Acad Dermatol. 2002;46:73–7.
18. Lauerma AI, Maibach HI, Granlund H, Erkoo P, Kartamaa M, Stubb S. Inhibition of contact allergy reactions by topical FK506. Lancet. 1992;340(8818):556.
19. Saripalli Y, Cradgia E, Belsito D. Tacrolimus ointment 0.1 % in the treatment of nickel-induced allergic contact dermatitis. J Am Acad Dermatol. 2003;49:477–82.
20. Belsito D, Wilson DC, Warshaw E, Fowler J, Ehrlich A, Anderson B, et al. A prospective randomized clinical trial of 0.1 % tacrolimus ointment in a model of chronic allergic contact dermatitis. J Am Acad Dermatol. 2006;55:40–6.
21. Nakada T, Iijima M, Maibach HI. Eyeglass frame allergic contact dermatitis: does tacrolimus prevent recurrences? Contact Dermatitis. 2005;53(4):219–21.
22. Thelmo MC, Lang W, Brooke E, Osborne B, McCarty M, Jorizzo J, et al. An open-label pilot study to evaluate the safety and efficacy of topically applied tacrolimus ointment for the treatment of hand and/or foot eczema. J Dermatol Treat. 2003;14:136–40.
23. Meingassner JG, Stutz A. Immunosuppressive macrolides of the type FK506: a novel class of topical agents for treatment of skin diseases. J Invest Dermatol. 1992;98(6):851–5.
24. Duncan JI. Differential inhibition of cutaneous T-cell-mediated reactions and epidermal cell proliferation by

cyclosporin A, FK-506, and rapamycin. J Invest Dermatol. 1994;102(1):84–8.

25. Katsarou A, Makris M, Papagiannaki K, Lagogianni E, Tagka A, Kalogeromitros D. Tacrolimus 0.1 % vs mometasone furoate topical treatment in allergic contact hand eczema: a prospective randomized clinical study. Eur J Dermatol. 2012;22(2):192–6.
26. Alomar A, Puig L, Crallardo CM, Valenzuela N. Topical tacrolimus 0.1 % ointment (Protopic©) reverses nickel contact dermatitis elucidated by allergen challenge to a similar degree to mometasone furoate 0.1 % with greater suppression of late erythema. Contact Dermatitis. 2003;49:185–8.
27. Grassberger M, Baumruker T, Enz A, Hiestand B, Hultsch Kalthoff F, Schuller W. A novel anti-inflammatory drug, SDZ ASM 981, for the treatment of skin diseases: in vitro pharmacology. Br J Dermatol. 1999;141:264–73.
28. Grassberger M, Steinhoff M, Schneider D, Luger TA. Pimecrolimus an anti-inflammatory drug targeting the skin. Exp Dermatol. 2004;13:721–30.
29. Hultsch T, Muller KD, Meingassner JG, Grassbergerv M, Schopf RE, Knop J. Ascomycin macrolactam derivative SDZ ASM 981 inhibits the release of granule-associated mediators and of newly synthesized cytokines in RBL 2H3 mast cells in an immunophilin-dependent manner. Arch Dermatol Res. 1998;290:501–7.
30. Zuberbier T, Chong SU, Grunow K, Guhl S, Welker P, Grassberger M, et al. The ascomycin macrolactam pimecrolimus (Elidel, SDZ ASM 981) is a potent inhibitor of mediator release from human dermal mast cells and peripheral blood basophils. J Allergy Clin Immunol. 2001;108(2):275–80.
31. Krummen M, Stuetz A, Luger T, Grabbe S. Effects of pimecrolimus on dendritic cell. J Invest Dermatol. 2003;121(1):1224.
32. Wolff B, Herzig G, Stuetz A. Pimecrolimus does not affect cytokine and chemokine secretion and adhesion molecule expression in primary human keratinocytes and dermal fibroblasts. J Invest Dermatol. 2003;121(1):1243.
33. Kalthoff F, Chung J, Musser P, Stuetz A. Pimecrolimus does not affect the differentiation, maturation, and function of human monocyte derived dendritic cells, in contrast to corticosteroids. Clin Exp Immunol. 2003;133(3):350–9.
34. Meingassner J, Grassberger M, Fahrngruber H, Moore HD, Schuurman H, Stutz A. A novel anti-inflammatory drug SDZ ASM 981, fort he topical and oral treatment of skin diseases: in vivo pharmacology. Br J Dermatol. 1997;137:568–76.
35. Stuetz A, Grassberger M, Meingassner J. Pimecrolimus preclinical pharmacological profile and selectivity. Semin Cutan Med Surg. 2001;20:233–41.
36. Gupta AK, Chow M. Pimecrolimus: a review. J Eur Acad Dermatol. 2003;17:493–503.
37. Harper J, Smith C, Rubins A, Green A, Jackson K, Ziqure S, et al. A multicenter study of the pharmacokinetics of tacrolimus ointment after first and repeated application to children with atopic dermatitis. J Invest Dermatol. 2005;124(4):695–9.
38. Thaci D, Salgo R. Malignancy concerns of topical calcineurin inhibitors for atopic dermatitis: facts and controversies. Clin Dermatol. 2010;28:52–6.
39. Van Leent EJ, Burtin P, Dorobek B, Spuls PI, Bos JD. Low systemic exposure after repeated topical application of pimecrolimus (Elidel, SDZ ASM981) in patients with atopic dermatitis. Dermatology. 2002;204:63–8.
40. Paul C, Cork M, Rossi AB, Papp KA, Barbier N, de Prosty Y. Safety and tolerability of 1 % pimecrolimus cream among infants: experience with 1133 patients treated for up to 2 years. Pediatrics. 2006;117:e118–28.
41. Mensing CO, Mensing CM, Mensing H. Treatment with pimecrolimus cream 1 % clears irritant dermatitis of the periocular region, face and neck. Int J Dermatol. 2008;47:960–4.
42. Schurmeyer F, Luger T, Bohm M. Long-term efficacy of occlusive therapy with topical pimecrolimus in severe dyshidrosiform hand and foot eczema. Dermatology. 2007;214:99–100.
43. Amrol D, Keitel D, Hagaman D, Murray J. Topical tacrolimus in the treatment of human allergic contact dermatitis. Ann Allergy Asthma Immunol. 2003;91(6):563–6.
44. Belsito D, Fowler J, Marks J, Pariser D, Hanifin J, Alzira Gomes Duarte A, et al. Pimecrolimus cream 1 %: a potential new treatment for chronic hand dermatitis. Cutis. 2004;73:31–8.
45. Hordinsky M, Fleischer A, Rivers J, Poulin Y, Belsito D, Hultsch T. Efficacy and safety of pimecrolimus cream 1 % in mild-to-moderate chronic hand dermatitis: a randomized double-blind trial. Dermatology. 2010;221:71–7.
46. Meingassner JG, Aschauer H, Stutz A, Billich A. Pimecrolimus permeates less than tacrolimus through normal, inflamed, or corticosteroid-pretreated skin. Exp Dermatol. 2005;14:752–7.
47. Kempers S, Boguniewicz M, Carter E, Jarratt M, Pariser D, Stewart D, et al. A randomized investigator-blinded study comparing pimecrolimus cream 1 % with tacrolimus ointment 0.03 % in the treatment of pediatric patients with moderate atopic dermatitis. J Am Acad Dermatol. 2004;51(4):515–25.
48. Bochelen D, Rudin M, Sauter A. Calcineurin inhibitors FK506 and DZ ASM 981 alleviate the outcome of focal cerebral ischemic reperfusion injury. J Pharmacol Exp Ther. 1999;288:653–9.
49. Patel RR, Vander Straten MR, Korman NJ. The safety and efficacy of tacrolimus therapy in patients younger than 2 years with atopic dermatitis. Arch Dermatol. 2003;139:1148–56.
50. Alaiti S, Kang S, Fielder VC, Ellis SN, Spurlin DV, Fader D, et al. Tacrolimus (FK 506) ointment for atopic dermatitis: a phase I study in adults and children. J Am Acad Dermatol. 1998;38:69–76.
51. Rubins A, Gutmare R, Valdmane N, Stevenson P, Foster C, Undre N. Pharmacokinetics of 0.1 % tacrolimus ointment after first and repeated application to

adults with moderate to severe atopic dermatitis. J Invest Dermatol. 2005;125:68–71.
52. Eichenfield LF, Thaci D, De Prost Y, Puig L, Paul C. Clinical management of atopic eczema with pimecrolimus cream 1 % in pediatric patients. Dermatology. 2007;215(1):3–17.
53. Allen BR, Lakhanpaul M, Morris A, Lateo S, Davies T, Scott G, et al. Systemic exposure, tolerability, and efficacy of pimecrolimus cream 1 % in atopic dermatitis patients. Arch Dis Child. 2003;88:969–73.
54. Wong WR, Tsai HJ, Hong HS. Efficacy and safety of topically applied Tacrolimus ointment in patients with moderate to severe atopic dermatitis. Chang Gung Med J. 2003;26(7):485–95.
55. Thaci D, Steinmeyer K, Ebelin ME, Scott G, Kaufmann R. Occlusive treatment of chronic hand dermatitis with pimecrolimus cream 1 % results in low systemic exposure, is well tolerated, safe and effective. An open study. Dermatology. 2003;207:37–42.
56. Neczyporenco F, Blondeel A. Allergic contact dermatitis to Elidel cream itself? Contact Dermatitis. 2010;63:171–2.
57. Andersen K, Broesby-Olsen S. Allergic contact dermatitis from oleyl alcohol in Elidel cream. Contact Dermatitis. 2006;55:354–6.
58. Saitta P, Brancaccio R. Allergic contact dermatitis to pimecrolimus. Contact Dermatitis. 2007;56:43–4.
59. Shaw DW, Maibach HI, Eichenfield LF. Allergic contact dermatitis from pimecrolimus in a patient with tacrolimus allergy. J Am Acad Dermatol. 2007;56:342–5.

Phototherapy in Hand Dermatitis 32

James L. Griffith Jr., Mark D.P. Davis, and Ali Alikhan

Contents

J.L. Griffith Jr., M.S.
School of Medicine, University of Mississippi,
2500 N. State Street, Jackson, MS 39216, USA
e-mail: 2griffijlg@gmail.com

M.D.P. Davis, M.D. • A. Alikhan, M.D. (✉)
Department of Dermatology, Mayo Clinic Rochester,
200 First St SW, Rochester, MN 55905, USA
e-mail: davis.mark2@mayo.edu;
alialikhan1@yahoo.com

32.1 Introduction

Ultraviolet light has been used to treat recalcitrant dermatologic diseases for over 3,500 years. Two of its historical highlights include the initial use by ancient Egyptian and Hindu healers, who combined herbal extracts containing 8-methoxypsoralen and 5-methoxypsoralen with sunlight to treat vitiligo, and the 1903 Nobel Prize in Medicine awarded to Neil Finsen for his work and initial publication on the treatment of lupus vulgaris with artificial ultraviolet radiation [1]. He remains the only dermatologist to receive this honor. Now refined beyond medicinal herbs and Finsen's carbon arc lamp, phototherapy has become the gold standard treatment for diffuse vitiligo and a standard of therapy for many other cutaneous conditions, including persistent hand dermatitis [2].

While dry skin care, contact avoidance, and topical steroidal or nonsteroidal therapies can successfully treat 96–98 % of compliant patients with hand dermatitis, the remaining 2–4 % of cases are recalcitrant to these treatments [3]. In this subset of cases, phototherapy may be incorporated into the treatment regimen: long-wave UV irradiation (UVA, 400–320 nm; UVA-1, 400–340 nm), topical or oral psoralen plus UVA irradiation (PUVA), and short-wave UV irradiation (UVB, 320–270 nm; narrowband UVB, 311–308 nm; monochromatic excimer light, 308 nm). The remainder of

A. Alikhan et al. (eds.), *Textbook of Hand Eczema*,
DOI 10.1007/978-3-642-39546-8_32, © Springer-Verlag Berlin Heidelberg 2014

this chapter will discuss these main modalities of UV therapy as they apply to chronic hand and foot dermatitis.[1]

32.2 Considerations Before CHD Phototherapy Treatment

32.2.1 Therapy Time Commitment

All ultraviolet phototherapy modalities require significant commitment by the patient to attend regular phototherapy treatments. Patients often must attend phototherapy sessions three to four times per week until maximum benefit is reached before possibly requiring less frequent maintenance treatments. If these frequent initial visits cannot be maintained, the efficacy of phototherapy will be limited. Several studies demonstrated equivalent efficacy of phototherapy administered at home compared to a hospital setting for both PUVA and UVB [4, 5]. Home light boxes may help reduce the burden of frequent visits and time off work [4], but a response to phototherapy generally is recommended before prescribing home use.

32.2.2 Short-Term Side Effects of Phototherapy

All modalities of phototherapy may induce local phototoxic effects ranging from mild erythema and transient hyperpigmentation to life-threatening burns if excessive exposure to ultraviolet radiation occurs. Tailoring of treatment regimens to the individual's Fitzpatrick skin type or minimal phototoxic dose along with incremental dosage adjustments at subsequent visits may reduce the frequency of phototoxic events. Photochemotherapy carries additional adverse effects and dosage considerations due to the administration of psoralen compounds. Further discussion of these topics may be found in the corresponding sections of this chapter.

32.2.3 Carcinogenic Risk

Ultraviolet radiation is a known carcinogen capable of inducing DNA damage either directly through the formation of cyclobutane pyrimidine dimers (UVB) or indirectly via the production of reactive oxygen species (UVA) [6, 7]. A recently published review of the US and European literature, which evaluated phototherapy's association with skin cancer, revealed an increased risk for both squamous and basal cell carcinomas following psoralen with UVA radiation (PUVA) [8]. Two out of three US studies assessing melanoma rates following phototherapy revealed more than twice the incidence of invasive and in situ melanoma in those with more than 200 PUVA treatments compared to those with lower doses [8]. However, similar findings were not identified in three European studies comparing PUVA's melanoma incidence to the general population via national cancer registries [8]. Although four studies evaluating the carcinogenic risk of narrowband UVB (NBUVB) included in this US and European review did not identify an increased risk of NBUVB-induced skin cancer [8], another publication assessing 1,908 NBUVB patients revealed a slight increased statistical association for developing basal cell carcinomas [9]. However, no association was identified with squamous cell carcinoma or malignant melanoma [9]. Animal studies estimate the carcinogenic risk of NBUVB to be equivalent to broadband UVB (BBUVB), which is less than PUVA [10, 11]. Altogether, phototherapy, regardless of UV spectrum, carries an inherent risk for inducing skin cancers, but BBUVB and NBUVB therapy may present a lower risk for the development of skin cancer than PUVA phototherapy.

[1] For the purpose of this chapter, treatment-resistant/recalcitrant, chronic hand dermatitis (CHD) is defined as an eczematous dermatitis (atopic, dyshidrotic, hyperkeratotic, nummular, allergic contact, or irritant contact dermatitis) limited to the hands and feet that has persisted for greater than 6 months without two continuous weeks of clearance despite adequate contact avoidance, dry skin care, and topical therapy (steroidal and nonsteroidal immunomodulatory agents) [3].

32.3 UVA and UVA-1 Phototherapy

Few studies have been published on the effects of UVA irradiation for palmoplantar eczema in contrast to the relatively large volume of literature on PUVA and UVB (Table 32.1). However, there is increasing evidence that long-wave irradiation alone has biologic effects on the skin. While the majority of UVB radiation is absorbed in the epidermis, 30–50 % of UVA radiation penetrates into the dermis [38]. This UVA radiation has been shown to induce T-cell apoptosis [39], reduce Langerhans and mast cell numbers in the dermis [40], as well as downregulate interferon-gamma expression [41]. The downregulation of interferon-gamma may be due to the enhanced expression of the anti-inflammatory, keratinocyte-derived cytokine IL-10 following irradiation [40]. In addition, fewer dendritic cells with high-affinity IgE receptors are found in UVA-irradiated dermis [40]. Thereby, UVA alone may yield therapeutic benefit through immunomodulation of inflammatory cytokine and cell-mediated pathways.

An open-pilot study evaluated UVA-1 chronic dyshidrotic hand dermatitis. Twelve patients received an irradiative dose of 40 J/cm^2 five times per week. After 3 weeks of therapy, 10 of 12 patients showed significant improvement with near to complete clinical resolution ($p=0.002$) [42]. Clinical improvement from irradiation persisted for 3 months in ten patients. Vesicles recurred in two subjects following a known contact allergen for one and bronchitis for the other. A subsequent double-blinded, placebo-controlled, randomized UVA-1 study and a 3-week UVA-1 case series supported these findings [15, 16]. However, they reported a lower mean improvement of clinical symptoms than Schmidt's pilot trial. The double-blinded trial noted a mean 50 % improvement in clinical symptoms compared to a slight worsening in the placebo group. The case series noted only 18.75 % and 31.25 % of patients achieving 50–75 % and greater than 75 % reduction of clinical symptoms, respectively. Further clinical improvements may be achieved by extending the treatment duration beyond 3 weeks. Grattan and colleagues observed continued clinical improvements throughout an 8-week trial consisting of three treatments of UVA each week [12]. While effective, UVA-1 alone may require a significant amount of cumulative irradiation compared to PUVA [14, 15].

32.4 PUVA Photochemotherapy

32.4.1 Psoralen

PUVA refers to the combination of a photosensitizing agent, psoralen, with UVA light. Upon photoactivation primarily by UVA (320–400 nm), psoralen forms monoadducts and cross-links between DNA strands [43]. Psoralen's actions enhance UVA's apoptotic effect and alter inflammatory cytokines secretion [13, 43]. The maximum erythematous reaction following oral and topical PUVA occurs 72–96 h after treatment [23, 44, 45]. Psoralen derivatives include 5-methoxypsoralen, 8-methoxypsoralen (8-MOP), and trioxsalen. However, 8-MOP is the only psoralen with approval by the US Food and Drug Administration (FDA), as trioxsalen no longer has FDA approval [46]. 8-MOP can be administered topically, as a cream, lotion, gel, or aqueous bath; orally; or via an injection [13, 46].

As a topical agent, psoralen concentrations vary greatly. While higher concentrations directly correlate with greater photosensitivity risks, a tenfold increase in concentration is associated with less than a threefold change in photosensitivity [47]. Higher concentrations of 8-MOP may offer better photosensitization potency, thereby requiring less cumulative irradiation for an equivalent therapeutic response [48]; not all authors agree with this view, as Behrens, Taylor, and colleagues did not observe additional efficacy from administering aqueous baths stronger than 0.0001 % 8-MOP [28, 30]. In comparison to the aqueous bath, other topical preparations generally contain higher concentrations of 8-MOP and

Table 32.1 Selected study findings for phototherapy in chronic hand dermatitis

	Lead author, date	Study type	CHD subtype	Modality of treatment	No. of CHD pts	Tx/week	Max tx. duration	Initial dose (J/cm^2)	Adjustment J/cm^2 per session (increase)	% Pts achieving X% clearance			Study findings
										>90	50–90	<50	
UVA and UVA1	Grattan et al. [12]	Double-blind, randomized, controlled, L/R comparison	Dyshidrotic	UVA PUVA: 8-MOP paint (0.1 %)	15	3x/week	8 weeks	0.5	0.5	– –	– –	– –	PUVA- and UVA-treated hands demonstrated reduction in severity scores by 8 weeks ($p<0.005$). The PUVA-treated side improved more rapidly and was less severe at the 8-week follow-up, but not statistically significant
	Engin and Oguz [13]	Open, randomized, placebo-controlled, L/R comparison	Hyperkeratotic	UVA PUVA:8-MOP gel (0.01 %)	6	3x/week	6 weeks	70 % MPD (*3 J/cm^2)	20 % weekly	– –	– –	– –	Statistical differences of mean clinical score and mean infiltration score were observed between PUVA gel and UVA alone in mixed palmoplantar diseases. Significant decrease in scaling for CHD at 6 weeks with 8-MOP ($p<0.02$), indicating at least 18 Tx are needed to induce significant disease improvement
	Petering et al. [14]	Open, L/R comparison	Dyshidrotic	UVA-1 PUVA: 8-MOP cream (0.0006 %)	27	5x/week (M-F)	3 weeks	30 2	30 2	– –	– –	– –	Approximately 60 % mean reduction in clinical Sx for both Tx by 6 weeks. No relapse in 23 of 27 pts at 3 weeks. UVA-1 is as effective as PUVA (c) therapy
	Polderman et al. [15]	Double-blind, randomized, placebo-controlled	Dyshidrotic	UVA-1 Placebo	28	5x/week	3 weeks	40 0	No dose adjustment 0	– –	– –	– –	Subjective and objective measures of dyshidrotic CHD significantly improve with UVA-1 ($p=0.005$). Elevated serum IgE in 4 pts of the Tx group did not change after UVA-1 therapy
	Tuchinda et al. [16]	Open, retro. case series	Palmoplantar dermatitis	UVA-1	19	–	–	–	–	–	–	50	37.25 % and 18.75 % of CHD pts showed >75 % and 50–75 % improvement, respectively. 75 % of CHD remained clear for 1.5 year

Oral PUVA	Morison et al. [17]	Open, controlled case series	Dyshidrotic, hyperkeratotic	PUVA: Oral 8-MOP (0.6 mg/kg)	5	4×/week, then maint.	–	2.5–4.5	0.5–1.0	100	0	0	All 5 pts cleared their CHD on the PUVA-treated side with no improvement in the untreated reciprocal area. Maintenance Tx helped patients who continued therapy remain clear for >6 months
	LeVine et al. [18]	Open, controlled, L/R comparison	Dyshidrotic	PUVA: Oral 8-MOP (0.6 mg/kg)	7	3×/week, then maint.	–	2.5	0.5 J/cm^2 for 1st 6 Tx, then 1 J/cm^2 until clear	100	0	0	Full clearance was achieved in PUVA-treated compared to untreated hand of all 7 dyshidrotic patients. 2 of 7 were relapse free at 4 months; remainder required maintenance
				Control (no UVA)				0	0	0	0	100	
	Tegner and Thelin [19]	Open, case series	ACD, chronic contact dermatitis, dyshidrotic	PUVA: Oral 8-MOP (0.6 mg/kg) Initial	38	3×/week (2×/ week in 1 case)	–	2.5 (usually)	0.5 every other Tx	H:50 F:36	H:36 F:46	H:14 F:18	Oral PUVA resolved 53 % of palmar and 41 % of plantar CHD cases and induced significant reduction of clinical symptoms in the majority of remaining cases. Maintenance may induce longer palmar remissions (8 months vs. 14 months), but the total UVA dose was more than twice as high as the initial course alone
				PUVA: Oral 8-MOP (0.6 mg/kg) initial and maintenance Tx						H:69 F:11	H:23 F:89	H:8 F:0	
	Hawk and Grice [20]	Open, retro. Case series	Eczema	PUVA: Oral 8-MOP (0.6 mg/kg)	7	2/week	–	0.5–4	0.5–2	40	20	40	Both topical and oral PUVA are effective in CHD with no major differences in improvement, duration, Tx number, or cumulative UVA exposure identified in this trial
				PUVA: 8-MOP emulsion (0.15 %)				0.25–1.5	0.25–1.05	50	0	50	
Oral PUVA	van Coevorden et al. [10]	Open, prospective, randomized, controlled	Eczema	PUVA: Oral 8-MOP (0.6 mg/kg) home	158	3×/week	10 weeks	0.54	15-step increase to max dose	–	–	–	Mean score reduction 72 %/61 % (home/ hospital). This reduction was significant ($p<0.001$) and generally persisted 8 weeks after Tx with ~20 % improving and ~20 % deteriorating. No difference b/w Tx groups
				PUVA: Trioxsalen bath (0.00002 %) hospital		2×/week		0.59 max (vary by MPD)	10–20 %	–	–	–	
	Tzameva et al. [21]	Single-blind, randomized, controlled	Dyshidrotic, hyperkeratotic	PUVA: Oral 8-MOP (0.6 mg/kg)	29	3–4×/ week, then taper	20 weeks	1.2–1.5/0.8–1 (palmar/dorsal)	20 %	–	–	–	Dyshidrotic eczema improved greater than hyperkeratotic with both treatments ($p=0.048$). Neither Tx was more effective for dyshidrotic pts ($p=0.64$). Oral PUVA was more effective than bath for hyperkeratotic eczema ($p=0.03$). For pts with >50 % improvement, 3/7 dyshidrotic and 6/7 hyperkeratotic relapsed <18 months (avg relapse ~7 months)
				PUVA: 8-MOP bath (0.0005 %)				0.8–1/0.55–0.7 (palmar/dorsal)		–	–	–	

(continued)

Table 32.1 (continued)

	Lead author, date	Study type	CHD subtype	Modality of treatment	No. of CHD pts	Tx/week	Max tx. duration	Initial dose (J/cm^2)	Adjustment J/cm^2 per session (increase)	% Pts achieving X% clearance			Study findings
										>90	50–90	<50	
Topical PUVA	Sheehan-Dare et al. [22]	Double-blind, controlled, L/R comparison	Eczema	PUVA: 8-MOP cream (1 %) Superficial radiotherapy (x-ray)	21	3×/week	6 weeks 18 weeks	2 0.9 Gy at 50KV	Gradual No dose adjustment	– –	– –	– –	Mean subjective symptom scores were lower for superficial x-ray than PUVA at 9 and 12 weeks (p=0.013). Clinical assessments of CHD noted greater improvements with superficial x-ray versus PUVA at 6 weeks (p=0.014), but no difference at 9 and 18 weeks
	De Rie et al. [23]	Open, case series	Hyperkeratotic	PUVA: psoralen gel (0.005 %)	2	2×/week	11 weeks	–	0.2–3.5	0	100	0	Relatively short (15 min) between psoralen application and UVA exposure is needed. Low-concentration (0.005 %) 8-MOP gel was effective for CHD treatment without detectable presence in serum and urine analysis
	Schempp et al. [24]	Open, case series	Dyshidrotic, hyperkeratotic	PUVA: 8-MOP bath (0.0001 %)	28	4×/week	8 weeks	0.5	0.5–1 q3Tx	53	36	11	93 % of dyshidrotic and 86 % of hyperkeratotic pts achieved good to excellent results with PUVA bath. Cumulative and single highest dose of UVA was higher for hyperkeratotic than dyshidrotic, but not statistically significant. Relapse rates b/w these CHD subtypes did not differ (avg 6 months)
	Davis et al. [25]	Open, retro. case series	Dyshidrotic, unspecified	PUVA: 8-MOP bath (0.0005 %)	17	3/week, then taper	–	0.5	0.5 per session after first 2–3 Tx	41	29	29	Clearance was achieved in 41 % of CHD. PUVA bath ensured distribution of psoralens on hands/ft to avoid ultraviolet burns from inadvertent painting of previously untreated skin. 18 % of patients did not complete trial due to inconvenience
	Gritiyarangsan et al. [26]	Open, case series	Eczema	PUVA: 8-MOP cream (0.1 %)	17	3×/week	8 weeks	1	0.25–0.5	0	82	18	The majority of CHD showed moderate to significant improvement. Clinical improvement was not associated with duration of CHD, atopic status, or patch test reactions. Relapse rates in the subsequent months were high; longer remission may require maintenance PUVA therapy
	Shephard et al. [27]	Open, randomized, controlled, L/R comparison	Eczema	PUVA: 8-MOP bath (0.0001 %) PUVA: 8-MOP lotion (0.15 %)	24	3×/week	4 weeks, then more effective modality	0.1	20 % every other Tx	– –	– –	– –	In mixed cohort of psoriasis and CHD, likely response to therapy can be determine in the first 12 treatments, as 88 % of initial responders in this trial reached 80+% clearance compared to less than 40 % of nonresponders. Ratio of CHD preference bath to lotion was 2:1. No difference in average relapse (3 months) identified between PUVA vehicles

Topical PUVA	Behrens et al. [28]	Open, case series	Atopic, dyshidrotic, hyperkeratotic	PUVA: 8-MOP bath (0.0001 %)	20	3–4×/week (M-F)	8 weeks	0.3	Unspecified increase q3Tx	55	25	20	55 % of CHD pts experienced >90 % resolution of clinical symptoms. CHD response rates by subtype to PUVA bath: atopic > dyshidrotic > hyperkeratotic. Mean clinical improvement was >50 % for each subtype. Slight remission in 2 dyshidrotic and 1 atopic CHD at 8 weeks
	Grundmann-Kollman et al. [29]	Open, prospective, randomized, L/R comparison	Atopic, hyperkeratotic	PUVA: 8-MOP bath (0.00005 %) PUVA: 8-MOP cream (0.0006 %)	8	4/week	8 weeks	0.3–0.5	Gradual increase q3Tx	12 25	38 25	50 50	50 % of hyperkeratotic pts showed no response to PUVA bath, while only 25 % did not respond to PUVA cream on the opposite hand. Overall, 4 of the 8 hyperkeratotic and atopic CHD cases showed >50 % clearance with either PUVA bath or cream. No remission at 8 weeks for good-excellent responders
	Taylor et al. [30]	Open, retro. case series	Atopic, dyshidrotic, unspecified	PUVA: 8-MOP bath (0.001–0.002 %)	38	*3/week	–	0.25	*0.125–0.5	20	–	–	18 % of CHD cases achieved >90 % clearance with PUVA bath. For CHD and other palmoplantar disorders, 3×/week 20 min PUVA baths (10 mg/L 8-MOP) at 0.25 J/cm2 initial dose and advanced to 0.125-0.25 J/cm2 per additional treatment can safely be given regardless of skin type
	Schiener et al. [31]	Single-blind, randomized, controlled, L/R comparison	Dyshidrotic, hyperkeratotic	PUVA: 8-MOP bath (0.0001 %) PUVA: 8-MOP gel (0.005 %)	11	3–4×/week	–	30 % MPD (*0.3–0.5 J/cm2)	0.3 q3Tx	45 64	36 27	18 9	PUVA gel and bath are comparable in efficacy for treating dyshidrotic and hyperkeratotic CHD as greater than 80 % of pts showed 50+% clinical improvement

(continued)

Table 32.1 (continued)

	Lead author, date	Study type	CHD subtype	Modality of treatment	No. of CHD pts	Tx/week	Max tx. duration	Initial dose (J/cm^2)	Adjustment J/cm^2 per session (increase)	% Pts achieving X% clearance			Study findings
										>90	50–90	<50	
UVB	Rosen et al. [32]	Open, randomized, L/R controlled	ACD, dyshidrotic, irrit., hyperkeratotic	UVB versus control (no UVB)	35	3×/week	12 weeks	0.03	0.015 J/cm^2, then 6 stepped increments to 0.18 J/cm^2	0	44	66	Both UVB and oral PUVA groups had statistically significant improvement versus the untreated hand. All PUVA pts cleared, with 64 % relapsing within 3 months. No pts cleared with UVB. Following the completion of the trial, 8 UVB pts were treated with PUVA; 6 achieved complete CHD clearance
				PUVA: oral 8-MOP (0.6 mg/kg) + UVA versus control (no UVA)				2	1, except half b/w 4–6 J	100	0	0	
	Sjovall and Christensen [11]	Case series	ACD, atopic, dyshidrotic, hyperkeratotic, irritant, nummular	UVB Clinic	26	4–5×/ week	10 weeks	0.10 (dorsal) 0.38 (palmar)	Palmar, 30–60s; dorsal, 10–20s	40	47	13	Clinic/home UVB Tx effective for CHD ($p<0.01$). 66 % of clinic pts and 33 % of home pts, who required the continued use of topical corticosteroids into the trial, did not require their use by the trial's end. Response may be due to UVA-UVB exposure rather than UVB alone as the device used emitted 3.23 mW/cm^2 and 4.26 mW/cm^2 of UVB and UVA, respectively. Peak emissions were 315–318 nm
				UVB Home						27	73	0	
	Simons et al. [33]	Open, randomized, L/R comparison	Dyshidrotic and hyperkeratotic	UVB	13	3×/week	6 weeks	40 % of MED or MPD in healthy volunteers	20 % × 5 Tx, then tapered increases	8	46	46	Statistically significant clinical improvement at 6 weeks for UVB and PUVA bath with 39 % and 25 % mean score reduction. No difference in reductions b/w Tx ($p>0.05$). Greater incidence of adverse effects occurred in PUVA than UVB
				PUVA: trioxsalen bath (0.00002 %)		2×/week			20 %	8	31	61	

UVB TL01	Nordal and Christensen [34]	Open, case series	Atopic, dyshidrotic, irritant	UVB-TL01	16	2–3×/ week	9 weeks	0.1–1 (dorsal) 0.2–.4 (palmar)	0.1–0.4 (dorsal) 0.2–1.4 (palmar)	0	69	31	UVB-TL01 appears to be less effective for dyshidrotic CHD than UVA-1; it is somewhat effective for CHD overall
	Sezer and Etikan [35]	Open, randomized, controlled, L/R comparison	Dry and dyshidrotic	UVB-TL01 PUVA: 8-MOP gel (0.1 %)	15	3×/week	9 weeks	0.15 1	20 % 0.5 every other Tx	17 8	75 75	8 17	Mean clinical score decreased for both Tx groups at 3, 6, and 9 weeks ($p<0.02$). No statistical difference between NBUVB and PUVA gel Tx at 9 weeks for dry and dyshidrotic CHD. 66 % (NBUVB) and 50 % (PUVA) showed no regression at 10 weeks following last Tx
	Jensen et al. [36]	Open, retro. case series	ACD, compositae, dyshidrotic, hyperkeratotic	UVB-TL01 PUVA: trioxsalen bath (0.000025 %)	68	–	24 weeks	0.1 0.1	0.1 0.05	– –	– –	– –	PUVA: 33 % ACD, 25 % compositae, 36 % dyshidrotic, and 50 % hyperkeratotic achieved >75 % clearance. UVB-TL01 group was very small (n=<4 pts/CHD type) but demonstrated 0 % ACD, 75 % compositae, 50 % dyshidrotic, and 50 % hyperkeratotic, reaching 75 % clearance
MEL	Aubin et al. [37]	Open, case series	Atopic, nonatopic	308 nm monochromatic excimer light (MEL)	18	1×/week	10 weeks	Multiples of predetermined MED	Response to Tx	11	–	–	Atopic and nonatopic CHD mean improvement 54 % and 46 %, respectively, with medium- and high-fluence MEL. Significant relapse occurred at 3 months for nonatopic and 6 months for atopic CHD ($p<0.05$). MEL may allow fewer Tx and a lower cumulative UV dose than NBUVB in CHD as this trend was seen in the trial's psoriasis group compared to psoriasis NBUVB literature (data presented in the table does not include those from psoriasis pts)

– not available or not specified, * mixed disease population + CHD, *8-MOP* methoxypsoralen, *ACD* allergic chronic hand dermatitis, *CHD* chronic hand dermatitis, *F* foot, *H* hand, *Irrit* irritant, *J* joules, *Maint* maintenance, *MED* minimal erythematous dose, *MPD* minimal phototoxic dose, *mW/cm²* milliwatts per centimeter², *No.* number, *Pts* patients, *Retro* retrospective, *UVA* ultraviolet-A (320–400 nm), *UVA-1* UVA (340–400 nm), *UVB-TL01* narrowband ultraviolet B (311 ± 2 nm)

Publications are arranged chronologically within each modality of phototherapy reviewed (UVA and UVA-1, oral PUVA, topical PUVA, UVB, UVB-TL01, and MEL) allow application to only affected areas. However, inconsistencies in covering the same areas raise the likelihood of local phototoxic effects, such as erythema, burns, hyperpigmentation, and blister formation at the lesion's borders [31]. In contrast, soaking the hands in aqueous psoralen (bath PUVA) allows a homogenous distribution of psoralen to the hands/feet, which is repeatable at subsequent treatments [49]. Serum analysis of 8-MOP concentrations 1 h after PUVA baths of the hands and feet demonstrated minimal systemic absorption, even at the high 8-MOP bath concentration of 0.0025 % [50]. Despite the minimal systemic concerns and choice of application vehicle, photoprecautions, such as sunscreen, protective clothing, and sun avoidance, should occur at least during the first 2 h following treatment [28]. Treated areas are the most photosensitive 30 min after topical applications but rapidly desensitize in the hours thereafter [28]. However, sensitivity may persist up to 72–96 h.

Oral dosing of 8-MOP is more uniform in published studies relating to chronic hand dermatitis than topical dosing. Of the studies listed in Table 32.1, all pertaining to oral PUVA dispensed a standard dose of 0.6 mg/kg of body weight. Although the time to peak serum levels following administration differs due to gastrointestinal absorption, the mean peak serum levels/maximum benefit of UVA exposure generally occurs 2 h after ingestion as compared to the relatively short period of time (15 min) for topical psoralens [1, 23]. Being systemic, oral psoralen requires greater photosensitivity precautions than topical formulations, as generalized photosensitivity, including ocular photosensitivity, may occur. Ocular photosensitivity may lead to the development of cataracts without the use of protective eyewear [51]. Additional adverse reactions reported in the literature include depression, dizziness, headache, transient hyperpigmentation, swelling, rash, leg cramps, possible premature aging, potential elevated risk of developing melanoma and nonmelanoma skin cancers, and the gastrointestinal symptoms of nausea and vomiting [51]. The incidence of nausea in the literature varies drastically, ranging from 0 % to 66.7 % [20, 52]. Concurrent drug ingestion with low-fat milk or food may prevent nausea, but high-fat meals can significantly lower absorption [51, 53]. Rare adverse reactions reported in the literature include psoralen-induced allergic reaction and punctate leukoderma [32, 54].

Photosensitivity precautions, which should be taken during and after oral PUVA therapy, include eye protection for the first 24 h, as well as skin and lip photoprotection for at least the first 8 h following treatment [46]. The FDA also recommends eye exams by an ophthalmologist at baseline, 1 year after therapy, and every 2 years thereafter [46]. Concurrent use while pregnant should be avoided, although no teratogenic effects have been reported [46, 53]. Similarly, the FDA advises mothers not to breast-feed while taking this drug, as it is not known whether 8-MOP passes into the mother's milk. Psoralen is metabolized by the liver and primarily eliminated by renal excretion. Therefore, a reduced dose of oral psoralen should be administered to those with stable renal impairment while avoided in severe liver disease [53].

Oral psoralen is absolutely contraindicated in the following nine diseases: Bloom syndrome, Cockayane syndrome, dermatomyositis, Gorlin syndrome, hereditary dysplastic nevus syndrome, prior malignant melanoma, trichothiodystrophy, systemic lupus erythematosus, and xeroderma pigmentosum [53].

32.4.2 PUVA's Efficacy

Of all the phototherapy options for treating recalcitrant, chronic hand dermatitis, PUVA is the most rigorously investigated. Published studies have demonstrated that all PUVA modalities, both oral and topical, are effective in the treatment of recalcitrant chronic hand eczema. Their findings are summarized in Table 32.1.

Response rates vary between clinical trials, with 38–100 % of patients experiencing at least a 50 % reduction of clinical symptoms. Of the studies delineating CHD response to PUVA treatment, approximately 42 % of cases achieved greater than 90 % clearance, 35 % between 50 % and 90 %, and 23 % less than 50 % (see

Table 32.1). Mixed evaluations of PUVA bath's effectiveness for the treatment of hyperkeratotic hand eczema were reported. Two studies, a randomized left-right comparison of PUVA cream versus bath and a single-blinded, randomized controlled trial of oral PUVA versus bath, observed PUVA bath as the less effective treatment modality in hyperkeratotic hand eczema but equivalent in dyshidrotic cases [29, 52]. The larger of these two studies, with 12 hyperkeratotic cases, found only a 33 % mean reduction in clinical symptoms for the bath compared to 70 % reduction for the cream ($p=0.03$) [52]. However, another equivalent-size trial ($n=11$) evaluating PUVA gel versus bath in a left-right comparison noted no difference between modalities with 80 % of patients achieving greater than 50 % clearance for each treatment group [31]. Two larger case series ($n=20$ and $n=28$) also observed a strong response to PUVA bath, but the trend of lower response rates for hyperkeratotic than dyshidrotic and atopic CHD was reported without being statistically significant [24, 28]. When compared to other wavelengths of radiation (superficial x-ray and broadband/narrowband UVB), PUVA is equally as effective in resolving the clinical symptoms of CHD [22, 33, 35].

CHD usually requires multiple PUVA sessions before significant clinical improvements are seen. However, in a mixed cohort of psoriasis and CHD, Shephard and colleagues identified that a patient's likely response to therapy can be determined in the first 12 treatments. Eighty-eight percent of initial responders (those who demonstrated clinical improvement in less than 12 treatments) reached greater than 80 % clearance compared to less than 40 % of noninitial responders [27].

Relapse in the subsequent months was frequently reported once phototherapy sessions ceased. The use of maintenance treatments or treatment taper after reaching the maximum benefit of initial therapy may delay CHD recurrence. Tegner and colleagues observed longer remission in patients receiving initial and maintenance treatments compared to initial treatment alone (14 months vs. 8 months). However, the mean total UVA dose of initial and maintenance treatments was more than twice the initial course alone [19].

Considering the small sample size in published studies and lack of standardized protocols for both phototherapy dosing regimens and assessment of CHD severity, limited conclusions concerning the superiority of one PUVA modality over another can be attained; fewer conclusions may be drawn comparing PUVA, UVA without psoralen, and UVB therapies to each other. In addition, several PUVA and UVB studies noted improvements in lesions lying beyond the treated area [18, 32, 55]. Although the improvement in untreated areas may be due to better compliance with contact avoidance and dry skin care, localized phototherapy may induce systemic immunomodulatory effects [32], which would confound left-right treatment comparisons aiming to assess the superiority of one modality over another. Larger randomized, controlled trials with a standardized means of assessment are needed before definitive conclusions can be ascertained.

32.5 UVB Phototherapy

Similar to UVA irradiation, UVB radiation modulates and suppresses the immune system via T-cell apoptosis, decreased antigen presentation, and alteration of inflammatory mediators and cytokines [56]. Although less UVB radiation penetrates into the dermis compared to UVA, UVB generates more extensive T-cell DNA damage in vitro than equivalent doses of UVA with the 308 nm wavelength inciting the greatest quantities of DNA breakage compared to longer wavelengths, 311–640 nm [7]. Once below 290 nm, the UVB spectrum primarily stimulates erythemogenic responses without significant therapeutic benefit based upon monochromator studies in psoriasis [57]. Based upon these and findings from psoriasis trials, several types of short-wave UVB phototherapies have been investigated in the treatment of CHD as an alternative to PUVA. These therapies include broadband UVB (BB-UVB, 270–320 nm), narrowband (NBUVB or UVB-TL01, 308–313 nm), and monochromatic excimer light (MEL, 308 nm).

32.5.1 Broadband UVB

Broadband UVB appears to be a useful tool in the treatment of CHD. Following an uncontrolled study in 1983 demonstrating significant improvements in 7 out of 10 patients with allergic contact dermatitis, Rosen and colleagues designed a randomized, controlled trial to compare the efficacy of PUVA and BB-UVB treatments [32]. Thirty-five patients of various CHD etiologies were randomly assigned to receive either oral PUVA or BB-UVB therapy with UV treatments administered to only one hand. The untreated hand served as a control. Despite equivalent pretreatment mean total scores, significantly greater clinical improvements were evident by 3 weeks in the PUVA treatment group compared to BB-UVB, with complete clearance by 12 weeks in all PUVA patients who completed the trial ($p<0.01$). No BB-UVB patients reached clearance by 12 weeks of treatment, with patients attaining only a 51 % mean reduction in CHD total clinical scores. Of note, the untreated hand in both the PUVA and BB-UVB treatment groups demonstrated a mean reduction of 49 % and 37 %, respectively. The reason for improvements in untreated areas was unable to be identified by the author, but may be due to greater compliance with dry skin care and contact avoidance or possibly due to systemic effects of phototherapy. The side effect profile of these therapies was significantly different ($p<0.001$). Half of PUVA patients experienced side effects, including nausea, pain, soreness, transient hyperpigmentation, and unprecedented spreading of allergic contact dermatitis to the arms and face. Thirteen percent of BB-UVB patients experienced side effects of bullae formation and *Staphylococcus aureus* infection. Following the trial, 10 of the 16 UVB patients were later treated with PUVA. Six completely cleared, two showed notable improvements, and two patients withdrew due to a trip and psoralen allergy [32]. However, PUVA's superiority over BB-UVB remains debatable, as no difference in treatment efficacy was identified during a 6-week left-right treatment comparison of BBUVB versus bath PUVA [33].

32.5.2 Narrowband UVB

Twenty years following the experimental use of a fluorescent lamp with 51 % of emitted wavelengths at 311 nm, the first clinical report of NBUVB's use as a treatment modality for CHD was published [34]. Sixteen patients with chronic dry and dyshidrotic hand eczema received two to three NBUVB treatments per week for up to 9 weeks. Since thickened epidermal layers would lower UVB's already limited penetrance to dermal lymphocytes compared to UVA radiation, hyperkeratotic CHD cases were excluded from the study. By the trial's end, 70 % of patients achieved a 50–90 % reduction in clinical symptoms, with no patients reaching complete clearance [34]. Similar results were published in a small, randomized left-right comparison of PUVA gel and NBUVB [35]. Both treatment arms reached 50–90 % clearance in 75 % of patients, with a small minority of both treatment groups clearing completely. No statistical difference in clinical improvement was evident between treatment groups. Relapse rates were comparable between NBUVB and PUVA, with 66 % and 50 % retaining clinical improvements 10 weeks following treatment, respectively [35]. Of note, one report exists in the literature on the novel use of a 308 nm xenon chloride monochromatic excimer light (MEL) as a treatment for CHD [37]. This case study noted approximately a 50 % mean reduction in clinical CHD symptoms following weekly exposure to MEL for up to 10 weeks. Further investigation is needed to deduce if MEL is therapeutically advantageous to other UVB and UVA therapies as indicated by monochromatic studies on T-cell DNA damage and apoptosis.

32.6 Phototherapy Administration

Due to a lack of randomized trials comparing different phototherapy dosing protocols, no consensus exists in the literature as to the optimal ultraviolet dosing regimen. Therefore, the initial dosing of UVA and UVB irradiation varies widely in published trials (see Table 32.1).

Three generalized approaches for administering the initial UVA or UVB dose are reported in the literature. The initial dose may be either uniformly administered to all patients or tailored to either the patient's Fitzpatrick skin type (fairer skin receiving less irradiation than darker skin) or a percentage of one's minimal phototoxic dose (MPD). MPD is predetermined by exposing unaffected skin to multiple doses of radiation (0.2–3.5 J/cm^2) and then examining the irradiated area 72 h later for the minimal dose required to induce erythema with a distinct border [23]. The two individualized approaches aim to minimize phototoxic events while delivering the greatest dose of UV radiation.

Although the exact initial dose used in each of the trial regimens varies drastically, topical PUVA should be administered at a lower dose than oral PUVA due to topical psoralen's greater tendency to burn [58]. The British Photodermatology Group recommends administering a lower dose of radiation (30–50 % MPD) with topical psoralen instead of the standard 70 % MPD with oral PUVA [58]. Similar energy reductions are observed in trials, which determined initial dosing based on skin type. In these trials, the maximum initial dose administered varied between 1 and 1.5 J/cm^2 and 4 and 4.5 J/cm^2 for topical and oral PUVA, respectively (see Table 32.1).

Most published studies, irrespective of the initial dosing approach, provided subsequent treatments two to five times per week with incremental dosage adjustments every one to three treatments until attaining the maximum dose. Dosage adjustments are based upon response to treatment. If erythema is noted, the dose is commonly altered in proportion to the erythema severity. For moderate and severe erythema, the dose is either held, decreased 20–30 %, or not administered until the next visit at a previous or lower dose.

In our practice, both NBUVB and bath PUVA (30-min soak time) are used for patients with CHD. These are typically started either twice or three times per week (with a minimum of 48 h in between treatments). The initial dose is generally determined by skin type (e.g., 70 mJ/cm^2 for NBUVB in Fitzpatrick skin type I patient), and dose increases are determined by response (e.g., 15 % increase at each session until 2,000 mJ is reached, and then increase by 10 % until 3,000 mJ is reached for NBUVB in a Fitzpatrick skin type I patient). Our practice employs specific guidelines in dealing with missed treatments and adverse response to treatments (e.g., erythema, pruritus) – these generally require holding phototherapy doses, skipping treatments, and/or decreasing phototherapy doses. Maintenance treatment occurs when the patient's skin is practically clear – the dose is usually held at the level at which the skin cleared, and the frequency of treatment is decreased. Minimum maintenance is once per every 6 weeks for bath PUVA and twice per week for NBUVB to prevent burning. If phototherapy is effective and the problem is persistent, we will occasionally complete paperwork to help patients obtain home hand/foot phototherapy units.

Conclusion

Phototherapy remains a very useful tool in the treatment of chronic hand dermatitis. UVA and the various UVB modalities of therapy may offer comparable clinical improvements to those of PUVA therapy. In the subset of hyperkeratotic CHD cases, oral 8-MOP PUVA or topical 8-MOP cream/gel PUVA may be preferred over bath PUVA. Similarly, NBUVB may not be the best modality for treating thick hyperkeratotic CHD due to lower penetrance to the deep epidermis and dermis than UVA radiation. However, the efficacy of NBUVB in hyperkeratotic CHD has not been investigated, rather only discussed as a justification for the exclusion of hyperkeratotic cases from an NBUVB trial citing the difference in wavelength skin penetration and lower response of hyperkeratotic CHD compared to other CHD subtypes in PUVA studies [35]. At present, PUVA remains the most investigated type of phototherapy and the standard for comparison. Home administration of oral PUVA and UVB offers similar therapeutic benefits to clinically administered therapy with less disruption of the patient's daily activities. Relapse rates are high for all phototherapy subtypes, but less frequent maintenance treatments may aid in sustaining prolonged clearance. Despite this high recurrence of symptoms, phototherapy is an important adjunctive therapy option for the management of CHD.

References

1. Roelandts R. The history of phototherapy: something new under the sun? J Am Acad Dermatol. 2002;46(6): 926–30.
2. Pacifico A, Leone G. Photo (chemo) therapy for vitiligo. Photodermatol Photoimmunol Photomed. 2011; 27(5):261–77.
3. Diepgen T, Agner T, Aberer W, Berth-Jones J, Cambazard F, Elsner P, et al. Management of chronic hand eczema. Contact Dermatitis. 2007;57(4):203–10.
4. van Coevorden A, Kamphof W, Sonderen E, Bruynzeel D, Coenraads P. Comparison of oral psoralen-UV-A with a portable tanning unit at home vs. hospital-administered bath psoralen-UV-A in patients with chronic hand eczema. Arch Dermatol. 2004;140(12):1463–6.
5. Sjovall P, Christensen O. Treatment of chronic hand eczema with UV-B Handylux in the clinic and at home. Contact Dermatitis. 1994;31(1):5–8.
6. WHO International Agency for Research on Cancer. IARC monographs on the evaluation of carcinogenic risks to humans [Internet]. 2012. Available from http://monographs.iarc.fr/ENG/Classification/index.php
7. de With A, Greulich K. Wavelength dependence of laser-induced DNA damage in lymphocytes observed by single-cell gel electrophoresis. J Photochem Photobiol B. 1995;30:71–6.
8. Archier E, Devaux S, Castela E, Gallini A, Aubin F, Le Maitre M. Carcinogenic risks of psoralen UV-A therapy and narrowband UV-B therapy in chronic plaque psoriasis: a systemic literature review. J Eur Acad Dermatol Venereol. 2012;26 Suppl 3:22–31.
9. Man I, Crombie I, Dawe R, Ibbotson S, Ferguson J. The photocarcinogenic risk of narrowband UVB (TL-01) phototherapy: early follow-up data. Br J Dermatol. 2005;152(4):755–7.
10. Flindt-Hansen H, McFadden N, Eeg-Larson T, Thune P. Effects of a new narrow-band UVB lamp on photocarcinogenesis in mice. Acta Derm Venereol. 1991;71(3):245–8.
11. Gibbs N, Traynor N, MacKie R, Campbell I, Johnson B, Ferguson J. The phototumorigenic potential of broad-band (270–250 nm) and narrow-band (311–313 nm) phototherapy sources cannot be predicted by their edematogenic potential in hairless mouse skin. J Invest Dermatol. 1995;104(3):359–63.
12. Grattan C, Carmichael A, Shuttleworth G, Foulds I. Comparison of topical PUVA with UVA for chronic vesicular hand eczema. Acta Derm Venereol. 1991;71(2):118–22.
13. Engin B, Oguz O. Evaluation of time-dependent response to psoralen plus UVA (PUVA) treatment with topical 8-methoxypsoralen (8-MOP) gel in palmoplantar dermatoses. Int J Dermatol. 2005;44(4):337–9.
14. Petering H, Breuer C, Herbst R, Kapp A, Werfel T. Comparison of localized high-dose UVA1 irradiation versus topical cream psoralen-UVA for treatment of chronic vesicular dyshidrotic eczema. J Am Acad Dermatol. 2004;50(1):68–72.
15. Polderman M, Govaert J, Cessie S, Pavel S. A double-blind placebo-controlled trial of UVA-1 in the treatment of dyshidrotic eczema. Clin Exp Dermatol. 2003;28(6):584–7.
16. Tuchinda C, Kerr H, Taylor C, Jacobe H, Bergamo B, Elmets C, et al. UVA1 phototherapy for cutaneous diseases: an experience of 92 cases in the United States. Photodermatol Photoimmunol Photomed. 2006;22(5):247–53.
17. Morison W, Parrish J, Fitzpatrick T. Oral methoxsalen photochemotherapy of recalcitrant dermatoses of the palms and soles. Br J Dermatol. 1978;99(3):297–302.
18. LeVine M, Parrish J, Fitzpatrick T. Oral methoxsalen photochemotherapy (PUVA) of dyshidrotic eczema. Acta Derm Venereol. 1981;61(6):570–1.
19. Tegner E, Thelin I. PUVA treatment of chronic eczematous dermatitis of the palms and soles. Acta Derm Venereol. 1985;65(5):451–3.
20. Hawk J, Grice P. The efficacy of localized PUVA therapy for chronic hand and foot dermatoses. Clin Exp Dermatol. 1994;19(6):479–82.
21. Tzameva S, Kittler H, Thallinger C, Honigsmann H, Tanew A. Oral vs. bath PUVA using 8-methoxypsoralen for chronic palmoplantar eczema. Photodermatol Photoimmunol Photomed. 2009;25(2):101–5.
22. Sheehan-Dare R, Goodfield M, Rowell N. Topical psoralen photochemotherapy (PUVA) and superficial radiotherapy in the treatment of chronic hand eczema. Br J Dermatol. 1989;121(1):65–9.
23. De Rie M, Van Eendenburg JP, Versnick A, Stolk L, Bos J, Westerhof W. A new psoralen-containing gel for topical PUVA therapy: development and treatment results in patients with palmoplantar and plaque-type psoriasis, and hyperkeratotic eczema. Br J Dermatol. 1995;132(6):964–9.
24. Schempp C, Muller H, Czech W, Schopf E, Simon J. Treatment of chronic palmoplantar eczema with local bath-PUVA therapy. J Am Acad Dermatol. 1997;36(5 Part I):733–7.
25. Gritiyarangsan P, Sukhum A, Tresukosol P, Kullavanijaya P. Topical PUVA therapy for chronic hand eczema. J Dermatol. 1998;25(5):299–301.
26. Davis M, McEvoy M, El-Azhary R. Topical psoralen-ultraviolet a therapy for palmoplantar dermatoses: experience with 35 consecutive patients. Mayo Clin Proc. 1998;73(5):407–11.
27. Shephard S, Schregenberger N, Dummer R, Panizzon R. Comparison of 8-MOP aqueous bath and 8-MOP ethanolic lotion (Meladinine) in local PUVA therapy. Dermatology. 1998;197(1):25–30.
28. Behrens S, von Kobyletzki G, Gruss C, Reuther T, Altmeyer P, Kerscher M. PUVA-bath photochemotherapy (PUVA-soak therapy) of recalcitrant dermatoses of the palms and soles. Photodermatol Photoimmunol Photomed. 1999;15(2):47–51.
29. Grundmann-Kollman M, Behrens S, Peter R, Kerscher M. Treatment of severe recalcitrant dermatoses of the

palms and soles with PUVA-bath versus PUVA-cream therapy. Photodermatol Photoimmunol Photomed. 1999;15(2):87–9.
30. Taylor C, Baron E. Hand and foot PUVA soaks: an audit of the Massachusetts General Hospital's experience from 1994 to 1998. Photodermatol Photoimmunol Photomed. 1999;15(5):188–92.
31. Schiener R, Gottlober P, Muller B, Williams S, Pillekamp H, Peter R, et al. PUVA-gel vs. PUVA-bath therapy for severe recalcitrant palmoplantar dermatoses A randomized, single-blinded prospective study. Photodermatol Photoimmunol Photomed. 2005;21(2): 62–7.
32. Rosen K, Mobacken H, Swanbeck G. Chronic eczematous dermatitis of the hands: a comparison of PUVA and UVB treatment. Acta Derm Venereol. 1987;67(1):48–54.
33. Simons J, Bohnen I, van der Valk P. A left-right comparison of UVB phototherapy and topical photochemotherapy in bilateral chronic hand dermatitis after 6 weeks' treatment. Clin Exp Dermatol. 1997;22(1):7–10.
34. Nordal E, Christensen O. Treatment of chronic hand dermatoses with UVB-TL01. Acta Derm Venereol. 2004;84(4):302–4.
35. Sezer E, Etikan I. Local narrowband UVB phototherapy vs. local PUVA in the treatment of chronic hand eczema. Photodermatol Photoimmunol Photomed. 2007;23(1):10–4.
36. Jensen L, Stensgaard A, Andersen K. Psoralen plus ultraviolet A (PUVA) soaks and UVB TL01 treatment for chronic hand dermatoses. Dermatol Rep. 2012;4(1):e3.
37. Aubin F, Vigan M, Puzenat E, Blanc D, Drobacheff C, Deprez P, et al. Evaluation of a novel 308-nm monochromatic excimer light delivery system in dermatology: a pilot study in different chronic localized dermatoses. Br J Dermatol. 2005;152(1): 99–103.
38. Beitner H. Clinical and experimental aspects of long-wave ultraviolet (UVA) irradiation of human skin. Acta Derm Venereol Suppl (Stockh). 1986;123:1–56.
39. Godar D. UVA1 radiation triggers two different final apoptotic pathways. J Invest Dermatol. 1999;112(1): 3–12.
40. Grabbe J, Wlker P, Humke S, Grewe M, Schopf E, Henz B, et al. High-dose ultraviolet A1 (UVA1), but not UVA/UVB therapy decreases IgE-binding cells in lesional skin of patients with atopic eczema. J Invest Dermatol. 1996;107(3):419–22.
41. Krutmann J. Phototherapy for atopic dermatitis. Clin Exp Dermatol. 2000;25(7):552–8.
42. Schmidt T, Abeck D, Boeck K, Mempel M, Ring J. UVA1 irradiation is effective in treatment of chronic vesicular dyshidrotic hand eczema. Acta Derm Venereol. 1998;78(4):318–9.
43. Bethea D, Fullmer B, Syed S, Seltzer G, Tiano J, Rischko C, et al. Psoralen photobiology and photochemotherapy: 50 years of science and medicine. J Dermatol Sci. 1999;19(2):78–88.
44. Behrens-Williams S, Gruss C, Grundmann-Kollmann M, Peter R, Kerscher M. Assessment of minimal phototoxic dose following 8-methoxypsoralen bath: maximal reaction on average after 5 days. Br J Dermatol. 2000;142(1):112–5.
45. Ibbotson S, Farr P. The time-course of psoralen ultraviolet A (PUVA) erythema. J Invest Dermatol. 1999;113(3):346–50.
46. FDA. Prescribing Information: 8-MOP Capsules [Internet]. 2012. Available from http://www.accessdata.fda.gov/drugsatfda_docs/label/2003/09048slr037_methoxsalen_lbl.pdf
47. Tanew A, Kipfelsperger T, Seeber A, Radakovic-Fijan S, Honigsmann H. Correlation between 8-methoxypsoralen bath-water concentration and photosensitivity in bath-PUVA treatment. J Am Acad Dermatol. 2001;44(4):638–42.
48. Grundmann-Kollman M, Leiter U, Behrens S, Gottlober P, Mooser G, Krahn G, et al. The time course of phototoxicity of topical PUVA: 8-methoxypsoralen cream-PUVA vs 8-methoxypsoralen gel-PUVA. Br J Dermatol. 1999;140(5):988–90.
49. Wainwright NJ, Mac Leod TM, Ferguson J. Bath PUVA – an investigation of the distribution of trioxsalen (TMP) and 8-methoxypsoralen (8-MOP) in bathwater. Photodermatol Photoimmunol Photomed. 1997;13(1–2):17–20.
50. Coleman W, Lowe N, David M, Halder R. Palmoplantar psoriasis: experience with 8-methoxypsoralen soaks plus ultraviolet A with the use of a high output metal halide. J Am Acad Dermatol. 1989;20:1078–82.
51. FDA. Drugs@FDA: FDA approved drugs [Internet] 2012. 8-MOP. Available from http://www.accessdata.fda.gov/scripts/cder/drugsatfda/index.cfm?fuseaction=Search.DrugDetailsTrisoralen. Available from: http://www.accessdata.fda.gov/scripts/cder/drugsatfda/index.cfm?fuseaction=Search.DrugDetails
52. Tzaneva S, Kittler H, Thallinger C, Honigsmann H, Tanew A. Oral vs. bath PUVA using 8-methoxypsoralen for chronic palmoplantar eczema. Photodermatol Photoimmunol Photomed. 2009;25(2):101–5.
53. Wakelin S, Maibach H, editors. Handbook of systemic drug treatment in dermatology. 1st ed. London: Manson Publishing; 2002. p. 196–200.
54. Park H, Lee M. Case of leukoderma punctata after topical PUVA treatment. Int J Dermatol. 2004;43(2): 138–9.
55. Jekler J, Larko O. UVB phototherapy of atopic dermatitis. Br J Dermatol. 1988;119(6):697–705.
56. Park K, Murase J. Ultraviolet B (UVB) phototherapy in the treatment of vitiligo. In: Park K, Murase J, editors. Vitiligo – management and therapy. New York: InTech; 2011. p. 69–79.
57. Parrish J, Jaenicke K. Action spectrum for phototherapy of psoriasis. J Invest Dermatol. 1981;76(5):359–62.
58. British Photodermatology Group guidelines for PUVA. Br J Dermatol. 1994;130(2):246–55.

Radiotherapy in the Treatment of Hand Eczema

33

Sarah Hannam, Michael R. Webster, and Rosemary L. Nixon

Contents

S. Hannam, M.B.B.S. • R.L. Nixon, B.Sc. (Hons), M.B.B.S., MPH, FACD, FAFOEM (✉)
Occupational Dermatology Research and Education Centre, Skin and Cancer Foundation, Inc, Level 1/80 Drummond Street, Carlton, Melbourne, VIC 3053, Australia
e-mail: sarahhan7@gmail.com; rnixon@occderm.asn.au

M.R. Webster, M.B.B.S., FACD
Radiotherapy Department, Skin and Cancer Foundation of Victoria, 80 Drummond St, Carlton, VIC 3053, Australia
e-mail: michaelrwebster@bigpond.com

33.1 Introduction

Low-dose external beam megavoltage radiotherapy has been used in the treatment of hand eczema for many years and is still used in the treatment of recalcitrant hand dermatitis today, although its use has declined over the years. This includes superficial x-ray, Grenz ray, and ultrasoft x-ray. Safe and effective use of these treatment modalities requires adequate training and knowledge of their special properties and risks. However, their use on localized areas of diseased skin may obviate the need for systemic therapy, with agents such as alitretinoin, acitretin, methotrexate, azathioprine, and cyclosporine all being associated with numerous side effects.

33.2 Background

Soon after the discovery of x-rays by Röentgen in the late nineteenth century, the therapeutic potential of radiation was discovered in the treatment of multiple benign inflammatory conditions [1]. By the 1950s, the use of radiation reduced considerably because of reports of its carcinogenic potential, as well as the development of alternative and more effective systemic and topical treatments, such as corticosteroids and phototherapy.

A. Alikhan et al. (eds.), *Textbook of Hand Eczema*,
DOI 10.1007/978-3-642-39546-8_33, © Springer-Verlag Berlin Heidelberg 2014

33.3 Basic Principles of Radiation Therapy

The basic unit of energy used in radiation therapy is the electron volt (eV): (103 eV = 1 keV, 106 eV = 1 MeV). The basic unit of radiation absorbed dose is known as the gray (Gy), which is the amount of energy absorbed per unit mass (kg), and has replaced the unit of rad (100 rads = 1 Gy) [2].

The quality of x-rays produced from an x-ray tube is also determined by any additional filtration to the beam that may be placed in its path. This is often described as half-value layer (HVL) of a certain material (usually aluminum – i.e., mm Al), that is, the thickness of material that reduces the amount of x-rays by 50 %. Grenz rays range from "soft" to "hard," with an HVL from up to 0.02 to 0.036 mm Al. Superficial x-ray radiation has an HVL of up to 0.7–2 mm Al [3].

33.3.1 Grenz Rays and Superficial X-Rays

In 1923, a German dermatologist, Gustav Bucky, developed a cathode vacuum tube that delivered ultrasoft/low energy x-rays in the form of long wavelength radiation. These became known as Grenz rays (Grenz translating to "border" in German), as he believed that their biological effects represented features bordering somewhere between ultraviolet light and traditional x-rays [4].

These are of low energy (<30 kV) and, thus, low skin penetration. Grenz rays are almost entirely absorbed within the first 2–3 mm of skin, with approximately 50 % of energy absorbed within the first 0.5 mm [3], limiting physiological effects mainly to the epidermis and superficial capillaries and sparing the reticular dermis [5]. Superficial x-rays are generated at 30–200 kV energy range and thus penetrate deeper. Both of these modalities are absorbed predominantly by the photoelectric effect, without a great deal of backscatter [6].

Because Grenz rays are significantly absorbed by air, the distance from which the tube is placed from the skin affects the quality of the beam; as a result, the machine must be calibrated specifically for the distance at which it is used for each individual. A cone may be used to help restrict exposure to the target areas and to ensure that this distance remains constant (usually approximately 10–20 cm) (Table 33.1).

Table 33.1 X-ray therapy voltage ranges

X-ray type	Voltage range
Grenz ray	<30 kV
Superficial x-ray (same as diagnostic x-ray)	30–150 kV
Orthovoltage x-ray	150–500 kV
Supervoltage x-ray	500–1,000 kV
Megavoltage x-ray	1–25 MV

33.4 Indications

33.4.1 Grenz Ray Therapy

Grenz ray therapy has been used in a variety of benign inflammatory skin conditions, where alternative therapies have been trialed and deemed unsuccessful or not tolerated:

- Hand eczema
- Allergic contact dermatitis
- Atopic dermatitis
- Psoriasis
- Palmoplantar pustulosis
- Mycosis fungoides
- Lichen planus
- Acne
- Hailey-Hailey disease
- Pruritus ani

33.4.2 Superficial X-Ray

Although superficial x-ray can be used for hand eczema, it is generally reserved for treatment of a variety of non-melanoma skin cancers (NMSC):

- Basal cell carcinoma (BCC)
- Squamous cell carcinoma (SCC)
- Cutaneous lymphomas
- Kaposi sarcoma
- Merkel cell carcinoma

33.5 Contraindications

Grenz rays and superficial x-rays should not be used in children or pregnant patients. Superficial x-rays in the treatment of cancer cannot be used in the same treatment area more than once. Although this is not the case for inflammatory skin conditions, repeated use is often limited due to risk of permanent skin changes.

33.6 Mechanism of Action

Although low-dose radiation therapy (LD-RT) has been documented clinically to exert an anti-inflammatory effect on benign disorders such as chronic hand eczema, the underlying cellular and molecular mechanisms are not yet fully identified. It is known that inflammatory diseases are due to multiple complex multicellular interactions, and it is thought that the effects of radiation also involve complex mechanisms, operating differentially at different dose levels [7, 8].

Grenz rays are thought to exert their predominant effect by reducing the number of Langerhans cells (dendritic lymphocytes) within the epidermis [9–13], which are responsible for the initiation of the innate and adaptive immune response, forming a major part of the immune system. Keratinocytes, stratum corneum, and other epidermal cells are thought to be unaffected [11, 12].

Other proposed immunomodulatory mechanisms of low-dose radiation have included hampered adhesion of peripheral blood mononuclear cells to the endothelium [14–16], a local increased rate of apoptosis [17, 18], modulation of cytokine expression [19], suppression of macrophage function [20, 21], and alteration of signal transduction pathways, DNA transcription, and repair [8, 10].

33.7 Equipment

Xstrahl (formerly Gulmay) makes Xstrahl 100 unit, which can provide superficial x-ray and Grenz ray. The unit can be set to give a number of x-ray qualities; at the Skin and Cancer Foundation, Victoria, the unit is set to deliver two ultrasoft qualities, HVL 0.033 mm Al and HVL0.047 mm Al, and three superficial ray qualities, HVL0.7 mm Al, HVL 1 mm Al, and 2 mm Al. It comes with a set of standard cones up to 15 cm in diameter, but custom cones can be made.

Progressus Medica AB makes new Grenz ray machines. The tube has a beryllium window that is 0.65 mm thick. Although the tube is rated for 50 kV, it operates at 9.95 kV. The unit has six cones, 1–12 cm in diameter. It produces Grenz rays only. These units are used extensively in Scandinavia.

Old units such as Philips Rt100 can be configured to deliver Grenz ray as well as superficial x-ray.

33.8 Delivery of Therapy

After an initial consultation to plan the treatment regimen and dose, the patient typically sits or lies on a treatment couch and the specifically calibrated Grenz ray machine is placed appropriately to direct radiation toward the affected area of skin. The trained operator should enforce strict radiation protection measures.

This procedure typically lasts no more than a few minutes and occurs on an outpatient basis, usually given over a number of sessions, based on the concept of fractionation, in which smaller, spaced-out doses ("fractions") of radiation, as opposed to the total dose at once, allow time for normal cells to heal and, as a result, improve clinical outcomes and reduce side effects. This biological explanation, which has been popularized in Sharma's textbook, refers to the "4 R's of radiobiology": repair of sublethal damage, reassortment (redistribution) of cells within the cell cycle, repopulation, and reoxygenation [2].

Therapeutic regimens for Grenz ray therapy generally include four to six treatments at 1–3-week intervals, with a 6-month rest between courses. Radiation dose should be adjusted for the treatment site's sensitivity to radiation as well as presence of hair on the skin. The palms, soles, and scalp are the least sensitive areas for irradiation, and it is generally recommended that they receive 2–4 Gy per treatment (fraction). Other sites generally tolerate 2 Gy, and a reduced dose of 0.5–2.0 Gy is recommended for the anogenital area. A maximal lifetime cumulative dose per treatment area is generally recommended up to 50–100 Gy [22, 23]. Nevertheless, there is relatively little published literature on this topic. Superficial x-ray treatment dose for benign inflammatory skin conditions is usually half to one quarter that of Grenz rays.

33.9 Clinical Effects

Multiple studies have assessed the effects of LD-RT in inflammatory skin conditions and specifically hand eczema. The majority of these have suggested at least some clinical improvement when treated with LD-RT [23–30]. Some, however, have shown minimal difference from placebo [31], particularly after 6 months [32]. It has been proposed, however, that even those who do not achieve a durable response to the radiation itself still experience a reduction in the severity and frequency of relapses of their symptoms [27].

In patients with allergic contact dermatitis to nickel, the application of Grenz rays has appeared to suppress the allergic response, as evidenced by a negative patch test in 83 % of patients in one study, lasting for 3 weeks posttreatment [33]. This suggests that Grenz rays inhibit the clinical expression of allergic contact dermatitis almost completely for a period of time. However, they have been found to have little effect on irritant contact dermatitis [34].

In some studies, conventional superficial x-rays have been shown to be superior to Grenz ray therapy in producing clinical improvement and patient satisfaction; however, as a result of deeper skin penetration, they have a limited ability to be repeated and carry an increased risk of carcinogenesis [24].

LD-RT has been shown to be efficacious in other inflammatory skin conditions, namely, psoriasis and specifically palmoplantar pustulosis, suggesting good clinical response from the radiation [35–38], and although recurrence was observed in these studies, so was a longer remission period compared to topical steroids alone [39].

Unfortunately, no study assessing the impacts of LD-RT on chronic eczema has followed patients long term, nor has patient selection criteria been identified, nor is there a standardized method for evaluating responses to treatments; thus, the validity of this form of therapy in clinical practice is unknown.

In regard to patient perception of the therapy, one study reported the patterns of use and perceived effectiveness of Grenz ray therapy in treating recalcitrant skin conditions at their center over a 10-year period. Approximately 64 % of patients reported decreased severity or clearing of disease and associated symptom relief, 54 % said the treatment was worthwhile and would choose it again, and 40 % reported mild side effects. In the subgroup of patients with a specific diagnosis of contact dermatitis (94 % with hand dermatitis), 64 % felt the treatment was worthwhile and 77 % indicated that they would choose this therapy again if needed [40]. A quality assurance analysis of a larger patient group over a 6-year period further supported these findings in 2011. One hundred fifty patients, of whom 35 % had hand dermatitis, responded to a standardized telephone questionnaire. This cohort described response to treatment as excellent (46.5 %), very good (21.3 %), and good (18.6 %), and approximately 50 % had more than 6 months' duration of response. Eighty-eight percent of patients reported that they would have the treatment again [41].

33.10 Side Effects

Side effects of LD-RT in the treatment of chronic hand eczema are relatively few and mild. No literature currently exists on the specific effects of low-dose radiation specifically to the hands.

Acute effects can include erythema, hyperpigmentation, mild burning sensation, and blistering. These are usually temporary, particularly with treatment involving low fractions. Overdose of radiation to the skin can lead to atrophy, telangiectasia, crusting, and erosions

[42]. Grenz ray erythema (usually requiring a dose of >3–4 Gy) has been shown to be inversely proportional to the thickness of the epidermis, particularly the stratum corneum [43], and has been shown to be reduced or inhibited by preceding treatment with application of hydrocortisone ointment [44]. However, concomitant application of any topical agents prior to treatment is not recommended.

Late side effects of LD-RT, more specifically superficial x-ray, include alopecia (>3–5 Gy), ongoing pigmentation changes, and chronic radiation dermatitis (>12 Gy). Perhaps the most important potential long-term consequence of any form of radiotherapy to consider is malignancy. The carcinogenic potential of Grenz rays was first reported in 1959, when a dermatologist developed an SCC on a finger after accidentally being exposed to high-dose Grenz irradiation [45]. This has been supported by further reports linking non-melanoma skin cancers to high-cumulative dose Grenz ray therapy [46, 47].

The carcinogenic effect of skin irradiation has been well documented in treatment of head and neck benign skin disease, both in the skin and other organs, such as thyroid, salivary gland, and brain [48, 49].

Multiple studies have been performed assessing the carcinogenic potential of LD-RT to the skin [44], including one large epidemiologic cancer linkage study [50] of over 14,000 patients treated with Grenz rays at the Karolinska Institutet with a mean follow-up of 15 years. This study found no significant increased incidence of melanoma, but a statistically significant increased incidence of SCC; however, the authors could not link this directly to Grenz ray treatment, as patients had been exposed to other known carcinogenic treatments, including tar, conventional x-rays, and immunosuppressive agents such as methotrexate and also UV light, which is often the case in refractory hand eczema. Additionally, the majority of these patients developed these lesions at sites that were not irradiated by Grenz therapy, and this subset of patients received lower-dose Grenz therapy than others in this cohort who remained cancer-free. As a result, it is widely concluded that while Grenz ray therapy cannot be excluded as a risk factor for the development of NMSC, the risk is small, if any [51].

Conclusion

Grenz rays, ultrasoft x-rays, and superficial x-rays are forms of ionizing radiation. Although labeled "unconventional" and somewhat controversial in many centers, these treatment modalities remain useful for the treatment of refractory benign dermatoses, including chronic hand eczema. The availability of new equipment now allows this treatment to be performed reliably and safely. Successful treatment and patient satisfaction relies on adequately educated and trained clinicians and technicians and patients counseled on the associated risks. There is, however, still a place for superficial radiation therapy, and when used appropriately, it can be safe and cost-effective and lead to good clinical outcomes in otherwise refractory chronic hand dermatitis. Further research into all aspects of treatment dosing; long-term impacts, including carcinogenic risk; and use in association with other treatment modalities is required to validate this currently underused treatment option.

References

1. Roentgen W. On a new kind of ray (first report) Munch Med Wochenschr 1959;101:1237–1239.
2. Sharma RA, Vallis KA, McKenna WG. Basics of radiation therapy. In: Abeloff MD, Armitage JO, Niederhuber JE, Kastan M, editors. Abeloff's clinical oncology. 4th ed. Philadelphia: Elsevier/Churchill Livingstone; 2008.
3. Warner JA, Cruz PD. Grenz ray therapy in the new millennium: still a valid treatment option? Dermatitis. 2008;19(2):73–80.
4. Bucky G. Grenz ray therapy. New York: Macmillan; 1929.
5. Olivo MP. Grenz ray treatment of benign skin diseases. In: Panizzon R, Cooper J, editors. Radiation treatment and radiation reactions in dermatology. Berlin: Springer; 2004.
6. Hollander MB. Ultrasoft x-rays, including Grenz rays. In: Goldschmidt H, editor. Physical modalities in dermatologic therapy. New York: Springer; 1978.

7. Marples B, Wouters BG, Collis SJ, Chalmers AJ, Joiner MC. Low-dose hyper- radiosensitivity: a consequence of ineffective cell cycle arrest of radiation-damaged G2-phase cells. Radiat Res. 2004; 161:247–55.
8. Rodel F, Frey B, Manda K, Hildebrandt G, Hehlgans S, Keilholz L, et al. Immunomodulatory properties and molecular effects in inflammatory diseases of low-dose X-irradiation. Front Oncol. 2012; 2(120):1–9.
9. Ek L, Lindelof B, Liden S. The duration of Grenz ray-induced suppression of allergic contact dermatitis and its correlation with the density of Langerhans cells in human epidermis. Clin Exp Dermatol. 1989;14: 206–9.
10. Jahns J, Anderegg U, Saalbach A, Rosin B, Patties I, Glasow A, et al. Influence of low dose irradiation on differentiation, maturation and T-cell activation of human dendritic cells. Mutat Res. 2011;709–710: 32–9.
11. Lindelof B, Linden C, Ros AM. Effect of Grenz rays on Langerhans' cells in human epidermis. Acta Derm Venereol. 1984;64:436.
12. Beitner H, Nakatani T, Lindelof B. An ultrastructural study of human epidermal Langerhans cells irradiated with Grenz rays and ultraviolet A. Photodermatol Photoimmunol Photomed. 1990;7:266–8.
13. Lindelof B, Forslind B. Electron microscopic observations of Langerhans' cells in human epidermis irradiated with Grenz rays. Photodermatology. 1985;2(6): 367–71.
14. Kern PM, Keilholz L, Forster C, Hallmann R, Herrmann M, Seegenschmiedt MH. Low-dose radiotherapy selectively reduces adhesion of peripheral blood mononuclear cells to endothelium in vitro. Radiother Oncol. 2000;54:273–82.
15. Hildebrandt G, Maggiorella L, Rödel F, Rödel V, Willis D, Trott KR. Mononuclear cell adhesion and cell adhesion molecule liberation after X-irradiation of activated endothelial cells in vitro. Int J Radiat Biol. 2002;78:315–25.
16. Rödel F, Kley N, Beuscher HU, Hildebrandt G, Keilholz L, Kern P, et al. Anti-inflammatory effect of low-dose X-irradiation and the involvement of a TGF-beta1- induced down-regulation of leukocyte/ endothelial cell adhesion. Int J Radiat Biol. 2002; 78:711–9.
17. Gaipl US, Meister S, Lödermann B, Rödel F, Fietkau R, Herrmann M, et al. Activation-induced cell death and total Akt content of granulocytes show a biphasic course after low- dose radiation. Autoimmunity. 2009;42:340–2.
18. Hengartner MO. The biochemistry of apoptosis. Nature. 2000;407:770–6.
19. Rodel F, Keilholz L, Herrmann M, Sauer R, Hildebrandt G. Radiobiological mechanisms in inflammatory diseases of low dose radiation therapy. Int J Radiat Biol. 2007;83(6):357–66.
20. Lödermann B, Wunderlich R, Frey S, Schorn C, Stangl S, Rödel F, et al. Low dose ionising radiation leads to a NF- kappaB dependent decreased secretion of active IL-1beta by activated macrophages with a discontinuous dose-dependency. Int J Radiat Biol. 2012;88(10):727–34.
21. Conrad S, Ritter S, Fournier C, Nixdorff K. Differential effects of irradiation with carbon ions and x-rays on macrophage function. J Radiat Res. 2009;50:223–31.
22. Jansen GT. Grenz rays: adequate or antiquated? J Dermatol Surg Oncol. 1978;4:67–9.
23. Lindelof B, Wrangsjo K, Liden S. A double-blind study of Grenz ray therapy in chronic eczema of the hands. Br J Dermatol. 1987;117:77–80.
24. Fairris GM, Jones DH, Mack DP, Rowell NR. Conventional superficial X ray versus Grenz ray therapy in the treatment of constitutional eczema of the hands. Br J Dermatol. 1985;112:339–41.
25. Lewis H. Grenz ray therapy: regimens and results. In: Goldschmidt H, editor. Physical modalities in dermatologic therapy. New York: Springer; 1978.
26. Hanfling S, Distelheim IH. Simultaneous symmetrical paired comparison method in evaluating results of Grenz ray and of X-ray therapy. J Inv Dermatol. 1951;16(1):65–70.
27. Duff M, Crutchfield 3rd CE, Moore J, Famick K, Potish RA, Gallego H. Radiation therapy for chronic vesicular hand dermatitis. Dermatitis. 2006;17(3):128–32.
28. Sumila M, Notter M, Itin P, Bodis S, Gruber G. Long-term results of radiotherapy in patients with chronic palmoplantar eczema or psoriasis. Strahlenther Onkol. 2008;4:218–23.
29. Sheehan-Dare RA, Goodfield MJ, Rowell NR. Topical psoralen photochemotherapy (PUVA) and superficial radiotherapy in the treatment of chronic hand eczema. Br J Dermatol. 1989;121:65–9.
30. Walling HW, Swick BL, Storrs FJ, Boddicker ME. Frictional hyperkeratotic hand dermatitis responding to Grenz ray therapy. Contact Dermatitis. 2008;58(1):49–51.
31. Cartwright PH, Rowell NR. Comparison of Grenz rays versus placebo in the treatment of chronic hand eczema. Br J Dermatol. 1987;117:73–6.
32. King CM, Chalmers RJG. A double blind study of superficial radiotherapy in chronic palmar eczema. Br J Dermatol. 1984;111:451–4.
33. Lindelof SL, Lagerholm B. The effect of Grenz rays on the expression of allergic contact dermatitis in man. Scand J Immunol. 1985;21:463–9.
34. Lindelof B, Lindberg M. The effect of Grenz rays on irritant skin reactions in man. Acta Derm Venereol. 1987;67:128–32.
35. Harber LC. Clinical evaluation of radiation therapy in psoriasis. Arch Dermatol. 1958;77:554–8.
36. Broderson I, Reymann F. Effect of Grenz rays on psoriasis treated with local corticosteroids. Dermatologica. 1981;162:327–9.

37. Lindelof B, Johannesson A. Psoriasis of the scalp treated with Grenz rays or topical corticosteroid combined with Grenz rays. A comparative randomized trial. Br J Dermatol. 1988;119:241–4.
38. Chalmers R, Hollis S, Leonardi-Bee J, Griffiths CEM, Marsland Bsc MRCP A. Interventions for chronic palmoplantar pustulosis. Cochrane Database of Systematic Reviews 2006, Issue 1. Art. No.: CD001433. DOI: 10.1002/14651858.CD001433.pub2.
39. Johannesson A, Lindelof B. Additional effect of Grenz rays on psoriasis lesions of the scalp treated with topical corticosteroids. Dermatologica. 1987; 175:290–2.
40. Schalock PC, Zug KA, Carter JC, Dhar D, MacKenzie T. Efficacy and patient perception of Grenz ray therapy in the treatment of dermatoses refractory to other medical therapy. Dermatitis. 2008;19(2):90–4.
41. Webster M. Quality assurance analysis of Grenz ray treatment at Skin and Cancer Foundation, Victoria. Aust J Dermatol. 2011;52 Suppl 1:1–40.
42. Laur W, Posey R, Waller J. Industrial Grenz ray overexposure report of a case. J Occup Med. 1978;20(2): 118–20.
43. Kalz F. Observations on Grenz ray reactions. Dermatologica. 1959;118:357–71.
44. Kalz F, Scott A. Inhibition of Grenz ray erythema by 1 single topical hormone application. J Inv Dermatol. 1956;26(3):165–8.
45. Frentz G. Grenz ray-induced nonmelanoma skin cancer. J Am Acad Dermatol. 1989;21(3 Pt 1):475–8.
46. Dabski K, StoU Jr HL. Skin cancer caused by Grenz rays. J Surg Oncol. 1986;31:87–93.
47. Mortensen AC, Kjeldsen H. Carcinomas following Grenz ray treatment of benign dermatoses. Acta Derm Venereol. 1987;67(6):523–5.
48. Paloyan E, Lawrence AM. Thyroid neoplasms after radiation therapy for adolescent acne vulgaris. Arch Dermatol. 1978;114(1):53–5.
49. Shore RE, Moseson M, Xue X, Tse Y, Harley N, Pasternack BS. Skin cancer after X-ray treatment for scalp ringworm. Radiat Res. 2002;157(4):410–8.
50. Lindelof B, Ekland G. Incidence of malignant skin tumors in 14,140 patients after Grenz ray treatment for benign skin disorders. Arch Dermatol. 1986;122:1391–5.
51. Hollander MB. Grenz rays. J Inv Dermatol. 1953; 21:15–26.

Treatment of Hand Eczema Caused by Hyperhidrosis

34

Majken G. Hougaard and Jacob P. Thyssen

Contents

M.G. Hougaard, M.D. (✉)
J.P. Thyssen, M.D., Ph.D., DmSci
The National Research Centre for Allergy, University Hospital Gentofte, Niels Andersens Vej 65DK-2900, Gentofte, Denmark
e-mail: majken.gabriel.hougaard@regionh.dk; jacob.p.thyssen@regionh.dk

34.1 Introduction

Hippocrates used the term "hidroa" for sweating, which was translated from Greek into Latin and English as sudamina. Both terms are used in modern day language as hidrosis and sudomotor function [1]. The main function of sweating is thermoregulation, which is achieved by evaporation of sweat. Perspiration exceeding physiological and environmental needs is termed hyperhidrosis. The degree of sweating in hyperhidrosis is variable, ranging from moderate moisture of the skin to severe dripping [2]. Hyperhidrosis is classified as general, involving the entire body surface, or focal, confined to one or more body areas, most often involving the palms (palmar hyperhidrosis), the soles of the feet (plantar hyperhidrosis), the arm pits (axillary hyperhidrosis), or the face (craniofacial hyperhidrosis). Several rare forms of focal hyperhidrosis occur with specific syndromes (e.g., Ross syndrome, Frey syndrome, and localized unilateral hyperhidrosis [LUH]).

Hyperhidrosis can be categorized according to the stimuli that trigger sweating. Emotional sweating (mental or sensory hyperhidrosis) originates from a cortical reflex (e.g., gustatory sweating, medullary origin), thermoregulatory sweating (hypothalamic origin), hyperhidrosis following spinal cord injury, disease, or transection (spinal origin); and local sweating (axonal reflex).

Hyperhidrosis may develop secondary to other medical conditions, such as drug abuse,

A. Alikhan et al. (eds.), *Textbook of Hand Eczema*,
DOI 10.1007/978-3-642-39546-8_34, © Springer-Verlag Berlin Heidelberg 2014

neurological, endocrine, infectious, or malignant disorders, or it may be primary or cryptogenic, with no apparent underlying cause. The focus of this chapter will be mainly on primary palmar hyperhidrosis, but keep in mind that generalized hyperhidrosis and palmoplantar hyperhidrosis can also affect the palms.

34.2 Hyperhidrosis and Hand Eczema

Excessive sweating of the palms results in chronic exposure to water, and, though not frequently, this may lead to the development of irritant contact eczema of the hands. Furthermore, some of the treatment modalities of hyperhidrosis, such as topical antiperspirants, iontophoresis, and sympathetic denervation, have hand eczema as an adverse effect because the skin is exposed to irritants and water. Hyperhidrosis may also increase the risk of allergic contact dermatitis of the hands to allergens such as metals, as metal ions are readily released from metallic items upon contact with sweat [3, 4]. Individuals with excessive sweating on the hands that causes metals to corrode are sometimes referred to as "rusters." The corrosion is caused by hyperhidrosis and not by elevated levels of sodium chloride concentrations [3]. Corrosion, and probably allergic contact dermatitis, can be limited by increasing copper concentrations in the alloy and by topical application of aluminum chloride hexahydrate in a 25 % solution in absolute ethyl alcohol [3].

Hyperhidrosis may also increase the risk of skin infections [5]. This is most likely due to increased skin moisture and may in some cases worsen preexisting hand eczema. A relationship between hyperhidrosis and atopic eczema has anecdotally been suggested [6].

34.3 Epidemiology of Hyperhidrosis

Hyperhidrosis is a relatively common disorder. The prevalence of the disease varies geographically. While 2.9 % of Americans suffer from primary focal hyperhidrosis [7], only 1 % of Israeli adolescents are affected [8]. The average age of onset of focal hyperhidrosis is 18–25 years [5, 7], but varies for the different body areas affected. Average age of onset for palmar hyperhidrosis is 13 years [7], and up to 82 % of patients with palmar hyperhidrosis appear to have childhood onset [7]. Men and women are equally affected by the condition [7, 9]. About 30–65 % of patients suffering from hyperhidrosis have a positive family history [10], which suggests a genetic predisposition [2]. One study suggested that genetic loci on chromosome 14 (locus 14q11.2-q13) were associated with the development of primary focal hyperhidrosis [11]. The genetic factor seems to be inherited in an autosomal dominant manner with a variable penetrance [12].

34.4 Pathophysiology of Hyperhidrosis

The nature of hyperhidrosis is complex and poorly understood. A feature common to the various types of hyperhidrosis is dysfunction and overstimulation of the sympathetic nervous system due to a deficiency in the hypothalamus limiting the regulatory feedback to peripheral thermoreceptors [13].

The human body contains about four to five million sweat glands, of which two-thirds are eccrine and the remaining apocrine or apoeccrine. Eccrine glands are distributed ubiquitously over the body surface, but the highest density is found in the soles and the forehead, followed by the palms and cheeks. They secrete an isotonic, odorless, clear fluid during thermoregulation. The apocrine glands, which are localized in the axillae, areola mammae, and perineum as of puberty, secrete a viscous liquid, which, owing to bacterial growth, has an unpleasant scent [14]. These glands are not involved in the pathogenesis of hyperhidrosis. The eccrine sweat glands are innervated by the sympathetic nervous system but utilize acetylcholine as the primary neurotransmitter. Ultimately, they are regulated by the thermoregulatory center in the preoptic area of the hypothalamus. No qualitative or quantitative histopathological changes have been found in the glands of patients with focal hyperhidrosis. Both physical and emotional stress are well-known exacerbating factors [5]. The excessive sweating in hyperhidrosis does not occur during sleep, indicating that emotional stimuli play an important role. However, hyperhidrosis is not considered to be an emotional disorder. Recently, a role of nitric oxide (NO) in the pathophysiology of primary focal hyperhidrosis was proposed [15]. Hyperhidrosis patients were found to have higher plasma values of NO when compared to healthy controls. NO synthase is found in eccrine glands [16], where it may act as a neurotransmitter or induce local vasodilatation, leading to excessive sweating [15].

34.5 Diagnosing Primary Palmar Hyperhidrosis

Patients with primary palmar hyperhidrosis complain of bilateral excessive sweating of the hands. The criteria for excessive sweating depend on location and gender. Although no standard definition for excessive sweat production exists, <1 mL/m^2 of sweat production per minute by eccrine sweat glands at rest in room temperature is considered normal [17]. For practical reasons, any degree of sweat production interfering negatively with daily activities should be viewed as abnormal. Although most cases of hyperhidrosis are idiopathic, health-care providers should consider that patients may have secondary hyperhidrosis due to malignancy, medication, infections, as well as endocrine and neurological disorders.

A diagnosis of primary palmar hyperhidrosis is based on the criteria according to Hornberg et al. [18].

Excessive visible sweating of the palms of at least 6 months' duration without apparent causes, plus a minimum of two of the following additional criteria:

- Bilateral and relatively symmetric sweating of the palms
- Frequency of at least one episode weekly
- Age of onset less than 25 years
- Positive family history
- Impairment of daily activities
- Cessation of focal sweating during sleep
- No evidence of underlying causes by history and physical examinations

34.6 Objective and Subjective Measures for Assessment of Hyperhidrosis

History and clinical examination are usually sufficient for diagnosing primary palmar hyperhidrosis, making additional testing unnecessary [18]. However, the Minor's starch iodine test and gravimetry can be used to assess the localization and quantity of excessive sweating. These tests quantifying sweat production are not routinely used in clinical practice, but are typically used for clinical research purposes. However, they may be helpful in establishing the diagnosis or directing therapy in selected patients. The degree of interference on quality of life can be assessed by different validated questionnaires, such as the Hyperhidrosis Impact Questionnaire (HHIQ), Dermatology Life Quality Index (DLQI), and the Hyperhidrosis Disease Severity Scale (HDSS).

34.6.1 Minor's Starch Iodine Test

The Minor's starch iodine test is often useful in assessing focal hyperhidrosis and to map areas of excessive sweating prior to the injection of botulinum toxin A (BTX-A) or local surgery. The skin is cleaned and dried, after which 3.5 % iodine in alcohol solution is applied to the affected surface. Starch flour is powdered after drying of the skin. The powder changes color to a dark-blue/violet tone as sweat comes into contact with the iodine-starch mixture. This indicates a positive sweat test and yields a diagram of the distribution of active eccrine glands.

34.6.2 Gravimetry

The "gold standard" of objective measurement of hyperhidrosis is gravimetry, most commonly used to assess axillary hyperhidrosis. Filter paper is weighed before and after exposure to the axillary skin for a defined period of time (60 s or 5 min). The weight difference quantifies the amount of sweat produced. Axillary hyperhidrosis is often defined as >50 mL/min.

The disadvantage of gravimetric measurements is that sweat production can vary over time and differ between patients and that there is no clearly established threshold level for severity with this method [19]. Results from the Minor's starch iodine test and gravimetry can be combined to assess the amount of sweating in 1 mg/cm^2 [20].

34.6.3 Pad Gloves

Bearing a resemblance to gravimetry, but intended for palmar hyperhidrosis, gloves made of gauze material and surgical gloves are prepared and weighed on an electronic scale. The patient puts on the pad gloves followed by the surgical gloves. After a defined period of time, the gloves are carefully removed, to avoid sweat evaporation, and immediately re-weighted [21]. Differences in initial and final measurements are noted in terms of gram per hour for sweat intensity of the hands [22].

34.6.4 Questionnaires

Hyperhidrosis is known to affect quality of life in a very negative way and has a significant impact on physical, social, professional, and daily activities [19, 23]. Measuring the functional limitations and health-related quality of life of patients with primary focal hyperhidrosis is important for clinicians in determining the need for treatment, the effectiveness of treatment, and informing patients about the expectations of treatments.

The Hyperhidrosis Impact Questionnaire (HHIQ) is a 41-item questionnaire used to assess hyperhidrosis characteristics, use of medical resources, and functional limitations in daily activities.

The Dermatology Life Quality Index (DLQI) is a dermatology-specific health-related quality of life (HRQOL) questionnaire. It is a reliable and validated 10-item questionnaire that is widely used to measure the effects of dermatological diseases on HRQOL [24].

The Hyperhidrosis Disease Severity Scale (HDSS) is another measure used to evaluate the effect of hyperhidrosis on the patient's life by quantifying the patient's symptoms on a 1-to-4 scale. A score of 1 or 2 indicates mild to moderate hyperhidrosis; 3 or 4 indicates severe hyperhidrosis.

34.7 Treatment of Primary Palmar Hyperhidrosis

In some patients, reassurance and explanation of the nature of the disorder are the only treatment required. In other patients, primary focal hyperhidrosis is a disabling condition, causing psychological stress and facilitating allergic and irritant contact dermatitis and/or cutaneous infections such as warts, dermatophytosis, and pitted keratolysis [5] and, therefore, requires treatment.

Since the underlying causes of hyperhidrosis remain partly unknown, most treatments only provide symptomatic relief. Different treatment modalities for primary focal hyperhidrosis were recently reviewed [13]. A critical analysis was performed according to the Oxford Centre for Evidence-Based Medicine (OCEBM) Levels of Evidence Working Group, designated as the Oxford 2011 level of evidence [25]. Results for primary palmar hyperhidrosis are presented in Table 34.1.

34.7.1 Topical Antiperspirants

Local treatment with aluminum salts is inexpensive, effective, and convenient and should be considered as first line of therapy for patients with mild primary palmar hyperhidrosis. Aluminum chloride hexahydrate is believed to temporarily block the epidermal ducts of the eccrine glands and induces atrophy and vacuolization at the level of the glandular secretory cell [13]. In addition, aluminum chloride hexahydrate induces necrosis of the cells lining the

Table 34.1 Current surgical and nonsurgical treatment options in a step-by-step approach for primary palmar hyperhidrosis

	Step 1	Step 2	Step 3	Step 4	Step 5
Palmar hyperhidrosis	Topical aluminum chloride hexahydrate 15–20 % (35 %) in ethyl alcohol (L2), salicylic acid gel (L3), or thermophobic foam (L3)	Iontophoresis, 15–20 mA, 20–30 min, TWI (L2), anticholinergics (L2), BTX-A (L3), dry type (L3)	Systemic anticholinergics (L2)	BTX-A injections (L2)	Sympathetic denervation (L2)

Adapted from Hoorens and Ongenae [13] , with permission from John Wiley and Sons

BTX-A botulinum toxin A, *TWI* tap water iontophoresis, *L* level of evidence according to the Oxford Centre for Evidence-Based Medicine 2011 [25], *L1* systematic review of randomized trials or n of trials, *L2* randomized trial or observational study with dramatic effect, *L3* nonrandomized, controlled cohort/follow-up study, *L4* case-series, case – control studies, or historically controlled studies, *L5* mechanism-based reasoning

glandular ducts [26]. An initial concentration of 10–12 % aluminum chloride hexahydrate in alcohol or salicylic acid gel may be tried to minimize irritation, although a 25 % solution is required to achieve euhidrosis in most patients. Unlike ethyl alcohol, salicylic acid does not affect skin hydration. In addition, salicylic acid gel has antiperspirant and keratolytic qualities that improve the absorption of aluminum chloride hexahydrate in hyperkeratotic skin [27, 28]. For hairy skin, a vehicle of 20 % aluminum sesquichlorohydrate thermophobic foam can be used to increase patient compliance. This formulation is also less irritating to the skin than an alcohol-based solution [29]. The main side effects of aluminum chloride hexahydrate treatment are local skin irritation accompanied by burning and stinging sensations. To minimize irritation, aluminum chloride salts should be applied to dry palms at bedtime and washed off after 6–8 h. Aluminum chloride is applied every 24–48 h until euhidrosis is achieved. Maintenance therapy is typically required once every 1–3 weeks. Skin irritation can be limited by reducing the frequency of application or by using weak topical corticosteroids [18]. Another notable disadvantage of treatment with aluminum salts is the short duration of the effect. Upon cessation, the condition reverts to near baseline state after 1 week [30].

34.7.2 Topical Methenamine

Methenamine is a polycyclic organic compound that releases ammonia and formaldehyde at acidic pH [31]. It can be used as a topical agent in the treatment of palmar hyperhidrosis [31–33]. The resultant anhidrosis is caused by precipitated protein plugs in the sweat duct [33]. No systemic absorption of formaldehyde has been documented.

34.7.3 Topical Anticholinergics

Treatment with topical anticholinergics such as glycopyrronium bromide (glycopyrrolate) in aqueous solution or cream preparation is primarily used for craniofacial hyperhidrosis [34, 35] and only infrequently for palmar hyperhidrosis. Interested readers can refer to Kavanagh et al. [35].

34.7.4 Iontophoresis

Iontophoresis is a method in which an electric current is passed through the tissue. It is a safe, effective, and noninvasive treatment for palmar hyperhidrosis and should be considered second-line treatment for primary palmar hyperhidrosis [13]. The inhibiting effects on sweating of iontophoresis were reported in 1938 by Ichihachi et al., and its clinical use was established in the 1960s [36].

Iontophoresis is traditionally performed with tap water, but can also be performed with anticholinergics, such as glycopyrronium bromide [37] and BTX-A [38–40] and recently also proposed as a dry type [41].

34.7.4.1 Tap Water Iontophoresis

The mechanism of action is not yet clear. It has been proposed that accumulation of hydrogen ions in glandular ducts, generated by hydrolysis of water in the anodal bath, leads to destructive changes in the eccrine glands [42]. However, when examining the glands of treated patients with an electron microscope, no structural changes are noted [43]. When performing the procedure, the patients' hands are placed in two separate reservoirs of tap water and an electrical current is directed through the water to the skin. Direct current (DC) is usually used, with each palm being treated for 20–30 min with 15–20 mA, initially three to four times per week. Once euhidrosis is achieved, maintenance treatment once a week or even once a month is sufficient. The main side effect of tap water iontophoresis is sensation of pins and needles, vesicles, papules, skin irritation, and excessive xerosis.

34.7.4.2 Administration of Anticholinergics Through Iontophoresis

Anticholinergics such as glycopyrronium bromide [37] and poldine methylsulfate [44] can also be administrated to the affected hands through iontophoresis and have been shown to be more effective than tap water iontophoresis [45, 46]. Systemic side effects such as dry mouth and throat, constipation, and urinary retention are common. In a recent report of patients treated for primary palmar hyperhidrosis, 45 % experienced dermatitis of the hands and 18 % develop vesiculation of the hands as an adverse effect to the treatment [37].

34.7.4.3 Administration of Botulinum Toxin A Through Iontophoresis

The BTX-A is a neurotoxin derived from *Clostridium botulinum*. It temporarily inhibits the release of acetylcholine from skeletal and autonomic cholinergic terminal nerve endings, preventing hyperstimulation of sweat glands and thus excessive sweating [47]. Several studies have investigated the effect of administered BTX-A through iontophoresis on palmar hyperhidrosis [38–40]. A quick reduction in sweating lasting up to 3 months has been reported. Administration of BTX-A with iontophoresis instead of injections is favorable because it is much less painful. Loss of muscle strength, a typical side effect of BTX-A injections, has not been observed using this modality [38]. At the moment, the role of BTX-A delivered through iontophoresis looks promising, but further studies should be performed to clarify the standard procedure for performing this treatment. Also, the costs should be considered.

34.7.4.4 Dry-Type Iontophoresis

In 2007 a new dry-type form of performing iontophoresis was proposed [41] and showed effects similar to that of tap water iontophoresis. The method basically utilizes the same mechanism as in tap water iontophoresis, but the conductive solution comprises the patient's own sweat production. The cylindrical dry-type iontophoretic device consists of a central insulating plastic tube and double-helix stainless wires directly connected with a current. The advantage of this method is that it enables the patient to administer treatment while performing other daily activities, such as jogging or watching TV. The results of the study are complemented by another study from 2011, in which conductive pads were applied to the volar side of the patient's wrists. This study reported immediate reduction in sweat production confirmed by the Minor starch iodine test [48]. The dry-type iontophoresis has at the moment only been proposed by one group [41], and a direct comparison of tap water iontophoresis is thus far lacking.

34.7.5 Systemic Anticholinergics

Systemic anticholinergics such as oxybutynin [49, 50], methantheline bromide [51, 52], and glycopyrronium bromide (glycopyrrolate) [53, 54] inhibit perspiration by antagonism of acetylcholine at the muscarinic receptors near the eccrine glands. Since muscarinic receptors are also present in the central and autonomic nervous system, the effects of anticholinergics are not limited to sweat glands. At least five subtypes of muscarinic receptors have been identified (M1–M5) [54]: M1 and M4 receptors are found predominantly in the neuronal tissue, M2 in the heart, M3 in glandular tissue, and the M5 receptors regulate cerebral blood flow. The use of anticholinergics in the treatment of hyperhidrosis is often limited by dose-dependent side effects [53, 54]. Common side effects include xerostomia, fatigue, urinary retention, erectile dysfunction, mydriasis, tachycardia, and constipation. Treatment of both focal and generalized hyperhidroses with anticholinergics has been described in several case reports, but not until recently tested in larger randomized controlled clinical trials [52, 55]. Glycopyrrolate might cause fewer side effects than the other anticholinergics [54], perhaps due to a highly polar quaternary ammonium group, which limits its passage across lipid membranes such as the blood – brain barrier and may be even the heart [54]. While a treatment success rate of about 53–63 % has been reported [54, 56], treatment-limiting adverse effects affect about 22–29 % [53, 54]. A total dose of 1–2 mg once or twice daily is sufficient in most patients to achieve symptom control [53, 54, 56], but it is the authors' experience that anticholinergics are often insufficient. Methantheline bromide, also containing a quaternary ammonium group, was recently tested in a multicenter randomized, double-blinded controlled trial [52] on 339 patients with axillary and/or palmar hyperhidrosis. The patients received 3×50 mg methantheline bromide daily or placebo, and the effects were assessed objectively and subjectively. The treatment showed a significant effect on axillary hyperhidrosis, while the treatment on palmar hyperhidrosis was less visible. The most frequent side effect was xerostomia, which was reported by almost 69 % (88/128) treated with methantheline. Oxybutynin is an antagonist of the muscarinic receptor M3 and is also thought to have fewer side effects than other anticholinergics. A prospective randomized, controlled study of 50 patients with palmar hyperhidrosis showed improvement in >70 % in patients receiving oxybutynin [55]. Frequency of side effects such as xerostomia was 47.8 % [55]. A dosage of 2.5–10 mg/day is usually recommended [55, 57, 58]. Systemic treatment of anticholinergics should be considered if topical treatment with aluminum salts and iontophoresis has proven unsuccessful. Therapy can be administered as monotherapy or in combination with other therapies. Further research is needed on the performance of commercially available anticholinergics to provide advice on which anticholinergic agent to select. Descriptions of other forms of systemic treatment, such as oral antiadrenergics (clonidine), have been sparse. Hence, information is limited to studies on generalized or craniofacial hyperhidrosis [56]. Further studies on the effects of antiadrenergic treatment on palmar hyperhidrosis are warranted.

34.7.6 Injections of Botulinum Toxin Type A

Studies have demonstrated BTX-A injections to be effective in treating palmar hyperhidrosis [59, 60]. Typically, 1 mL of saline is mixed for every 25 U of BTX-A [61]. In general, 60–100 U of BTX-A are injected into each palm [62]. The cumulative dose should not exceed 360 U during a 3-month period [61]. The injection field can be defined as a grid on the palm, and injections are placed subdermally or intradermally into each 1-cm square area of the palm and at three sites in the digits [59]. No compensatory sweating has been reported [50], but recurrent sweating of the treated area has occurred and can be treated with reinjections. The duration of the effect of the treatment is usually about 6–12 months [62]. Treatment with injections of BTX-A is costly and painful. It should only be considered when other less invasive treatment options have failed. The main side effects include muscle weakness, which is often transient, lasting a few weeks after injections, and hematomas at injection sites. Owing to the rich nerve endings in the palms and the digits, many patients associate the procedure with pain. This can be reduced by various measures, such as oral or intravenous sedation, topical lidocaine, nerve blocks, or cryoanalgesia.

34.7.7 Sympathetic Denervation/ Video-Assisted Thoracic Surgery (VATS)

Surgical interruption (sympathotomy) or surgical removal (sympathectomy) of the thoracic ganglia on the upper sympathetic chain (ganglions T2 to T4) running alongside the spine leads to sympathetic denervation of the eccrine glands of the palms and thereby termination of excessive sweating in this area. Surgery is the most invasive of therapeutic options and should only be considered for patients with moderate to severe hyperhidrosis who have not responded to medical treatment options and where treatment is warranted. The procedure is performed under general anesthesia. Pneumothorax is induced and an operating endoscope inserted into the thorax via a small axillary incision, allowing visualization of the sympathetic trunk. The sympathetic chain can either be removed by resection or cauterization (sympathectomy), or interrupted by transection or clipping (sympathotomy) [63]. The procedure can be performed on different levels, depending on localization of the affected area and the patient's demands. Generally, the larger the segment interrupted or removed, the higher the risk of compensatory sweating [63]. The overall success rate of the different forms of the operation is 95–99 % in patients with palmar hyperhidrosis [64, 65]. Like any type of surgery, the procedure is subject to risks and potential side effects. The most common side effect is compensatory sweating in another body area, bradycardia, gustatory sweating, and Horner's syndrome [63]. Postoperative Horner's syndrome is due to direct or indirect damage of the stellate ganglion [66]. Compensatory sweating occurs in 50.5–86 % [64, 67–69]. Severe compensatory sweating is reported in 1–2 % [68]. Excessively dry palms leading to irritant eczema after surgical denervation has been reported [70].

Conclusion

This chapter provides an update on the relationship between hyperhidrosis and hand eczema and summarizes different treatment modalities for primary palmar hyperhidrosis.

Hyperhidrosis of the palms can be a cofactor for hand eczema. The excessive sweating of the palms can facilitate the development of allergic contact dermatitis or act in concert with irritants in the development of irritant contact dermatitis. Hand eczema may also be an adverse effect of the treatment of palmar hyperhidrosis.

Decisions on available treatments should be made in consultation with the patient and take into account the severity of the disease. The decision process should be performed in a step-wise manner, and less invasive treatment modalities should be chosen first. The first step is usually application of topical antiperspirants or methenamine, followed by iontophoresis, systemic anticholinergics, botulinum toxin A injections, and, finally, surgical denervation of the thoracic sympathetic chain.

References

1. Renbourn ET. The history of sweat and the sweat rash from earliest times to the end of the 18th century. J Hist Med Allied Sci. 1959;14(2):202–27.
2. Ro KM, Cantor RM, Lange KL, Ahn SS. Palmar hyperhidrosis: evidence of genetic transmission. J Vasc Surg. 2002;35(2):382–6.
3. Jensen O. 'Rusters'. The corrosive action of palmar sweat: I. Sodium chloride in sweat. Acta Derm Venereol. 1979;59(2):135–8.
4. Jensen O, Nielsen E. "Rusters". The corrosive action of palmar sweat: II. Physical and chemical factors in palmar hyperhidrosis. Acta Derm Venereol. 1979; 59(2):139–43.
5. Walling HW. Primary hyperhidrosis increases the risk of cutaneous infection: a case – control study of 387 patients. J Am Acad Dermatol. 2009;61(2):242–6.
6. Lee HJ, Ha SJ, Ahn WK, Kim D, Park YM, Byun DG, et al. Clinical evaluation of atopic hand-foot dermatitis. Pediatr Dermatol. 2001;18(2):102–6.

7. Strutton DR, Kowalski JW, Glaser DA, Stang PE. US prevalence of hyperhidrosis and impact on individuals with axillary hyperhidrosis: results from a national survey. J Am Acad Dermatol. 2004;51(2):241–8.
8. Adar R, Kurchin A, Zweig A, Mozes M. Palmar hyperhidrosis and its surgical treatment: a report of 100 cases. Ann Surg. 1977;186(1):34–41.
9. Hashmonai M, Kopelman D, Assalia A. The treatment of primary palmar hyperhidrosis: a review. Surg Today. 2000;30(3):211–8.
10. Lear W, Kessler E, Solish N, Glaser DA. An epidemiological study of hyperhidrosis. Dermatol Surg. 2007;33(1 Spec No):S69–75.
11. Higashimoto I, Yoshiura K, Hirakawa N, Higashimoto K, Soejima H, Totoki T, et al. Primary palmar hyperhidrosis locus maps to 14q11.2-q13. Am J Med Genet A. 2006;140(6):567–72.
12. Kaufmann H, Saadia D, Polin C, Hague S, Singleton A, Singleton A. Primary hyperhidrosis – evidence for autosomal dominant inheritance. Clin Auton Res. 2003;13(2):96–8.
13. Hoorens I, Ongenae K. Primary focal hyperhidrosis: current treatment options and a step-by-step approach. J Eur Acad Dermatol Venereol. 2012;26(1):1–8.
14. Kippenberger S, Havlicek J, Bernd A, Thaci D, Kaufmann R, Meissner M. "Nosing Around" the human skin: what information is concealed in skin odour? Exp Dermatol. 2012;21(9):655–9.
15. Karaca S, Kulac M, Uz E, Barutcu I, Yilmaz HR. Is nitric oxide involved in the pathophysiology of essential hyperhidrosis? Int J Dermatol. 2007;46(10):1027–30.
16. Shimizu Y, Sakai M, Umemura Y, Ueda H. Expression of endothelial nitric oxide synthase in human eccrine clear cells. Br J Dermatol. 1997;136(4):572–4.
17. Sato K, Kang WH, Saga K, Sato KT. Biology of sweat glands and their disorders. I. Normal sweat gland function. J Am Acad Dermatol. 1989;20(4):537–63.
18. Hornberger J, Grimes K, Naumann M, Glaser DA, Lowe NJ, Naver H, et al. Recognition, diagnosis, and treatment of primary focal hyperhidrosis. J Am Acad Dermatol. 2004;51(2):274–86.
19. Hamm H, Naumann MK, Kowalski JW, Kutt S, Kozma C, Teale C. Primary focal hyperhidrosis: disease characteristics and functional impairment. Dermatology. 2006;212(4):343–53.
20. Bahmer FA, Sachse MM. Hyperhidrosis area and severity index. Dermatol Surg. 2008;34(12):1744–5.
21. Ambrogi V, Campione E, Mineo D, Paterno EJ, Pompeo E, Mineo TC. Bilateral thoracoscopic T2 to T3 sympathectomy versus botulinum injection in palmar hyperhidrosis. Ann Thorac Surg. 2009;88(1):238–45.
22. Aydemir EH, Kalkan MT, Karakoc Y. Quantitative effect of anodal current in the treatment of primary hyperhidrosis by direct electrical current. Int J Dermatol. 2006;45(7):862–4.
23. Amir M, Arish A, Weinstein Y, Pfeffer M, Levy Y. Impairment in quality of life among patients seeking surgery for hyperhidrosis (excessive sweating): preliminary results. Isr J Psychiatry Relat Sci. 2000;37(1):25–31.
24. Finlay AY. Quality of life measurement in dermatology: a practical guide. Br J Dermatol. 1997;136(3):305–14.
25. OCEBM. The Oxford 2011 level of evidence. www.cebm.net/index.aspx?o=5653. 2012. 9-6-2012. Ref Type: Online Source
26. Holzle E, Braun-Falco O. Structural changes in axillary eccrine glands following long-term treatment with aluminium chloride hexahydrate solution. Br J Dermatol. 1984;110(4):399–403.
27. Benohanian A, Dansereau A, Bolduc C, Bloom E. Localized hyperhidrosis treated with aluminum chloride in a salicylic acid gel base. Int J Dermatol. 1998;37(9):701–3.
28. Flanagan KH, Glaser DA. An open-label trial of the efficacy of 15 % aluminum chloride in 2 % salicylic acid gel base in the treatment of moderate-to-severe primary axillary hyperhidrosis. J Drugs Dermatol. 2009;8(5):477–80.
29. Innocenzi D, Ruggero A, Francesconi L, Lacarrubba F, Nardone B, Micali G. An open-label tolerability and efficacy study of an aluminum sesquichlorohydrate topical foam in axillary and palmar primary hyperhidrosis. Dermatol Ther. 2008;21 Suppl 1:S27–30.
30. Goh CL. Aluminum chloride hexahydrate versus palmar hyperhidrosis. Evaporimeter assessment. Int J Dermatol. 1990;29(5):368–70.
31. Bergstresser PR, Quero R. Treatment of hyperhidrosis with topical methenamine. Int J Dermatol. 1976;15(6):452–5.
32. Pagliarello C, Paradisi M, Paradisi A. Reply to: "Primary focal hyperhidrosis: current treatment options and a step-by-step approach.". J Eur Acad Dermatol Venereol. 2012;26(9):1172.
33. Cullen SI. Topical methenamine therapy for hyperhidrosis. Arch Dermatol. 1975;111(9):1158–60.
34. Seukeran DC, Highet AS. The use of topical glycopyrrolate in the treatment of hyperhidrosis. Clin Exp Dermatol. 1998;23(5):204–5.
35. Kavanagh GM, Burns C, Aldridge RD. Topical glycopyrrolate should not be overlooked in treatment of focal hyperhidrosis. Br J Dermatol. 2006;155(2):487.
36. Levit F. Simple device for treatment of hyperhidrosis by iontophoresis. Arch Dermatol. 1968;98(5):505–7.
37. Chia HY, Tan AS, Chong WS, Tey HL. Efficacy of iontophoresis with glycopyrronium bromide for treatment of primary palmar hyperhidrosis. J Eur Acad Dermatol Venereol. 2012;26(9):1167–70.
38. Davarian S, Kalantari KK, Rezasoltani A, Rahimi A. Effect and persistency of botulinum toxin iontophoresis in the treatment of palmar hyperhidrosis. Australas J Dermatol. 2008;49(2):75–9.
39. Kavanagh GM, Shams K. Botulinum toxin type A by iontophoresis for primary palmar hyperhidrosis. J Am Acad Dermatol. 2006;55(5 Suppl):S115–7.

40. Kavanagh GM, Oh C, Shams K. BOTOX delivery by iontophoresis. Br J Dermatol. 2004;151(5):1093–5.
41. Na GY, Park BC, Lee WJ, Park DJ, Kim DW, Kim MN. Control of palmar hyperhidrosis with a new "dry-type" iontophoretic device. Dermatol Surg. 2007;33(1):57–61.
42. Sato K, Timm DE, Sato F, Templeton EA, Meletiou DS, Toyomoto T, et al. Generation and transit pathway of H+ is critical for inhibition of palmar sweating by iontophoresis in water. J Appl Physiol. 1993;75(5): 2258–64.
43. Hill AC, Baker GF, Jansen GT. Mechanism of action of iontophoresis in the treatment of palmar hyperhidrosis. Cutis. 1981;28(1):69–70. 72.
44. Hill BH. Poldine iontophoresis in the treatment of palmar and plantar hyperhidrosis. Australas J Dermatol. 1976;17(3):92–3.
45. Abell E, Morgan K. The treatment of idiopathic hyperhidrosis by glycopyrronium bromide and tap water iontophoresis. Br J Dermatol. 1974;91(1):87–91.
46. Dolianitis C, Scarff CE, Kelly J, Sinclair R. Iontophoresis with glycopyrrolate for the treatment of palmoplantar hyperhidrosis. Australas J Dermatol. 2004;45(4):208–12.
47. Swartling C, Naver H, Pihl-Lundin I, Hagforsen E, Vahlquist A. Sweat gland morphology and periglandular innervation in essential palmar hyperhidrosis before and after treatment with intradermal botulinum toxin. J Am Acad Dermatol. 2004;51(5):739–45.
48. Shams K, Kavanagh GM. Immediate reduction in sweat secretion with electric current application in primary palmar hyperhidrosis. Arch Dermatol. 2011;147(2):241–2.
49. Maillard H, Fenot M, Bara C, Celerier P. Therapeutic value of moderate-dose oxybutynin in extensive hyperhidrosis. Ann Dermatol Venereol. 2011;138(10): 652–6.
50. Krogstad AL, Skymne A, Pegenius G, Elam M, Wallin BG. No compensatory sweating after botulinum toxin treatment of palmar hyperhidrosis. Br J Dermatol. 2005;152(2):329–33.
51. Hund M, Sinkgraven R, Rzany B. Randomized, placebo-controlled, double blind clinical trial for the evaluation of the efficacy and safety of oral methantheliniumbromide (Vagantin) in the treatment of focal hyperhidrosis. J Dtsch Dermatol Ges. 2004;2(5):343–9.
52. Muller C, Berensmeier A, Hamm H, Dirschka T, Reich K, Fischer T, et al. Efficacy and safety of methantheline bromide (Vagantin(®)) in axillary and palmar hyperhidrosis: results from a multicenter, randomized, placebo-controlled trial. J Eur Acad Dermatol Venereol. 2013;27(10):1278–84.
53. Paller AS, Shah PR, Silverio AM, Wagner A, Chamlin SL, Mancini AJ. Oral glycopyrrolate as second-line treatment for primary pediatric hyperhidrosis. J Am Acad Dermatol. 2012;67(5):918–23.
54. Bajaj V, Langtry JA. Use of oral glycopyrronium bromide in hyperhidrosis. Br J Dermatol. 2007;157(1): 118–21.
55. Wolosker N, De Campos JR, Kauffman P, Puech-Leao P. A randomized placebo-controlled trial of oxybutynin for the initial treatment of palmar and axillary hyperhidrosis. J Vasc Surg. 2012;55(6):1696–700.
56. Walling HW. Systemic therapy for primary hyperhidrosis: a retrospective study of 59 patients treated with glycopyrrolate or clonidine. J Am Acad Dermatol. 2012;66(3):387–92.
57. Wozniacki L, Zubilewicz T. Primary hyperhidrosis controlled with oxybutynin after unsuccessful surgical treatment. Clin Exp Dermatol. 2009;34(8): e990–1.
58. Schollhammer M, Misery L. Treatment of hyperhidrosis with oxybutynin. Arch Dermatol. 2007;143(4): 544–5.
59. Wollina U, Karamfilov T. Botulinum toxin A for palmar hyperhidrosis. J Eur Acad Dermatol Venereol. 2001;15(6):555–8.
60. Solomon BA, Hayman R. Botulinum toxin type A therapy for palmar and digital hyperhidrosis. J Am Acad Dermatol. 2000;42(6):1026–9.
61. Doft MA, Hardy KL, Ascherman JA. Treatment of hyperhidrosis with botulinum toxin. Aesthet Surg J. 2012;32(2):238–44.
62. de Almeida AR, Kadunc BV, de Oliveira EM. Improving botulinum toxin therapy for palmar hyperhidrosis: wrist block and technical considerations. Dermatol Surg. 2001;27(1):34–6.
63. Cerfolio RJ, De Campos JR, Bryant AS, Connery CP, Miller DL, DeCamp MM, et al. The society of thoracic surgeons expert consensus for the surgical treatment of hyperhidrosis. Ann Thorac Surg. 2011;91(5):1642–8.
64. Reisfeld R, Nguyen R, Pnini A. Endoscopic thoracic sympathectomy for treatment of essential hyperhidrosis syndrome: experience with 650 patients. Surg Laparosc Endosc Percutan Tech. 2000;10(1):5–10.
65. Inan K, Goksel OS, Ucak A, Temizkan V, Karaca K, Ugur M, et al. Thoracic endoscopic surgery for hyperhidrosis: comparison of different techniques. Thorac Cardiovasc Surg. 2008;56(4):210–3.
66. Vorkamp T, Foo FJ, Khan S, Schmitto JD, Wilson P. Hyperhidrosis: evolving concepts and a comprehensive review. Surgeon. 2010;8(5):287–92.
67. Gossot D, Kabiri H, Caliandro R, Debrosse D, Girard P, Grunenwald D. Early complications of thoracic endoscopic sympathectomy: a prospective study of 940 procedures. Ann Thorac Surg. 2001;71(4): 1116–9.
68. Zacherl J, Huber ER, Imhof M, Plas EG, Herbst F, Fugger R. Long-term results of 630 thoracoscopic sympathicotomies for primary hyperhidrosis: the Vienna experience. Eur J Surg Suppl. 1998;580:43–6.
69. Lin TS. Transthoracic endoscopic sympathectomy for palmar and axillary hyperhidrosis in children and adolescents. Pediatr Surg Int. 1999;15(7):475–8.
70. Hofbauer GF, Nestle FO. Irritant contact dermatitis of the hands following thoracic sympathectomy. Contact Dermatitis. 2000;42(2):119–20.

Systemic Treatment of Hand Eczema: Retinoids

35

Tove Agner

Contents

35.1 Introduction

When the decision is made to start systemic treatment for hand eczema (HE), it means that the patient has a severe chronic HE. The patient typically has undergone a thorough diagnostic workup, including patch testing, and has been educated with respect to skin care [1, 2]. Changes have been made to diminish irritant exposure, and possible relevant contact allergens have been omitted from the environment. First-line therapy with topical corticosteroids has failed, and second-line therapy (UV therapy, topical tacrolimus/pimecrolimus) has been attempted without an enduring effect. The patient has often suffered from HE for more than 6 months, and at this stage of the disease, the patient's quality of life (QoL) is most often significantly disturbed; even the patient's social life may be threatened by the disease [3, 4]. For a significant number of HE patients, it is difficult to remain in their jobs, and the social consequences of this are often overwhelming.

Patients may react in different ways to this situation. Some patients are highly motivated to try a third-line therapy and are ready to accept possible side effects, as well as blood tests at regular intervals. However, other patients are so depressed or exhausted with the situation that they refuse systemic treatment, since they have no faith in a successful outcome, and are afraid of side effects or that the treatment may even worsen the situation. The concerns of the patients in this group should not be ignored, and they should be motivated for optimized therapy by an

T. Agner, M.D., M.Sc.
Department of Dermatology, Bispebjerg Hospital, University of Copenhagen, Copenhagen 2900, Denmark
e-mail: t.agner@dadlnet.dk

A. Alikhan et al. (eds.), *Textbook of Hand Eczema*,
DOI 10.1007/978-3-642-39546-8_35, © Springer-Verlag Berlin Heidelberg 2014

open dialog and information about exactly what should be expected from the treatment (e.g., efficacy and tolerability).

Which systemic treatment to choose depends on the lifestyle of the patient, concomitant diseases, and on the subclassification of the HE [5]. At the moment, we have only clinical experience to guide us with respect to which kind of treatment is the best choice for specific subclasses of HE, but a scenario for the future is that evidence will be provided for a tailor-made treatment for the various subclasses. In the following sections, focus will be on the treatment with retinoids.

35.2 Evidence for Systemic Therapy

Today, randomized controlled trials (RCTs) are mandatory to have a new drug licensed. Efficacy must be evidence based, and side effects must be acceptable and thoroughly investigated. Such studies are demanding and expensive to perform, and most RCTs performed today are driven by pharmaceutical companies. This means that many old drugs traditionally used for treatment of HE will never be investigated with respect to evidence for efficacy or safety, since no companies will have financial interest in initiating such studies. Alitretinoin is a "new" drug, and it is an example of a drug for which the efficacy is documented by RCTs; therefore, today it is the only drug licensed in Europe for treatment of HE. However, this does not mean that older traditionally used drugs are useless. From a clinical standpoint, it is the impression of this author that many HE patients may benefit from treatment with traditional systemic immunosuppressive drugs [1, 6]. In the future, research grants should be directed at RCTs that are performed independently of industry and that compare the efficacy and tolerability of various systemic drugs used for HE ("head-to-head-studies").

35.2.1 Retinoids: Mechanisms

Two retinoids relevant for treatment of HE are on the market: acitretin and alitretinoin. Both are vitamin A derivatives that influence cell differentiation, proliferation, and apoptosis. There are two families of retinoid nuclear receptors (RNR), the RA receptors (RAR) and the retinoid X receptors (RXR). Acitretin is a ligand of the RAR, and alitretinoin is a ligand of both RAR and RXR. As opposed to acitretin, alitretinoin has an anti-inflammatory and immunomodulatory mechanism of action. Acting as a pan-agonist, it binds to both acid receptors and directly affects cytokine production in keratinocytes and downregulates leukocyte activity. However, the exact mechanisms for the effects on eczema are not known. In target cells, retinoids not utilized are degraded by enzymes of cytochrome P450. Absorption of retinoids will not be satisfactory if the tablet is not taken with a meal, and this should be emphasized to patients [7].

35.2.2 Acitretin: Clinical Efficacy and Side Effects

Acitretin is currently not licensed for the treatment of HE, but has traditionally been used for treatment of hyperkeratotic HE, as well as eczema on the feet. Clinical evidence is best provided in a paper including 29 patients with hyperkeratotic HE in an open-label study [8]. Patients with psoriasis were not excluded. Patients were randomized to 30 mg acitretin daily for 4 weeks or placebo. A 51 % reduction was found in the treatment group compared to only a 9 % reduction in the placebo group [8]. Acitretin is only recommended for hyperkeratotic HE, and an effect on vesicular hand eczema is not to be expected.

The dosage most often used is 25 mg daily, but if this is not tolerated due to side effects, a positive treatment effect may also be obtained from 25 mg every other day. The treatment period for most patients is 3–6 months. If no response is obtained after 2–3 months, the treatment should be discontinued.

An important side effect, as for other retinoids, is teratogenicity, and precautions for pregnancy must be taken and should be continued until 2 years after the completion of treatment, which makes acitretin treatment unsuitable for women of childbearing age. Increase in serum cholesterol and triglycerides during treatment should be expected, and patients with diabetes mellitus or cardiac risk factors should be carefully monitored. Mucosal dryness and hair loss are side effects of which patients often complain. Mood disturbances have been reported as a side effect of all retinoids, and the patients should be observed in this regard.

35.2.3 Alitretinoin: Clinical Efficacy and Side Effects

Several studies have provided clinical evidence that oral alitretinoin is effective in the treatment of severe chronic hand eczema. Alitretinoin is licensed for use in adults with severe chronic HE that does not respond to treatment with topical corticosteroids. The first clinical study reporting the effect of alitretinoin on chronic HE was published in 1999 [9], and since then others have followed [10–15] (Table 35.1).

In the first randomized, controlled study [10], 319 patients with moderate or severe refractory chronic hand dermatitis were randomized to placebo or 10, 20, or 40 mg alitretinoin daily, respectively. Alitretinoin led to a significant and dose-dependent improvement in disease status in up to 53 % of patients, and treatment was generally well tolerated. In a later RCT study [11], 1,032 patients with severe chronic HE were included. Response to treatment was statistically significantly higher in the treatment group (48 %) than in the placebo group (17 %), and the response was dose dependent.

Criticism directed at this study has included that a subclassification of the patients had not been attempted. Eighty-seven percent of the patients were reported to have had a hyperkeratotic morphology of the HE, and almost all had inflammation. The results indicate that patients with a hyperkeratotic eczema should be expected to respond better to treatment than those with vesicular eczema. However, this finding was not supported by a recent study [15], including 680 patients, where hyperkeratotic eczema, fingertip eczema, and vesicular eczema were found to respond almost equally to treatment.

Intermittent long-term treatment has been reported to be successful, and efficacy and toxicity have been reevaluated in recent studies [15, 16]. Relapse of HE should be expected in a significant portion of the patients [15]; however, when re-treated with alitretinoin 30 mg daily, 80 % of those who had a relapse were reported to have a significantly positive effect of re-treatment [12].

The recommended dosage is 30 mg daily, and the treatment period for most patients is 3–6 months. If no response is obtained after 3 months, the treatment should be stopped. In patients with cardiac risk factors or diabetes mellitus, one should consider starting the treatment at a lower dose (i.e., 10 mg daily), and possible toxicity should be carefully monitored.

An important side effect, as for other retinoids, is teratogenicity, and in women of childbearing age, precautions for pregnancy must be taken and should be continued until 1 month after treatment completion. Headache and flushing are the most commonly reported side effects of alitretinoin; they are both reversible and dose dependent, and lowering the dose may often solve the problem.

Increase in serum cholesterol and triglycerides during treatment should be expected; sometimes this effect on lipid metabolism may lead to cessation of treatment [10, 11]. Thyroid function may be influenced, and a slight reduction in thyroid hormones may be seen during the treatment period [13]; however, this is often not of clinical relevance. Mucosal dryness and hair loss, which are frequently found during treatment with acitretin, seem to be much less pronounced during alitretinoin treatment, although data on this are sparse. Mood disturbances have been reported as a side effect of all retinoids, and patients should be observed in this regard.

Table 35.1 Clinical efficacy and side effects of alitretinoin in hand eczema

Authors	Year	Number of participants	Study design	Efficacy	Side effect	Reference
Bollag et al.	1999	38	Pilot study	89 % showed either a very good or good response	Mild	[9]
Ruzicka et al.	2004	319	Randomized, double-blind, placebo-controlled multicenter study	Response in 53 % of patients	24 withdrew owing to adverse events (headache, flushing, mucocutaneous events, hyperlipidemia, and decreased hemoglobin and decreased free thyroxine levels)	[10]
Ruzicka et al.	2008	1,032	Randomized, double-blind, placebo-controlled, multicenter study	"Clear" or "almost clear" hands were achieved in up to 48 % of patients treated with alitretinoin, compared with 17 % for placebo	Headache, mucocutaneous events, hyperlipidemia, and decreased free thyroxine and thyroid-stimulating hormone	[11]
Bissonette et al.	2010	117	Double-blind study including patients previously treated with alitretinoin	Response rates were 80 % in patients *re-treated* with 30 mg alitretinoin compared with 8 % for placebo	Typical retinoid class effects and no late-arising side effects were observed	[12]
Aguayo-Leiva et al.	2011	15	Prospective, observational, descriptive study	"Clear" or "almost clear" hands were obtained in 80 % 54 % relapsed within 6 months	Headache, elevated lipid levels, slightly elevated transaminase levels, and epigastric pain. One patient had a substantial reduction in thyroid-stimulating hormone levels	[13]
Dirschka et al.	2011	249	Open-label study	"Clear" or "almost clear" hands were reported for 47 % of patients	Mild side effects, mostly headache leading to treatment interruption in 16 %	[14]
Diepgen et al.	2011	680	Prospective, observational open study	"Clear" or "almost clear" hands were obtained in 57 %, with only small differences in patients with different morphological forms: hyperkeratotic-rhagadiform (59.2 %), fingertip (52.2 %), and vesicular (47.9 %)	Mild side effects	[15]

Conclusion

Onset of systemic treatment of HE is a decision that should be made after topical treatment has failed and after the patient has been thoroughly informed about expectations, including efficacy, side effects, and expected duration of therapy. The patient must be motivated to start systemic treatment and accept regular blood tests to monitor treatment. If these steps are taken before the systemic treatment is initiated, the chances for a successful outcome will be significantly increased.

Treatment with retinoids (acitretin and alitretinoin) can be quite effective and is generally well tolerated. It is generally accepted that retinoids (acitretin, in particular) are more effective for treatment of hyperkeratotic HE than other subclasses of HE. Acitretin has only been shown effective in patients with hyperkeratotic eczema, while all subclasses of HE patients have been reported to respond to alitretinoin, but with the best response in patients with hyperkeratotic eczema. Clinical efficacy of alitretinoin is better documented than for acitretin, and alitretinoin is licensed for treatment of HE. Side effects of alitretinoin are generally much more acceptable for patients than the side effects of acitretin. For women of childbearing age, acitretin should not be considered, owing to the slow elimination time of the drug, and the patient must adhere to a pregnancy precaution program for 2 years after treatment completion. However, it should be kept in mind that clinical experience with alitretinoin is still limited, and although carefully surveyed, new and unanticipated side effects may still occur. The prices of the two drugs differ significantly; alitretinoin is significantly more expensive than acitretin, as well as other drugs used for systemic treatment of HE, and this should also be taken into consideration.

References

1. Lynde C, Guenther L, Diepgen TL, Sasseville D, Poulin Y, Gulliver W, et al. Canadian hand dermatitis management guidelines. J Cutan Med Surg. 2010; 14:267–84.
2. Agner T, Held E. Skin protection programmes. Contact Dermatitis. 2002;47:253–6.
3. Agner T, Andersen KE, Brandao FM, Bruze M, Bruynzeel DP, Frosch P, EECDRG, et al. Hand eczema severity and quality of life: a cross-sectional, multicentre study of hand eczema patients. Contact Dermatitis. 2008;59(1):43–7.
4. Diepgen T, Agner T, Aberer W, Berth-Jones J, Cambazard F, Elsner P, et al. Management of chronic hand eczema. Contact Dermatitis. 2007;57(4): 203–10.
5. Diepgen TL, Andersen KE, Brandao FM, Bruze M, Bruynzeel DP, Frosch P, et al. Hand eczema classification: a cross-sectional, multicentre study of the aetiology and morphology of hand eczema. Br J Dermatol. 2009;160(2):353–8.
6. Veien NK, Menne T. Treatment of hand eczema. Skin Ther Lett. 2003;8(5):4–7.
7. Schmitt-Hoffmann AH, Roos B, Sauer J, Schleimer M, Kovăcs P, Stoeckel K, et al. Influence of food on the pharmacokinetics of oral alitretinoin (9-cis retinoic acid). Clin Exp Dermatol. 2011;36 Suppl 2:18–23.
8. Thestrup-Pedersen K, Andersen KE, Menne T, Veien N. Treatment of hyperkeratotic dermatitis of the palms (eczema keratoticum) with oral acitretin. A single-blind placebo controlled study. Acta Derm Venereol. 2001;81:353–5.
9. Bollag W, Ott F. Successful treatment of chronic hand eczema with oral 9-cis-retinoic acid. Dermatology. 1999;199(4):308–12.
10. Ruzicka T, Larsen FG, Galewicz D, Horváth A, Coenraads PJ, Thestrup-Pedersen K, et al. Oral alitretinoin (9-cis-retinoic acid) therapy for chronic hand dermatitis in patients refractory to standard therapy: results of a randomized, double-blind, placebo-controlled, multicenter trial. Arch Dermatol. 2004; 140(12):1453–9.
11. Ruzicka T, Lynde CW, Jemec GB, Diepgen T, Berth-Jones J, Coenraads PJ, et al. Efficacy and safety of oral alitretinoin (9-cis retinoic acid) in patients with severe chronic hand eczema refractory to topical corticosteroids: results of a randomized, double-blind, placebo-controlled, multicentre trial. Br J Dermatol. 2008;158(4):808–17.
12. Bissonnette R, Worm M, Gerlach B, Guenther L, Cambazard F, Ruzicka T, et al. Successful retreatment with alitretinoin in patients with relapsed chronic hand eczema. Br J Dermatol. 2010;162(2): 420–6.
13. Aguayo-Leiva IR, Urrutia S, Jaén-Olasolo P. Response to treatment with oral alitretinoin in patients with chronic hand eczema that is refractory to treatment with potent topical corticosteroids: experience in 15 patients. Actas Dermosifiliogr. 2011;102(8): 616–22.
14. Dirschka T, Reich K, Bissonnette R, Maares J, Brown T, Diepgen TL. An open-label study assessing the safety and efficacy of alitretinoin in patients with severe chronic hand eczema unresponsive to topical corticosteroids. Clin Exp Dermatol. 2011;36(2): 149–54.

15. Diepgen TL, Pfarr E, Zimmermann T. Efficacy and tolerability of alitretinoin for chronic hand eczema under daily practice conditions: results of the TOCCATA open study comprising 680 patients. Acta Derm Venereol. 2012;92:251–5.
16. Lynde C, Cambazard F, Ruzicka T, Sebastian M, Brown TC, Maares J. Extended treatment with oral alitretinoin for patients with chronic hand eczema not fully responding to initial treatment. Clin Exp Dermatol. 2012;37(7):712–7.

Systemic Treatment of Hand Eczema: Methotrexate

36

Cooper C. Wriston and Mark R. Pittelkow

Contents

C.C. Wriston, M.D. (✉)
Department of Dermatology,
Mayo Clinic College of Medicine,
200 1st St S.W, Rochester, MN 55905, USA
e-mail: wriston.cooper@mayo.edu

M.R. Pittelkow, M.D.
Departments of Dermatology and Biochemistry and Molecular Biology,
Mayo Clinic College of Medicine,
200 1st St S.W, Rochester, MN 55905, USA
e-mail: pittelkow.mark@mayo.edu

36.1 Introduction

Methotrexate, a folic acid antagonist, remains one of the most widely used antimetabolites in dermatology [1]. In 1951, Gubner and colleagues recognized the role of the folic acid antagonist aminopterin for the treatment of psoriasis [2]. In 1971, methotrexate was finally approved for the treatment of psoriasis. In more recent years, methotrexate has gained widespread recognition for its role in the treatment of many dermatologic diseases. Methotrexate has been found to be helpful in the "off-label" treatment of many dermatoses, including connective tissue diseases, autoimmune blistering skin diseases, vasculitis, neutrophilic dermatoses, disorders of keratinization, and dermatitis. Very limited evidence exists for the use of methotrexate in the treatment of hand dermatitis, and its use may be complicated by hematologic or hepatic toxicity.

36.2 Mechanism of Action

Methotrexate has antiproliferative effects, immunosuppressive effects, and anti-inflammatory effects. It competitively inhibits dihydrofolate reductase, preventing the conversion of dihydrofolate to tetrahydrofolate. Methotrexate also partially inhibits thymidylate synthase. Consequently, less reduced folate and thymidylate are available, and RNA and DNA synthesis is impaired [1]. Methotrexate inhibits cell division, and it is specific for the S phase (DNA synthesis) [3]. This

A. Alikhan et al. (eds.), *Textbook of Hand Eczema*,
DOI 10.1007/978-3-642-39546-8_36, © Springer-Verlag Berlin Heidelberg 2014

results in reduced keratinocyte proliferation and (to a higher degree) reduced lymphocyte proliferation [4]. Methotrexate has also been shown to block T-cell migration [5].

Methotrexate's anti-inflammatory properties likely result from an increase in intracellular and extracellular adenosine secondary to inhibition of aminoimidazole-carboxamide-ribonucleoside (AICAR) transformylase [6]. Adenosine, a purine nucleoside, has anti-inflammatory effects on various cells (e.g., neutrophils, monocytes), processes (e.g., chemotaxis, adherence), and cytokines (e.g., IL-10, TNF-α) [6].

36.3 Metabolism

Methotrexate is primarily excreted by the kidneys, with 60–95 % excreted unchanged [1]. As a weak organic acid, renal excretion is susceptible to interactions with other weak acids such as salicylates, probenecid, and sulfonamides [3].

36.4 Interactions

NSAIDs, salicylates, sulfonamides, chloramphenicol, phenothiazines, phenytoin, and tetracyclines may increase methotrexate levels and drug toxicity. Probenecid and dipyridamole may increase the intracellular accumulation of methotrexate. The concurrent use of these medications should be avoided [3, 7].

Trimethoprim, sulfonamides, and dapsone inhibit the folate metabolic pathway. Concurrent use of these medicines significantly increases the risk of severe hematologic toxicity. Concomitant use of systemic retinoids or alcohol may increase the risk of hepatotoxicity [3].

36.5 Contraindications

Absolute contraindications to therapy include lactation and pregnancy. Relative contraindications include renal impairment, active infection, immunodeficiency, hepatic disease or dysfunction, hematologic abnormality, excessive alcohol consumption, diabetes, obesity, or contemplating impending conception [8]. Those with hematologic abnormality or renal impairment may be able to pursue methotrexate therapy at reduced dose [1, 3].

36.6 Adverse Effects

Hepatotoxicity and myelosuppression are the most important adverse effects complicating methotrexate use. Anemia, thrombocytopenia, and neutropenia may occur. Identifiable risk factors for hematologic toxicity include advanced age, renal impairment, and drug interactions (including trimethoprim/sulfamethoxazole combinations, dapsone, and NSAIDs). The risk of cytopenia is significantly reduced by routine folic acid supplementation [1, 3].

Liver toxicity is an important consideration with methotrexate use. Methotrexate is hepatotoxic, and some elevation of transaminases is expected near dose administration. Liver fibrosis may occur in patients treated with long-term methotrexate. The gold standard for assessing methotrexate-induced liver fibrosis is periodic liver biopsy, but magnetic resonance elastography represents an emerging diagnostic tool.

Lymphoma has been reported among patients with connective tissue disease treated with methotrexate; however, there is no statistical evidence that methotrexate increases the risk of malignancy among psoriasis patients [3, 9, 10].

Nausea, anorexia, oral ulceration, and stomatitis may be noted with methotrexate. Folic acid supplementation may improve methotrexate-associated nausea.

Rarely, pneumonitis and pulmonary fibrosis may follow methotrexate use. Pneumonitis may be life-threatening. Unfortunately, routine chest x-rays and pulmonary function testing do not enhance the detection or prevention of pulmonary toxicity [3, 11].

Methotrexate is a pregnancy category X medication. Women of childbearing potential should use reliable birth control. Men should wait 3 months after stopping methotrexate before attempting conception [1].

36.7 Baseline Assessment and Monitoring

When considering methotrexate therapy, patients should be thoroughly counseled regarding the nature of methotrexate therapy, the initial evaluation of methotrexate treatment candidates, and the necessary clinical follow-up and screening evaluations. Prior to initiating therapy, patients should undergo a thorough history and physical examination. The presence of preexisting medical conditions should be documented. The clinician should identify risk factors, medical conditions, and medicines that may limit methotrexate use. Baseline measurements should include, at minimum, a complete blood count including platelet count, liver function studies, renal function studies, and serologic screening for hepatitis B and C. HIV and pregnancy screening should be conducted when indicated. Screening for tuberculosis with purified protein derivative (PPD) should be considered. A complete blood count and liver function studies are reassessed 7 days after an initial 5–10-mg test dose [1, 3].

Ongoing laboratory assessment includes complete blood count and liver function studies every 1–2 weeks for the first month of therapy or during dose escalations. The frequency may then be slowly decreased to every 3 months. Renal function studies should be repeated every 3 months or if alterations in renal function are suspected [1].

36.8 The Role of Liver Biopsy

The role of routine liver biopsies for patients treated with methotrexate is controversial. Liver biopsies for non-psoriasis patients without risk factors for hepatic toxicity may not be indicated, or the frequency of such biopsies may be markedly reduced [7]. Risk factors for hepatotoxicity include history of liver disease, alcohol consumption, family history of heritable liver disease, diabetes, obesity, dyslipidemia, history of hepatotoxin exposure, and lack of folate supplementation. A baseline liver biopsy for patients at low risk of hepatotoxicity may be deferred until 1.5-g cumulative dose of methotrexate. Magnetic resonance elastography may represent an effective, safer, less expensive, and less invasive alternative to liver biopsy in assessing hepatic fibrosis [12–17].

36.9 Use in Hand Dermatitis

Although methotrexate has been used by dermatologists for recalcitrant hand dermatitis for many years, very limited published evidence is available demonstrating efficacy of methotrexate for hand dermatitis. In particular, Egan and colleagues reported a series of five patients with recalcitrant palmoplantar pompholyx who did not respond to or were unable to tolerate conventional therapy [18]. Methotrexate was added to their regimen. All five patients responded to the addition of methotrexate at doses between 15 mg/week and 22.5 mg/week required for initial control. Methotrexate was stopped in one patient due to gastrointestinal intolerance. Two of five patients stopped methotrexate and maintained satisfactory control of their pompholyx with oral or topical steroids only.

While published data for hand dermatitis are minimal, there is strong evidence for the use of methotrexate in chronic and/or severe eczema [19–23]; it should be considered as a steroid-sparing agent for patients with recalcitrant hand eczema unresponsive to nonsystemic modalities. It appears to be safe in both children and the elderly [24–27].

36.10 Initiation and Dose Titration

Based on limited available evidence, recalcitrant pompholyx responds to methotrexate as an adjunctive treatment at doses between 15 mg/week and 22.5 mg/week. Other subtypes of hand eczema may also respond to hand eczema, though published data are limited. Methotrexate is available in 2.5-mg tablets and should be given in a single weekly dose or divided into three portions, given 12 h apart over 24 h. Following an initial test dose of 5–10 mg, the dose may be slowly increased by 2.5–5 mg every 2–4 weeks until an adequate response is attained or toxicity intercedes. Once adequate control is achieved, methotrexate may be tapered by 2.5 mg every 1–2 weeks until the lowest adequate dosage is achieved. Of note, methotrexate is also available in a liquid form, which may be less expensive. Daily supplementation with 1–5 mg of folate may reduce gastrointestinal intolerance, transaminitis, and hematologic toxicity [1].

Conclusion

Methotrexate is effective in various dermatoses and should be considered in hand eczema recalcitrant to nonsystemic therapies. A thorough discussion with patients regarding comorbidities, adverse effects, and monitoring is imperative. Of note, methotrexate can be used safely with other treatments for cutaneous disorders, including phototherapy and various topical and systemic agents [6].

References

1. Goldsmith LA, Katz SI, Gilchrest BA, Paller AS, Leffell DJ, Wolff K. Fitzpatrick's dermatology in general medicine. New York: McGraw-Hill; 2012.
2. Gubner R, August S, Ginsberg V. Therapeutic suppression of tissue reactivity. II. Effect of aminopterin in rheumatoid arthritis and psoriasis. Am J Med Sci. 1951;221(2):176–82.
3. Wolverton SE. Comprehensive dermatologic drug therapy. E-Book. Philadelphia: Elsevier/Saunders; 2007.
4. Jeffes 3rd EW, McCullough JL, Pittelkow MR, McCormick A, Almanzor J, Liu G, et al. Methotrexate therapy of psoriasis: differential sensitivity of proliferating lymphoid and epithelial cells to the cytotoxic and growth-inhibitory effects of methotrexate. J Invest Dermatol. 1995;104(2):183–8.
5. Sigmundsdottir H, Johnston A, Gudjonsson JE, Bjarnason B, Valdimarsson H. Methotrexate markedly reduces the expression of vascular E-selectin, cutaneous lymphocyte-associated antigen and the numbers of mononuclear leucocytes in psoriatic skin. Exp Dermatol. 2004;13(7):426–34.
6. Shen S, O'Brien T, Yap LM, Prince HM, McCormack CJ. The use of methotrexate in dermatology: a review. Australas J Dermatol. 2012;53(1):1–18.
7. Rapini RP, Bolognia JL, Jorizzo JL. Dermatology. St. Louis: Mosby; 2007.
8. Montaudie H, Sbidian E, Paul C, Maza A, Gallini A, Aractingi S, et al. Methotrexate in psoriasis: a systematic review of treatment modalities, incidence, risk factors and monitoring of liver toxicity. J Eur Acad Dermatol Venereol. 2011;25 Suppl 2:12–8.
9. Bailin PL, Tindall JP, Roenigk Jr HH, Hogan MD. Is methotrexate therapy for psoriasis carcinogenic? A modified retrospective-prospective analysis. JAMA. 1975;232(4):359–62.
10. Nyfors A, Jensen H. Frequency of malignant neoplasms in 248 long-term methotrexate-treated psoriatics. A preliminary study. Dermatologica. 1983;167(5):260–1.
11. Verdich J, Christensen AL. Pulmonary disease complicating intermittent methotrexate therapy of psoriasis. Acta Derm Venereol. 1979;59(5):471–3.
12. Venkatesh SK, Yin M, Ehman RL. Magnetic resonance elastography of liver: technique, analysis, and clinical applications. J Magn Reson Imaging. 2013;37(3):spcone.
13. Godfrey EM, Mannelli L, Griffin N, Lomas DJ. Magnetic resonance elastography in the diagnosis of hepatic fibrosis. Semin Ultrasound CT MR. 2013;34(1):81–8.
14. Dzyubak B, Glaser K, Yin M, Talwalkar J, Chen J, Manduca A, et al. Automated liver stiffness measurements with magnetic resonance elastography. J Magn Reson Imaging. 2013;38(2):371–9
15. Mitsufuji T, Shinagawa Y, Fujimitsu R, Urakawa H, Inoue K, Takano K, et al. Measurement consistency of MR elastography at 3.0 T: comparison among three different region-of-interest placement methods. Jpn J Radiol. 2013;31(5):336–41
16. Barbero-Villares A, Mendoza J, Trapero-Marugan M, Gonzalez-Alvaro I, Daudén E, Gisbert JP, et al. Evaluation of liver fibrosis by transient elastography in methotrexate treated patients. Med Clin (Barc). 2011;137(14):637–9.
17. Bray AP, Barnova I, Przemioslo R, Kennedy CT. Liver fibrosis screening for patients with psoriasis taking methotrexate: a cross-sectional study comparing transient elastography and liver biopsy. Br J Dermatol. 2012;166(5):1125–7.
18. Egan CA, Rallis TM, Meadows KP, Krueger GG. Low-dose oral methotrexate treatment for recalcitrant palmoplantar pompholyx. J Am Acad Dermatol. 1999;40(4):612–4.
19. De D, Sarangal R, Handa S. The comparative efficacy and safety of azathioprine vs methotrexate as steroid-sparing agent in the treatment of airborne-contact dermatitis due to Parthenium. Ind J Dermatol Venereol Leprol. 2013;79(2):240–1.
20. Patel AN, Langan SM, Batchelor JM. A randomized trial of methotrexate vs. azathioprine for severe atopic eczema: a critical appraisal. Br J Dermatol. 2012;166(4):701–4. discussion 704.
21. Schram ME, Roekevisch E, Leeflang MM, Bos JD, Schmitt J, Spuls PI. A randomized trial of methotrexate versus azathioprine for severe atopic eczema. J Allergy Clin Immunol. 2011;128(2):353–9.

22. Lyakhovitsky A, Barzilai A, Heyman R, Baum S, Amichai B, Solomon M, et al. Low-dose methotrexate treatment for moderate-to-severe atopic dermatitis in adults. J Eur Acad Dermatol Venereol. 2010;24(1):43–9.
23. Weatherhead SC, Wahie S, Reynolds NJ, Meggitt SJ. An open-label, dose-ranging study of methotrexate for moderate-to-severe adult atopic eczema. Br J Dermatol. 2007;156(2):346–51.
24. Park YW, Yeom KB, Kim KH. Refractory atopic dermatitis in childhood: improvement with methotrexate? Ann Dermatol. 2013;25(1):114–6.
25. Tetart F, Joly P. Low doses of methotrexate for the treatment of chronic eczema in the elderly. J Eur Acad Dermatol Venereol. 2011;25(11):1364–5.
26. El-Khalawany MA, Hassan H, Shaaban D, Ghonaim N, Eassa B. Methotrexate versus cyclosporine in the treatment of severe atopic dermatitis in children: a multicenter experience from Egypt. Eur J Pediatr. 2013;172(3):351–6.
27. Roberts H, Orchard D. Methotrexate is a safe and effective treatment for paediatric discoid (nummular) eczema: a case series of 25 children. Australas J Dermatol. 2010;51(2):128–30.

Systemic Treatment of Hand Eczema: Cyclosporine

37

Cooper C. Wriston and Mark R. Pittelkow

Contents

C.C. Wriston, M.D. (✉)
Department of Dermatology,
Mayo Clinic College of Medicine,
200 1st St SW, Rochester, MN 55905, USA
e-mail: wriston.cooper@mayo.edu

M.R. Pittelkow
Departments of Dermatology and Biochemistry and Molecular Biology,
Mayo Clinic College of Medicine,
200 1st St SW, Rochester, MN 55905, USA
e-mail: pittelkow.mark@mayo.edu

37.1 Introduction

Cyclosporine has been used in clinical practice for four decades, originally in renal transplant recipients for the prevention of graft rejection [1]. Its application in dermatology was discovered in 1979 by Mueller and colleagues, who noted improvement in cutaneous psoriasis during a pilot study of cyclosporine efficacy for inflammatory arthritis [2]. In more recent years, it has gained recognition as a potent treatment for many dermatologic diseases. While only FDA approved for the treatment of severe or recalcitrant psoriasis in dermatologic practice, cyclosporine has been helpful in the "off-label" treatment of many dermatoses, including connective tissue disease, autoimmune blistering skin diseases, neutrophilic dermatoses, urticaria, and dermatitis. Limited evidence exists for the use of cyclosporine in the treatment of hand dermatitis, and its use may be complicated by systemic toxicity.

37.2 Mechanism of Action

Cyclosporine is a neutral cyclic peptide of ten amino acids originally isolated from the soil fungus *Tolypocladium inflatum* in 1970 [3]. Cyclosporine is T-cell selective, forming a complex with cyclophilin that inhibits the activity of calcineurin. As a result, calcineurin is unable to dephosphorylate nuclear factor of activated T-cells (NFAT), a transcription factor with phosphorylation-dependent nuclear translocation. Decreased transcription of

A. Alikhan et al. (eds.), *Textbook of Hand Eczema*,
DOI 10.1007/978-3-642-39546-8_37, © Springer-Verlag Berlin Heidelberg 2014

NFAT-target genes, including interleukin-2 (IL-2), results in decreased lymphocytes and macrophages in the epidermis and dermis and inhibition of T-cell, natural killer cell, and antigen-presenting cell activation [1].

37.3 Metabolism

The microemulsion-based formulation of cyclosporine, Neoral, has improved bioavailability and a more predictable absorption [4]. Cyclosporine is metabolized in the liver cytochrome P_{450} 3A4 (CYP3A4) pathway and is primarily excreted in bile. Monitoring therapeutic blood levels of cyclosporine is not necessary, as evidence-based target levels do not exist for dermatologic indications [5].

37.4 Interactions

Drugs that compete for CYP3A4 will increase cyclosporine levels, whereas drugs that induce P_{450} will decrease cyclosporine levels [4]. Grapefruit juice inhibits the metabolism of cyclosporine by inhibiting the cytochrome P_{450} enzymes in the intestinal wall and should be avoided [5]. Macrolide antibiotics should be used with caution, and erythromycin should be avoided. Additionally, care must be taken in the use of nephrotoxic drugs such as nonsteroidal anti-inflammatory drugs (NSAIDs), aminoglycosides, ciprofloxacin, ketoconazole, clotrimazole, and fibrates that can impair renal function during cyclosporine treatment and should be avoided, if possible [5]. Cyclosporine can increase the concentration of digoxin, statins, prednisolone, diclofenac, methotrexate, colchicine, phosphodiesterase inhibitors, and benzodiazepines, leading to toxicity. A full drug history should be taken in any patient starting cyclosporine.

37.5 Contraindications

Absolute contraindications to therapy include significant renal impairment, uncontrolled hypertension, and hypersensitivity to cyclosporine [3]. Cyclosporine is also contraindicated in patients with serious infections and in those with a previous history of malignancy, excluding basal cell carcinoma [5]. Antimicrobial therapy should be started for patients with superficial skin infections affecting eczematous skin before cyclosporine is initiated. Cyclosporine may increase cutaneous malignancy among patients with an extended treatment history of psoralen plus ultraviolet A light (PUVA) photochemotherapy [6], with marked photodamage, or who have been exposed to ionizing radiation.

37.6 Adverse Effects

One in four patients taking cyclosporine develops clinical and laboratory evidence of altered renal function, including hypertension [4]. Nephrotoxicity is the most important adverse effect common to cyclosporine, and the risk for nephrotoxicity increases with higher doses and longer courses of cyclosporine therapy [7]. Many of these effects are reversible upon therapy cessation. Adherence to current guidelines for use of cyclosporine considerably reduces the risk of side effects (the American Academy of Dermatology published consensus guidelines for the use of cyclosporine in 2010 [8]). Most persistent renal dysfunction is related to duration of therapy longer than 2 years or doses greater than 5 mg/kg/day. Indeed, no cases of clinically significant kidney damage from cyclosporine use adhering to dermatological guidelines have been reported [7].

Hypertension is a common occurrence during cyclosporine therapy. It is generally mild and reversible. Hypertension is not a contraindication to continued therapy, as long as it can be controlled. The incidence ranges from 0 % to 54 % among different studies of cyclosporine use and from 0 % to 24 % among studies of short-course cyclosporine therapy [5].

While the risk of malignancy associated with long-term cyclosporine use among transplant recipients is well described, internal cancer risk among patients treated with cyclosporine under proper dermatological guidelines has not been clearly demonstrated [7, 9]. However, a sixfold increased risk of cutaneous squamous cell carcinoma among psoriasis patients treated with long-term cyclosporine therapy has been observed [9].

Other common adverse effects of cyclosporine include tremor, headache, dysesthesia, nausea, diarrhea, myalgia, arthralgia, and laboratory derangements (hyperkalemia, hypomagnesemia, hyperlipidemia, hyperuricemia).

Skin-specific cyclosporine adverse effects include hypertrichosis, gingival hypertrophy, and acneiform eruptions [5].

37.7 Baseline Assessment and Monitoring

When considering cyclosporine treatment, patients should be thoroughly counseled regarding the nature of cyclosporine therapy, the initial evaluation for cyclosporine-treatment candidates, and the frequency and importance of follow-up clinical and laboratory evaluations during ongoing therapy. A thorough history and clinical examination should be conducted to evaluate for preexisting medical conditions; cardiovascular, renal, or liver disease; infection; and malignancy. The physical examination should assess the presence and degree of actinic damage and the presence of skin cancers and skin infections. Patients should be instructed to be thorough in oral hygiene and to visit their dentist at 6-month intervals to assess for gingival hypertrophy. Contraception and pregnancy status should be addressed in women of childbearing potential. Before therapy is started, patients should complete age-appropriate cancer screening and, ideally, required vaccinations. Baseline measurements should include, at least, blood pressure on two separate occasions, serum creatinine on two separate occasions, complete blood count, blood urea nitrogen, potassium, magnesium, uric acid, liver function tests, fasting lipid panel, and urinalysis (for proteinuria) [5].

Blood pressure, blood urea nitrogen, and serum creatinine should be assessed at weeks two, four, six, eight, and then every 4–6 weeks thereafter. Complete blood count, potassium, liver function studies, uric acid, fasting lipid panel, and magnesium should be assessed monthly initially and periodically thereafter. Weights should be recorded at every visit [5].

A serum cyclosporine level may be useful to assess medication adherence in non-responders if clinically indicated.

37.8 Managing Renal Function and Hypertension

Serum creatinine should be monitored routinely. If the creatinine rises >30 % above baseline, the level should be rechecked in 2 weeks. If creatinine returns to <30 % elevation above baseline, treatment may be continued at the current dose; otherwise, cyclosporine should be reduced by at least 1 mg/kg/day for at least 1 month, with the creatinine rechecked at that time. If the creatinine at the reduced dose remains elevated >30 % above baseline, cyclosporine should be stopped until the serum creatinine returns to <10 % above baseline. Once the creatinine has normalized to <10 % of baseline, restarting therapy at a lower dose may be considered. Any patient who experiences a serum creatinine >50 % above baseline should be discontinued from therapy until the creatinine returns to baseline [10].

If blood pressure monitoring reveals >140 mmHg systolic or >90 mmHg diastolic, the blood pressure should be rechecked in 2 weeks. If these values persist, the cyclosporine dose should be reduced by 25–50 %, or a dihydropyridine calcium channel blocker such as nifedipine, amlodipine, or isradipine should be started.

37.9 Use in Hand Dermatitis

Similar to methotrexate, there is good evidence for the use of cyclosporine in dermatitis [10–16], but limited evidence and anecdotal reports confirm the efficacy of cyclosporine in hand eczema specifically. Reitamo reported a series of seven patients with chronic vesiculobullous or hyperkeratotic hand dermatitis treated with cyclosporine [17]. Low-dose treatment was initiated at

1.25–2.5 mg/kg/day. Six patients (86 %) responded to doses between 2.5 and 5.0 mg/kg/day within several weeks. No response was observed with a starting dose of 1.25 mg/kg/day. Three patients were in remission for at least 4 months after stopping cyclosporine.

Granlund and colleagues [18] performed a randomized, double-blind crossover study of patients with severe chronic hand eczema comparing treatment with cyclosporine (3.0 mg/kg/day) with betamethasone dipropionate 0.05 % cream. After 6 weeks, no statistically significant improvement in total disease activity was observed for cyclosporine compared to betamethasone dipropionate cream; however, each group had improved compared to baseline measurements. Granlund and colleagues later reported similar quality-of-life indices between these treatment groups [19]. Long-term assessment of 27 patients treated with cyclosporine for 6 weeks for severe chronic hand eczema showed significant improvement of disease activity at 1-year follow-up [20]. Twenty-one of 27 evaluable patients were still in remission. In 1992, Petersen reported a case of recalcitrant chronic vesicular hand eczema with dramatic improvement within 2 weeks of initiating cyclosporine (5.0 mg/kg/day), followed by rapid recurrence after cyclosporine was stopped due to increased blood pressure [21].

Cyclosporine was reported effective in Dogger Bank itch, an allergic contact dermatitis to *Alcyonidium diaphanum* (a marine bryozoan) seen in fishermen and dock laborers which frequently affects the hands [22].

37.10 Initiation and Dose Titration

Based on limited available evidence, chronic hand dermatitis responds to cyclosporine at doses between 2.5 and 5.0 mg/kg/day. An initial dose of 2.5–3.0 mg/kg/day, administered in two divided doses, is a reasonable starting dose. If improvement is not realized after 1 month, cyclosporine may be increased by 0.5–1.0 mg/kg/day every 2–3 weeks as necessary. Cyclosporine should not exceed a maximum dose of 5.0 mg/kg/day (but if needed, then trough levels should be measured – in our experience, most dermatological patients display a good response to cyclosporine with trough whole blood levels of 100–250 ng/mL). Typically, if no improvement is noted after 3 months on the maximum dose of 5.0 mg/kg/day, cyclosporine should be discontinued.

Once control has been achieved, cyclosporine may be tapered to the minimum effective maintenance dose or an alternative therapy may be instituted. If maintenance therapy with cyclosporine is desired, the dose may be tapered by 1 mg/kg/day every 2 weeks until the minimum effective maintenance dose is achieved. If maintenance with an alternative therapy is desired, the cyclosporine dose may be tapered by 1 mg/kg/day every month until the patient is receiving the alternative therapy only [3]. All cyclosporine dosing is based on ideal body weight.

Conclusion

Cyclosporine is a very effective short-term immunosuppressive agent for many dermatological conditions, including hand dermatitis. An appreciation of its adverse effects is crucial, and appropriate monitoring of patients is necessary. It is important to consider a long-term plan for patients on cyclosporine as many will be slowly transitioned to other safer agents once acute control is achieved.

References

1. Amor KT, Ryan C, Menter A. The use of cyclosporine in dermatology: part I. J Am Acad Dermatol. 2010;63(6):925–46. quiz 947–8.
2. Mueller W, Herrmann B. Cyclosporin A for psoriasis. N Engl J Med. 1979;301(10):555.
3. Rapini RP, Bolognia JL, Jorizzo JL. Dermatology. St. Louis: Mosby; 2007.
4. Goldsmith LA, Katz S, Gilchrest B, Paller A, Leffell D, Wolff K. Fitzpatrick's dermatology in general medicine. 8th ed. New York: McGraw-Hill; 2012.
5. Ryan C, Amor KT, Menter A. The use of cyclosporine in dermatology: part II. J Am Acad Dermatol. 2010;63(6):949–72. quiz 973–4.
6. Marcil I, Stern RS. Squamous-cell cancer of the skin in patients given PUVA and cyclosporin: nested

cohort crossover study. Lancet. 2001;358(9287):1042–5.
7. Wolverton SE. Comprehensive dermatologic drug therapy E-Book. Philadelphia: Saunders; 2007.
8. Rosmarin DM, Lebwohl M, Elewski BE, Gottlieb AB, National Psoriasis Foundation. Cyclosporine and psoriasis: 2008 National Psoriasis Foundation Consensus Conference. J Am Acad Dermatol. 2010;62(5):838–53.
9. Paul CF, Ho VC, McGeown C, Christophers E, Schmidtmann B, Guillaume JC, Lamarque V, et al. Risk of malignancies in psoriasis patients treated with cyclosporine: a 5 y cohort study. J Invest Dermatol. 2003;120(2):211–6.
10. Munro CS, Levell NJ, Shuster S, Friedmann PS. Maintenance treatment with cyclosporin in atopic eczema. Br J Dermatol. 1994;130(3):376–80.
11. Schmitt J, Schäkel K, Fölster-Holst R, Bauer A, Oertel R, Augustin M, et al. Prednisolone vs. cyclosporin for severe adult eczema. An investigator-initiated double-blind placebo-controlled multicentre trial. Br J Dermatol. 2010;162(3):661–8.
12. Salek MS, Finlay AY, Luscombe DK, Allen BR, Berth-Jones J, Camp RD, et al. Cyclosporin greatly improves the quality of life of adults with severe atopic dermatitis. A randomized, double-blind, placebo-controlled trial. Br J Dermatol. 1993;129(4):422–30.
13. van Joost T, Heule F, Korstanje M, van den Broek MJ, Stenveld HJ, van Vloten WA. Cyclosporin in atopic dermatitis: a multicentre placebo-controlled study. Br J Dermatol. 1994;130(5):634–40.
14. Harper JI, Ahmed I, Barclay G, Lacour M, Hoeger P, Cork MJ, et al. Cyclosporin for severe childhood atopic dermatitis: short course versus continuous therapy. Br J Dermatol. 2000;142(1):52–8.
15. Atakan N, Erdem C. The efficacy, tolerability and safety of a new oral formulation of Sandimmun–Sandimmun Neoral in severe refractory atopic dermatitis. J Eur Acad Dermatol Venereol. 1998;11(3):240–6.
16. Berth-Jones J, Graham-Brown RA, Marks R, Camp RD, English JS, Freeman K, et al. Long-term efficacy and safety of cyclosporin in severe adult atopic dermatitis. Br J Dermatol. 1997;136(1):76–81.
17. Reitamo S, Granlund H. Cyclosporin A in the treatment of chronic dermatitis of the hands. Br J Dermatol. 1994;130(1):75–8.
18. Granlund H, Erkko P, Eriksson E, Reitamo S. Comparison of cyclosporine and topical betamethasone-17,21-dipropionate in the treatment of severe chronic hand eczema. Acta Derm Venereol. 1996;76(5):371–6.
19. Granlund H, Erkko P, Reitamo S. Comparison of the influence of cyclosporine and topical betamethasone-17,21-dipropionate treatment on quality of life in chronic hand eczema. Acta Derm Venereol. 1997;77(1):54–8.
20. Granlund H, Erkko P, Reitamo S. Long-term follow-up of eczema patients treated with cyclosporine. Acta Derm Venereol. 1998;78(1):40–3.
21. Petersen CS, Menne T. Cyclosporin A responsive chronic severe vesicular hand eczema. Acta Derm Venereol. 1992;72(6):436–7.
22. Bowers PW, Julian CG. Dogger Bank Itch and cyclosporin. J Dermatol Treat. 2001;12(1):23–4.

Systemic Treatment of Hand Eczema: Mycophenolate Mofetil

38

Denis Sasseville

Contents

38.1 Introduction

Mycophenolic acid was initially used in the treatment of psoriasis in the 1970s [1–4] but fell into disfavor because of its high rate of gastrointestinal side effects and the concern for carcinogenicity [5, 6]. The development of mycophenolate mofetil, which displays greater bioavailability and a lower rate of side effects, led to renewed interest in this potent immunosuppressant. The Food and Drug Administration (FDA) of the United States has approved the use of mycophenolate mofetil for the prevention of renal allograft rejection. Since the 1990s, however, the drug has found numerous off-label applications in dermatology, mostly in the treatment of autoimmune blistering diseases, and a reappraisal of its role in psoriasis management [7–10]. It has been successfully used to control severe atopic dermatitis and could theoretically be of benefit in the management of chronic hand dermatitis refractory to standard therapy.

38.2 Pharmacology

Isolated in 1896, mycophenolic acid (Fig. 38.1) is derived from the fungus *Penicillium stoloniferum* [6]. This weak organic acid is rapidly absorbed after oral administration and conjugated in the liver to mycophenolic acid glucuronide. This metabolite cannot penetrate cell membranes and is thus inactive. It is reactivated by the enzyme β-glucuronidase, which is

D. Sasseville, M.D., FRCPC
Division of Dermatology, Department of Medicine, McGill University Health Centre, Royal Victoria Hospital, Room A4.17, 687 Pine Avenue West, Montreal, Quebec H3A 1A1, Canada
e-mail: denis.sasseville@mcgill.ca

A. Alikhan et al. (eds.), *Textbook of Hand Eczema*,
DOI 10.1007/978-3-642-39546-8_38, © Springer-Verlag Berlin Heidelberg 2014

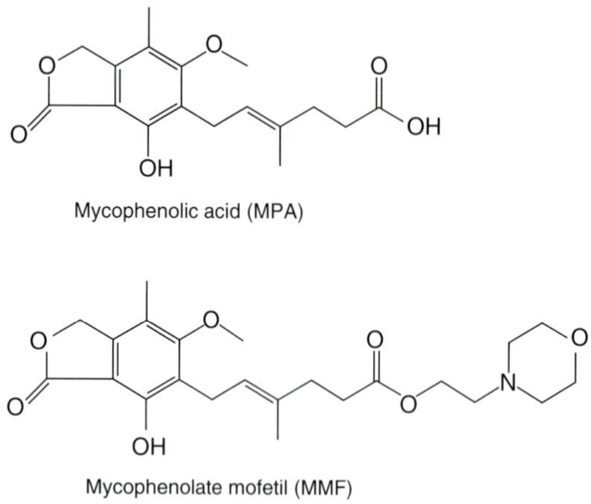

Fig. 38.1 Chemical structure of mycophenolic acid and its prodrug, mycophenolate mofetil

present in cells of the epidermis, the gastrointestinal tract, the urinary tract, and certain tumors [2, 11].

The prodrug mycophenolate mofetil (see Fig. 38.1) is a morpholinoester of mycophenolic acid with greater bioavailability than its active metabolite. It is cleaved by plasma esterases into mycophenolic acid after oral absorption [6]. Both mycophenolic acid and its inactive glucuronide metabolite are 97 % and 82 % albumin bound, respectively [12]. Over 95 % of an administered dose of mycophenolate mofetil is excreted in the urine as mycophenolic acid glucuronide. Renal insufficiency increases the plasma levels of mycophenolic acid glucuronide, but not of mycophenolic acid, and dosage adjustments do not appear necessary, given the lack of activity of the glucuronide metabolite [12].

38.3 Mechanism of Action

Mycophenolic acid is an antimetabolite that inhibits the de novo pathway of purine nucleotides synthesis. It acts as a noncompetitive and reversible inhibitor of inosine monophosphate dehydrogenase (IMPDH), thus blocking the conversion of inosine monophosphate into xanthine monophosphate. This leads to downstream depletion of guanosine triphosphate (GTP), the building block of DNA, RNA, and protein synthesis [6].

Most cells possess a salvage pathway of purine synthesis, but T and B lymphocytes are strictly dependent on the de novo pathway. In addition, proliferating lymphocytes harbor the type II isoform of IMPDH, which is four times more sensitive to inhibition by mycophenolic acid than the type I expressed in other cells [13]. Mycophenolic acid, therefore, selectively affects lymphocyte proliferation, activation, and antibody production.

It has also been demonstrated that mycophenolic acid-mediated depletion of GTP inhibits glycosylation of adhesion molecules such as selectins and their ligands, thereby impeding lymphocyte and monocyte recruitment at sites of inflammation [13]. This effect further increases the immunosuppressive and anti-inflammatory properties of mycophenolic acid and its prodrug mycophenolate mofetil.

Quéméneur et al. investigated in a mouse model the effect of various immunosuppressive drugs on the sensitization and elicitation phases of contact hypersensitivity [14]. Through blockage of clonal expansion of cycling CD8+ T lymphocytes, mycophenolate mofetil effectively suppressed contact hypersensitivity when administered during the sensitization phase, but had no effect when given immediately before challenge in already sensitized mice. In another study involving a murine model, Mehling et al. have shown that, in addition to its effect on T lymphocytes, mycophenolate mofetil also moderately impairs the maturation and function of dendritic cells [15].

38.4 Side Effects

At the usual daily dose of 1–3 g, mycophenolate mofetil appears to have a better safety profile than other equipotent immunosuppressive drugs, being much less myelotoxic, nephrotoxic, and hepatotoxic.

The most common and troublesome side effects involve the gastrointestinal tract. Diarrhea and abdominal cramps occur in more than 30 % of patients, but constipation has also been reported. The pathophysiology of mycophenolate mofetil-induced diarrhea is unknown, but in one case, villous atrophy of the small intestine was demonstrated by duodenal biopsy, with a return to normal histology upon withdrawal of the drug [16]. Nausea and vomiting affect 20–50 % of patients who receive the higher daily dose of 3 g. Less common manifestations include oral ulcers, gastritis, duodenitis, and gastrointestinal bleeding.

Genitourinary symptoms will develop in approximately 40 % of patients [5]. Dysuria, urgency, frequent micturition, hematuria, sterile pyuria, and at times frank urinary infection may occur, most often during the first year of treatment, and tend to decrease afterwards [6].

Hematologic abnormalities include anemia, leukopenia, and thrombocytopenia. They are usually mild and dose related, with an occurrence that ranges between 5 % and 35 % of patients, and are reversible upon discontinuation of the drug or reduction of the dose. Severe leukopenia has been reported in organ transplantation patients who were receiving other immunosuppressive drugs in addition to mycophenolate mofetil. In addition, as of February 2008, 41 cases of pure red cell aplasia had come to the attention of the manufacturer of the drug. Here, also, some of these patients were treated with other immunosuppressive medicaments that may have contributed to their hematologic condition.

With the exception of progressive multifocal leukoencephalopathy (PML), discussed below, neurologic symptoms are uncommon and usually not severe enough to warrant withdrawal of the drug. Tiredness, tremor, weakness, and headache are the symptoms most commonly reported [11].

Approximately 40 % of organ transplant recipients treated with mycophenolate mofetil develop infectious complications, mostly cytomegalovirus, herpes simplex, and herpes zoster infections [5]. In 2 % of renal and cardiac patients and 5 % of hepatic transplantation recipients, these infections were fatal. Baudard et al. have used mycophenolate mofetil with success in the treatment of 21 patients with acute or chronic graft-versus-host reaction but also reported a total of 22 viral or bacterial infections in ten patients [17]. It is likely that patients on mycophenolic acid or mycophenolate mofetil monotherapy for dermatologic diseases will have a lower incidence and a milder course of infections. Investigators treating psoriasis with mycophenolic acid reported an increased frequency of herpes zoster infections [18]. Likewise, in patients treated with mycophenolate mofetil, herpesvirus infections, both zoster and simplex, staphylococcal cutaneous infections and septicemia, mycobacterial abscess, and bronchopulmonary legionella and blastomycosis infections have been documented [6, 19–21]. Of greater concern, however, is the possible reactivation of latent viruses. Progressive multifocal leukoencephalopathy is a demyelinating disease caused by reactivation of the John Cunningham polyomavirus, present in 70–90 % of adult population. As of June 2008, ten confirmed and seven possible cases had been reported, and six had a fatal outcome related to the infection. No treatment is available except reducing the degree of immunosuppression. All reported cases were receiving other immunosuppressive agents. This prompted Roche Pharmaceuticals to issue a warning letter advising health care professionals who prescribe mycophenolate mofetil to be on the lookout for neurologic symptoms and signs such as apathy, confusion, ataxia, and hemiparesis.

Animal studies have shown that mycophenolate mofetil is not carcinogenic, is not incorporated in DNA, and does not cause chromosomal breakage [11]. However, in transplant-recipient populations, some patients will develop lymphomas, nonmelanoma skin cancer, or other solid organ tumors [6]. This is thought to be due to the degree and duration of immunosuppression and is more likely to occur when patients are treated with a combination of immunosuppressive drugs. By comparison with regimens that include azathioprine instead of mycophenolate mofetil, the latter drug is associated with a lower incidence of malignancies [19].

The FDA has assigned mycophenolate mofetil to pregnancy category D. Its use in pregnancy is recommended only when there is no alternative and benefit outweighs risk. Animal studies have shown malformations of the head and eyes [19].

Spontaneous abortions and fetal malformations have been documented in humans. Observed malformations included facial dysmorphism such as microtia and cleft lip or palate, shortened fingers, hypoplastic nails, congenital heart defects, and malformations of the esophagus and kidney. No data are available concerning the excretion of mycophenolic acid in human milk, but mycophenolate mofetil has been measured in the milk of lactating rats.

38.5 Mycophenolate Mofetil in the Treatment of Eczema

38.5.1 Atopic Dermatitis

In 1999, Grundmann-Kollmann et al. reported the successful use of mycophenolate mofetil in two patients with severe atopic dermatitis who had failed PUVA phototherapy, as well as oral corticosteroids and cyclosporin [22]. They used a dose of 1 g twice daily. Both patients had a rapid response to treatment and cleared after 2 and 4 weeks, respectively. Tolerated without side effect, mycophenolate mofetil was stopped 4 weeks after clearance, and no relapse was seen in the following 12 weeks. The patient of Satchell and Barnetson, a 50-year-old woman with generalized dermatitis, cleared almost completely on a daily dose of 1,250 mg, increased to 2 g daily after 5 months of treatment because of worsening of her condition. She again experienced some improvement but then developed staphylococcal septicemia and the drug was stopped [21]. Benez and Fierlbeck treated three patients with generalized dermatitis or erythroderma with 2 g daily [23]. The dermatitis cleared almost completely within 3–5 weeks of therapy. Mycophenolate mofetil was administered for periods ranging from 12 to 29 months without major side effects or infectious complication.

In an open-label study conducted in Hamburg, ten patients with severe atopic dermatitis were treated for 12 weeks with mycophenolate mofetil 2 g daily [24]. The baseline median score of disease severity, as measured by the Scoring of Atopic Dermatitis scale (SCORAD index), was 68.3 and decreased to 22.0 at the end of the treatment period. One patient cleared completely, three had 75 % improvement, and the rest were >50 % better. Side effects were mild and no infection was reported. Another open-label study also enrolled ten patients who were treated for 4 weeks with a daily dose of 2 g, followed by 4 weeks at 1 g daily [25]. After 4 weeks, the SCORAD index had decreased from a baseline of 49.2 down to 27.5. Seven patients had cleared completely, but two eventually relapsed while on mycophenolate mofetil, and one patient developed herpes retinitis. Six of the seven responders showed a lasting remission during a 20-week follow-up.

In contrast with the excellent results of the early case reports and studies, Hansen et al. were unable to substantiate beneficial effects in six of seven patients that they treated with a daily dose of 2 g for up to 12 weeks [26]. More recent studies, however, confirm the usefulness of mycophenolate mofetil in the management of atopic dermatitis. In 2007 Murray and Cohen published a retrospective chart review of 20 patients diagnosed with moderate to severe atopic dermatitis, who had failed topical or systemic therapy [20]. Improvement was seen in 18 patients at or before 4 weeks, and treatment was continued for periods that ranged from 5 to 200 weeks. Four patients developed herpes zoster, one had widespread genital herpes, and two acquired *Staphylococcus aureus* cellulitis and folliculitis, respectively [20]. Ballester et al. treated eight patients with severe atopic dermatitis, five of which improved in the first 4 weeks of treatment [27]. One patient eventually cleared and was able to stop mycophenolate mofetil. The remaining four remained controlled on maintenance therapy. In an open-label study, Jackson et al. enrolled 16 patients with chronic dermatitis refractory to topical therapy [28]. Patients were divided into three groups based on dosage of mycophenolate mofetil: 1 g, 1.5 g, or 2 g daily. Over the 30-week study period, patients in cohort three displayed rapid and constant improvement as measured by global severity assessment. Subjects in the other groups improved markedly after the daily dose of mycophenolate mofetil was increased to 2.5 g in cohort 2 and 3 g in cohort 1. Fourteen patients improved, three cleared completely, and six were almost clear. One patient was diagnosed with pancreatic cancer at week 12 of the study, but his tumor was probably present before initiation of treatment for his dermatitis [28].

Mycophenolate mofetil has also been studied in the pediatric population. Heller et al. performed a retrospective analysis of 14 patients treated with mycophenolate mofetil monotherapy for severe atopic dermatitis [29]. A daily dose of 45–50 mg kg^{-1} was used in younger children, while teenagers were treated with 30–40 mg kg^{-1}. Maximal effects were seen between 8 and 12 weeks of therapy. Four patients cleared completely, four were almost clear, and five reached 60–90 % improvement. No infection or other complication supervened. Waxweiler et al. reviewed the medical records of 28 children with atopic dermatitis who were treated with either mycophenolate mofetil or azathioprine [30]. Twelve patients were treated with mycophenolate mofetil at a daily dose ranging from 20 to 40 mg kg^{-1}. Of these 12 patients, eight reported significant improvement and four reported no improvement. There was no statistical difference in the response rates in the group treated with azathioprine or mycophenolate mofetil. The incidence of side effects was less in the mycophenolate group, but the rates of infections were similar [30].

38.5.2 Hand Eczema

Very few of the reports dealing with treatment of atopic dermatitis with mycophenolate mofetil specifically mention the presence of hand eczema and the effect of treatment on this anatomical area. The first patient of Grundmann-Kollmann et al. had involvement of the hands in addition to widespread dermatitis. We can only presume that her hand dermatitis responded to treatment [22]. Among the patients of Hansen et al. who failed to improve was a 58-year-old atopic man with hand eczema, whose SCORAD actually worsened from 42.3 to 44.6 while under treatment [26]. The only patient who showed some degree of improvement was a 45-year-old woman with severe chronic vesicular hand dermatitis and contact sensitization to nickel and Compositae mix. The authors state that "at entrance to the study she had bilateral volar hand dermatitis with numerous vesicles, erythema, infiltration, crusts, and scaling." After 12 weeks of treatment, only a few vesicles and mild scaling were present [26].

Pickenäcker et al. used mycophenolate mofetil to treat a 39-year-old man with a 4-year history of severe, relapsing dyshidrosis [31]. Unable to work for 1 year, the patient was dependent on systemic corticosteroid. Cyclosporin had exerted some beneficial effect but was stopped because of marked hypertension. The initial dose of mycophenolate mofetil was 3 g daily, and the dermatitis cleared in 4 weeks, allowing the patient to return to work. The dosage was reduced to 2 g daily and further tapered over 12 months.

Abreu-Velez et al. reported the case of a 58-year-old African American woman with a clinical history of rheumatoid arthritis and chronic, vesicular dermatitis of the palms and soles evolving for 5 years [32]. Histological examination from a skin biopsy showed spongiotic dermatitis. Treatment was initiated with mycophenolate mofetil, and the lesions eventually cleared. Unfortunately, the article, focusing on the immunological abnormalities found in this patient, failed to mention the course of the disease, the dose of mycophenolate mofetil, and the presence or absence of side effects.

Strangely, the administration of mycophenolate mofetil has also been associated with the development of dyshidrosis [33]. A 45-year-old female liver transplant recipient was treated with cyclosporin and prednisolone. When nephrotoxicity supervened, mycophenolate mofetil was administered at a dose of 2 g daily in order to wean her off cyclosporin. Three days later, the patient suddenly developed a vesiculobullous eruption of the hands and feet. The drug was immediately stopped and the lesions cleared. Three months later, a relapse of the same eruption occurred within 24 h of mycophenolate mofetil reintroduction. A skin biopsy was consistent with dyshidrotic eczema, and allergy testing with mycophenolate mofetil reproduced the lesions [33]. This publication, however, remains the only one to report this type of adverse effect.

Conclusion

In the past decade, dermatologists have increasingly added mycophenolate mofetil in their therapeutic armamentarium, mostly to treat inflammatory conditions such as psoriasis and autoimmune bullous diseases. Its unique mechanism of action that specifically targets lymphocytes makes it relatively safer than other immunosuppressive agents. In view of the pathophysiology of eczema, the use of mycophenolate mofetil to treat chronic hand eczema makes sense, especially if there are contraindications or side effects with more conventional systemic agents. Well-conducted clinical studies are needed to firmly establish its role in the management of this condition.

References

1. Jones EL, Epinette WW, Hackney VC, Menendez L, Frost P. Treatment of psoriasis with oral mycophenolic acid. J Invest Dermatol. 1975;111:853–6.
2. Marinari R, Fleischmajer R, Schragger AH, Rosenthal AL. Mycophenolic acid in the treatment of psoriasis. Arch Dermatol. 1977;113:930–2.
3. Lynch WS, Roenigk Jr HH. Mycophenolic acid for psoriasis. Arch Dermatol. 1977;113:1203–8.
4. Gomez EC, Menendez L, Frost P. Efficacy of mycophenolic acid for the treatment of psoriasis. J Am Acad Dermatol. 1979;1:531–7.
5. Mydlarski PR. Mycophenolate mofetil: a dermatologic perspective. Skin Therapy Lett. 2005;10(3):1–6.
6. Orvis AK, Wesson SK, Breza Jr TS, Church AA, Mitchell CL, Watkins SW. Mycophenolate mofetil in dermatology. J Am Acad Dermatol. 2009;60:183–99.
7. Enk AH, Knop J. Mycophenolate is effective in the treatment of pemphigus vulgaris. Arch Dermatol. 1999;135:54–6.
8. Grundmann-Kollmann M, Korting HC, Behrens S, Kaskel P, Leiter U, Krähn G, et al. Mycophenolate mofetil: a new therapeutic option in the treatment of blistering autoimmune diseases. J Am Acad Dermatol. 1999;40:957–60.
9. Davison SC, Morris-Jones R, Powles AV, Fry L. Change of treatment from cyclosporin to mycophenolate mofetil in severe psoriasis. Br J Dermatol. 2000;143:405–7.
10. Zhou Y, Rosenthal D, Dutz J, Ho V. Mycophenolate mofetil (CellCept®) for psoriasis: a two-center, prospective, open-label clinical trial. J Cutan Med Surg. 2003;7:193–7.
11. Kitchin JE, Pomeranz MK, Pak G, Washenik K, Shupack JL. Rediscovering mycophenolic acid: a review of its mechanism, side effects, and potential uses. J Am Acad Dermatol. 1997;37:445–9.
12. Bullingham RE, Nicholls AJ, Kamm BR. Clinical pharmacokinetics of mycophenolate mofetil. Clin Pharmacokinet. 1998;34:429–55.
13. Allison AC, Eugui EM. Immunosuppressive and other effects of MPA and an ester prodrug, mycophenolate mofetil. Immunol Rev. 1993;136:5–28.
14. Quémeneur L, Michallet MC, Ferraro-Peyret C, Saint-Mézard P, Benetière J, Ducluzeau MT, et al. Immunosuppressive antimetabolites inhibit induction of contact hypersensitivity while lymphoablative drugs also prevent its expression. Eur J Dermatol. 2003;13:540–7.
15. Mehling A, Grabbe S, Voskort M, Schwarz T, Luger TA, Beissert S. Mycophenolate mofetil impairs the maturation and function of murine dendritic cells. J Immunol. 2000;165:2374–81.
16. Ducloux D, Ottignon Y, Semhoun-Ducloux S, Labbé S, Saint-Hillier Y, Miguet JP, et al. Mycophenolate mofetil-induced villous atrophy. Transplantation. 1998;66:1115–6.
17. Baudard M, Vincent A, Moreau P, Kergueris MF, Harousseau JL, Milpied N. Mycophenolate mofetil for the treatment of acute and chronic GVHD is effective and well tolerated but induces a high risk of infectious complications: a series of 21 BM or PBSC transplant patients. Bone Marrow Transplant. 2002;5:287–95.
18. Epinette WW, Parker CM, Jones EL, Greist MC. Mycophenolic acid for psoriasis. A review of pharmacology, long-term efficacy, and safety. J Am Acad Dermatol. 1987;17:962–71.
19. Buell C, Koo J. Long-term safety of mycophenolate mofetil and cyclosporine: a review. J Drugs Dermatol. 2008;7:741–8.
20. Murray ML, Cohen JB. Mycophenolate mofetil therapy for moderate to severe atopic dermatitis. Clin Exp Dermatol. 2007;32:23–7.
21. Satchell AC, Barnetson RS. Staphylococcal septicaemia complicating treatment of atopic dermatitis with mycophenolate. Br J Dermatol. 2000;143:202–3.
22. Grundmann-Kollmann M, Korting HC, Behrens S, Leiter U, Krähn G, Kaufmann R, et al. Successful treatment of severe refractory atopic dermatitis with mycophenolate mofetil. Br J Dermatol. 1999;141:175–6.
23. Benez A, Fierlbeck G. Successful long-term treatment of severe atopic dermatitis with mycophenolate mofetil. Br J Dermatol. 2001;144:638–9.
24. Neuber K, Schwartz I, Itschert G, Dieck AT. Treatment of atopic eczema with oral mycophenolate mofetil. Br J Dermatol. 2000;143:385–91.
25. Grundmann-Kollmann M, Podda M, Ochsendorf F, Boehncke WH, Kaufmann R, Zollner TM. Mycophenolate mofetil is effective in the treatment of atopic dermatitis. Arch Dermatol. 2001;137:870–3.
26. Hansen ER, Buus S, Deleuran M, Andersen KE. Treatment of atopic dermatitis with mycophenolate mofetil. Br J Dermatol. 2000;143:1324–6.
27. Ballester I, Silvestre JF, Pérez-Crespo M, Lucas A. Severe adult atopic dermatitis: treatment with

mycophenolate mofetil in 8 patients. Actas Dermosifiliogr. 2009;100:883–7.
28. Jackson JM, Fowler Jr FJ, Callen JP, Lorenz DJ. Mycophenolate mofetil for the treatment of chronic dermatitis: an open-label study of 16 patients. J Drugs Dermatol. 2010;9:356–62.
29. Heller M, Shin HT, Orlow SJ, Schaffer JV. Mycophenolate mofetil for severe childhood atopic dermatitis: experience in 14 patients. Br J Dermatol. 2007;157:127–32.
30. Waxweiler WT, Agans R, Morrell DS. Systemic treatment of pediatric atopic dermatitis with azathioprine and mycophenolate mofetil. Pediatr Dermatol. 2011;28:689–94.
31. Pickenäcker A, Luger TA, Schwarz T. Dyshidrotic eczema treated with mycophenolate mofetil. Arch Dermatol. 1998;134:378–9.
32. Abreu-Velez AM, Pinto Jr FJ, Howard MS. Dyshidrotic eczema: relevance to the immune response in situ. N Am J Med Sci. 2009;1:117–20.
33. Semhoun-Ducloux S, Ducloux D, Miguet JP. Mycophenolate mofetil-induced dyshidrotic eczema. Ann Intern Med. 2000;132:417.

Systemic and Topical Treatment of Hand Eczema: Less Well-Established Agents

39

Richard R. Winkelmann and Ali Alikhan

Contents

R.R. Winkelmann, DO (✉)
Intern, O'Bleness Memorial Hospital,
Athens, OH, USA
e-mail: rrwink@gmail.com

A. Alikhan, M.D.
Department of Dermatology, Mayo Clinic,
200 1st St SW, Rochester, MN 55905, USA
e-mail: alialikhan1@yahoo.com

39.1 Introduction

Despite advances in the treatment of refractory chronic hand eczema, many patients remain burdened with recalcitrant disease. Patients with limited therapeutic options may use several atypical agents to achieve control of symptoms. There is little support in the literature for using these interventions, and none are licensed for the treatment of chronic hand eczema. Evidence for the use of these atypical agents is only supported by smaller studies, anecdotal evidence, or single case reports.

39.2 Topical Bexarotene

A gel formulation of bexarotene was approved in the United States for cutaneous T-cell lymphoma in 2000. Bexarotene is a rexinoid, part of a new class of medications that act as ligands for retinoid X receptors and, in turn, on other important receptors in skin physiology [1]. The therapeutic potential of bexarotene for inflammatory skin disorders is attributed to its interaction with peroxisome proliferation-activating receptors [2]. A phase I–II open-label randomized clinical study of 55 patients with severe chronic hand dermatitis evaluated the safety, tolerability, and efficacy of topical bexarotene alone or in combination with a low-mid potency topical steroid [3]. Of the 55 patients receiving 1.0 % bexarotene gel two or three times daily, 20 (36 %) reached ≥90 % clearance of hand dermatitis and 39 (71 %) experienced ≥50 %

A. Alikhan et al. (eds.), *Textbook of Hand Eczema*,
DOI 10.1007/978-3-642-39546-8_39, © Springer-Verlag Berlin Heidelberg 2014

improvement after 22 weeks. The efficacy of bexarotene monotherapy was not improved in combination with topical steroids. Bexarotene gel may be a promising new therapeutic alternative for patients with chronic severe hand dermatitis.

39.3 Systemic Corticosteroids

Oral corticosteroids are suitable for treating acute exacerbations of hand eczema recalcitrant to topical therapy. In general, doses range from 0.5 to 1 mg/kg/day with subsequent tapering [4]. For recurrent dyshidrotic hand eczema, one author recommends short bursts of 60 mg daily for 3–4 days, repeated every 2–4 months as needed [5]. No randomized controlled trials exist studying the effectiveness of this well-established therapeutic agent. Following rapid control of symptoms, dermatitis can re-flare after cessation of therapy. Long-term use is generally not appropriate owing to the risk of osteoporosis, glaucoma, cataracts, hypothalamic-pituitary-adrenal axis suppression, hyperglycemia, hypertension, and immunosuppression [6].

39.4 Ranitidine

Ranitidine has been studied as an adjuvant to topical steroid therapy in patients with chronic hand dermatitis. The beneficial effects of ranitidine are attributed to the blockade of H2 receptors on immunoactive cells [7]. A randomized, controlled trial of 47 patients found that those on 300 mg of ranitidine twice daily, in addition to topical betamethasone valerate, had a statistically significant reduction of disease activity after 16 weeks of therapy [8]. No side effects were observed in the study from ranitidine or placebo.

39.5 Vitamin E

Oral preparations of vitamin E have been reported to effectively treat palmar dermatitis refractory to topical and systemic steroid therapy. On one account, a patient was taking 400 mg of vitamin E daily for prevention of coronary disease and serendipitously experienced complete clearance of his chronic hand dermatitis [9]. Vitamin E is known as an antioxidant with a safe side-effect profile and may benefit some patients with recalcitrant dermatitis [10]. Additional clinical studies on the therapeutic benefits of vitamin E supplementation are needed to establish its routine use.

39.6 Azathioprine

Azathioprine is a steroid-sparing agent shown to successfully treat hand eczema in patients with parthenium dermatitis and atopic dermatitis [11–14]. The immunosuppressive effects of azathioprine are attributed to its ability to alter the synthesis and function of RNA and DNA in lymphocytes. Doses of azathioprine range from 1 to 2 mg/kg/day for the treatment of parthenium dermatitis and generally take 2–3 months to attain clinical results [11]. In a case series of nine patients with upper limb lymphedema associated with hand dermatitis, six patients improved on azathioprine, although three stopped the drug owing to side effects [13]. Limitations of azathioprine therapy include slow onset of activity and potential to cause bone-marrow suppression, hepatotoxicity, and malignancy [14].

39.7 Treatment Options in Nickel-Induced Hand Dermatitis

Chelating agents, like disulfiram, have proven useful in allergic contact dermatitis to nickel. Nickel sensitivity is common in the general population, and its ingestion can provoke or aggravate existing hand eczema in allergic individuals [15]. Dyshidrotic and vesicular eczema are the most common variants of hand eczema associated with sensitivity to nickel ingestion [15]. Several studies have examined the treatment of nickel-sensitive hand eczema with the nickel chelating agent disulfiram [15–17]. In general, patients treated with 200–400 mg disulfiram daily for 4 weeks achieved significant reductions in disease activity. However, there are reports of hepatotoxicity in patients following long-term disulfiram therapy [18–20]. Therefore, short courses of oral disulfiram may be considered in patients with chronic, recalcitrant nickel-sensitive hand eczema.

Other agents, including disodium cromoglycate (DSCG), zinc sulfate, and iron, have demonstrated effectiveness in nickel-sensitive hand dermatitis by interfering with intestinal nickel absorption. DSCG inhibits intestinal uptake of nickel by reducing movement of nickel through small aqueous pores. In 24 patients with dyshidrotic hand eczema, patients taking 1,500–2,000 mg of DSCG three times daily exhibited improvement in clinical disease compared with low-nickel diet and control groups [21]. Intestinal permeability tests demonstrated diminished nickel uptake after 15 days of DSCG treatment.

Cases of nickel dermatitis have improved following oral administration of zinc sulfate ($ZnSO_4$) [22, 23]. One clinical study of 15 $NiSO_4$-positive patients demonstrated 300 mg $ZnSO_4$ daily for 30 days improves clinical manifestations of nickel dermatitis [22]. No adverse effects were reported, indicating that $ZnSO_4$ is a safe and efficacious alternative for nickel-sensitive hand dermatitis.

Oral iron therapy has also been studied for its use in nickel-sensitive hand eczema [24]. Adequate levels of iron in the diet are associated with reduced dietary uptake of nickel [25]. In a study of 23 patients with chronic vesicular hand eczema, 10 of 12 patients taking 30-mg elemental iron daily showed complete clearance of their hand dermatitis following 12 weeks of therapy [24]. Only moderate improvement was noted in 5 of 11 patients in the control group over a 12-week period.

39.8 Biologic Agents

With the success of biologic therapies for the treatment of psoriasis, several case reports suggest additional therapeutic benefits in patients with hand dermatitis. Etanercept, a recombinant human TNF-receptor fusion protein, antagonizes the effects of TNF-α on cell-surface receptors [26]. According to one report, etanercept successfully induced remission in a woman with recalcitrant endogenous hand pompholyx for 4 months following 25-mg subcutaneous injections twice weekly [27]. The drug was well tolerated and suggests that the anti-inflammatory properties of etanercept may prove beneficial in patients with severe, refractory hand eczema.

Alefacept is a recombinant human leukocyte-function-associated antigen 3 (LFA-3) IgG1 fusion protein effective in the treatment of severe psoriasis [28]. The interaction between LFA-3 on antigen presenting cells and CD2 on all T-lymphocyte subgroups activates the proliferation and effector functions of T-lymphocytes. By interfering with this interaction in patients with psoriasis, alefacept suppresses CD45RO+ memory T-cell activity [29]. CD45RO+ cells also play an important role in the pathogenesis of acute hand dermatitis [30]. One patient with a 5-month history of hand dermatitis refractory to standard therapy dramatically improved after 16 weeks of 15 mg of alefacept administered intramuscularly once weekly [31]. No side effects were reported, suggesting that alefacept might be another safe and effective option in patients with refractory chronic hand dermatitis.

Conclusion

Whether a treatment intervention is newer or supported by decades of anecdotal evidence, it is important to stress the need for powerful clinical studies proving their efficacy and safety. Due to the current climate of health care and increasing emphasis on practicing evidence-based medicine, physicians will likely be required to make clinical judgments based on the strength of evidence from the literature. With better-designed trials on a sufficient number of patients with recalcitrant hand eczema, clinicians will be able to offer atypical treatment options more confidently under the aegis of evidence-based medicine.

References

1. Mangelsdorf DJ, Evans RM. The RXR heterodimers and orphan receptors. Cell. 1995;83:841–50.

2. Cheng S, Kupper T. A new rexinoid for cutaneous T-cell lymphoma. Arch Dermatol. 2001;137:649–52.
3. Hanifin JM, Stevens V, Sheth P, Breneman D. Novel treatment of chronic severe hand dermatitis with bexarotene gel. Br J Dermatol. 2004;150(3):545–53.
4. Alavi A, Skotnicki S, Sussman G, Sibbald RG. Diagnosis and treatment of hand dermatitis. Adv Skin Wound Care. 2012;8:381–2.
5. Warshaw E, Lee G, Storrs FJ. Hand dermatitis: a review of clinical features, therapeutic options, and long-term outcomes. Am J Contact Dermatol. 2003; 14(3):119–37.
6. Nesbitt Jr LT. Minimizing complications from systemic glucocorticoid use. Dermatol Clin. 1995;13:925–39.
7. Nielsen HJ, Nielsen H, Georgsen J. Ranitidine for improvement of treatment resistant psoriasis: mechanisms and speculations. Dan Med Bull. 1991;38: 478–80.
8. Veien NK, Kaaber K, Larsen PO, Nielsen AO, Thestrup-Pedersen K. Ranitidine treatment of hand eczema in patients with atopic dermatitis: a double blind placebo controlled trial. J Am Acad Dermatol. 1995;32:1056–7.
9. Olson PE, Torp EC, Mahon RT, Weiss PJ, Wallace MR. Oral vitamin E for refractory hand dermatitis. Lancet. 1994;343(8898):672–3.
10. Kappus H, Diplock AT. Tolerance and safety of vitamin E: a toxicological position report. Free Radic Biol Med. 1992;13:55–74.
11. Lakshmi C, Srinivas CR. Parthenium the terminator: an update. Indian Dermatol Online J. 2011;3:89–100.
12. Berth-Jones J, Takwale A, Tan E, Barclay G, Agarwal S, Ahmed I. Azathioprine in severe adult atopic dermatitis: a double-blind, placebo-controlled, crossover trial. Br J Dermatol. 2002;147:324–30.
13. Pearce VJ, Mortimer PS. Hand dermatitis and lymphoedema. Br J Dermatol. 2009;161(1):177–80.
14. Meggitt SJ, Reynolds NJ. Azathioprine for atopic dermatitis. Clin Exp Dermatol. 2001;26:369–75.
15. Christensen OB, Moller H. Nickel allergy and hand eczema. Contact Dermatitis. 1975;1:136–42.
16. Sharma AD. Disulfiram and low nickel diet in the management of hand eczema: a clinical study. Indian J Dermatol Venereol Leprol. 2006;72:113–8.
17. Kaaber K, Menne T, Tjell JC. Low nickel diet in the treatment of patients with chronic nickel dermatitis. Br J Dermatol. 1978;98:197.
18. Kaaber K, Menne T, Tjell JC, Veien N. Antabuse treatment of nickel dermatitis. Chelation- a new principal in the treatment of nickel dermatitis. Contact Dermatitis. 1979;5:221–8.
19. Kaaber K, Menne T, Veien N, Hougaard P. Treatment of nickel dermatitis with Antabuse; a double blind study. Contact Dermatitis. 1983;9:297–9.
20. Christensen OB, Kristensen M. Treatment with disulfiram in chronic nickel hand dermatitis. Contact Dermatitis. 1982;8:59–63.
21. Pigatto PD, Gibelli E, Fumagalli M, Bigardi A, Morelli M, Altomare GF. Disodium cromoglycate versus diet in the treatment and prevention of nickel-positive pompholyx. Contact Dermatitis. 1990;22:27–31.
22. Santucci B, Cristaudo A, Mehraban M, Valenzano C, Camera E, Picardo M. ZnSO4 treatment of NiSO4-positive patients. Contact Dermatitis. 1999;40:281–2.
23. Weissmann K, Menne T. Nickel allergy and drug interaction. In: Maibach HI, Menne T, editors. Nickel and the skin: immunology and toxicology. 1st ed. Boca Raton: CRC Press; 1989.
24. Sharma AD. Iron therapy in hand eczema: a new approach for management. Indian J Dermatol. 2011;56(3):295–9.
25. Tallkvist J, Bowlus CL, Lonnerdal B. Effect of iron treatment on nickel absorption and gene expression of the divalent metal transporter (DMT1) by human intestinal Caco-2 cells. Pharmacol Toxicol. 2003;92: 121–4.
26. Leonardi CL, Powers JL, Matheson RT, Goffe BS, Zitnik R, Wang A, Gottlieb AB, Etanercept Psoriasis Study Group. Etanercept as monotherapy in patients with psoriasis. N Engl J Med. 2003;349(21): 2014–22.
27. Ogden S, Clayton TH, Goodfield MJ. Recalcitrant hand pompholyx: variable response to etanercept. Clin Exp Dermatol. 2006;31(1):145–6.
28. Ellis CN, Krueger GG, Alefacept Clinical Study Group. Treatment of chronic plaque psoriasis by selective targeting of memory effector T lymphocytes. N Engl J Med. 2001;345(4):248–55.
29. Gribetz GH, Blum R, Brady C, Cohen S, Lebwohi M. An extended 16-week course of alefacept in the treatment of chronic plaque psoriasis. J Am Acad Dermatol. 2005;53:73–5.
30. Moed H, Boosma DM, Stoof TJ, von Blomberg BM, Bruynzeel DP, Scheper RJ, et al. Nickel-responding T cells are CD4+, CLA+, CD45RO45+ and express chemokine receptors CXCR3, CCR4, and CCRIO. Br J Dermalol. 2004;151:32–41.
31. Aronson PJ, Yeung-Yue KA. Treatment of hand dermatitis with alefacept. Dermatitis. 2008;19(3):161–2.

Approaches to the Management of Hand Eczema

40

Tove Agner

Contents

T. Agner, M.D., M.Sc.
Department of Dermatology,
Bispebjerg Hospital, University of Copenhagen,
Copenhagen 2900, Denmark
e-mail: t.agner@dadlnet.dk

40.1 Introduction

The diagnosis "hand eczema" (HE) is used to describe a disease in which the symptom is eczema localized to the hand(s). The disease may be acute, lasting for less than 3 months, or chronic or appear as recurrent flares in between periods with normal skin. The morphology may be dominated by vesicles, erythema, and inflammation (mostly seen in acute eczema) or by scaling, hyperkeratosis, and fissures (as seen in more chronic eczema), and both forms are pruritic [1]. The location of the eczema may vary, sometimes including all parts of the hands, but often limited to either the palmar side or the dorsal side of the hand and fingers. Tips of the fingers, as well as the wrists, may sometimes also be affected. The eczema is, in most cases, limited to the hands but sometimes spreads to the forearms or even to the upper arms, legs, and trunk. Spreading to the feet without spreading to the rest of the skin is also quite common. Severity of HE varies from mild to very severe. A high degree of severity at the onset of the disease is an important marker for a poor prognosis [2], but all cases of HE should be taken seriously, since mild eczema may later develop into more serious cases. Chronicity often occurs, and for occupational hand eczema, it has been demonstrated that symptoms were still present in 72 % of all HE patients when reinvestigated after 12 years [3]. Current data indicate that chronicity is best avoided by rapid onset of effective treatment [4].

HE is often caused by exposure to environmental factors, sometimes due to vocation, and in

A. Alikhan et al. (eds.), *Textbook of Hand Eczema*,
DOI 10.1007/978-3-642-39546-8_40, © Springer-Verlag Berlin Heidelberg 2014

these cases legal precautions may be taken (i.e., notification of the disease to the appropriate authorities). Some subclasses of HE are not caused by any (known) external factors. These endogenous eczemas are often quite severe and chronic types of HE [5, 6], and the morphology is either hyperkeratotic or vesicular [7].

As the management of HE is complex and dependent on many factors, all cases of HE should undergo a thorough examination, aiming at a subclassification of each case [8–10], and a generally accepted subclassification of HE is badly needed. The ultimate goal for the treatment of HE would be a tailor-made treatment for each subdiagnosis, supported by evidence from clinical trials including specific subclasses of HE. At the moment, however, there are few randomized controlled trials investigating the evidence for the treatment of HE and even fewer trials trying to subclassify HE. Some limitations of the evidence for the treatment of HE today are that the data obtained are far from perfect and that the treatment results are based on populations with a mixture of subclasses of HE and are, therefore, not directly comparable to other populations, where the composition may differ.

Management of HE includes much more than just medical treatment. In this chapter, issues regarding the examination and treatment of HE patients will be discussed. Although there is a need for further clinical trials in relation to the *medical treatment* of HE, there is, nevertheless, considerable evidence for successful initiatives in the *prevention* of HE. These will be emphasized in the following sections.

40.2 Management of Hand Eczema in the Acute Phase

The first medical consultation with HE patients often takes place when the eczema is in an acute phase, and issues in relation to approaches to HE in this phase are important. Acute eczema needs an immediate onset of treatment to avoid complications and to influence the prognosis in a positive direction [4]. In the acute phase of HE, the symptoms will, in most cases, be vesicles, erythema, and inflammation. The eczema will be wet, and infection with *Staphylococcus aureus* is often an important complication [11]. Rapid onset of treatment focusing on inflammation and infection should be initiated. Topical corticosteroids and/or, in severe cases, systemic prednisolone is the anti-inflammatory drug of choice in this situation. If topical treatment is chosen, an emollient with a higher water content than emollients used for more chronic and dry eczema should be chosen. Additional treatment of infection is important, and bacterial swabs should be obtained to identify bacteria and to test for antimicrobial resistance. To avoid development of sensitization or resistance to antibiotics, treatment with systemic antibiotics is generally preferred. An alternative to antibiotics is disinfection of the skin, either by potassium permanganate or aluminum acetate baths, which have traditionally been used, and there are other similar options available. Additionally, this topical disinfective treatment is reported by most patients to give relief from their pruritus. The acute flare of HE is often healed after 1–2 weeks, and after this, long-term treatment can begin.

In the acute situation, focus should be on treatment, but a short medical history, including current exposures that may have led to the situation and should be avoided, is important. Work-related issues should also be discussed with the patient; sick leave may sometimes be necessary to protect the skin but sometimes also to avoid spreading the infection (i.e., if the patient is in a food-related job or in health care). General advice about skin protection should be given [12]. In the acute situation, it is not recommended to start patch testing, because this may lead to flare-up of the eczema. A new appointment with the patient should be made within a month, where an extended medical examination and testing should take place.

40.3 Long-Term Management of Hand Eczema

When meeting the patient in a chronic state of the disease, a number of important factors need to be considered prior to starting treatment (in order to

Table 40.1 Factors to be considered before onset of treatment

Has sufficient patch testing been performed?
In case of contact allergies, has allergen avoidance been effective?
Have irritant exposures been identified?
Have measures been taken to avoid irritant exposures?
Has a subclassification of HE been obtained?
Has reporting/notifying this case as occupational been considered?
Has the patient received full information/education about skin care, including information about protective devices and use of emollients?
Is sick leave advisable?

obtain a good long-term result). A list of the most important issues is given in Table 40.1.

40.3.1 Medical History

A medical history must be obtained to acquire information about physical characteristics and the social situation of the patient. This history should include questions about previous or current atopic eczema or other atopic diseases (asthma or rhinitis). Questions about psoriasis, in the patient or in close family, and previous attacks of HE also should be included.

Epidemiological studies have shown that there is a greatly increased risk for patients with atopic eczema of developing HE [13], probably due to an impaired skin barrier function. The skin barrier is of extreme importance for the protection of the skin, and in the case of an impaired barrier, the risk of developing HE is increased. About 50 % of patients with atopic dermatitis have a mutation in the filaggrin genes [14], and the mutations have been shown to correlate with severe HE [15]. In tertiary centers treating HE patients with moderate and severe HE, a genetic analysis for this defect may be considered.

40.3.2 Exposure Assessment

Since the majority of HE is caused by external factors, detailed information about exposures should be obtained. For patients who are currently working, exposures should be defined. Possible contact allergens should be discussed with the patient. However, knowledge about which contact allergens are commonly found in different job situations is crucial in order to be able to ask appropriate questions. The patient's work situation should be discussed in detail, since the job title can sometimes cover many different functions. Use of gloves must be clarified. For irritant exposures, the quantity and frequency of exposure should be assessed. In wet-work situations, which are frequent irritant exposures, it is necessary to obtain information about daily number of hours with wet hands or wearing gloves, number of hand washes and disinfections daily, and number of gloves used.

Exposures during leisure hours are also important. It is a well-established fact that having children less than 4 years of age and the lack of a dishwasher in the household are both risk factors for the development of HE [16]. New data indicate that behavior with respect to skin care and especially hand washing is highly individual [17], probably learned in childhood, and therefore not easily changed. One should inquire about the patient's hobbies and activities during leisure hours, in case these may pose risk factors for the development of eczema. Information about exposures to contact allergens and irritants in the patient's private life is important to obtain the full picture for each individual.

40.3.3 Severity

It is important to determine the severity of the HE, since this will influence the treatment strategy and is probably also related to the prognosis [2].

Severity can be assessed by the following:

- Severity assessment of the current eczema by the medical personnel. Different scoring instruments for HE severity have been developed [18–20]. One of the most commonly used systems is the HECSI score, based on six different symptoms, which can each have a score from 0 to 3, and five different locations, each scored from 0 to 4 [18]. Another and more simple system is the PGA (physician's global assessment) [21, 22], where the physician indicates his/her overall impression of severity on a scale from 0 to 3. These symptoms are objective, and a high degree of reproducibility can be obtained. However, these instruments only evaluate the current situation, and do not include any information about fluctuation in the severity.

- Counting numbers of flares over a period of time gives some important information about eczema activity.
- Severity assessment by the patient may be obtained using instruments specifically designed for this purpose or by use of a VAS (visual analog scale) score [22]. These instruments may, however, not be unbiased, as the total lifestyle of the patient may be reflected in a nonspecific way rather than just eczema severity.
- HR-QoL (health-related quality of life) instruments, either generic or dermatology specific, have become increasingly popular and frequently used in recent years, since these instruments, by asking specific questions about lifestyle, clarify the effect of the skin disease/eczema on the patient's private life as well as working life [23–25]. For the patient, this may be more relevant in the clinical situation than just assessing the severity of the eczema; thus, HR-QoL instruments are increasingly used in clinical trials.

40.3.4 Morphology and Location

It is important to register the morphology of the eczema, although it may sometimes change significantly over months/years. Some cases may be dominated by vesicles and inflammation, while others are predominantly of the hyperkeratotic type. Some cases may involve the palmar side of the hand and fingers only; others may involve only the fingertips, while still others may be more widespread. The morphology helps to differentiate between acute and chronic cases and may also give a hint as to whether the HE is due to exposures (irritant and allergic HE) or is endogenous (hyperkeratotic eczema) [8, 10]. However, subclassification cannot be made from the morphology alone, and patch testing should be considered in all cases.

40.3.5 Patch Testing

If the HE does not disappear within a few weeks after the start of the treatment, patch testing should be considered to identify possible contact allergens of relevance for the HE. Before patch testing, the patient should be informed about the procedure, including the fact that in only about 20 % of cases will it reveal a contact allergen as the culprit causing the disease. Patch testing should, as a minimum, include the European Baseline Series [26] (other baseline series can be considered in different parts of the world), but in many cases, other series relating to the job situation also may be relevant. The patient's own products and cosmetic ingredients should also be included in the test [27]. If an HE patient has been tested more than 2 years ago and the eczema is still ongoing, repeated patch testing may be considered, and allergens previously causing positive reactions may then be omitted.

The physician must determine if positive patch test reactions are currently relevant and related to the HE. The next step is to inform the patient about allergen avoidance. This information may sometimes be quite complex, since it often includes long chemical names and different sources of exposure. It is therefore recommended that a follow-up appointment with the patient be planned about 3 month later, to make sure that the information has been understood and that recommendations are being followed by the patient. This is particularly important for patients with several (relevant) contact allergies.

40.3.6 Subclassification

On the basis of the information obtained about medical history, exposures, morphology, and/or the results of patch testing, it is recommended that a subclassification be made (i.e., irritant HE, allergic HE, atopic HE, or endogenous HE [vesicular or hyperkeratotic HE]) [8–10]. A subclassification is helpful when giving the necessary information to the patient and also facilitates the choice of treatment.

40.3.7 Legal Implications

If the HE is suspected to be either due to or exacerbated by occupational exposures, the eczema should be notified to the appropriate authorities. Different rules apply in different countries and different professions, however; in many countries, the patient will be entitled to paid time off or financial compensation while they recover. It is the responsibility of the doctor to inform the patient of this right.

40.3.8 Sick Leave

For HE patients of working age, the possibility of sick leave for a short period of time should be considered. In some cases of severe eczema, a sick-leave period of 2–3 weeks may help to facilitate onset of the healing process. It is important from the start to have an agreement with the patient about the length of the sick-leave period, since the expectation is that the eczema will have improved but most often not totally cleared at the end of the sick-leave period. It is also necessary that the patient understands and respects that all kinds of harmful exposures to the skin are to be avoided during the sick-leave period and that the patient should be relieved from his/her daily duties at home during this period.

Another situation in which sick leave should be considered is when the patient is handling food. Previous studies have shown that 50 % of all HE patients have *Staphylococcus aureus* on the skin [11], and in these cases contact with food should be avoided.

40.3.9 Information About Skin Care: Skin Care Programs

All patients with HE should be offered information about skin care, since this has been documented to improve the prognosis of the disease, as well as improve the QoL of the patients [28]. This information is best given as a structured program, including specific evidence-based advice to the patient (Table 40.2), and the teaching time should not exceed 20–30 min [29, 30]. The skin care program focuses on the use of protective equipment, disinfectants, and emollients. However, specific information relating to the specific job situation of each patient should also be included. The information can be given by the doctor, specially trained nurses, or other specially trained medical staff [31–33]. In tertiary clinics, in particular, where the patients may often have had their HE for a number of years, patients may sometimes state that they are not interested in receiving further information, implying that they are already well aware of how to treat the eczema. However, clinical experience shows that although patients may know a great deal, there is, in almost all cases, room for improvement. Interestingly, patients at the top of the educational ladder seem to need the information most [34]. We have therefore found it useful to offer a skin care information/skin care program as a "mandatory" part of our program for HE patients; it is given to all patients, regardless of their job or level of education. In addition to

Table 40.2 Skin care program

Skin care program
Use gloves when performing wet work
Protective gloves should be used appropriately and for as short a time as possible
Protective gloves should be intact, clean, and dry inside
When protective gloves are used for more than 10 min, cotton gloves should be worn underneath
Wash hands in lukewarm water. Rinse and dry hands thoroughly after washing
Hand washing with soaps should be substituted with alcohol disinfectant when hands are not visibly dirty
Do not wear finger rings at work
Apply moisturizers on your hands during the working day but especially after work and before bedtime. It may be advisable to use a lighter moisturizing lotion during the day and a greasier fragrance-free, lipid-rich moisturizer before bedtime
Moisturizers should be applied all over the hands, including the webs, fingertips, and dorsal aspects
Take care when doing domestic work. Use protective gloves for dishwashing, and wear insulating gloves in the winter

the advice shown in Table 40.2, we also include information about the use of topical corticosteroids in the skin care program, since most HE patients are using this treatment.

40.3.10 Treatment of HE

When all the above mentioned factors have been considered, long-term treatment can be started. Which treatment to choose depends on whether the eczema is acute or chronic and the severity of the eczema, and, in the longer term, it will also depend on the subclassification of the eczema. The treatment should be chosen after consultation with the patient. Quite often, patients have strong opinions on which treatment they prefer. Some patients find it easier to have a systemic treatment and find messy topical treatments too much of a hassle, while other patients approach the treatment from a more "organic" angle and may prefer a "natural treatment," whatever that may be.

40.3.11 First-Line Therapy

First-line therapy includes topical corticosteroids, together with general skin care, as given in the skin care program. Topical corticosteroids have been on the market for more than 50 years, and their efficacy and side effects are well documented. Moderately potent products should be preferred, since mild topical corticosteroids are not sufficiently effective, and very strong topical corticosteroids may rapidly induce atrophy of the dermis, as well as the epidermis [35]. In most cases, a satisfying result can be obtained with moderately potent topical corticosteroids; stronger products will not, in most cases, bring any accelerated healing and may cause more side effects in the long run.

Treatment with topical corticosteroids will successfully lead to clearance of HE in most cases. However, there is still widespread insecurity and unwillingness among patients to use these products, due to a biased focus on side effects and confusing up side effects of systemic and topical treatments. Some patients may choose not to use the products or to use them for a short time only and sometimes for too short a period to obtain a long-term effect. It is therefore important to discuss the potential side effects of the product with the patient at the onset of the treatment.

Misunderstandings about the side effects of topical corticosteroids occur frequently and may sometimes be surprising to health-care personnel if time is taken to listen to the patients' concerns. Important information to stress to the patient is that topical corticosteroids are recommended worldwide as a first-line therapy due to their high effectiveness and few side effects, that topical treatment limited to the hands will not influence their whole system/body, that the hormones in the product should not be confused with sex hormones, and that the side effects do not include skin cancer. Such basic information will, in most cases, diminish the concerns of the patient and improve compliance.

Topical corticosteroids are first-line therapy for treatment of HE, and most patients will have tried this treatment before they are referred to a secondary or tertiary center. The patients may have had eczema for several years and will often report that they have tried topical corticosteroids to little or no avail, or that they helped for a short while, but that the symptoms reappeared after treatment cessation. Sometimes the patient will say that he/she uses topical corticosteroids once in a while, but that the treatment is not sufficient. Treatment failure is often due to either lack of information about the use of topical corticosteroids or to lack of adherence. In these cases, it is very helpful to start the treatment with topical corticosteroids again, giving very precise instructions about how to use the treatment and for how long a period. Information to the patient about use of topical treatment should include that treatment should be used only once daily (no evidence that twice is better), that only eczematous skin should be treated (and not healthy adjacent skin), and that products should not be blended with or applied to the skin at the same time as emollients. Since topical corticosteroids are known to cause skin atrophy everyday, treatment should be limited to a period of 6 weeks.

It is useful for the doctor to obtain information about the exact amount of topical corticosteroid that is being used. The expression "I use the treatment every day" may cover everything from use of 10 g up to 500 g over a 1-year period. The patients should be asked to bring their medication, and they should be instructed to obtain prescriptions from one source only. The response should then be evaluated at a consultation after 2–6 weeks (depending on local variations), during which period the treatment should continue. In many cases, the treatment will be sufficiently effective, and instructions for future maintenance therapy are then warranted. If the patients, after improvement, disregard treatment with topical corticosteroids (and, at the same time, forget all about skin care measures), the eczema will most likely return. Even if a specific cause of the eczema has been found – for example, an allergic contact dermatitis in which the culprit allergen has been identified and removed – the eczema may, unfortunately, take a chronic course if it is not carefully treated for some time. A rational choice in these cases will be to instruct the patient to keep using topical corticosteroids as a maintenance therapy, either twice or three times weekly, for some time; or to introduce second-line treatment.

However, in some cases maintenance therapy is insufficient, and second-line therapy should be started. In a minority of cases, the treatment will not have had any effect at all, in spite of acceptable adherence. These patients most often benefit from systemic therapy only.

40.3.12 Second-Line Therapy

When a satisfying result cannot be obtained by first-line therapy, the next step is either UV treatment or use of tacrolimus/pimecrolimus. The effect of UV therapy for HE is well documented; however, this treatment is time-consuming for the patient, who will have to attend the clinic several times a week in order to receive the treatment. Use of topical tacrolimus [36, 37] and pimecrolimus [38] was found to be effective in some studies, and tacrolimus, in particular, is currently used for treatment of HE. The product is, however, not licensed for this use (except in the case of atopic HE), and the patient should be informed of this fact.

40.3.13 Third-Line Therapy (Systemic Treatment)

When topical treatment (and potentially UV treatment) is not sufficient to obtain a satisfying result, systemic treatment is the next step. For many years, immunosuppressive drugs have been used, but retinoids (e.g., acitretin) have also proven effective, and recently a new retinoid, alitretinoin, has been registered for treatment of chronic HE. Randomized controlled trials support the evidence of this new drug [21, 39], while the use of the immunosuppressive drugs mostly relies on anecdotal and clinical experience [40–42]. Prednisolone treatment should be restricted to a period not longer than 3 weeks, and long-term treatment, or frequently repeated short-term treatments, should be avoided due to side effects.

Before starting systemic treatment, data on previous diseases and blood tests relating to the relevant drug should be obtained. In tertiary centers, where the disease severity is often quite high, it may be helpful to obtain baseline laboratories at the patient's first visit. Medical history and test results provide information on which systemic drug is best tolerated by the patient. In the case of prior malignancies, retinoids may be preferred over immunosuppressive agents, while in patients with increased cholesterol values and/or a history of heart disease, immunosuppressive drugs may be preferred. Some systemic drugs are only recommended for specific subclasses of HE (i.e., acitretin for hyperkeratotic HE) [43].

Mutual agreement between the patient and the doctor should be ensured before starting systemic treatment of HE. Before onset of treatment, the patient should be informed about possible side effects (oral and in writing) and also about expectations for efficacy (how many patients will benefit from the treatment, and when is the benefit expected to occur). Patients should be informed about the planned duration of the treatment, about precautions relating to each treatment, and about maintenance blood laboratories to monitor toxicity. If the patient has not accepted these limitations of the treatment before onset, there is an increased risk of dropout. After the end of systemic treatment, the patients should be followed up for 3–6 months, since relapses may occur, and new treatment or a refill of the previous treatment may be needed.

Conclusion

Management of HE includes more than medical treatment alone, and many factors should be taken into consideration before onset of therapy. However, in the acute phase, focus should be on the initiation of an effective short-term treatment, and investigations must be postponed until a calm phase is reached.

A thorough examination, including medical history, patch testing, and severity assessment, leading to subclassification, is mandatory. Information about skin care should be given to all HE patients regardless of subdiagnosis and level of education, and the information should comprise skin protection at the workplace. The patients should be counselled on expectations of allergy testing. When medical treatment is started, it is important to give full information about the efficacy, expectations, and side effects before onset of treatment to obtain good adherence and a strong relationship between the patient and the doctor.

References

1. Lynde C, Guenther L, Diepgen TL, Sasseville D, Poulin Y, Gulliver W, et al. Canadian hand dermatitis management guidelines. J Cutan Med Surg. 2010; 14:267–84.
2. Meding B, Wrangsjo K, Jarvholm B. Hand eczema extent and morphology–association and influence on long-term prognosis. J Invest Dermatol. 2007; 127:2147–51.
3. Meding B, Lantto R, Lindahl G, Wrangsjo K, Bengtsson B. Occupational skin disease in Sweden–a 12-year follow-up. Contact Dermatitis. 2005;53:308–13.
4. Hald M, Agner T, Blands J, Johansen JD, Danish Contact Dermatitis Group. Delay in medical attention to hand eczema: a follow-up study. Br J Dermatol. 2009;161:1294–300.
5. Menne T, Johansen JD, Sommerlund M, Veien NK, Danish Contact Dermatitis Group. Hand eczema guidelines based on the Danish guidelines for the diagnosis and treatment of hand eczema. Contact Dermatitis. 2011;65:3–12.
6. Menne T. Hyperkeratotic dermatitis of the palms. In: Menne T, Maibach H, editors. Hand eczema. Boca Raton: CRC Press; 2000.
7. Wilkinson DS. Introduction, definition and classification. In: Menne T, Maibach H, editors. Hand eczema. Boca Raton: CRC Press; 2000.
8. Diepgen TL, Andersen KE, Brandao FM, Bruze M, Bruynzeel DP, Frosch P, et al. Hand eczema classification: a cross-sectional, multicentre study of the aetiology and morphology of hand eczema. Br J Dermatol. 2009;160:353–8.
9. Johansen JD, Hald M, Andersen BL, Laurberg G, Danielsen A, Avnstorp C, et al. Classification of hand eczema: clinical and aetiological types. Based on the guideline of the Danish Contact Dermatitis Group. Contact Dermatitis. 2011;65(1):13–21.
10. Molin S, Diepgen TL, Ruzicka T, Prinz JC. Diagnosing chronic hand eczema by an algorithm: a tool for classification in clinical practice. Clin Exp Dermatol. 2011;36(6):595–601.
11. Haslund P, Bangsgaard N, Jarlov JO, Skov L, Skov R, Agner T. Staphylococcus aureus and hand eczema severity. Br J Dermatol. 2009;161:772–7.
12. Agner T, Held E. Skin protection programs. Contact Dermatitis. 2002;47:253–6.
13. Rystedt I. Hand eczema and long-term prognosis in atopic dermatitis. Acta Derm Venereol Suppl (Stockh). 1985;117:1–59.
14. Palmer CN, Irvine AD, Terron-Kwiatkowski A, Zhao Y, Liao H, Lee SP, et al. Common loss-of-function variants of the epidermal barrier protein filaggrin are a major predisposing factor for atopic dermatitis. Nat Genet. 2006;38:441–6.
15. Thyssen JP, Carlsen BC, Menne T, Linneberg A, Nielsen NH, Meldgaard M, et al. Filaggrin null mutations increase the risk and persistence of hand eczema in subjects with atopic dermatitis: results from a general population study. Br J Dermatol. 2010;163:115–20.
16. Meding B, Swanbeck G. Predictive factors for hand eczema. Contact Dermatitis. 1990;23:154–61.
17. Ibler KS, Jemec GB, Agner T. Exposures related to hand eczema: a study of healthcare workers. Contact Dermatitis. 2012;66(5):247–53.
18. Held E, Skoet R, Johansen JD, Agner T. The hand eczema severity index (HECSI): a scoring system for clinical assessment of hand eczema. A study of inter- and intraobserver reliability. Br J Dermatol. 2005;152(2):302–7.
19. Coenraads PJ, Van Der Walle H, Thestrup-Pedersen K, Ruzicka T, Dreno B, De La Loge C, et al. Construction and validation of a photographic guide for assessing severity of chronic hand dermatitis. Br J Dermatol. 2005;152(2):296–301.
20. Dulon M, Skudlik C, Nübling M, John SM, Nienhaus A. Validity and responsiveness of the Osnabrück Hand Eczema Severity Index (OHSI): a methodological study. Br J Dermatol. 2009;160(1):137–42.
21. Ruzicka T, Lynde CW, Jemec GBE, Diepgen T, Berth-Jones J, Coenraads PJ, et al. Efficacy and safety

of oral alitretinoin (9-cis retinoic acid) in patients with severe chronic hand eczema refractory to topical corticosteroids: results of a randomized, double-blind, placebo-controlled, multicentre trial. Br J Dermatol. 2008;158:808–17.
22. Agner T, Jungersted JM, Coenraads PJ, Diepgen T. Comparison study of four methods for assessment of severity of hand eczema. Contact Dermatitis. 2013;69:10–11.
23. Finlay AY, Khan GK. Dermatology life quality index (DLQI)–a simple practical measure for routine clinical use. Clin Exp Dermatol. 1994;19:210–6.
24. Chren MM, Lasek RJ, Quinn LM, Mostow EN, Zyzanski SJ. SKINDEX: a quality of life measure for patients with skin disease. Reliability, validity and responsiveness. J Invest Dermatol. 1996;107(5):707–13.
25. Wallenhammar L-M, Nyfjäll M, Lindberg M, Meding B. Health-related quality of life and hand eczema – a comparison of two instruments, including factor analysis. J Invest Dermatol. 2004;122:1381–9.
26. Wahlberg JE. Patch testing. In: Frosch P, Menne T, Lepoittevin J, editors. Contact dermatitis. 4th ed. Berlin: Springer; 2006. p. 366–90.
27. Held E, Johansen JD, Agner T, Menné T. Contact allergy to cosmetics: testing with patients' own products. Contact Dermatitis. 1999;40(6):310–5.
28. Ibler KS, Jemec GB, Diepgen TL, Gluud C, Lindschou Hansen J, et al. Skin care education and individual counselling versus treatment as usual in healthcare workers with hand eczema: randomised clinical trial. BMJ. 2012;345:e7822.
29. Held E, Wolff C, Gyntelberg F, Agner T. Prevention of work-related skin problems in student auxiliary nurses. An intervention study. Contact Dermatitis. 2001;44:297–303.
30. Held E, Mygind K, Wolff C, Gyntelberg F, Agner T. Prevention of work related skin problems: an intervention study in wet work employees. Occup Environ Med. 2002;59:556–61.
31. Weisshaar E, Radulescu M, Soder S, Apfelbacher CJ, Bock M, Grundmann JU, et al. Secondary individual prevention of occupational skin diseases in health care workers, cleaners and kitchen employees: aims, experiences and descriptive results. Int Arch Occup Environ Health. 2007;80:477–84.
32. van Gils RF, Boot CR, Knol DL, Rustemeyer T, van Mechelen W, van der Valk PG, et al. The effectiveness of integrated care for patients with hand eczema: results of a randomized, controlled trial. Contact Dermatitis. 2012;66(4):197–204.
33. Weisshaar E, Skudlik C, Scheidt R, Matterne U, Wulfhorst B, Schönfeld M, et al., for the ROQ Study Group. Multicentre study 'rehabilitation of occupational skin diseases -optimization and quality assurance of inpatient management (ROQ)'-results from 12-month follow-up. Contact Dermatitis. 2012 Oct 10 2013;68:169–74
34. Fisker MH, Jungersted JM, Ebbehøj N, Agner T. What do patients with occupational hand eczema know about skin care? Accepted for publication in Contact Dermatitis 2013;69:93–98.
35. Kao JS, Fluhr JW, Man MQ, Fowler AJ, Hachem JP, Crumrine D, et al. Short-term glucocorticoid treatment compromises both permeability barrier homeostasis and stratum corneum integrity: inhibition of epidermal lipid synthesis accounts for functional abnormalities. J Invest Dermatol. 2003;120(3):456–64.
36. Schnopp C, Remling R, Mohrenschlager M, Weigl L, Ring J. Topical tacrolimus (FK506) and mometasone furoate in treatment of dyshidrotic palmar eczema: a randomized, observer-blinded trial. J Am Acad Dermatol. 2002;46:73–6.
37. Krejci-Manwaring J, McCarty MA, Camacho F, Manuel J, Hartle J, Fleischer Jr A, et al. Topical tacrolimus 0.1% improves symptoms of hand dermatitis in patients treated with a prednisone taper. J Drugs Dermatol. 2008;7:643–6.
38. Belsito DV, Fowler Jr JF, Marks Jr JG, Pariser DM, Hanifin J, Duarte IA, et al. Pimecrolimus cream 1%: a potential new treatment for chronic hand dermatitis. Cutis. 2004;73:31–8.
39. Bissonnette R, Worm M, Gerlach B, Guenther L, Cambazard F, Ruzicka T, et al. Successful retreatment with alitretinoin in patients with relapsed chronic hand eczema. Br J Dermatol. 2010;162:420–6.
40. Verma KK, Manchanda Y, Pasricha JS. Azathioprine as a corticosteroid sparing agent for the treatment of dermatitis caused by the weed Parthenium. Acta Derm Venereol. 2000;80:31–2.
41. Granlund H, Erkko P, Eriksson E, Reitamo S. Comparison of cyclosporine and topical betamethasone-17,21-dipropionate in the treatment of severe chronic hand eczema. Acta Derm Venereol. 1996;76:371–6.
42. Granlund H, Erkko P, Reitamo S. Long-term follow-up of eczema patients treated with cyclosporine. Acta Derm Venereol. 1998;78:40–3.
43. Thestrup-Pedersen K, Andersen KE, Menne T, Veien N. Treatment of hyperkeratotic dermatitis of the palms (eczema keratoticum) with oral acitretin. A single-blind placebo controlled study. Acta Derm Venereol. 2001;81:353–5.

41 Prognosis of Hand Eczema

Richard Brans and Swen Malte John

Contents

R. Brans, M.D. (✉) • S.M. John, M.D. (✉)
Department of Dermatology, Environmental Medicine and Health Theory, University of Osnabrueck, Sedanstr. 115, Osnabrueck 49090, Germany
e-mail: rbrans@uos.de; sjohn@uos.de

41.1 Background

Hand eczema (HE) is a common disease that is often associated with a poor prognosis. Prognosis of HE refers to the course of the disease, taking into account the extent of healing over time. Although HE can be transient or improved by adequate treatment, a chronic course with continual or intermittent symptoms over years is frequently seen. There are only a few prognostic follow-up studies giving limited evidence-based insight into the long-term course of HE. In these studies, the assessment of prognosis differs widely. Some studies prefer complete clearance of the dermatitis as their endpoint, whereas others use improvement. Moreover, measurements may vary from patient-administered postal questionnaires to clinical review by a dermatologist [1]. Healing rates of HE in these studies range from 18 % to 41 % [2–7]. A 15-year follow-up of patients with HE in a general population in Sweden showed that 66 % of the responders ($n=868$) still reported periods of HE, and 44 % reported continuous eczema during the previous year [2]. In a 5-year follow-up of patients with HE in a general population in Denmark, 65 % of the participants ($n=353$) still had constant or intermittent hand eczema after 5 years, despite treatment and dermatological instructions. However, 48 % stated that their dermatitis had improved [5]. In a study from the Netherlands, a cohort of patients ($n=105$) with dermatitis of the hands and forearms was reexamined after 3 years, finding a clearance rate of 41 % [6]. The mean

A. Alikhan et al. (eds.), *Textbook of Hand Eczema*,
DOI 10.1007/978-3-642-39546-8_41, © Springer-Verlag Berlin Heidelberg 2014

duration of HE was reported to be 11.6 years in a general population in Sweden, depending on the cause [8]. Irritant contact dermatitis, allergic contact dermatitis, and atopic HE had a mean duration of 9.0 years, 12.0 years, and 16.3 years, respectively.

HE is the most common variant of occupational contact dermatitis, comprising up to 90 % of all cases [9]. Occupational HE, in particular, is associated with a poor prognosis, resulting in detrimental socioeconomic consequences, including prolonged absences from work, retraining, relocation, job loss, and long-term unemployment [10, 11]. The course of occupational HE varies widely depending on the occupational settings and the potential to control aggravating factors. Occupational HE has been reported to heal in 21–72 % of all cases [12–18]. In working populations, the percentage of patients with HE who have relapses varies between 35 % and 80 %, depending on the severity, period of follow-up, and intensity of exposures [19]. Often occupational HE is a chronic condition, despite all efforts in education [20]. A 1-year follow-up of 564 patients with occupational HE in Denmark showed that 25 % of all patients had persistently severe or aggravated disease, 41 % improved, and 34 % had unchanged minimal or mild to moderate disease [21]. In many reports, more than a third of patients with occupational HE changed either job or occupation, but the reasons for the change were not always clearly stated [21, 22]. In two studies from Sweden and Finland, about 20 % of patients with occupational HE had been retrained at the expenses of insurance companies at a follow-up of 12 years and 10 years, respectively [12, 18]. However, the majority of people with occupational contact dermatitis manage to continue working in some capacity, albeit sometimes in altered employment [10].

41.2 Factors Influencing Prognosis

HE is influenced by internal and external factors. The prognosis depends on the cause of the disease and the potential to eliminate irritants and allergens. Avoidance of these factors may be achieved in some cases, but often this is a difficult task, especially in occupational HE. Moreover, individual susceptibility can worsen prognosis.

41.2.1 Age

Older age has been associated with severity [8] and a poorer prognosis of occupational HE [20–22]. Holness and Nethercott reported that workers over 40 years of age were less likely to be working 2 years after diagnosis (65 %) than those under 40 years (90 %). Older workers were also more likely to have applied for workers' compensation than those under 40 years (52 % and 36 %, respectively) [22]. In another study, age below 20 years at onset of HE influences the prognosis negatively [23]. However, others suggest that age of onset does not significantly influence the prognosis of occupational HE [24].

41.2.2 Sex

Studies report both a less favorable [25, 26] and a more favorable prognosis [14] for HE in females. Another study did not find a gender influence on the course of HE at all [23]. The effect of gender on the prognosis of occupational skin disease is similarly uncertain. Some studies report that male sex is a risk factor for a poor prognosis for occupational contact dermatitis [22], whereas other studies could not confirm this effect [21, 27].

41.2.3 Atopic Dermatitis

Association between atopic eczema and severe HE has been reported [8, 28]. In a 5-year follow-up study of Danish patients with HE, a history of atopy did not correlate with poor healing, but a diagnosis of atopic HE did. Previous or present atopic dermatitis was associated with long-standing HE [5, 29]. In a Swedish study, a history of childhood eczema doubled the risk of persistent HE at follow-up after 15 years [23].

Similarly, atopy is associated with a poorer prognosis of occupational HE [12, 13, 18, 21, 27, 28, 30].

41.2.4 Genetics

Filaggrin null-alleles causing structural defects in the skin barrier are major predisposing factors for atopic dermatitis. Subsequently, they have been associated with irritant HE [31, 32]. Recently, they have been reported to predispose for sensitization to nickel and fragrances [33, 34]. The presence of filaggrin null-alleles in combination with atopic dermatitis has been shown to have a negative impact on the course of occupational HE [35]. Other studies have reported that polymorphisms in genes encoding for cytokines may influence the individual risk to develop HE [36–38]. All these findings highlight the importance of genetics and the complexity of the susceptibility of the individual HE patient to various external factors. However, the influence of genetic factors on the clinical severity and prognosis of HE needs further exploration.

41.2.5 Contact Allergy

Contact allergy is frequent among those who suffer from HE, with a prevalence of 21–48 % [39, 40]. In 1990, a population-based study of 1,238 individuals with HE living in a Swedish city was published reporting that patients with allergic contact dermatitis had a greater number of medical consultations and were more likely to have had absence from work because of their dermatitis compared to those with irritant contact dermatitis [8]. At a 15-year follow-up, a positive patch test was significantly related to current HE [8, 23]. In line with that, in a population-based study from the Netherlands, positive patch test reactions were found more frequently in persons with persistent HE [6]. However, a Danish study of 799 patients with HE demonstrated that contact sensitization was associated with the severity of disease, but not with a poor prognosis [4]. A high frequency of contact sensitization in those suffering from HE is frequently explained by the impaired skin barrier in severe eczema, which may facilitate the penetration of contact allergens. Moreover, the associated proinflammatory milieu may induce sensitization. However, the presence of multiple contact allergies may be the consequence of severe HE rather than the cause of it. With regard to occupational HE, some studies found an association between contact allergies and a poorer prognosis [12, 13, 41], whereas others could not confirm this association [13, 18, 21]. Some studies even suggest that allergic contact dermatitis is associated with a better prognosis of occupational HE [14, 22].

The impact of contact allergy on the course of HE is influenced by the potential to avoid the causative allergen, which differ greatly depending on the individual allergen, its distribution, chances for replacement, and access to preventive measures and their practicability. Among the work-related contact allergies analyzed in a Finish population of patients with occupational HE, allergies to chromate, rubber chemicals, and formaldehyde were associated with lower frequency of healing, whereas allergies to acrylates and epoxy chemicals were associated with a high percentage of healing [18]. This is in line with the hypothesis that prognosis is better in patients who have work-related allergies to substances that are easily avoided compared with substances that are ubiquitous at work or in everyday life. Chromate allergy is often related to poor prognosis and persistent HE even in the absence of continuing occupational exposure [13, 42, 43]. In a Danish study, chromate allergy was a risk factor for poor prognosis with regard to HE being unchanged/aggravated at follow-up after 6 months by an OR of 4.18, whereas other contact allergies had no effect [4].

41.2.6 Morphology and Extent

Frequent eruptions during the previous 12 months were associated with a poor prognosis in a Danish study of 799 patients with HE. With respect to morphology, fissures and scaling were identified as risk factors for a poor prognosis [4].

Fissures and scaling may reflect a more chronic stage of the disease, which is difficult to treat. In a Swedish follow-up study, the severity of HE at the initial examination was the individual factor with the strongest relation to the prognosis [23]. A moderate/severe extension of the dermatitis doubled the risk of HE at follow-up after 15 years. The presence of vesicles or erythema was the only morphological feature that had a negative influence on the prognosis [44]. Others found a correlation between involvement of a large area of the hands and a poor prognosis [5]. Hyperkeratotic dermatitis of the palms has been reported to have a low healing rate. In a follow-up study, it had only cleared in 2 of 32 patients at the time of reexamination after 10 years [45].

41.2.7 Socioeconomic Factors

Being unskilled is a risk factor for a poor prognosis of HE [4]. This may be explained by poorer working conditions and more contact to irritants and allergens. In addition, it may be related to lower compliance. Individuals from a lower social position have more difficulty in reading ingredient labels and, accordingly, more difficulty in complying with the medical instructions [46]. A study of 230 patients with occupational contact dermatitis demonstrated that only 33 % of the participants could correctly identify their diagnosis 2–9 years after the initial assessment. These patients were more likely to report clearance (OR 1.95, $p=0.03$) or improvement (OR 2.14, $p=0.04$) of their symptoms [47]. It is possible that people with less education have more difficulties in understanding medical conditions and their prevention, resulting in a worse prognosis. The authors conclude that further efforts should be directed at the patient's education. Patients with occupational HE coming from a high to medium socioeconomic background have a tendency to change jobs less often than patients with lower socioeconomic status, suggesting that job modification is easier for this group [21]. In the same study by Cvetkovksi et al., it was demonstrated that patients with occupational HE with high to medium socioeconomic status in Denmark have a better prognosis than those with a lower socioeconomic status. This may be related to better access to medical care and protective equipment, better adherence, and a better understanding of preventive strategies in those with a higher socioeconomic status.

41.2.8 Change of Occupation

There are controversial opinions about the effect of a change of occupation on the prognosis of occupational HE. In a 10-year follow-up study, Fregert did not find a better result in healing of the dermatitis for those who changed their occupation compared to those who continued their jobs [25]. It was noted that most of those who changed their work had the most severe dermatitis, which might explain its persistence. Also other studies suggest that a change of work does not necessarily make a difference to prognosis [15, 16, 21]. However, most authors report that a change of work significantly improves prognosis of occupational HE [13, 17, 18, 22, 27, 48, 49]. Holness and Nethercott found that 35 % of individuals who had changed work still had active dermatitis compared to 46 % of those who had not changed [22]. Susitaival and Hannuksela reported that 50 % of farmers with a history of dermatitis had changed their job or retired from farming. This group was significantly more likely to have clearance of symptoms than those still farming ($p<0.001$) [27].

41.2.9 Duration of Disease Before Diagnosis

In a Finnish long-term follow-up study, a short duration (less than a year) of occupational HE before diagnosis was associated with favorable prognosis, whereas a duration of occupational HE for over 10 years before the diagnosis was the strongest risk factor for the continuation of disease [18]. These results were congruent with other findings of longer delays before diagnosis leading to worse prognosis [3, 5, 7]. Hald et al. reported a significant association between longer patient delay and a poor prognosis of HE, which was most evident for patients seeking medical attention immediately compared with those who waited more than 12 months [50]. This may suggest that people who seek help at an early stage are more likely to have better compliance to treatment and suggested interventions. Thus, it emphasizes the importance of early diagnosis and intervention, especially as another study showed that 33 % of persons with HE had never sought medical advice [51].

41.2.10 Prevention

Adisesh et al. analyzed a group of patients with occupational dermatitis and found a poor prognosis associated with a longer exposure to the causative agent [20]. There is good evidence that preventive initiatives for occupational HE are successful [52, 53]. However, the efficacy of such prevention programs is difficult to evaluate because of the lack of no-intervention control groups, which are often not constituted for legal and ethical reasons [54, 55]. A recent multicenter study from Germany demonstrated that individuals with severe occupational HE taking part in a tertiary rehabilitation program had a significant improvement with regard to severity of the disease, quality of life, and absence from work at the 1-year follow-up [56]. However, more long-term trials are needed to evaluate links between prognosis of HE and prevention.

Conclusion

The fact that the prognosis of HE is often poor emphasizes the importance of prevention and risk management. Relevant allergens and irritants potentially initiating or maintaining HE need to be detected and preferably eliminated, replaced, or diminished. However, complete avoidance can be difficult, expensive, and sometimes impossible. Thus, often consequent usage of personal protective equipment is indicated, especially in work settings [10]. In addition, interventions need to be accompanied by regulatory efforts to limit the overall exposure to hazardous substances.

Other factors that have the potential to improve the prognosis of HE are early diagnosis and treatment. Frequently, HE develops from a more reversible phase at the beginning into chronic stages. Minor symptoms of HE, especially at work places, must be considered as potential precursors of a more severe disease. Thus, persons who develop initial signs of HE should be encouraged to seek medical advice as early as possible. It can be assumed, and is corroborated by several studies, that early medical intervention would impede the progression, leading to a better prognosis. It is generally acknowledged that the more a patient knows about relevant irritants and allergens, the better the prognosis [19]. Therefore, in addition to dermatological interventions, teaching is considered as pivotal, particularly in occupational HE [53]. Patients and employers who are aware of risk factors may take an active role in implementation of substitution and avoidance measures, and use of personal protective equipment. Thus, it is important to provide specific vocational guidance in risky professions, especially for atopics [29]. More prospective and standardized studies are needed to describe more accurately the prognosis of HE and its predictive factors [1], as well as to evaluate the role of treatment, education, and other preventive strategies [23]. This preferably should be performed in coordinated transnational, multicenter studies, which may then form the basis for common guidelines and standards of all aspects of patient management in HE.

References

1. Cahill J, Keegel T, Nixon R. The prognosis of occupational contact dermatitis in 2004. Contact Dermatitis. 2004;51(5–6):219–26.
2. Meding B, Wrangsjo K, Jarvholm B. Fifteen-year follow-up of hand eczema: persistence and consequences. Br J Dermatol. 2005;152(5):975–80.
3. Lerbaek A, Kyvik KO, Ravn H, Menne T, Agner T. Clinical characteristics and consequences of hand eczema – an 8-year follow-up study of a population-based twin cohort. Contact Dermatitis. 2008;58(4):210–6.

4. Hald M, Agner T, Blands J, Veien NK, Laurberg G, Avnstorp C, et al. Clinical severity and prognosis of hand eczema. Br J Dermatol. 2009;160(6):1229–36.
5. Veien NK, Hattel T, Laurberg G. Hand eczema: causes, course, and prognosis II. Contact Dermatitis. 2008;58(6):335–9.
6. Lantinga H, Nater JP, Coenraads PJ. Prevalence, incidence and course of eczema on the hands and forearms in a sample of the general population. Contact Dermatitis. 1984;10(3):135–9.
7. Li LF, Liu G, Wang J. Etiology and prognosis of hand eczema in a dermatology clinic in China: a follow-up study. Contact Dermatitis. 2008;58(2):88–92.
8. Meding B. Epidemiology of hand eczema in an industrial city. Acta Derm Venereol Suppl (Stockh). 1990;153:1–43.
9. Nicholson PJ. Evidence-based guidelines: occupational contact dermatitis and urticaria. Occup Med (Lond). 2010;60(7):502–4.
10. Nicholson PJ, Llewellyn D, English JS. Evidence-based guidelines for the prevention, identification and management of occupational contact dermatitis and urticaria. Contact Dermatitis. 2010;63(4):177–86.
11. Thyssen JP, Johansen JD, Linneberg A, Menne T. The epidemiology of hand eczema in the general population–prevalence and main findings. Contact Dermatitis. 2010;62(2):75–87.
12. Meding B, Lantto R, Lindahl G, Wrangsjo K, Bengtsson B. Occupational skin disease in Sweden – a 12-year follow-up. Contact Dermatitis. 2005; 53(6):308–13.
13. Rosen RH, Freeman S. Prognosis of occupational contact dermatitis in New South Wales, Australia. Contact Dermatitis. 1993;29(2):88–93.
14. Nethercott JR, Holness DL. Disease outcome in workers with occupational skin disease. J Am Acad Dermatol. 1994;30(4):569–74.
15. Keczkes K, Bhate SM, Wyatt EH. The outcome of primary irritant hand dermatitis. Br J Dermatol. 1983;109(6):665–8.
16. Wall LM, Gebauer KA. A follow-up study of occupational skin disease in Western Australia. Contact Dermatitis. 1991;24(4):241–3.
17. Malkonen T, Jolanki R, Alanko K, Luukkonen R, Aalto-Korte K, Lauerma A, et al. A 6-month follow-up study of 1048 patients diagnosed with an occupational skin disease. Contact Dermatitis. 2009; 61(5):261–8.
18. Malkonen T, Alanko K, Jolanki R, Luukkonen R, Aalto-Korte K, Lauerma A, et al. Long-term follow-up study of occupational hand eczema. Br J Dermatol. 2010;163(5):999–1006.
19. Hogan DJ, Dannaker CJ, Maibach HI. The prognosis of contact dermatitis. J Am Acad Dermatol. 1990;23(2 Pt 1):300–7.
20. Adisesh A, Meyer JD, Cherry NM. Prognosis and work absence due to occupational contact dermatitis. Contact Dermatitis. 2002;46(5):273–9.
21. Cvetkovski RS, Zachariae R, Jensen H, Olsen J, Johansen JD, Agner T. Prognosis of occupational hand eczema: a follow-up study. Arch Dermatol. 2006;142(3):305–11.
22. Holness DL, Nethercott JR. Work outcome in workers with occupational skin disease. Am J Ind Med. 1995;27(6):807–15.
23. Meding B, Wrangsjo K, Jarvholm B. Fifteen-year follow-up of hand eczema: predictive factors. J Invest Dermatol. 2005;124(5):893–7.
24. Burrows D. Prognosis in industrial dermatitis. Br J Dermatol. 1972;87(2):145–8.
25. Fregert S. Occupational dermatitis in a 10-year material. Contact Dermatitis. 1975;1(2):96–107.
26. Yngveson M, Svensson A, Johannisson A, Isacsson A. Hand dermatosis in upper secondary school pupils: 2-year comparison and follow-up. Br J Dermatol. 2000;142(3):485–9.
27. Susitaival P, Hannuksela M. The 12-year prognosis of hand dermatosis in 896 Finnish farmers. Contact Dermatitis. 1995;32(4):233–7.
28. Cvetkovski RS, Rothman KJ, Olsen J, Mathiesen B, Iversen L, Johansen JD, et al. Relation between diagnoses on severity, sick leave and loss of job among patients with occupational hand eczema. Br J Dermatol. 2005;152(1):93–8.
29. Veien NK, Hattel T, Laurberg G. Hand eczema: causes, course, and prognosis I. Contact Dermatitis. 2008;58(6):330–4.
30. Shmunes E, Keil J. The role of atopy in occupational dermatoses. Contact Dermatitis. 1984;11(3):174–8.
31. Palmer CN, Irvine AD, Terron-Kwiatkowski A, Zhao Y, Liao H, Lee SP, et al. Common loss-of-function variants of the epidermal barrier protein filaggrin are a major predisposing factor for atopic dermatitis. Nat Genet. 2006;38(4):441–6.
32. de Jongh CM, Khrenova L, Verberk MM, Calkoen F, van Dijk FJ, Voss H, et al. Loss-of-function polymorphisms in the filaggrin gene are associated with an increased susceptibility to chronic irritant contact dermatitis: a case–control study. Br J Dermatol. 2008;159(3):621–7.
33. Thyssen JP, Linneberg A, Engkilde K, Menne T, Johansen JD. Contact sensitization to common haptens is associated with atopic dermatitis: new insight. Br J Dermatol. 2012;166(6):1255–61.
34. Novak N, Baurecht H, Schafer T, Rodriguez E, Wagenpfeil S, Klopp N, et al. Loss-of-function mutations in the filaggrin gene and allergic contact sensitization to nickel. J Invest Dermatol. 2008;128(6):1430–5.
35. Landeck L, Visser M, Skudlik C, Brans R, Kezic S, John SM. Clinical course of occupational irritant contact dermatitis of the hands in relation to filaggrin genotype status and atopy. Br J Dermatol. 2012;167(6):1302–9.
36. de Jongh CM, John SM, Bruynzeel DP, Calkoen F, van Dijk FJ, Khrenova L, et al. Cytokine gene polymorphisms and susceptibility to chronic irritant contact dermatitis. Contact Dermatitis. 2008;58(5):269–77.
37. Landeck L, Visser M, Kezic S, John SM. IL1A-889 C/T gene polymorphism in irritant contact

dermatitis. J Eur Acad Dermatol Venereol. 2013; 68(3):169-74.
38. Landeck L, Visser M, Kezic S, John SM. Impact of tumour necrosis factor-alpha polymorphisms on irritant contact dermatitis. Contact Dermatitis. 2012;66(4):221–7.
39. Nielsen NH, Linneberg A, Menne T, Madsen F, Frolund L, Dirksen A, et al. The association between contact allergy and hand eczema in 2 cross-sectional surveys 8 years apart. Contact Dermatitis. 2002;47(2):71–7.
40. Lerbaek A, Kyvik KO, Menne T, Agner T. Retesting with the TRUE Test in a population-based twin cohort with hand eczema – allergies and persistence in an 8-year follow-up study. Contact Dermatitis. 2007;57(4):248–52.
41. Lammintausta K, Kalimo K, Aantaa S. Course of hand dermatitis in hospital workers. Contact Dermatitis. 1982;8(5):327–32.
42. Avnstorp C. Prevalence of cement eczema in Denmark before and since addition of ferrous sulfate to Danish cement. Acta Derm Venereol. 1989; 69(2):151–5.
43. Halbert AR, Gebauer KA, Wall LM. Prognosis of occupational chromate dermatitis. Contact Dermatitis. 1992;27(4):214–9.
44. Meding B, Wrangsjo K, Jarvholm B. Hand eczema extent and morphology–association and influence on long-term prognosis. J Invest Dermatol. 2007;127(9):2147–51.
45. Hersle K, Mobacken H. Hyperkeratotic dermatitis of the palms. Br J Dermatol. 1982;107(2):195–201.
46. Noiesen E, Larsen K, Agner T. Compliance in contact allergy with focus on cosmetic labelling: a qualitative research project. Contact Dermatitis. 2004;51(4):189–95.
47. Holness DL, Nethercott JR. Is a worker's understanding of their diagnosis an important determinant of outcome in occupational contact dermatitis? Contact Dermatitis. 1991;25(5):296–301.
48. Nielsen J. The occurrence and course of skin symptoms on the hands among female cleaners. Contact Dermatitis. 1996;34(4):284–91.
49. Rystedt I. Long term follow-up in atopic dermatitis. Acta Derm Venereol Suppl (Stockh). 1985;114:117–20.
50. Hald M, Agner T, Blands J, Johansen JD. Delay in medical attention to hand eczema: a follow-up study. Br J Dermatol. 2009;161(6):1294–300.
51. Hald M, Berg ND, Elberling J, Johansen JD. Medical consultations in relation to severity of hand eczema in the general population. Br J Dermatol. 2008;158(4):773–7.
52. Skudlik C, Weisshaar E, Scheidt R, Elsner P, Wulfhorst B, Schonfeld M, et al. First results from the multicentre study rehabilitation of occupational skin diseases–optimization and quality assurance of inpatient management (ROQ). Contact Dermatitis. 2012;66(3):140–7.
53. Wulfhorst B, Bock M, Skudlik C, Wigger-Alberti W, John SM. Prevention of hand eczema – gloves, barrier creams and workers' education. In: Duus Johansen J, Frosch PJ, Lepoittevin JP, editors. Contact dermatitis. Berlin: Springer; 2011. p. 985–1028.
54. van Gils RF, Boot CR, van Gils PF, Bruynzeel D, Coenraads PJ, van Mechelen W, et al. Effectiveness of prevention programmes for hand dermatitis: a systematic review of the literature. Contact Dermatitis. 2011;64(2):63–72.
55. Wilke A, Gediga K, Weinhoppel U, John SM, Wulfhorst B. Long-term effectiveness of secondary prevention in geriatric nurses with occupational hand eczema: the challenge of a controlled study design. Contact Dermatitis. 2012;66(2):79–86.
56. Weisshaar E, Skudlik C, Scheidt R, Matterne U, Wulfhorst B, Schonfeld M, et al. Multicentre study 'rehabilitation of occupational skin diseases -optimization and quality assurance of inpatient management (ROQ)'-results from 12-month follow-up. Contact Dermatitis. 2013;68(3):169–74.

42 Educational Interventions to Improve Hand Eczema

John Hassani and Ali Alikhan

Contents

J. Hassani, BA, MA (✉)
New York Institute of Technology College of Osteopathic medicine, Northern Boulevard 8000, Old Westbury, NY 11568, USA
e-mail: john.hassani@gmail.com

A. Alikhan, M.D.
Department of Dermatology, Mayo Clinic, 200 1st St SW, Rochester, MN 55905, USA
e-mail: alialikhan1@yahoo.com

42.1 Introduction

Though hand eczema may be easily diagnosed by a dermatologist, effective management typically requires altered individual behavior, knowledge of the disease, patient self-determination, and safer domestic and working environments. Patient education is an underemphasized method to help address issues of treatment and prevention. One of the main reasons why dermatitis treatment may be unsuccessful is that poor patient education leads to lower levels of adherence [1]. Furthermore, the frequency and outcome of contact dermatitis are typically correlated to causal factors. Thus, success in disease prevention requires adequate knowledge about basic risks, protection, and therapy for eczema.

Hand eczema education is especially needed in the workplace, as hand eczema alone can lead to high turnover in at-risk professions [2–4]. Workplace education is a powerful tool, which can decrease the occurrence of occupational contact dermatitis (OCD) [5]. Early education is necessary, as half of all OCD cases occur in the first 2 years of employment, particularly during employee training [6]. Currently, the prevention of OCD is not a major priority in most workplaces. A low number of confectioners, bakers, and caterers with hand disease regularly used gloves, particularly before skin protection procedures were implemented [7]. Bakers' apprentices found protective gloves to be less acceptable than other forms of protective measures (barrier creams and skin care) [8],

A. Alikhan et al. (eds.), *Textbook of Hand Eczema*,
DOI 10.1007/978-3-642-39546-8_42, © Springer-Verlag Berlin Heidelberg 2014

although the use of gloves increased after the benefits were demonstrated in bakers [9] and automobile engineers [10]. In the metalworking industry, less than half of apprentices thought they were working with agents harmful to their skin. However, they did express the desire to get more information about the problem and considered it possible to protect themselves by appropriate preventative measures [11].

42.2 Aims of Educational Interventions

The goals of educational interventions are simple: an ideal educational program should increase knowledge about skin care, as well as help modify behavior to decrease clinical symptoms. Patients should know the treatments available, proper application of these treatments, and have the opportunity to select treatments that suit them best. Treatment dissatisfaction will eventually lead to poor adherence. Patients may need reassurance that therapies are safe (e.g., some patients may possess a fear "steroid" usage) [1]. The core principle of basic skin education for laypersons can be conveyed via pamphlets, lectures, audio, video, Internet resources, diagrams, posters, live demonstrations (e.g., model dirt can be washed off easily if skin protection cream has been applied) [12], mini-courses, plastic skin models, and other ways. With this in mind, educators should not be limited to written or verbal methods of informing patients. Passing rote knowledge does not automatically lead to changes in behavior or attitude. A variety of teaching methods helps to avoid boredom and accounts for the fact that patients have different preferences and different ways of learning. Armstrong et al. showed that online video education was superior to written pamphlets in improving clinical outcomes, with the benefit of having combined audiovisual appeal [13].

There are other elements of a well-rounded education that the educator should be aware of to make a long-lasting impact on patient education and behavior. To maximize educational effectiveness, there needs to be an emphasis on primary prevention. Health education is particularly effective for primary (unexposed apprentice or trainee) prevention, as compared to secondary (detection of disease while subject is already working) and tertiary (reducing symptoms in subjects who are already afflicted) prevention. First-hand education is needed but does not necessarily need to be provided by a dermatologist; other qualified professionals (e.g., trained dermatology nurse) are generally sufficient.

Another factor that must be addressed is patient motivation, as not all patients desire skin protection measures (i.e., they do not consider themselves at risk or do not consider themselves exposed). Measures to enhance self-motivation must consider different lifestyles and dispel such misconceptions as "only women get rashes, not men," "I've never had it before, so there's no reason to worry," or "I'm immune; I'm not an allergic-type person" [14]. Some patients may require proof that they are at risk for hand eczema (e.g., a fluorescent tracer can be added to the source of skin exposure and then illuminated on the patient's skin with a black light). Seven hundred sixty-four patients with severe occupational skin disease (OSD) that underwent an interdisciplinary tertiary prevention program and successfully returned to work reported that individual motivation to use skin protection is needed to avoid job loss due to severe OSD [15]. A key element for sustained motivational efforts is the support of unions, health officials, and upper management in the workplace. Managers of workplaces can be motivated themselves to increase safety, as safe working conditions increase employee satisfaction and productivity and decrease costs (e.g., decreased costs of workers' compensation).

Ultimately, the meticulous care and time required to educate individuals with eczema is unlikely to be practical in every dermatology setting. The average appointment with a general practitioner in Britain lasts 10 min, which is likely insufficient to thoroughly educate patients about hand eczema [1]. Increasing the number of general practitioners or other medical professionals with dermatologic training in the community would improve the management of dermatitis.

Online video education is an alternative that may increase accessibility and ease of distribution of educational materials [13]. Institutes dedicated to eczema may offer an opportunity to educate groups of patients [1]. An "eczema school" model in Finland, implemented at the beginning of the 1990s, was a program with a trained nurse who gave lessons (30 min to 2 h long) about skin care, allergen avoidance, and skin protection to patients [16]. Outcomes of patients who participated in such eczema schools proved to be significantly better than those of the control group. In particular, patients with multiple contact allergies to metals benefited from the eczema school.

Hand eczema can bring about tremendous psychosocial stress [17]. OCD mostly affects the hands of young people. It may have an impact on self-esteem, body image, daily activities, professional life, social life, and ability to practice hobbies. A population-based study of 1,000 people with hand eczema demonstrated that 74 % of men and 85 % of women experienced some degree of negative impact on their everyday lives [18]. Nearly half of the respondents described their hand eczema as interfering with their work and hobbies, and approximately one-third reported that it resulted in a change of their daily activities [18]. One-third of respondents reported mood and sleep disturbances and a negative influence of hand eczema on social interactions. Additionally, there are some patients with self-inflicted dermatitis (e.g., excessive hand washing secondary to obsessive-compulsive disorder) [19]. Therefore, educational interventions should keep in mind the short-term and potential long-term (chronic cases of hand eczema have a mean duration of 10 years) [3] psychosocial aspects of eczema. Psychologist-led support groups can mediate conversation regarding emotional stress and personal experience between patients and experts.

42.3 Effectiveness of Educational Interventions

Most trials have shown a positive effect of education on patients' perspectives about the course of the disease, their ability to cope with the disease, as well as the clinical outcome of disease treatment (Table 42.1). Only one study from Table 42.1 reported a negative impact of hand education on both clinical and self-reported signs of eczema. Primary and secondary prevention were more effective than tertiary prevention interventions.

There are limitations to current research, as most of these trials are not randomized, double-blinded, and/or controlled. Many of these studies do not indicate the etiologies of the hand eczema. All studies were done in Denmark, Germany, or Sweden; thus, additional studies are needed to account for different geographic, cultural, and ethnic settings. Additionally, self-assessment of hand eczema, which is a commonly used method in these studies, may lead to an inaccurate estimation of hand eczema.

42.4 Education in Children

Additional steps must be taken in the education of children with eczema. Communication skills are particularly applicable to parents and their children who have eczema. Improving parents' knowledge will improve the outcome of their child's eczema [35]. This can be achieved by going beyond solely disseminating information about eczema. Acknowledging a parent's role in managing their child's care will help empower parents and improve management of eczema in their children. Jowett and Ryan surveyed a dermatology department, and a major complaint of most patients was the paucity of information and short time for explaining eczema and its treatment [36]. Many parents are generally dissatisfied with the information they receive, find difficulty in obtaining information, are given insufficient information, receive information too quickly, and are given inaccurate information [37]. Cork et al. observed that 86 % of parents of children with atopic dermatitis (AD) received minimal, if any, information about the mechanism of action or proper application techniques for topical therapy. Furthermore, 96 % of parents reported receiving no explanation as to the cause of AD [38]. In the same study, after a dermatology nurse

Table 42.1 Hand eczema educational interventions trials

Author, year	Patient population, duration, and location	Educational intervention	Measurement method of eczema	Results	Type of study
Bauer et al. (2002) [8]	Bakers' apprentices IG: 39 subjects CG: 55 subjects 4 months Germany	IG: Bakers' apprentices received two, 60-minute seminars in 4 weeks. The seminars included a standardized 15-min video lecture, a 15-min oral lecture, and 30 min of practical training in the proper use of gloves and barrier creams CG: These bakers' apprentices received no intervention	Participants received a standardized interview	Participants who engaged in regular skin care protection and maintenance: IG (%) / CG (%) Baseline: 67.6 / 61.7 Follow up: 90 / 83.9 Note: $n = 61$ for 4-month follow-up period Glove use of participants: IG (%) / CG (%) Baseline: 7.7 / 14.5 Follow up: 43.3 / 32.3 Note: $n = 61$ for 4-month follow-up period	CT Primary prevention
Bregnhoj et al. (2012) [20]	Hairdresser apprentices IG: 148 subjects CG: 136 subjects 18 months Denmark	IG: Teachers in hairdresser training schools were educated about skin protection. These teachers received a 2-day course of training in skin physiology, allergy and prevention of hand eczema. Subsequently, these trained teachers provided an evidence-based educational program to hairdresser apprentices during their initial vocational training. The apprentices received oral presentations, pamphlets, group exercises, hands on training and a glove fitting guide CG: Apprentices received normal hairdresser training without an educational program intervention	Participants received a self-administered questionnaire, and underwent a clinical examination for hand eczema	Hand eczema prevalence At follow up: IG: 20.4 % CG: 29.4 % Of those apprentices who experienced hand eczema, 40.6 % from the IG versus 19.6 % from CG had visited their general practitioner, and 15.6 % in the IG compared to 10.8 % in the CG consulted a dermatologist	CT Primary prevention Multicenter

Dulon et al. (2009) [21]	Geriatric nurses IG: 146 subjects CG: 242 subjects 12 months Germany	IG: Nurses were given 3–5 educational sessions about risk factors and skin care instructions. They were encouraged to develop a workplace skin protection program. In addition, senior nurses received a 1-day seminar and training in skin protection methods CG: These nurses received no intervention	Participants received a self-administered questionnaire, and underwent a clinical examination for hand eczema	The frequency of hand dermatitis: IG (%) / CG (%) Baseline: 26 / 19 Follow up: 17 / 17	RCT Primary prevention

Held et al. (2001) [22]	Student auxiliary nurses
	IG: 61 subjects
	CG: 46 subjects
	10 weeks
	Denmark
		IG: During nurse practical training, students were given two teaching sessions including skin physiology, contact dermatitis, proper glove use, hand hygiene, and utilization of disinfectants and moisturizers. In between both teaching sessions, students were asked to study an educational video and a pamphlet
		CG: Students received normal nurse practical training without an educational program intervention
			Participants received self-administered questionnaires, were clinically examined, and measurements of TEWL[a] were taken	Clinical examination of skin problems:
				  IG / CG
				Baseline: 25 % / 20 %
				Follow up: 39 % ($n=16$) / 17 % ($n=15$)
				Self-reported skin problems:
				  IG (%) / CG (%)
				Baseline: 39 / 32
				Follow up: 56 / 44
				TEWL[a] (%) was greater in the CG than the IG
					CT
					Primary prevention

(continued)

Table 42.1 (continued)

Author, year	Patient population, duration, and location	Educational intervention	Measurement method of eczema	Results	Type of study
Held et al. (2002) [23]	Nurses, kitchen staff, and cleaning staff in homes for the elderly with self-reported skin problems IG: 156 subjects CG: 131 subjects 5 months	IG: The subjects were given a 4-hour course twice, with 14 days in between. The education consisted of the basic physiology of eczema, use of disinfectants and moisturizers, glove use, and basic skin hygiene. Subjects met with instructors after 6 weeks for reinforcement. Thereafter, the subjects passed on the knowledge to their colleagues in any form they chose. However, at a minimum, it was mandatory to give written instructions to colleagues	Participants completed an exam as well as questionnaires on behavior and symptoms; they also underwent a clinical examination for hand eczema	Clinical examination of skin at baseline: No significant difference between the IG and CG	RCT
	Denmark	CG: This group was given no educational intervention		Clinical examination of skin at follow up: Fewer symptoms were found in the IG but not in the CG Self-reported skin problems: IG (%) / CG (%) Baseline: 25 / 30 Follow up: 27 / 34	Tertiary prevention
Flyvholm et al. (2005) [24]	Gut cleaners in slaughterhouses IG: 136 subjects CG: 280 subjects 1 year	IG: The group included 2–5 gut cleaners who were given lectures, discussions, homework, and feedback. A 2-day educational course was administered with one month in between. Afterwards, subjects acted as role models, practicing proper skin protection and supervising their colleagues	Participants received a telephone interview questionnaire based on the NOSQ-2002	Frequency of eczema within the past 3 months:	RCT
	Denmark	CG: This group was given no educational intervention		IG (%) / CG (%) Baseline: 56.2 / 45.9 Follow up: 41 / 50.2 Usage of skin care products during work: IG (%) / CG (%) Baseline: 69.1 / 55 Follow up: 72.1 / 60.2	Tertiary prevention

<table>
<tr><td>Ibler et al. (2012) [25]</td><td>Health care workers with self-reported eczema in the last year
IG: 123 subjects
CG: 132 subjects
5 months
Denmark</td><td>IG: The intervention for health care workers included prick and patch testing, identification of hand eczema subtype, individual counseling, and teaching of hand washing and emollient use
CG: This group was given no educational intervention</td><td>Clinical severity of disease measured by scores on the HECSI[b], scores on the DLQI[c], self-evaluated severity of hand eczema, skin protective behaviors, and knowledge of hand eczema was evaluated</td><td>The mean score on the HECSIb at follow up:
IG: 4.97
CG: 8.53
The mean score on the DLQIc at follow up:
IG: 1.22
CG: 2.00
The mean score of self-evaluated severity and skin protective behavior:
IG: Higher probability of reporting “mild” disease
CG: Higher probability of reporting “moderate” or “severe” disease
The mean score of knowledge of hand eczema and skin protection at follow up: There was no difference between the IG and CG</td><td>RCT
Secondary prevention</td></tr>
<tr><td>Loffler et al. (2006) [26]</td><td>Nurse trainees at nursing schools
IG: 156 subjects
CG: 169 subjects
3 years
Germany</td><td>IG: The trainees received lectures regarding skin structure and function, use of emollients, hand washing, and hand disinfection. The trainees were given these lecture three times in their first year of nurse training, and two times in their second year of nurse training
CG: This group was given no educational intervention</td><td>Participants underwent a clinical examination for hand dermatitis</td><td>Development of irritant skin changes:
<table><tr><td></td><td>IG (%)</td><td>CG (%)</td></tr><tr><td>Baseline</td><td>17.3</td><td>17.2</td></tr><tr><td>Follow up</td><td>46.8</td><td>66.3</td></tr></table></td><td>RCT
Primary prevention</td></tr>
</table>

(continued)

Table 42.1 (continued)

Author, year	Patient population, duration, and location	Educational intervention	Measurement method of eczema	Results	Type of study
Nilsson et al. (1999) [27]	Seven patients with severe eczema for greater than 6 years, who had at least some symptoms during the previous year. Six of seven patients had hand eczema IG: 7 subjects CG: none Time period not mentioned Sweden	IG: Teaching lessons were given to patients and contained practical instruction for self-care treatment. One-hour teaching lessons were given individually 2–4 times. The patients read through an educational pamphlet between the first and second lessons CG: N/A	Participants received a self-administered questionnaire	Four of seven patients felt that their eczema improved. Three of the patients stated that they would be more conscious about their emollient use in the future	Not randomized; not controlled Tertiary prevention
Schurer et al. (2005) [28]	Geriatric Nurses IG: 102 subjects CG: 109 subjects 6 months Germany	IG: Nurses completed a 6-month training program including hands on training, skin physiologic measurements, individualized protective measures, interview focused on attitudes and motivation of the patient, a dermatology evaluation and treatment strategy session. A seminar about skin health, disease, and protective measures was also given handouts. A final reinforcement seminar was given at the end of the 6 months CG: Nurses had access to dermatology consultation on demand and therapeutic medical management	Participants received a self-administered questionnaire, were clinically examined, and measurements of TEWL[a] were taken	Self-assessment questionnaire (indicating if eczema was present): — IG (%) / CG (%) Baseline: 89 / 90 Follow up (3 months after study completion): 53 / 82 TEWL[a] measurements: — IG / CG Baseline: 9.27 ± 8.94 g/m²/h / N/A Follow up: 3.47 ± 5.13 g/m²/h / N/A Clinical skin examination revealing hand eczema: — IG (%) / CG Baseline: 90 / N/A Follow up: 59 / N/A	Partially CT Secondary prevention

Schwanitz et al. (2003) [29]	Hairdressers' apprentices IC: 41 subjects CG: 56 subjects 3 years Germany	IG: During hairdresser vocational training, apprentices participated in 6 seminars (lessons totaling 15 hours) educating them about skin care and prevention of OSD. They were given gloves, protective creams and consultations regarding their work environment CG: N/A	Participants received a self-administered questionnaire and underwent a standardized clinical examination for hand eczema	After 4 weeks the IG increased glove use and practice of skin protection measures, while little to no changes was reported in the CG	CT
				Resignation from employment due to severity of skin changes: IG: 0 % CG: 10 % Year by year skin incidence of OSD during vocational training period: – IG (%) / CG (%) Year 1: 44 / 43.8 Year 2: 10 / 25 Year 3: 19.5 / 33.9	Primary intervention
Schwanitz et al. (2003) [29]	Hairdressers' apprentices IG: 134 subjects CG: 80 subjects 3 years Germany	IG: During hairdresser vocational training, apprentices participated in a seminar on skin protection and OSD that concentrated on the barriers to the practicality of skin protection measures in the workplace CG: This group was supervised medically	Participants were administered a semi-standardized interview	Hairdressers who remained in their occupation 3 months after study completion:	Not randomized; not controlled
				IG: 79.9 % CG: 60 % The use of protective gloves: – IG (%) / CG Baseline: 26.9 / N/A Follow up: 51.1 / N/A	Secondary prevention

(continued)

Table 42.1 (continued)

Author, year	Patient population, duration, and location	Educational intervention	Measurement method of eczema	Results	Type of study
Schwanitz et al. (2003) [29]	Inpatients with OSDs recalcitrant to outpatient treatments admitted over a course of 2–3 weeks. These patients were identified as being at risk for job loss due to OSD IG: 136 subjects CG: N/A 1 year Germany	IG: An interdisciplinary team provided an individualized skin protection program and general information about OSD for 2–3 weeks. Preventive strategies, personal consultations, seminars, and ergotherapy were also offered. During this intervention period, the patients did not work CG: N/A	Questionnaires regarding their OSD and employment 1 year after inpatient treatment	Inpatients unable to retain their employment due to OSD: IG: 31 % CG: N/A Inpatients that continued to protect their skin as advised: IG: 78 % CG: N/A Inpatients that started to receive gloves from their employer: IG: 49 % CG: N/A	Not randomized; not controlled Tertiary prevention
Sell et al. (2005) [30]	Employees at cheese dairies. Two dairies were the IG, and two were the CG IG: 335 subjects CG: 247 subjects 1 year Denmark	IG: Over the course of 8 months, two educational sessions and one follow-up session was given to employees. The sessions consisted of the latest evidence-based recommendations (e.g., avoid manual wet working, don't wear jewelry, wear protective gloves, etc.) CG: No information given	Participants received a telephone interview questionnaire based on the NOSQ-2002	Eczema of the hands or forearms in the last 3 months: (blank) / IG (%) / CG (%) Baseline / 9.8 / 8.0 Follow up / 9.8 / 6.9 A minimum of 2 skin symptoms on the hands or forearms in the last 12 months: (blank) / IG (%) / CG (%) Baseline / 35.5 / 33.8 Follow up / 24.8 / 15.4	CT Secondary prevention

Skudlik et al. (2011) [31]	Patients with OSD, of which 93.4 % ($n = 1{,}670$) had hand eczema IG: 1,788 subjects CG: N/A 10 weeks	IG: patients underwent a 3-week inpatient period, including treatment, education, and counseling. Afterwards, patients remained absent from work for 3 weeks and received outpatient treatment from a dermatologist. At the conclusion of the combined 6-week period of inpatient and outpatient care, the patients return to work with outpatient dermatological support. Four weeks after the patient returned to work, the OSD was clinically re-evaluated	Clinical outcomes were determined by the standardized OHSI[d]	93.2 % of patients refrained from using topical steroids before returning to work. 88 % of patients were able to return to work. 4 weeks after returning to work, 81.3 % (1,250 out of 1,537) were steroid free	Not randomized; not controlled
	Germany	CG: N/A		OHSI[d] score at baseline: IG: 6.3 CG: N/A OHSI[d] score at follow up: IG: 3.7 CG: N/A	Tertiary prevention Multicenter
Wilke et al. (2011) [32]	Geriatric nurses with occupational hand eczema IG: 72 subjects CG: 44 subjects 6 years	IG: During a 6-month period, Geriatric nurses were offered a visit by a health educator to aid in application of skin protective measures at work. Nurses were individually counseled on use and disposal of gloves, and the correct application of skin care products. Nurses attended skin protection course in groups of 8–10 nurses for 1 day. Topics for discussion included the anatomy of skins, the pathophysiology of contact dermatitis, and the application of effective skin protection. The nurses underwent 3 or 4 consultations involving diagnosis and treatment strategies. At the conclusion of the 6 month period, a seminar was conducted to discuss the methods of workplace implementation of skin protection	Participants received a standardized self-administered questionnaire	Job loss due to hand eczema at follow up:	CT
	Germany	CG: These nurses were simply treated medically by dermatologists		IG: 6.9 % CG:13.6 % Presence of skin lesions: (IG / CG) Baseline: 88.2 % ($n = 90$) / 89.7 % ($n = 96$) Follow up: 61.7 % ($n = 29$) / 72 % ($n = 18$) Participants that experienced minimal or no inconvenience due to skin protection during everyday life: IG: 76.6 % ($n = 36$) CG: 72 % ($n = 18$)	Secondary prevention

(continued)

Table 42.1 (continued)

Author, year	Patient population, duration, and location	Educational intervention	Measurement method of eczema	Results	Type of study
Wilke et al. (2012) [33]	Workers with OHE IG: 84 subjects CG: N/A 5 years	IG: Patients were given dermatological consultation and examination, and two outpatient educational seminars. During the second seminar, which took place 3 months after the first seminar, participants exchanged experiences, and were retrained with a focus their current skin protection needs. In addition, the IG also participated in a day-long skin protection seminar, as well as individual counseling and recommendations concerning the proper usage of protective gloves and skin care products	Participants received a semi-standardized interview and standardized questionnaires	At follow up, 71.4 % of patients remained in their occupation, and 13.1 % did not report to work because of OHE	Not randomized; not controlled
	Germany	CG: N/A		Self-reported presence of OHE was 83.7 % ($n=36$) at baseline and 58.1 % ($n=25$) at follow up	Secondary prevention
Wulfhorst et al. (2010) [34]	Hairdressers suffering OSD IG: 172 subjects CG: 55 subjects 5 years	IG: Patients were given a dermatology consultation (semi-standardized interview sheet), skin protection seminar, work consultations, and a final seminar/consultation 6 months after the first consultation	Participants received a standardized questionnaire	Patients who had stopped working because of OSD:	CT
	Germany	CG: These patients received dermatology treatment only		IG:12.8 % CG: 27.3 %	Secondary prevention

OHE occupational hand eczema, *OSD* occupational skin disease, *NOSQ-2002* Nordic Occupational Skin Questionnaire, *CT* controlled trial, *RCT* randomized controlled trial, *IG* intervention group, *CG* control group

[a]*TEWL* Transepidermal water loss. An increase in TEWL is secondary to impaired barrier function of the skin

[b]*HECSI* Hand eczema severity index. A higher score on the HECSI indicates a more severe eczema

[c]*DLQI* Dermatology life quality index. A higher score on the DLQI indicates a worsening quality of life

[d]*OHSI* Osnabruck hand eczema severity index. A higher OHSI score indicates higher severity hand eczema

demonstrated proper topical therapy application to parents during patient visits over the course of a year, there was an 89 % reduction in the degree of eczema. The primary change in treatment was an 800 % increase in the use of emollients and little to no overall increase in the use of topical steroids. Greater confidence in managing eczema was reported in all respondents after the trial. A year-long multicenter trial with six once-weekly educational group sessions for parents of children experiencing AD showed a subjective improvement in children aged 3 months to 18 years [39]. It had a greater effect on the quality of life for the 3-month to 7-year group than the other age groups [39].

Specific steps can be taken to aid in eczema education for children and adults (Table 42.2). Diagrams can be particularly helpful in explaining eczema to children. Standardized video education has been shown to be better than behavior-based parental education groups in enhancing parents' education about their children's atopic eczema [55]. Parents should be given written instructions to reinforce the therapies that have been explained and demonstrated, such as where and how to apply creams. Videos and information booklets available from many children's hospitals may assist parents with techniques such as wet dressings. A letter to the child's school can be helpful in management (e.g., requesting seating away from heaters). School visits and the use of liaison educators can be of great help in managing and improving the child's self-esteem. A combination of both a specialist nurse and a dermatologist may augment the impact of education on childhood eczema [35]. Adhering to the most up-to-date practice guidelines should provide control in the majority of children.

42.5 Suggestions for a Skin Protection Program

Table 42.2 is a list of practical steps that can be implemented right away for patients with hand eczema. Topics patients should be educated about include (1) normal skin versus disease pathogenesis, (2) early recognition of skin symptoms, (3) legislation relating to skin protection (e.g., the European Union Nickel Directive limits the concentration of nickel to no more than 0.05 % in posts used for body piercings) [56], (4) how skin barriers/creams work, (5) contact information if they have problems or questions, (6) warning signs and what to do about them, (7) the importance of caring for skin, (8) feeling responsible for skin, (9) regarding skin protection as a regular part of work, (10) understanding methods of applying skin protection the right way and with the right frequency, and (11) where to access the most up-to-date evidence-based recommendations.

A skin protection program is most useful in working environments. It must include occupational health support modification of work habits, hazard identification, and risk awareness. Job training should teach proper use of protective gloves, clothing, moisturizers, and emollients. In professions with a higher risk for irritant exposure, employee education should begin before job initiation, and should be repeated regularly. Employers who receive training can act as teachers, reinforcing safety protocols and identifying potentially dangerous irritants or chemicals [42].

A way to emphasize employee involvement in skin care is to initially train a group of employees that can subsequently develop guidelines (written guidelines are strongly recommended) about skin protection and environmental hazard management tailored for the needs of their colleagues. A team effort incorporating managers, safety officials, and employees will improve the success rate of a skin protection program. A skin protection program should be integrated into the daily workplace routine. Limited information should be taught to employees during each training session, as too much information at one time will lead to poor retention. Introspective homework assignments for employees allows for self-reflection on their daily activities, which may influence their skin exposure and skin care [27]. The main potential barrier to implementing these guidelines in the workplace is the achievement of effective cooperation between doctors in primary or specialty care and employers. It is important to address concerns about job security, and

Table 42.2 Hand eczema prevention tips

Tips on how to reduce hand eczema		Rationale/details
Limit wet work to less than 2 h		Wet work of more than 2 h per day is associated with 2.3 times risk of developing hand dermatitis [40, 41]
Maintain personal hygiene with hand washing and cleansers, as needed		Rinsing skin with water (with or without mild soap) can remove allergens, fats, oils, irritants, and other foreign matter [7]. Do not use disinfectants, unless specifically required
		The cleanser should be water soluble and should not remove lipids from the skin [42]. Furthermore, hot water causes more irritation than lukewarm or cold water
Avoid further aggravating stimuli		Avoid activities such as scratching of the affected areas
Be careful of polish removers		Polish removers containing toluene and other organic solvents can remove lipids from the skin (fingertips) [43]
Advice for parents of children with eczema	Parents should apply a moisturizer before swimming and a cool rinse after swimming, with reapplication of moisturizer	These steps will help prevent exacerbation of the eczema due to chlorine irritation
	Apply cool compresses rather than nag children to stop scratching	This approach will make treatment more pleasant to children
	Warm the emollient in warm water prior to use	This approach will make treatment more pleasant to children [38]
Health surveillance	Identify susceptible individuals or perform preemployment screening	Patch testing or preemployment screening questionnaires can be performed to establish a history, help identify higher-risk individuals, and provide the necessary job counseling
		Workers with underlying predisposing factors (e.g., AD) should avoid wet work and work duties that expose them to irritants [7]
	Perform regular skin checks	A physician or qualified employee can perform skin checks to identify early signs of dermatitis
Environmental (work or industrial) awareness	Use preventative measures in hostile environments	Workers may be accidentally exposed to allergens and irritants on contaminated work surfaces. To avoid these exposures, cover work surfaces with protective towels, sheets, or other coverings. Work surfaces can be cleaned with an industrial cleaner, and dusts and other particles can be vacuumed [14]
		Workers responsible for environmental hygiene will help prevent accumulation of harmful contaminants
	Perform technical control of hazardous material	Control measures depend on the form and route of exposure. If exposure occurs from a solid or liquid, protective equipment for the employee is necessary (e.g., splash guards). If the exposure occurs from an airborne form (e.g., mist, dust, fume or vapor), then ventilation methods (e.g., damp dusts or ventilation extraction) can reduce exposure [43]
		Cement dust [43], sawdust [43], and paper dust [7] produce a dry dermatitis. Be aware of professions exposed to these dusts (e.g., carpenters, woodworkers, and printers)
Allergens/ irritants	Investigate any patient allergens	If a patient or employee is suspected of having a skin allergy, patch testing should be performed. A physician can provide the patient/employee with a list of items that contain the pertinent allergen(s) to which they reacted on patch testing, and the patient/ employee should avoid all items that contain the allergen(s). A list may also be provided (using the CARD database) of products that do not contain the allergen(s) and that the patient can safely use

(continued)

Table 42.2 (continued)

Tips on how to reduce hand eczema		Rationale/details
Psychosocial	Manage stress properly	Eczema can flare up when one is under stress [44]. Patients should learn how to cope with stress, such as changing something in one's activities to reduce daily stress [45]
	Use the habit reversal technique	Introducing an alternative behavior incompatible with scratching will allow the skin to heal. This therapy can be taught by a therapist and/or dermatologist [45]
Hand hygiene	Avoid using alkaline soaps	Alkaline soaps disrupt the stratum corneum by degrading corneodesmosomes and activating serine proteases [46]
	Conventional soap bars are preferred over liquid soaps	Patients usually use too much liquid soap; thus, conventional soap bars are better [47]
	Only rinse hands with soap and water when they are visibly dirty; otherwise, use hand sanitizer, particularly in healthcare workers	Soap/cleansing agents can change the pH of the skin and remove lipids from the skin [48]
		Alcohol-based sanitizers may be used as alternatives to soap and water but cannot eliminate visible contaminants such as dirt, blood, or other fluids [49]
	Regulate hand washing temperature	Wash hands in lukewarm water; if the water temperature is too high, protective lipids may be depleted from the skin [49]
Gloves	Gloves should be used when necessary and for short time periods; they should be clean and should not cause an allergic or irritant dermatitis	Gloves are important in protecting the skin against allergens, irritants, and toxic substances. However, prolonged and excessive use of protective gloves can weaken the skin barrier, especially if the hands have had prior exposure to detergents [3]. Wearing gloves can occasionally result in irritant dermatitis for several reasons (e.g., material on hands prior to wearing gloves, unclean gloves, allergy to one or more glove components)
	Use protective gloves for housework (e.g., dishwashing)	Exposure to irritants over time can eventually result in contact dermatitis. Therefore, domestic exposure to irritants can contribute to the risk of contracting hand dermatitis at work and vice versa [3]
	The importance of glove use must be emphasized	Patients typically use gloves less during low-risk procedures. Gloves should always be worn, because frequent low-risk procedures may inflict as much damage as infrequent high-risk procedures [50]
	Use proper glove type	Cotton gloves can be used alone for dry work. In cases of wet work, cotton gloves can be worn inside rubber or vinyl gloves (the cotton gloves will absorb moisture and sweat)
	Gloves need to be maintained	Protective gloves should be clean and dry inside. They should be monitored periodically and replaced if perforations or signs of deterioration are seen [3]
		Some petroleum-based moisturizers (that may contain petrolatum and mineral oil) may cause deterioration of latex gloves [49]
	Once gloves are removed, wash hands	Gloves have an imperfect barrier to infectious material; thus, hands must be washed after glove removal [49]
	Avoid glove allergens	Glove allergens are common (e.g., rubber gloves are known to cause delayed allergy and contact urticaria due to latex protein). Hand dermatitis in patients who wear gloves regularly should prompt patch testing for possible allergy to glove components. A dermatologist can assist in finding alternative glove types using specialized databases [3]
		The powder used to lubricate the interior of gloves can irritate the skin. Additionally, there is a potential additional risk of contact allergy from powders that have absorbed the glove allergen (e.g., latex protein) [3]

Table 42.2 (continued)

Tips on how to reduce hand eczema		Rationale/details
Emollients	Use lipid-rich emollients, especially those containing ceramide	Levels of ceramide correlate with skin barrier protection [51, 52]. Ceramide aids in regeneration of the stratum corneum by forming a protective layer preventing water loss [51, 52]
		Eczematous skin has been shown to regenerate quicker once a moisturizer is applied for multiple days [52]
		Use an oil-based emollient for severely dry skin [53]; otherwise, use a water-based emollient for normal skin (if the first ingredient of an emollient is listed as water, then it can be assumed that it is not an oil-based emollient)
	Apply emollient correctly	Moisturizers should be smeared over the entire surface of the hands (e.g., fingertips, palms, web spaces, and dorsal hands) prior to, during, and after work [3]
	Be aware that there may be limitations	The benefit of emollients in the prevention of eczema in the workplace has not yet been fully evaluated [7]. The long-term use of emollients may possibly decrease the integrity of the stratum corneum, enhancing the skin's susceptibility to irritants [7]
	Be aware of their limitations in the healthcare setting	Some emollients that contain anionic substances may interfere with chlorhexidine gluconate (common antimicrobial agent used in healthcare settings) [53]
		Oil-based emollients may cause breakdown of latex gloves [53]
Barrier creams/ protective creams	Can provide a protective layer in between the skin and possible irritants (e.g., zinc oxide, silicone, dimethicone)	Barrier creams are protective against many irritants and allergens (e.g., paints, cutting oils, epoxy resins, and metals) [7]. They should be used only for handling nontoxic, noncarcinogenic, and nonsensitizing low-grade irritants such as water and detergents [7]
	Be aware of their limitations	They should not be applied to irritated skin, as they may potentially exacerbate dermatitis [7]. It is inconclusive if barrier creams alone protect against contact with irritants (irritants and allergens could possibly adhere to the cream and be transmitted into the skin) [54]
		Some barrier creams have limited short-term protective effects against irritating and toxic solvents [54]. It is unsettled if barrier creams are effective against cutting fluids (used in metalworking) [7]
		There are practical drawbacks to using barrier creams. They require sufficient and frequent application, and many vulnerable areas of skin are commonly missed. These issues may be addressed with education, and improvements in proper barrier cream application can be achieved [54]

to ensure that employees have given consent for treating clinicians to share medical information.

Group sessions are a powerful tool that can be used in a skin protection program. Groups allow individuals to exchange experiences and emotional stresses with people in similar situations who overcame their eczema [29]. Schwanitz et al. report that patients felt that group sessions allowed them "not to be laughed at" and "helped a great deal to see that others have the same problems." Patients' skepticism regarding use of gloves or other protective gear can be reduced significantly. Groups with psychologists can clarify conversations between participants and experts, and help development of possible solutions and strategies.

Awareness about hand eczema can also be aimed at the general public. A large-scale public protection program was successful in Germany in 2007 and 2008 [57]. In this campaign, a motto ("Your Skin. The Most Important 2 m^2 of Your Life") was printed on posters and hung at different workplaces. Trade fairs and city festivals contained booths featuring topics of skin cancer, sun protection, tinea pedis, and skin protection. In addition, videos showing correct skin protection behavior at the workplace were distributed. In conjunction with these activities, there were also sporting (marathon teams ran wearing the campaign motto) and music events (rap bands performed songs dealing with dermatologic topics).

Conclusion

For success, a strategy should utilize a collaborative effort between physicians, patients, and other relevant parties (e.g., nurses, employers, safety officials, unions, parents) and encompass several elements of the measures described above. Hand eczema can usually be prevented with relatively simple proactive measures. Evidence suggests that early hand eczema can be reversed with careful hand care and proper treatment [58]. The education should be a perpetual and a constantly evolving process. The concept of instilling and reinforcing education on a regular basis is required for long-term prevention of eczema. A study with 757 respondents using the contact allergen replacement database (CARD), which can provide patients with a list of over 8,000 allergens and cross-reactors and over 5,500 prescreened skin care products, demonstrated that when patients were informed both verbally and with printouts about the allergen content of products using CARD, more than 50 % reported improved contact dermatitis. In spite of that, patients later forgot 40 % of the identified allergens [59]. Additionally, it must be stressed that greater patient participation in their care improves satisfaction, adherence, and outcome of treatment. Patients require consistent and follow-up care, as exemplified by the fact that adherence to topical therapy in patients with AD increases on the few days before and immediately after office visits [60].

Current evidence is favorable for the use of educational interventions in hand eczema (see Table 42.1), but there are still insufficient formal intervention studies. Moreover, many of the studies use self-reporting outcomes to determine the clinical outcome of the educational interventions. Larger, long-term studies are needed to confirm the effectiveness of skin protection programs and to investigate the cost-effectiveness of these programs.

References

1. Lapsley P. Commentary: the double benefits of educational programmes for patients with eczema. BMJ. 2006;332:923–4.
2. Leino T, Tuomi K, Paakkulainen H, Klockars M. Health reasons for leaving the profession as determined among Finnish hairdressers in 1980–1995. Int Arch Occup Environ Health. 1999;72:56e9.
3. Agner T, Held E. Skin protection programmes. Contact Dermatitis. 2002;47:253e6.
4. Lysdahl SH, Sosted H, Andersen KE, Johansen JD. Hand eczema in hairdressers: a Danish register-based study of the prevalence of hand eczema and its career consequences. Contact Dermatitis. 2011;65:151–8.
5. Heron RJ. Worker education in the primary prevention of occupational dermatoses. Occup Med (Lond). 1997;47:407–10.
6. Dickel H, Kuss O, Blesius CR, Schmidt A, Diepgen TL. Occupational skin diseases in Northern Bavaria between 1990 and 1999: a population-based study. Br J Dermatol. 2001;145:453–62.
7. Brown T. Strategies for prevention: occupational contact dermatitis. Occup Med (Lond). 2004;54:450–7.
8. Bauer A, Kelterer D, Bartsch R, Pearson J, Stadeler M, Kleesz P, et al. Skin protection in Bakers' apprentices. Contact Dermatitis. 2002;46:81–5.
9. Bauer A, Kelterer D, Bartsch R, Schlegel A, Pearson J, Kleesz P, et al. Prevention of hand dermatitis in bakers' apprentices: different efficacy of skin protection measures and UVB hardening. Int Arch Occup Environ Health. 2002;75:491–9.
10. Kristensen O. A prospective study of the development of hand eczema in an automobile manufacturing industry. Contact Dermatitis. 1992;26:341–5.
11. Itschner L, Hinnen U, Elsner P. Prevention of hand eczema in the metal-working industry: risk awareness and behavior of metal worker apprentices. Dermatology. 1996;196:226–9.

12. Pohrt U. Skin protection training. Curr Probl Dermatol. 2007;34:161–70.
13. Armstrong AW, Kim RH, Idriss NZ, Larsen LN, Lio PA. Online video improves clinical outcomes in adults with atopic dermatitis: a randomized controlled trial. J Am Acad Dermatol. 2011;64:502–7.
14. Mathias CG. Prevention of occupational contact dermatitis. J Am Acad Dermatol. 1990;23:742–8.
15. Skudlik C, Wulfhorst B, Gediga G, Bock M, Allmers H, John SM. Tertiary individual prevention of occupational skin diseases: a decade's experience with recalcitrant occupational dermatitis. Int Arch Occup Environ Health. 2008;81:1059–64.
16. Kalimo K, Kautiainen H, Niskanen T, Niemi L. "Eczema school" to improve compliance in an occupational dermatology clinic. Contact Dermatitis. 1999;41:315–9.
17. Schwanitz HJ, Wulfhorst B. Workers education. In: Kanerva L, Elsner P, Wahlberg JE, Maibach HI, editors. Occupational dermatoses handbook. Berlin: Springer; 2000. p. 441–3.
18. Meding B, Swanbeck G. Consequences of having hand eczema. Contact Dermatitis. 1990;23:6–14.
19. Fowler J. Chronic hand eczema: a prevalent and challenging skin condition. Cutis. 2008;82:4–8.
20. Bregnhoj A, Menne T, Johansen JD, Sosted H. Prevention of hand eczema among Danish hairdressing apprentices: an intervention study. Occup Environ Med. 2012;69:310–6.
21. Dulon M, Pohrt U, Skudlik C, Nienhaus A. Prevention of occupational skin disease: a workplace intervention study in geriatric nurses. Br J Dermatol. 2009;161:337–44.
22. Held E, Wolff C, Gyntelberg F, Agner T. Prevention of work-related skin problems in student auxiliary nurses: an intervention study. Contact Dermatitis. 2001;44:297–303.
23. Held E, Mygind K, Wolff C, Gytelberg F, Agner T. Prevention of work related skin problems: an intervention study in wet work employees. Occup Environ Med. 2002;59:556–61.
24. Flyvholm MA, Mygind K, Sell L, Jensen A, Jepsen KF. A randomised controlled intervention study on prevention of work related skin problems among gut cleaners in swine slaughterhouses. Occup Environ Med. 2005;62:642–9.
25. Ibler KS, Jemec GB, Diepgen TL, Gluud C, Hansen JL, Winkel P, et al. Skin care education and individual counseling versus treatment as usually in healthcare workers with hand eczema: randomised clinical trial. BMJ. 2012;345:e7822.
26. Loffler H, Bruckner T, Diepgen T, Effendy I. Primary prevention in health care employees: a prospective intervention study with a 3-year training period. Contact Dermatitis. 2006;54:202–9.
27. Nilsson T, Klang B, Berg M. Patient education for adults with chronic eczema. Dermatol Nurs. 1999;11:117–22.
28. Schurer NY, Klippel U, Schwanitz HJ. Secondary individual prevention of hand dermatitis in geriatric nurses. Int Arch Occup Environ Health. 2005;75:149–57.
29. Schwanitz HJ, Riehl U, Schlesinger T, Bock M, Skudlik C, Wulhorst B. Skin care management: educational aspects. Int Arch Occup Environ Health. 2003;76:374–81.
30. Sell L, Flyvholm MA, Lindhard G, Mygind K. Implementation of an occupational skin disease prevention programme in Danish cheese dairies. Contact Dermatitis. 2005;53:155–61.
31. Skudlik C, Weisshaar E, Scheidt R, Elsner P, Wulfhorst B, Schonfeld M, et al. First results from the multicenter study rehabilitation of occupational skin disease – optimization and quality assurance of inpatient management (ROQ). Contact Dermatitis. 2011;66:140–7.
32. Wilke A, Gediga K, Weinhoppel U, John SM, Wulfhorst B. Long-term effectiveness of secondary prevention in geriatric nurses with occupational hand eczema: the challenge of a controlled study design. Contact Dermatitis. 2011;66:79–86.
33. Wilke A, Gediga G, Schlesinger T, John SM, Wulfhorst B. Sustainability of interdisciplinary secondary prevention in patients with occupational hand eczema:a 5-year follow-up survey. Contact Dermatitis. 2012;67:208–16.
34. Wulfhorst B, Bock M, Gediga G, Skudlik C, Allmers H, John SM. Sustainability of an interdisciplinary secondary prevention program for hairdressers. Int Arch Occup Environ Health. 2010;83:165–71.
35. Broberg A, Kalimo K, Lindblad B, Swanbeck G. Parental education in the treatment of childhood atopic eczema. Acta Derm Venereol. 1990;70:495–9.
36. Jowett S, Ryan T. Dermatology patients and their doctors. Clin Exp Dermatol. 1985;10:246–54.
37. Lawton S, Roberts A, Gibb C. Supporting the parents of children with atopic eczema. Br J Nurs. 2005;14:693–6.
38. Cork MJ, Britton J, Butler L, Young S, Murphy R, Keohane SG. Comparison of parent knowledge, therapy utilization and severity of atopic eczema before and after explanation and demonstration of topical therapies by a specialist dermatology nurse. Br J Dermatol. 2003;149:582–9.
39. Staab D, Diepgen TL, Fartasch M, Kupfer J, Lob-Corzilius T, Ring J, et al. Age related, structured educational programmes for the management of atopic dermatitis in children and adolescents: multicentre, randomised controlled trial. BMJ. 2006;332:933–8.
40. Uter W, Pfahlberg A, Gefeller O, Schwanitz HJ. Hand dermatitis in a prospectively-followed cohort of hairdressing apprentices: final results of the POSH study. Prevention of occupational skin disease in hairdressers. Contact Dermatitis. 1999;41:280e6.
41. Uter W, Pfahlberg A, Gefeller O, Schwanitz HJ. Occupational dermatitis in hairdressing apprentices. Early-onset irritant skin damage. Curr Probl Dermatol. 1995;23:49–55.
42. English J. Current concepts of irritant contact dermatitis. Occup Environ Med. 2004;61:722–6.
43. Nanko H. Treatment of housewives' hand eczema. JMAJ. 2004;47:44–51.

44. American Academy of Family Physicians. Eczema. Am Fam Physician. 2003;68:1603–4.
45. Grillo M, Long R, Long D. Habit reversal training for the itch-scratch cycle associate with pruritic skin conditions. Dermatol Nurs. 2007;19:243–8.
46. Hachem JP, Crumrine D, Fluhr J, Brown BE, Feingold KR, Elias PM. pH directly regulates epidermal permeability barrier homeostasis, and stratum corneum integrity/cohesion. J Invest Dermatol. 2003;121:345–53.
47. Andersen KE. Atopic hand eczema and treatment strategies. Acta Derm Venereol. 2005;215:45–8.
48. Kampf G, Loffler H. Prevention of irritant contact dermatitis among health care workers by using evidence-based hand hygiene practices: a review. Ind Health. 2007;45:645–52.
49. Marino C, Cohen M. Prevention of hand dermatitis in the health care setting. Olympia (WA): Safety and Health Assessment and Research for Prevention (SHARP) program. Report No.66-6-2001. Olympia: Washington Department of Labor and Industries. 2001 July. Available from: http://www.lni.wa.gov/Safety/Research/Dermatitis/files/prevent_hcw.pdf
50. Ling TC, Coulson IH. What do trainee hairdressers know about hand dermatitis? Contact Dermatitis. 2002;47:227–31.
51. Di Nardo A, Sugino K, Wertz P, Ademola J, Maibach HI. Sodium lauryl sulfate (SLS) induced irritant contact dermatitis: a correlation study between ceramides and in vivo parameters of irritation. Contact Dermatitis. 1996;35:86–91.
52. Draelos ZD. The effect of ceramide-containing skin care products on eczema resolution duration. Cutis. 2008;81:87–91.
53. Hand dermatitis in health care workers. Olympia (WA): Safety and Health Assessment and Research for Prevention (SHARP) program. Report No. 66-1-2001. Olympia: Washington Department of Labor and Industries. 2001 July. Available from: http://www.lni.wa.gov/Safety/Research/Dermatitis/files/derm_hcw.pdf
54. Wigger-Alberti W, Maraffio B, Wernli M, Elsner P. Training workers at risk for occupational contact dermatitis in the application of protective creams: efficacy of a fluorescence technique. Dermatology. 1997;195:129–33.
55. Niebel G, Kallweit C, Lange I, Folster-Holst R. Direct versus video-aided parent education in atopic eczema in childhood as a supplement to specialty physician treatment. A controlled-pilot study. Hautarzt. 2000;51:401–11.
56. Linh KL, Warshaw E, Dunnick C. Prevention of nickel allergy: the case for regulation? Dermatol Clin. 2009;27:155–61.
57. Seyfarth F, Schliemann S, Antonov D, Elsner P. Teaching interventions in contact dermatitis. Dermatitis. 2011;22:8–15.
58. Van Der Walle HB. Dermatitis in hairdressers (II). Management and prevention. Contact Dermatitis. 1994;30:265–70.
59. Scalf LA, Genebriera J, Davis MD, Farmer SA, Yiannias JA. Patients' perceptions of the usefulness and outcome of patch testing. J Am Acad Dermatol. 2007;56:928–32.
60. Feldman SR, Camacho FT, Krejci-Manwaring J, Carroll CL, Balkrishnan R. Adherence to topical therapy increases around the time of office visits. J Am Acad Dermatol. 2007;57:81–3.

Appendix 1. Hand Dermatitis Treatment

1. The most important part of your treatment is to apply a lubricating, unscented cream (your doctor will provide suggestions depending on local availability) or ointment (white petrolatum) to your hands several times a day. You should apply this hand lubricant after each handwashing and as often as possible at other times – at least ten times each day. Apply the hand lubricant very thinly to your whole hand and massage it in well. Plain white petrolatum under white cotton skin gloves overnight for several weeks at a time is also a valuable treatment.
2. If a steroid cream is prescribed, this should be applied as many times as recommended by the prescribing physician. It should ideally be left on for at least a few hours prior to any handwashing. Also, it should be ideally applied to clean, dry skin and prior to any moisturizers.
3. When washing your hands, use lukewarm water and a very small amount of mild soap. Rinse the soap off well and dry gently. Then apply either a little medicated cream or moisturizing cream (depending on doctor's recommendation) and massage it in well. Hand sanitizers, particularly those with moisturizers, represent another way to cleanse hands during the day with potentially fewer drying and irritating effects of handwashing; that said, some hand sanitizers can also be drying and irritating.
4. When your rash is much better, you can slowly wean down usage of the topical medication(s) but continue using the hand lubricant indefinitely.
5. Pampering your hands with frequent use of a gentle hand moisturizer should become part of your daily hygiene regimen even after your hands have healed. This behavior will be important preventatively. Furthermore, it takes a long time for skin to recover from prolonged inflammation.
6. Hand dermatitis is stubborn and often recurs. If your hand rash clears but then comes back or worsens, it usually means that you need to use your medication again (as prescribed) and continue to pamper your hands with good sensitive skin care.
7. If your rash does not clear or is worsening, please return to your doctor's office so we can reevaluate your treatment.

Appendix 2. Hand Protection for Hand Dermatitis

Hand dermatitis is common. Hand rashes usually result from a combination of (1) sensitive skin and (2) irritation or allergy from materials touched. Our hands routinely touch irritating soaps and detergent several times a day, in addition to raw foods, solvents, paints, oils, greases, acids, glues, and so on that most of us touch at work or in the home. Furthermore, many people have their hands in water during work or at home,

A. Alikhan et al. (eds.), *Textbook of Hand Eczema*,
DOI 10.1007/978-3-642-39546-8, © Springer-Verlag Berlin Heidelberg 2014

which can be quite irritating over time. Some people have "tough" skin, but others have skin that's easily damaged. The result is dermatitis.

Skin protection is an important part of treatment. This instruction sheet gives you detailed directions on how to protect your hands. Please read it carefully every day for a week to cement these instructions in your mind.

1. Protect your hands from direct contact with soaps, detergents, scouring powders, and similar irritating chemicals by wearing waterproof, heavy-duty vinyl gloves. Heavy-duty vinyl gloves such are better than rubber gloves, because you may become allergic to rubber (glove material should be selected based on the hazard and contact allergens in the glove itself – please consult with your doctor if you have questions). Heavy-duty vinyl gloves are usually available at paint and hardware stores. Buy four or five pairs so they can be conveniently located throughout your house. If a glove develops a hole or mildew, discard it immediately.
2. The waterproof, heavy-duty vinyl gloves may be lined or unlined. You should have enough waterproof gloves so that the insides of the gloves can dry between wearings. Try not to contaminate the inside of the gloves.
3. Wear waterproof gloves while peeling and squeezing lemons, oranges, or grapefruit, while peeling potatoes, and while handling tomatoes.
4. Wear leather or heavy-duty fabric gloves when doing dry work and gardening (be aware that these, like other gloves, can cause contact eczema in certain people). If you are in charge of cleaning your house, scatter a dozen pairs of cheap cotton gloves about your home and use them while doing dry housework. When they get dirty, put them in the washing machine (try to use a fragrance-free laundry detergent like all® free clear).
5. If you have an automatic dishwasher, use it as much as possible. If you do not, let a member of your family do the dishes. Do your laundry by machine, not by hand.
6. Avoid direct contact with turpentine, paint thinner, paints, and floor, furniture, metal, or shoe polishes. They contain irritating solvents. When using them, wear heavy-duty vinyl gloves.
7. If your hands are frequently exposed to solvents and other irritating chemicals, especially at work, ask an industrial hygienist about protective gloves.
8. Rings often worsen dermatitis by trapping irritating materials beneath them. Remove your rings when doing housework and before washing your hands.
9. When you are outdoors in cold or windy weather, wear leather gloves to protect your hands from drying and chapping.
10. Use only the prescribed medicines and recommended lubricants. Do not use other lotions, creams, or medications – they may irritate your skin.
11. Protect your hands for the rest of your life, even after your rash has healed. Note that it takes a long time for skin to recover. Also, dermatitis has a tendency to recur, especially if good skin care measures are not followed.

Appendix 3. Overnight Vinyl Occlusion for Hand Dermatitis

Covering skin overnight with vinyl increases the penetration and effectiveness of cortisone medications. For hand dermatitis, you should wear vinyl gloves overnight after applying a cortisone cream to your rash. Please carefully follow the instructions given to you by your doctor as to which cortisone to use, how often to use it, and how long to use it. For the overnight vinyl occlusion, please follow these directions carefully:

1. At bedtime, apply a cortisone cream thinly to the rash areas only. Do not apply it to normal skin. Then put on the vinyl gloves; take them off in the morning. The vinyl gloves recommended are disposable vinyl examining gloves; they can be reused for a few nights or until they develop holes. If your drugstore does not stock them, your doctor's office can tell you where to buy them.

Important: Use only vinyl (plastic) gloves. Do not use latex (rubber) gloves.

2. At first, wearing the vinyl gloves may be a bit uncomfortable. It may take a few days to get used to them.
3. The cortisone cream-vinyl glove treatment can make your skin become thin. You should use it exactly as directed on this sheet and by your doctor. It's important to apply the cortisone medicine only to the rash when using vinyl gloves. Do not apply the cortisone medicine to normal skin. If your fingertips are normal, cut the fingertips off your gloves, because the vinyl covering softens skin. If your rash is on only one or two fingers, cut the proper number of fingers from a vinyl glove and hold them in place with nonirritating paper tape.
4. During the day, follow the patient instruction sheets "Hand Dermatitis Treatment" and "Hand Protection for Hand Dermatitis." Apply the daytime lubricant thinly and often to the entire skin of both hands.
5. Keep your follow-up appointment. You will need an appointment 14–28 days after starting the cortisone-vinyl covering treatment.

Note: This treatment can also be done with white cotton skin gloves rather than vinyl gloves, though it may be somewhat less effective. It may be better for milder hand dermatitis in this case.

Index

A. Alikhan et al. (eds.), *Textbook of Hand Eczema*,
DOI 10.1007/978-3-642-39546-8, © Springer-Verlag Berlin Heidelberg 2014